KT-130-124

Evidence-Based Infectious Diseases

Edited by

Mark Loeb BSc, MD, MSc, FRCPC

Professor, Department of Pathology and Molecular Medicine &
Department of Clinical Epidemiology and Biostatistics
McMaster University
Hamilton, Ontario
Canada

Fiona Smaill MB, ChB, FRCPC

Department Chair & Professor of Pathology and Molecular Medicine
McMaster University
Hamilton, Ontario
Canada

Marek Smieja MD, DIP, MSc, PhD, FRCPC

Department of Pathology and Molecular Medicine
McMaster University
Hamilton, Ontario
Canada

Second Edition

BMJ Books

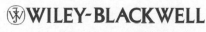
WILEY-BLACKWELL

A John Wiley & Sons, Ltd., Publication

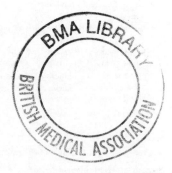
BMA LIBRARY
BRITISH MEDICAL ASSOCIATION

This edition first published 2009, © 2009 by Blackwell Publishing Ltd
Previous editions: 2004

BMJ Books is an imprint of BMJ Publishing Group Limited, used under licence by Blackwell
Publishing which was acquired by John Wiley & Sons in February 2007. Blackwell's publishing
programme has been merged with Wiley's global Scientific, Technical and Medical business to form
Wiley-Blackwell.

Registered office: John Wiley & Sons Ltd, The Atrium, Southern Gate, Chichester,
West Sussex, PO19 8SQ, UK

Editorial offices:
9600 Garsington Road, Oxford, OX4 2DQ, UK
    The Atrium, Southern Gate, Chichester, West Sussex, PO19 8SQ, UK
    111 River Street, Hoboken, NJ 07030-5774, USA

For details of our global editorial offices, for customer services and for information about how to apply
for permission to reuse the copyright material in this book please see our website at www.wiley
.com/wiley-blackwell

The right of the author to be identified as the author of this work has been asserted in accordance with
the Copyright, Designs and Patents Act 1988.

All rights reserved. No part of this publication may be reproduced, stored in a retrieval system, or
transmitted, in any form or by any means, electronic, mechanical, photocopying, recording or
otherwise, except as permitted by the UK Copyright, Designs and Patents Act 1988, without the prior
permission of the publisher.

Wiley also publishes its books in a variety of electronic formats. Some content that appears in print
may not be available in electronic books.

Designations used by companies to distinguish their products are often claimed as trademarks. All
brand names and product names used in this book are trade names, service marks, trademarks or
registered trademarks of their respective owners. The publisher is not associated with any product or
vendor mentioned in this book. This publication is designed to provide accurate and authoritative
information in regard to the subject matter covered. It is sold on the understanding that the publisher
is not engaged in rendering professional services. If professional advice or other expert assistance is
required, the services of a competent professional should be sought.

The contents of this work are intended to further general scientific research, understanding, and
discussion only and are not intended and should not be relied upon as recommending or promoting
a specific method, diagnosis, or treatment by physicians for any particular patient. The publisher and
the author make no representations or warranties with respect to the accuracy or completeness of the
contents of this work and specifically disclaim all warranties, including without limitation any implied
warranties of fitness for a particular purpose. In view of ongoing research, equipment modifications,
changes in governmental regulations, and the constant flow of information relating to the use of
medicines, equipment, and devices, the reader is urged to review and evaluate the information
provided in the package insert or instructions for each medicine, equipment, or device for, among
other things, any changes in the instructions or indication of usage and for added warnings and
precautions. Readers should consult with a specialist where appropriate. The fact that an organization
or Website is referred to in this work as a citation and/or a potential source of further information does
not mean that the author or the publisher endorses the information the organization or Website may
provide or recommendations it may make. Further, readers should be aware that Internet Websites
listed in this work may have changed or disappeared between when this work was written and when it
is read. No warranty may be created or extended by any promotional statements for this work. Neither
the publisher nor the author shall be liable for any damages arising herefrom.

Library of Congress Cataloging-in-Publication Data

Evidence-Based infectious diseases / edited by Mark Loeb, Fiona Smaill, Marek Smieja. — 2nd ed.
    p. ; cm.
  Includes bibliographical references and index.
  ISBN 978-1-4051-7026-0
1. Communicable diseases. 2. Evidence-Based medicine. I. Loeb, Mark. II. Smaill, Fiona.
III. Smieja, Marek.
  [DNLM: 1. Communicable Diseases—diagnosis. 2. Communicable Diseases—therapy.
3. Evidence-Based Medicine. WC 100 E93 2009]
RC112.L637 2009
616.9—dc22

                                       2009009650

ISBN: 978-1-4051-7026-0

A catalogue record for this book is available from the British Library.

Set in 9.5/12pt Minion by Macmillan Publishing Solutions, Chennai, India

Printed and bound in Singapore by Ho Printing Singapore Pte Ltd

1   2009

Contents

Contributors, vii

Preface to the First Edition, ix

Preface to the Second Edition, xi

1 Introduction to evidence-based infectious diseases, 1
Mark Loeb, Marek Smieja & Fiona Smaill

Part 1: Specific diseases, 9

2 Skin and soft-tissue infections, 11
Douglas Austgarden & Guilio DiDiodato

3 Bone and joint infections, 26
William J. Gillespie

4 Infective endocarditis, 42
Scott D. Halpern, Elias Abrutyn & Brian L. Strom

5 Meningitis and encephalitis, 55
Kara B. Mascitti & Ebbing Lautenbach

6 Management of community-acquired pneumonia, 73
David C. Rhew

7 Tuberculosis, 83
Peter Daley & Marek Smieja

8 Diarrhea, 98
Guy De Bruyn & Alain Bouckenooghe

9 Urinary tract infections, 115
Thomas Fekete

10 Sexually transmitted infections, 136
Kaede Ota, Darrell H.S. Tan, Sharmistha Mishra & David N. Fisman

11 Human immunodeficiency virus, 177
Ravindra K. Gupta & Brian J. Angus

12 Influenza, 206
Ashley Roberts & Joanne M. Langley

13 Critical care, 213
Jocelyn A. Srigley & Maureen O. Meade

Part 2: Special populations, 227

14 Infection control, 229
Graham M. Snyder, Eli N. Perencevich & Anthony D. Harris

15 Infections in neutropenic hosts, 250
Stuart J. Rosser & Eric J. Bow

16 Infections in general surgery, 270
Christine H. Lee

17 Infections in the thermally injured patient, 280
Edward E. Tredget, Robert Rennie, Robert E. Burrell & Sarvesh Logsetty

18 Infections in healthcare workers, 291
Gregory Rose & Virginia R. Roth

19 Infections in long-term care, 302
Lindsay E. Nicolle

Index, 315

Contributors

Elias Abrutyn, MD (deceased)
Drexel University College of Medicine, Philadelphia, PA, USA

Brian J. Angus BSc, MD
Reader in Infectious Diseases, University of Oxford, Nuffield Department of Medicine, John Radcliffe Hospital, Oxford, UK

Douglas Austgarden MD
Division of Infectious Diseases, The Hospital for Sick Children, Toronto, ON, Canada

Alain Bouckenooghe MD
Clinical R & D, Head Asia Pacific, Sanofi Pasteur, Singapore

Eric J. Bow MD, MSc
Professor and Head, Section of Haematology/Oncology, Professor, Department of Medical Microbiology and Infectious Diseases, University of Manitoba; *and* Head, Department of Medical Oncology and Haematology, Director, Infection Control Services, CancerCare Manitoba, Winnipeg, MB, Canada

Robert E. Burrell MD
Department of Surgery, University of Alberta, Edmonton, Alberta, Canada

Peter Daley MD
Lecturer, Infectious Diseases Training and Research Center, Vellore, India

Guy De Bruyn MBBCh, BCh, MPH
Programme Director, HIV Prevention Studies, Perinatal HIV Research Unit, University of the Witwatersrand, Johannesburg, South Africa

Guilio DiDiodato MD
Division of Infectious Diseases, The Hospital for Sick Children, Toronto, ON, Canada

Thomas Fekete MD
Section Chief, Infectious Diseases, Professor of Medicine, Temple University School of Medicine, Philadelphia, PA, USA

David N. Fisman MD, MPH
The Research Institute of the Hospital for Sick Children, Toronto, ON, Canada; The University of Toronto, Toronto, ON, Canada

William J. Gillespie BSc, MB, ChB, ChM
Emeritus Professor of Medicine, Hull York Medical School, University of Hull, Hull, UK

Ravindra K. Gupta MD
Centre for Tropical Medicine, Nuffield Department of Medicine, University of Oxford, Oxford, UK

Scott D. Halpern, MD, PhD
Assistant Professor of Medicine and Epidemiology, University of Pennsylvania, Philadelphia, PA, USA

Anthony D. Harris MD, MPH
Department of Epidemiology and Preventive Medicine, University of Maryland School of Medicine, Baltimore, MD, USA

Joanne M. Langley MD, MSc
Professor of Pediatrics; Professor, Community Health and Epidemiology, Canadian Centre for Vaccinology, Halifax, Dalhousie University, Halifax, NS, Canada

Ebbing Lautenbach MD, MPH, MSCE
Associate Professor of Medicine and Epidemiology, Department of Biostatics and Epidemiology, Center for Clinical Epidemiology and Biostatistics, Center for Education and Research of Therapeutics, University of Pennsylvania, School of Medicine, Philadelphia, PA, USA

Christine H. Lee MD
Department of Pathology and Molecular Medicine, McMaster University, St. Joseph's Healthcare, Hamilton, ON, Canada

Mark Loeb BSc, MD, MSc
Professor, Department of Pathology and Molecular Medicine, Department of Clinical Epidemiology and Biostatistics, McMaster University, Hamilton, ON, Canada

Sarvesh Logsetty MD
Department of Surgery, University of Alberta, Edmonton, Alberta, Canada

Kara B. Mascitti MD
Division of Infectious Diseases, University of Pennsylvania, School of Medicine, Philadelphia, PA, USA

Maureen O. Meade MD, MSc
Critical Care Consultant, Hamilton Health Sciences; Associate Professor of Medicine, McMaster University Hamilton, ON, Canada

Sharmistha Mishra MD
The Research Institute of the Hospital for Sick Children, Toronto, ON, Canada

Lindsay E. Nicolle MD
Professor of Internal Medicine and Medical Microbiology, University of Manitoba, Winnipeg, MB, Canada

Kaede Ota MD
The Research Institute of the Hospital for Sick Children, Toronto, ON, Canada

Eli N. Perencevich MD, MSc
Department of Epidemiology and Preventive Medicine, University of Maryland School of Medicine, Baltimore, MD, USA; Veterans Affairs Maryland Health Care System, Baltimore, MD, USA

Robert Rennie MD
Department of Surgery, University of Alberta, Edmonton, Alberta, Canada

David C. Rhew MD
Zynx Health Incorporated, Los Angeles, CA, USA; Associate Clinical Professor, UCLA David Geffen School of Medicine; Division of Infectious Diseases, Veterans Affairs Greater Los Angeles Healthcare System, Los Angeles, CA, USA

Ashley Roberts MD
Pediatric Infectious Diseases, Hospital for Sick Children, Toronto, ON, Canada

Gregory Rose MD
Infectious Prevention and Control Program, Division of Infectious Diseases, The Ottawa Hospital, Ottawa, ON, Canada

Stuart J. Rosser MD, MPH
Assistant Professor, Department of Medicine, University of Alberta, Edmonton, AB, Canada

Virginia R. Roth MD
Director, Infectious Prevention and Control Program, The Ottawa Hospital; Associate Professor of Medicine, Division of Infectious Diseases, University of Ottawa, Ottawa, ON, Canada

Fiona Smaill MB, ChB
Department Chair & Professor Pathology and Molecular Medicine, Faculty of Health Sciences, McMaster University, Hamilton, ON, Canada

Marek Smieja MD
Associate Professor, Department of Pathology and Molecular Medicine, Department of Clinical Epidemiology and Biosatistics, Department of Medicine, McMaster University, Hamilton, Ontano, Canada

Graham M. Snyder MD
Fellow, Division of Infectious Diseases, Beth Israel Deaconess Medical Center, Boston, MA, USA

Jocelyn A. Srigley MD
Infectious Diseases and Medical Microbiology Fellow, McMaster University, Hamilton, ON, Canada

Brian L. Strom MD, MPH
George S. Pepper Professor of Public Health and Peventive Medicine in Biostatistics and Epidemiology, University of Pennsylvania, School of Medicine; Vice Dean for Institutional Affairs, Philadelphia, PA, USA

Darrell H.S. Tan MD
The Research Institute of the Hospital for Sick Children, Toronto, ON, Canada

Edward E. Tredget MD, MSc
Department of Surgery, University of Alberta, Edmonton, Alberta, Canada

Preface to the First Edition

As busy academic physicians we are often approached about assuming new roles and responsibilities, and frankly are sometimes hesitant about placing yet another item on the "to do" list. However, when we were first approached about editing this book, our reaction was different. The idea of editing the first book about evidence-based infectious diseases was exciting. Although there are many standard textbooks on infectious diseases, none that we were aware of use an "evidence-based" approach.

We emphasize in this book both the methodological issues in assessing the quality of evidence, as well as the "best evidence" for practicing infectious diseases. We have divided the book into two parts. In Part I, we focus on specific infections, including skin and soft tissue infections, bone and joint infections, infective endocarditis, meningitis and encephalitis, community-acquired pneumonia, tuberculosis, diarrhea, urinary tract infections, sexually transmitted infections, and human immunodeficiency virus (HIV). In Part II, we focus on infections that occur in specific populations and settings. These include infection control, infections in the neutropenic host, surgical infections, the thermally injured patient, and infection in healthcare workers. We have asked chapter authors to begin with a clinical scenario, to help focus on relevant clinical questions, and then to briefly summarize the burden of illness or background epidemiology. The remainder of each chapter summarizes the best evidence with respect to diagnosis, prognosis, treatment, and prevention, with a focus, where possible, on systematic reviews.

As we discuss in the introductory chapter, we believe that important clinical questions that arise should be approached in a systematic fashion. The chapters in this book will never be as up to date as the information that you can derive by searching the most recent literature. This is particularly relevant when we are faced with new emerging infections, such as severe acute respiratory syndrome (SARS). However, browsing through these chapters will give a good context and will provide you with key evidence that you can update by conducting a search to see if there is any useful new information. While evidence from well-designed studies informs the decision-making process, it obviously does not replace it. The outcomes of a clinical trial, for example, may suggest a default antibiotic to use for pneumonia, but does not preclude our individualizing treatment based on patient allergies, the biology of the responsible organism, or the pharmacokinetics and pharmacodynamics of the drugs to be administered in that patient.

We hope that our approach will help to emphasize aspects of diagnosis, prognosis, treatment, or prevention in which there is already excellent evidence, while highlighting areas in which more compelling evidence is needed. In these latter areas in which our confidence is limited, the reader should be particularly careful to look for newer published data when faced with a similar clinical problem.

We are grateful to the chapter authors who made this book possible. We appreciate the guidance (and patience) of Christina Karaviotis and Mary Banks from BMJ Books. We thank our families (Andrea, Julia, and Nathalie Loeb; Cathy Marchetti and Daniel, Nicole, and Benjamin Smieja; Peter Seary) for their patience and support.

We hope you find this book informative and stimulating, and we shall certainly appreciate any feedback.

Mark Loeb
Marek Smieja
Fiona Smaill
Hamilton, 2004

Preface to the Second Edition

Following the success of our original edition in 2004, we are privileged to have this opportunity to edit an updated version of *Evidence-Based Infectious Diseases*. We have targeted this book to general internists and to trainees in infectious diseases, as feedback from the first edition indicated that our textbook was particularly helpful to these groups.

We hope that this new edition will bring added value, while continuing to serve as an evidence-based resource for physicians who manage patients with infections. Along with major updates in chapters on HIV, febrile neutropenia, bone and joint infections, sexually transmitted infections, urinary tract infections, and tuberculosis, there are three brand new chapters in this edition: Influenza, Critical care, and Infections in long-term care.

We are grateful to the chapter authors for all of their hard work. We would like to thank Mirjana Misina, Heather Addison, Rob Blundell, Laura Quigley, Beckie Brand, Lauren Brindley, and Mary Banks for their assistance in preparing this updated edition. We thank our families Andrea, Julia, and Nathalie Loeb; Cathy Marchetti and Benjamin, Nicole, and Daniel Smieja; and Peter Seary for their support.

We hope that you will find this edition informative and we welcome any feedback.

Mark Loeb
Marek Smieja
Fiona Smaill
Hamilton

CHAPTER 1

Introduction to evidence-based infectious diseases

Mark Loeb, Marek Smieja & Fiona Smaill

Our purpose in this chapter is to provide a brief overview of evidence-based infectious diseases practice and to set the context for the chapters which follow. We highlight evidence-based guidelines for assessing diagnosis, treatment, and prognosis, and discuss the application of evidence-based practice to infectious diseases, as well as identifying areas in which such application must be made with caution.

What is evidence-based medicine?

Evidence-based medicine was born in the writings of clinical epidemiologists at McMaster University, Yale, and elsewhere. Two series of guidelines for assessing the clinical literature articulated these, then revolutionary, ideas and found a wide audience of students, academics, and practitioners alike [1,2]. These guidelines emphasized the randomized clinical trial (RCT) for assessing treatment, now a standard requirement for the licensing of new drugs or other therapies. David Sackett, the founding chair of the Department of Clinical Epidemiology and Biostatistics at McMaster University, defined evidence-based medicine as "the conscientious, explicit and judicious use of current best evidence in making decisions about the care of patients" [3].

These guidelines, which we summarize later in the chapter, were developed primarily to help medical students and practicing doctors find answers to

clinical problems. The reader was guided in assessing the published literature in response to a given clinical scenario, to find relevant clinical articles, to assess the validity and understand the results of the identified papers, and to improve their clinical practice. Aided by computers, massive databases, and powerful search engines, these guidelines and the evidence-based movement empowered a new generation of practitioners and have had a profound impact on how studies are conducted, reported, and summarized. The massive proliferation of randomized clinical trials, the increasing numbers of systematic reviews and evidence-based guidelines, and the emphasis on appropriate methods of assessing diagnosis and prognosis, have affected how we practice medicine.

Evidence-based infectious diseases

The field of infectious diseases, or more accurately the importance of illness due to infections, played a major role in the development of epidemiological research in the 19th and early 20th centuries. Classical observational epidemiology was derived from studies of epidemics – infectious diseases such as cholera, smallpox, and tuberculosis. Classical epidemiology was nevertheless action-oriented. For example, John Snow's observations regarding cholera led to his removal of the Broad Street pump handle in an attempt to reduce the incidence of cholera. Pasteur, on developing an animal vaccine for anthrax, vaccinated a number of animals with members of the media in attendance [4]. When unvaccinated animals subsequently died, while vaccinated animals did not,

Evidence-Based Infectious Diseases, 2nd edition. Edited by
Mark Loeb, Fiona Smaill and Marek Smieja. © 2009
Wiley-Blackwell Publishing, ISBN: 978-1-4051-7026-0

the results were immediately reported throughout Europe's newspapers.

In the era of clinical epidemiology, it is notable that the first true randomized controlled trial is widely attributed to Sir Austin Bradford Hill's 1947 study of streptomycin for tuberculosis [5]. In subsequent years, and long before the "large simple trial" was rediscovered by the cardiology community, large-scale trials were carried out for polio prevention, and tuberculosis prevention and treatment.

Having led the developments in both classical and clinical epidemiology, is current infectious diseases practice evidence-based? We believe the answer is "somewhat". We have excellent evidence for the efficacy and side effects of many modern vaccines, while the acceptance of before-and-after data to prove the efficacy of antibiotics for treating bacterial meningitis is ethically appropriate. In the field of HIV medicine we have very strong data to support our methods of diagnosis, assessing prognosis and treatment, as well as very persuasive evidence supporting causation. However, in treating many common infectious syndromes – from sinusitis and cellulitis to pneumonia – we have many very basic diagnostic and therapeutic questions that have not been optimally answered. How do we reliably diagnose pneumonia? Which antibiotic is most effective and cost-effective? Can we improve on the impaired quality of life that often follows such infections as pneumonia?

While virtually any patient presenting with a myocardial infarction will benefit from aspirin and thrombolytic therapy, there may not be a single "best" antibiotic for pneumonia. Much of the "evidence" that guides therapy in the infectious diseases, particularly for bacterial diseases, may not be clinical, but exists in the form of a sound biologic rationale, the activity of the antimicrobial against the offending pathogen, and the penetration at the site of infection (pharmacodynamics and pharmacokinetics). Still, despite having a sound biologic basis for choice of therapy, there are many situations where better randomized controlled trials need to be conducted and where clinically important outcomes, such as symptom improvement and health-related quality, are measured.

How, then, can we define "evidence-based infectious diseases" (EBID)? Paraphrasing David Sackett, EBID may be defined as "the explicit, judicious and conscientious use of current best evidence from infection diseases research in making decisions about the prevention and treatment of infection of individuals and populations". It is an attempt to bridge the gap between research evidence and the clinical practice of infectious diseases. Such an "evidence-based approach" may include critically appraising evidence for the efficacy of a vaccine or a particular antimicrobial treatment regimen. However, it may also involve finding the best evidence to support (or refute) use of a diagnostic test to detect a potential pathogen. Additionally, EBID refers to the use of the best evidence to estimate prognosis of an infection or risk factors for the development of infection. EBID therefore represents the application of research findings to help answer a specific clinical question. In so doing, it is a form of knowledge transfer, from the researcher to the clinician. It is important to remember that use of research evidence is only one component of good clinical decision-making. Experience and clinical skills are essential components. EBID serves to inform the decision-making process. For the field of infectious diseases, a sound knowledge of antimicrobials and microbiologic principles are also needed.

Posing a clinical question and finding an answer

The first step in practicing EBID is posing a clinically driven and clinically relevant question. To answer a question about diagnosis, therapy, prognosis, or causation, one can begin by framing the question [2]. The question usually includes a brief description of the patients, the intervention, the comparison, and the outcome (a useful acronym is "PICO"). For example, if asking about the efficacy of antimicrobial-impregnated catheters in intensive care units [6], the question can be framed as follows: "In critically ill patients, does use of antibiotic-impregnated catheters reduce central line infections?" After framing the question, the second step is to search the literature. There are increasingly a number of options for finding the best evidence. The first step might be to assess evidence-based synopses such as *Evidence-Based Medicine* or *ACP Journal Club* (we admit to bias – two of the editors [ML, FS] are associate editors for these journals). These journals regularly report on high-quality studies that can impact practice. The essential components of the studies are abstracted and the papers are reviewed in an accompanying commentary by knowledgeable clinicians. However, since these journals are geared to a general internal medicine audience, many questions faced by clinicians practicing infectious diseases may not be addressed.

The next approach that we would recommend is to search for systematic reviews. Systematic reviews can be considered as concise summaries of the best available evidence that address sharply defined clinical questions [7]. Increasingly, the Cochrane Collaboration is publishing high-quality infectious diseases systematic reviews (http://www.cochranelibrary.com). Another source of systematic reviews is the *DataBase of Abstracts of Reviews of Effects* (DARE) (http://www.crd.york.ac.uk/crdweb). To help find systematic reviews, MEDLINE can be searched using the systematic review clinical query option in PubMed (http://www.ncbi.nlm.nih.gov/pubmed/). If there are no synopses or systematic reviews that can answer the clinical question, the next step is search the literature itself by accessing MEDLINE through PUBMED. After finding the evidence the next step is to critically appraise it.

Evidence-based diagnosis

Let us consider the use of a rapid antigen detection test for group A streptococcal infection in throat swabs. The first question to ask is whether there was a blinded comparison against an accepted reference standard. By blinded, we mean that the measurements with the new test were done without knowledge of the results of the reference standard.

Next, we would assess the results. Traditionally, we are interested in the sensitivity (proportion of reference-standard positives correctly identified as positive by the new test) and specificity (the proportion of reference-standard negatives correctly identified as negative by the new test).

Ideally, we would also like to have a measure of the precision of this estimate, such as a 95% confidence interval on the sensitivity and specificity, although such measures are rarely reported in the infectious diseases literature.

Note, however, that while the sensitivity and specificity may help a laboratory to choose the best test to offer for routine testing, they do not necessarily help the clinician. Thus, faced with a positive test with known 95% sensitivity and specificity, we cannot infer that our patient with a positive test for group A streptococcal infection has a 95% likelihood of being infected. For this, we need a positive predictive value, which is calculated as the percentage of true positives among all those who test positive. If the positive predictive value is 90%, then a positive test would suggest a 90% likelihood that the person is truly infected. Similarly, the negative predictive value is the percentage of true negatives among all those who test negative. Both positive and negative predictive value change with the underlying prevalence of the disease, hence such numbers cannot be generalized to other settings.

A more sophisticated way to summarize diagnostic accuracy, which combines the advantages of positive and negative predictive values while solving the problem of varying prevalence, is to quantify the results using likelihood ratios. Like sensitivity and specificity, likelihood ratios are a constant characteristic of a diagnostic test, and independent of prevalence. However, to estimate the probability of a disease using likelihood ratios, we additionally need to estimate the probability of the target condition (based on prevalence or clinical signs). Diagnostic tests then help us to shift our suspicion (pretest probability) about a condition depending on the result. Likelihood ratios tell us how much we should increase the probability of a condition for a positive test (positive likelihood ratio) or reduce the probability for a negative test (negative likelihood ratio). More formally, likelihood ratio positive (LR+) and negative (LR−) are defined as:

$$LR+ = \frac{\text{odds of a positive test in an individual with the condition}}{\text{odds of a positive test in an individual without the condition}}$$

$$LR- = \frac{\text{odds of a negative test in an individual with the condition}}{\text{odds of a negative test in an individual without the condition}}$$

A positive likelihood ratio is also defined as follows: sensitivity/(1 – specificity). Let us assume, hypothetically, that the sensitivity of the rapid antigen test is 80% and the specificity 90%. The positive likelihood ratio for the antigen test is (0.8/0.1) or 8. This would mean that a patient with a positive antigen test would have 8 times the odds of being positive compared with a patient without group A streptococcal infection. The tricky part in using likelihood ratios is to convert the pretest probability (say 20% based on our expected prevalence among patients with pharyngitis in our clinic) to odds: these represent 1:4 odds. After multiplying by 8, we have odds of 8:4, or a 67% post-test probability of disease. Thus, our patient probably has group A streptococcus, and it would be reasonable to treat with antibiotics.

The negative likelihood ratio, defined as (1 – sensitivity)/specificity, tells us how much we should reduce the probability for disease given a negative test. In this case, the negative likelihood ratio is 0.22, which can be interpreted as follows: a patient with pharyngitis and a negative antigen test would have their odds of disease multiplied by 0.22. In this case, a pretest probability of 20% (odds 1:4) would fall to an odds of 0.22 to 4, or about 5%, following a negative test. Nomograms have been published to aid in the calculation of post-test probabilities for various likelihood ratios [8].

Having found that the results of the diagnostic test appear favorable for both diagnosing or ruling out disease, we ask whether the results of a study can be generalized to the type of patients we would be seeing. We might also call this "external validity" of the study. Here we are asking the question: "Am I likely to get the same good results as in this study in my own patients?" This includes such factors as the severity and spectrum of patients studied versus those we will encounter in our own practice, and technical issues in how the test is performed outside the research setting.

To summarize, to assess a study of a new diagnostic test, we identify a study in which the new test is compared with an independent reference standard; we examine its sensitivity, specificity, and positive and negative likelihood ratios; and we determine whether the spectrum of patients and technical details of the test can be generalized to our own setting.

In applying these guidelines in infectious diseases, there are some important caveats.

- There may be no appropriate reference standard.
- The spectrum of illness may dramatically change the test characteristics, as may other co-interventions such as antibiotics.

For example, let us assume that we are interested in estimating the diagnostic accuracy of a new commercially available polymerase chain reaction (PCR) test for the rapid detection of *Neisseria meningitidis* in spinal fluid. The reference standard of culture may not be completely sensitive. Therefore, use of an expanded reference ("gold") standard might be used. For example, the reference standard may be growth of *N. meningitidis* from the spinal fluid, demonstration of an elevated white blood cell count in the spinal fluid along with gram-negative bacilli with typical morphology on Gram stain, or elevated white blood cell count along with isolation of *N. meningitidis* in the blood.

It is also important to know in what type of patients the test was evaluated, such as the inclusion and exclusion criteria, as well as the spectrum of illness. Given that growth of microorganisms is usually progressive, test characteristics in infectious diseases can change depending when the tests are conducted. For example, PCR conducted in patients who are early in their course of meningitis may not be sensitive as compared to patients that presented with late-stage disease. This addresses the issue of spectrum in test evaluation.

Evidence-based treatment

The term "evidence-based medicine" has become largely synonymous with the dictum that only randomized, double-blinded clinical trials give reliable estimates of the true efficacy of a treatment. For the purposes of guidelines, "levels of evidence" have been proposed, with a hierarchy from large to small RCTs, prospective cohort studies, case–control studies, and case series. In newer iterations of these "levels of evidence", a metaanalysis of RCTs (without statistical heterogeneity, indicating that the trials appear to be estimating the same treatment effect), are touted as the highest level of evidence for a therapy.

In general, clinical questions about therapy or prevention are best addressed through randomized controlled trials. In observational studies, since the choice of treatment may have been influenced by extraneous factors which influence prognosis (so-called "confounding factors"), statistical methods are used to "adjust" for identified potentially confounding variables. However, not all such factors are known or accurately measured. An RCT, if large enough, deals with such extraneous prognostic variables by equally apportioning them to the two or more study arms by randomization. Thus, both known and unknown confounders are distributed roughly evenly between the study arms.

For example, a randomized controlled trial would be the appropriate design to assess whether dexamethasone administered prior to antibiotics reduces mortality in adults who have bacterial meningitis [9]. We would evaluate the following characteristics of such a study: who was studied; was there true random assignment; were interventions and assessments blinded; what was the outcome; and can we generalize to our own patients?

When evaluating clinical trials it is important to ensure that assignment of treatment was truly randomized. Studies should describe exactly how the patients were randomized (e.g., random numbers table, computer generating). It is also important to assess whether allocation of the intervention was truly concealed. It is especially important here to distinguish allocation concealment from blinding. Allocation of an intervention can always be concealed even though blinding of investigators, participants or outcome assessors may be impossible. Consider an RCT of antibiotics versus surgery for appendicitis (improbable as this is). Blinding participants and investigators after patients have been randomized would be difficult (sham operations are not considered ethical). However, allocation concealment occurs before randomization. It is an attempt to prevent selection bias by making certain that the investigator has no idea to what arm (antibiotics versus surgery) the next patient enrolled will be randomized. In many trials this is done through a centralized randomized process whereby the study investigator is faxed the assignment after the patient has been enrolled. In some trials, the assignment is kept in envelopes. The problem with this is that, if the site investigator (or another clinician) has a preference for one particular intervention over another, the possibility for tampering exists. For example, if a surgeon who is a site investigator is convinced that the patient he has just enrolled would benefit most from surgery, the

surgeon might be tempted to hold the envelope up to a strong light, determine the allocation, and then select another if the contents of the envelope do not indicate surgery as the allocation. This would lead to selection bias and distort the result of the clinical trial. This type of tampering has been documented [10].

The degree of blinding in a study should also be considered. It is important to recognize that blinding can occur at six levels: the investigators, the patients, the outcome assessors, adjudication committee, the data monitoring committee, the data analysts, and even the manuscript writers (although in practice few manuscripts are written blinded of the results) [11]. Describing a clinical trial as "double-blinded" is vague if in fact blinding can occur at so many different levels. It is better to describe who was blinded than using generic terms.

Similarity of groups at baseline should also be considered when evaluating randomized controlled trials to assess whether differences in prognostic factors at baseline may have had an impact on the result. A careful consideration of the intervention is also important. One can ask what actually constitutes the intervention – was there a co-intervention that really may have been the "active ingredient"?

Follow-up is another important issue. It is important to assess whether all participants who were actually randomized are accounted for in the results. A rule of thumb is that the potential for the results to be misleading occurs if fewer than 80% of individuals randomized are not accounted for at the end (i.e., loss to follow-up of over 20% of participants). More rigorous randomized controlled trials are analyzed on an intention-to-treat basis. That is, all patients randomized are accounted for and are analyzed with respect to the group to which they were originally allocated. For example, an individual in our hypothetical appendicitis trial who was initially randomized to antibiotics but later received surgery would be considered in the analysis to have received antibiotics.

Having assured ourselves that the study is randomized, the randomization allocation was not prone to manipulation, and the randomized groups have ended up as comparable on major prognostic factors, we next examine the actual results. Consider a randomized controlled trial of two antibiotics A and B for community-acquired pneumonia. If the mortality rate with antibiotic A is 2% and that with B is

4%, the absolute risk reduction is the difference between the two rates (2%), the relative risk of A versus B is 0.5, and the relative risk reduction is 50%, that is the difference between the control and intervention rate (2%) divided by the control rate (4%). In studies with time-to-event data, the hazard ratio is measured rather than the relative risk, and can be thought of as an averaged relative risk over the duration of the study. Absolute risk reduction, relative risk, and hazard ratios are all commonly reported with a 95% confidence interval (CI) as a measure of precision. A 95% CI that does not cross 1.0 (for a relative risk or hazard ratio) or 0 (for the absolute risk reduction) has the same interpretation as a P value of < 0.05: we declare these results as "statistically significant". Unlike the P value, the 95% CI gives us more information regarding the size of the treatment effect. Note that statistical significance simply tells us whether the results were likely due to chance; the CI also tells us the precision of the estimate (helpful especially for underpowered studies, in which the wide CI warns us that a larger study may be required to more precisely determine the effect). It is important to be aware that statistical significance and clinical importance are not synonymous. A small study may miss an important clinical effect, whereas a very large study may reveal a small but statistically significant difference of no clinical importance. In well-designed studies, researchers prespecify the size of a postulated "minimum clinically important difference" rather than solely relying on statistical significance.

Measures of relative risk, hazard ratios, or absolute risk reduction may be difficult to apply in clinical practice. A more practical way of determining the size of a treatment effect is to translate the absolute risk reduction into its reciprocal, the number needed to treat (NNT). In this example, the number needed to treat is the number of patients who need to be treated to prevent one death. It is the inverse of the absolute risk reduction (1/0.02), which is 50. Therefore, if 50 patients are treated with antibiotic B instead of A, one death would be prevented. A 95% CI can be calculated on the NNT, although we would only recommend such calculations for statistically significant treatment effects. This recommendation is based on the curious mathematical property that, as the absolute risk reduction crosses 0, the NNT becomes infinite, and thereafter crosses over into the bounds of a "number needed to harm".

It is important to determine if all important outcomes were considered in the randomized controlled trial. For example, a clinical trial of a novel immunomodulating agent for patients with severe West Nile virus disease would need not only to consider neurologic signs and symptoms but also to assess functional status and health-related quality of life. When deciding whether the results of a randomized trial can be applied to your patients, the similarity in the setting and patient population needs to be considered. Finally, you must consider whether the potential benefits of the therapy outweigh the potential risks.

Rather than relying on individual RCTs, it is generally preferable to try to identify systematic reviews on the topic. Systematic reviews, however, also need to be critically evaluated. First, one must ensure that the stated question of the review addresses the clinical question that you are asking. The methods section should describe how all relevant studies were found: that is, including the specific search strategy as well as the inclusion and exclusion criteria. Study validity should be assessed, although there is no universally accepted method for scoring validity in systematic reviews. Both size and precision of treatment effects need to be considered. Similar to evaluating randomized controlled trials, whether all important outcomes were assessed in the review is important. Asking whether the findings are generalizable to your patients and whether the likely benefits are worth the potential harms and benefits is also important.

In summary, to assess a treatment we would find a systematic review or clinical trial; assess whether patients were properly randomized; whether various components of the study were blinded; whether there was a high proportion followed up for all clinically relevant outcomes. We then consider the actual results, and express these ideally as a "number needed to treat" to appreciate the importance (or lack thereof) for individual patients. Finally, we consider whether these results are applicable to the type and severity of disease that we may see in our clinics.

In examining a treatment in infectious diseases, a few caveats to these guidelines are in order.
- For many infections there may be a very strong historic and biologic rationale to treat; in such cases an RCT using placebo will be unethical.
- Many infections may be too rare to study in RCTs, and some infected populations (such as injection

drug users) may be difficult to enrol into treatment studies. Observational methods, such as case–control or cohorts to examine therapies or durations associated with cure or relapse, may be the most appropriate methods in these circumstances.

- While the individually randomized clinical trial is held up as an ideal, it may be more sensible to study many infections through so-called "cluster randomization" in which the unit of randomization may be the hospital, a school, neighborhood, or family. Such studies may detect a treatment effect where herd immunity is important, and may be more feasible to run. However, the confidence intervals for a cluster-randomized study are somewhat wider than if individuals are randomized.
- Even when individually randomized, the infection itself may represent a "cluster". Thus, a highly effective therapy for one strain of multidrug resistant (MDR) *M. tuberculosis* may be useless against another MDR strain. Hence, biologic knowledge of the pathogen and therapy need to be considered when the results of an RCT are generalized to a particular clinical setting.

Evidence-based assessment of prognosis

Many studies about risk factors and outcomes for infectious diseases are published but the quality is variable. The best designs for assessing these are cohort studies in which a representative sample of patients is followed, either prior to developing the infection (to determine risk) or after being infected (to determine outcome). Patients should be assembled at a similar point in their illness (the so-called "inception cohort"), and follow-up should be sufficiently long and complete. Important prognostic factors should be measured, and adjusted for in the analysis. As with clinical trials, the outcome measures are a relative risk, absolute risk, or hazard ratio associated with a particular infection or prognostic factor. For example, to assess the outcome of patients with severe acute respiratory syndrome (SARS), one would optimally want an inception cohort of individuals who meet the case definition within several days of onset of symptoms. These individuals would then be followed prospectively. One of the challenges with SARS was the lack of a "realtime" diagnostic test with high sensitivity and

specificity. In general, as diagnostic tests improve, our ability to detect early disease will improve. If SARS re-emerges and therapeutic agents are developed, this will change the natural history, hence the importance of noting whether therapy was administered in the cohort study. If strains of SARS coronavirus mutate as immunity to the virus builds, this may reduce the virulence of the agent. Therefore, it is important to keep in mind that estimates of risk and outcome may change with changes in the infectious agent.

Summary

We hope that the approaches described in this chapter will prove useful for evaluating articles about diagnosis, prognosis, treatment, or prevention in the infectious diseases literature. Using the principles described in this chapter, the chapters that follow attempt to summarize the best evidence for key clinical issues about infectious diseases.

References

1 Department of Clinical Epidemiology and Biostatistics. How to read clinical journals: I. why to read them and how to start reading them critically. CMAJ 1981;124:555–8.
2 Oxman A, Sackett DL, Guyatt GH. Users' guides to the medical literature. I. How to get started. JAMA 1993;270: 2093–5.
3 Sackett DL, Rosenberg WM, Gray JA, Haynes RB, Richardson WS. Evidence-based medicine: what it is and what it isn't. BMJ 1996;312:71–2.
4 Dubos R. Pasteur and Modern Science. Washington: ASM Press 1998.
5 Daniels M, Hill AB. Chemotherapy of pulmonary tuberculosis in young adults: an analysis of the combined results of three medical research council trials. BMJ 1952;1:1162–8.
6 Darouriche RO, Raad II, Heard SO et al. A comparison of two antimicrobial-impregnated central venous catheters. N Engl J Med 1999;340:1–8.
7 Cook DJ, Mulrow CD, Haynes RB. Systematic reviews: synthesis of best evidence for clinical decisions. Ann Intern Med 1997;126:376–80.
8 Detsky AS, Abrams HB, Forbath N, Scott JG, Hilliard JR. Cardiac assessment for patients undergoing noncardiac surgery. A multifactorial clinical risk index. Arch Intern Med 1986;146:2131–4.
9 de Gans J, van de Beek D. Dexamethasone in adults with bacterial meningitis. N Engl J Med 2002;347:1549–56.
10 Schulz KF, Grimes DA. Allocation concealment in randomized trials: defending against deciphering. Lancet 2002;359:614–18.
11 Devereau PJ, Manns BJ, Ghali WA et al. Physician interpretations and textbook definitions of blinding terminology in randomized controlled trials. JAMA 2001;285:2000–3.

PART 1
Specific diseases

Skin and soft-tissue infections

Douglas Austgarden & Guilio DiDiodato

Impetigo

Impetigo is a common skin infection distributed worldwide. *Staphylococcus aureus* and β-hemolytic streptococci are invariably the pathogens [1]. Typically, streptococcal impetigo (nonbullous impetigo) starts as papules, turning to pustules that break down to form the characteristic "honey-coloured" crust. Bullous impetigo is more commonly associated with staphylococci. In this form, vesicles first appear that then evolve to larger bullae and eventually rupture leaving a shiny thin brown "varnish-like" crust. Usually the lesions are on exposed areas of the body, typically face and extremities. Generally streptococci have recently colonized the skin and then subsequently been inoculated into the dermis by a minor trauma, whereas staphylococcal impetigo is associated with colonization of the nares [2]. There can be transmission to other persons with close personal contact, such as athletes [3]. Infection occurs most frequently in children of lower socioeconomic groups. Impetigo is seen year round in warmer climates and in the summer months in northern climates [2]. Patients with impetigo rarely have systemic signs of infection.

There is evidence from a systematic review and metaanalysis that treatment with topical antibiotics is more effective than placebo (odds ratio [OR] 2.69, 95% confidence interval [CI] 1.49–4.86) [4]. There is no significant difference between the effects of mupirocin and fusidic acid (OR 1.7, 95% CI 0.77–4.03) [4]; however, strains of *S. aureus* resistant to mupirocin are

Evidence-Based Infectious Diseases, 2nd edition. Edited by Mark Loeb, Fiona Smaill and Marek Smieja. © 2009 Wiley-Blackwell Publishing, ISBN: 978-1-4051-7026-0

being found [5]. A Cochrane review concluded that topical mupirocin was superior to oral erythromycin (OR 1.22, 95% CI 1.05–2.97), but in most other comparisons topical and oral antibiotics did not show different cure rates [6]. A penicillinase-resistant penicillin, a first-generation cephalosporin or a macrolide are recommended for oral therapy [7] but local resistance patterns, for example, prevalence of erythromycin-resistant *S. aureus* and *Streptococcus pyogenes*, should be taken into account in the choice of antibiotic. In cases of a nonresolving impetigo, infection may be with community-acquired methicillin resistant *S. aureus* (MRSA). See later in this chapter for further discussion on community-acquired MRSA infections.

Cellulitis and erysipelas

Case presentation 1

A healthy 45-year-old man hit his forearm while doing some house renovations, causing a minor abrasion 3 days prior to his presentation to the Emergency Department. He noted some minor swelling, pain, and erythema yesterday, but this morning he noted much more pain. His right forearm was swollen and erythema covered most of the dorsal surface from wrist to elbow. The emergency physician refers him for consideration of parenteral therapy and inpatient treatment with concerns about the area of involvement and rate of spread. His health is otherwise excellent.

On examining the patient, he is afebrile, pulse rate of 78 per minute and blood pressure of 134/75 mmHg. He has a small abrasion on his dorsal wrist with erythema extending to the elbow. The erythema is not raised, has indistinct borders, with no vesicles or bullae. The lesion is warm, tender to palpation, but there is no increase in pain on movement.

Cellulitis is a common problem in primary care but only a minority are referred to consultants or admitted for inpatient treatment. A review of a patient database in five urban hospitals showed 3929 diagnoses of cellulitis representing 1·3% of Emergency Department visits; 7% required inpatient treatment [8].

Cellulitis usually presents with pain, erythema with typically indistinct borders, and swelling. Fever and regional lymphadenitis are occasionally seen. In a predominately outpatient population, pain, erythema, and swelling were described in 69%, 78%, and 69% of cases, respectively, while fever and lymphadenitis occurred in only 7% and 10% of patients [8]. For an inpatient population, pain, erythema, and swelling were seen in 87%, 79%, and 90%, respectively, and fever occurred in 63% of patients [9]. Unfortunately, these signs and symptoms are not specific and many other processes can present with similar clinical findings, for example superficial or deep vein thrombophlebitis, fasciitis, hematoma, dermatitis, and local reaction to a bite or sting.

Most commonly *S. aureus* and *S. pyogenes* are the pathogens. Less often and usually associated with underlying chronic disease, immunosuppression, or infection at a particular site (e.g., periorbital cellulitis with sinusitis), pathogens can include *Haemophilus influenzae*, *Pseudomonas aeruginosa*, other *Streptococcus* spp., gram-negative bacilli, *Clostridium* spp., and other anaerobes [10,11]. In a data registry of hospitalized patients in Canada and the USA, 1562 bacterial isolates were identified over 1 year in a wide variety of patients with skin and soft-tissue infections: *S. aureus* accounted for 42·6% of isolates, with 24% being MRSA, *P. aeruginosa* (11·3%), *Enterococcus* spp. (8·1%), *Escherichia coli* (7·2%), *Enterobacter* spp. (5·2%), and β-hemolytic streptococci (5·1%) [12]. Essentially the same rank was seen in both countries with the exception of *Enterococcus* spp. which was third in the USA and seventh in Canada [12]. If there is a concern with exposure to water, certain specific organisms should be considered. In salt water, *Vibrio vulnificus* can cause a cellulitis and a potentially life-threatening infection in patients with liver disease. In fresh water, *Aeromonas hydrophilia* is a possible pathogen.

Erysipelas is a distinctive form of cellulitis. The lesion is typically bright red, warm, painful (which differentiates it from more superficial infections) with a raised, clearly demarcated border (usually not seen in other forms of cellulitis). Facial erysipelas with the often described malar "butterfly" rash actually represents only 15–20% of cases and most infections involve the lower extremity [10,11]. Systemic symptoms, for example fever, chills, sweats and rigors, are common. Infants, young children, and older adults are most commonly affected [13]. Erysipelas has a predisposition for areas of impaired lymphatic drainage and in these patients recurrent episodes can occur [11]. Group A streptococcus (*S. pyogenes*) is primarily responsible for erysipelas but groups B, C, and G, as well as *S. aureus* have been described [12]. Only 5% of blood cultures are positive [10].

Surface cultures, aspiration, and blood cultures all have low diagnostic yield in identifying the infecting organism causing cellulitis. Surface cultures are not recommended because of low yield and contamination with skin flora. Some advocate culturing an intact pustule if present [10]. Several studies have described varying techniques to aspirate from the lesion, resulting in positive cultures from 10% to 100% of the time [14–17]. In a large retrospective study of over 750 patients with cellulitis and 553 blood cultures, only 2% of blood cultures yielded a pathogen, and 73% of these were β-hemolytic streptococci [18]. In the healthy patient without an unusual exposure, microbiologic testing is neither necessary nor cost-effective.

Routine laboratory investigations have little diagnostic role in managing the healthy patient with cellulitis but may be required in the management of patients with chronic diseases, such as diabetes, liver disease, or renal failure, where an infection may lead to acute deterioration of the underlying disease, influencing the choice and dose of antibiotics and the decision whether to admit. Plain radiographs to rule out a foreign body are sometimes needed. Often radiographs are obtained to screen for tissue air if necrotizing fasciitis is a concern, or for osteomyelitis in an infected diabetic foot ulcer.

In mild and localized cellulitis in otherwise healthy patients presenting to the Emergency Department, an oral agent covering *S. aureus* and *Streptococcus* spp. is sufficient, and there is no advantage to agents with broader spectrum antimicrobial activity [19]. A penicillinase-resistant penicillin, first- or second-generation cephalosporin, or macrolide have

Case presentation 1 (continued)

After careful review you decide this patient has cellulitis and unlikely has a fasciitis. Since he is otherwise healthy with no history of unusual exposure you feel no extra tests are required. You are, however, concerned about the size and the rapidity of spread and decide this patient needs parenteral antibiotics, but which one(s) and does he need to be admitted?

appropriate activity, although no studies demonstrating superiority of one agent over another have been done. While a 7- to 10-day course of therapy with the agent at its higher dose range is recommended, there is little evidence on which to base the duration of therapy or the optimal dose. In a randomized controlled trial of levofloxacin 500 mg/day in patients with uncomplicated cellulitis, 5 days of therapy was as effective as 10 days of therapy [20]. Cellulitis recurs in some patients and in a retrospective, population-based cohort study, tibial involvement, history of cancer, and dermatitis predicted recurrence (hazard ratios of 5.02, 3.87, and 2.99 respectively) [21]. Prophylactic penicillin is recommended for patients with recurrent episodes, although one study showed that this approach was only effective in patients without predisposing factors [22,23].

In patients with more severe cellulitis, it is generally accepted that parenteral antibiotics are required. What is not well defined is in which patients cellulitis should be deemed moderate or severe. Studies of moderate or severe cellulitis have included patients with cellulitis and one or more of the following: extensive area, ulceration, abscess, signs of toxicity or sepsis, associated with surgical site, bite, foreign body, trauma, intravenous drug injection site, diabetic foot or pressure ulcer, immunosuppression (e.g. HIV), diabetes, chronic corticosteroid use, or failure of previous therapy [24–30].

Many antibiotic regimens evaluated in methodologically sound studies have demonstrated similar efficacy with inpatient populations and complicated skin infections: pipercillin-tazobactam [24], ticarcillin-clavulanate [24,25], levofloxacin [25,31], teicoplanin [32,33], meropenem [26], imipenem/cilastin [26],

ceftriaxone [30,33–36], ciprofloxacin [28], ofloxacin [27], cefotaxime [27,28], linezolid [29], oxacillin [29], and cefazolin [35,36]. Clinical cure rates ranged from 84% to 98·4% and microbiological cure rates from 71% to 94%. In a metaanalysis that compared the effectiveness and safety of fluoroquinolones versus β-lactams for the empirical treatment of skin and soft-tissue infections that included 20 randomized controlled trials, fluoroquinolones were more effective than β-lactams for the clinically evaluable patients (OR 1.29, 95% CI 1.00–1.66) but not for patients with moderate to severe infections (OR 1.12, 95% CI 0.80–1.55) [37]. However, the authors concluded that because of the high proportion of successfully treated patients in both groups and more adverse effects associated with fluoroquinolones, fluoroquinolones did not have a substantial advantage compared with β-lactams. In a randomized controlled trial of patients with lower limb cellulitis requiring intravenous antibiotics, there was no evidence to support the addition of intravenous benzylpenicillin to intravenous flucloxacillin (difference in mean number of doses −0.24, 95% CI −2.48 to 2.01, $P = 0.83$) [38].

Many patients may choose to be treated with parenteral therapy on an outpatient basis. Prospective evaluations of outpatient antibiotic programs have shown that they are safe and effective [30,33–36,39] and a randomized controlled trial of intravenous antibiotics at home or in hospital for treatment of cellulitis demonstrated no difference in outcome between the two groups (mean difference in days to no advancement of cellulitis 0.01 days, 95% CI −0.3 to 0.28) [40]. Patient satisfaction was greater in patients treated at home.

Intravenous ceftriaxone has been widely recommended for outpatient therapy owing to its once daily dosing [30,34]. Two randomized studies have demonstrated that cefazolin and probenecid have equivalent efficacy to ceftriaxone in an outpatient setting [35,36]. Brown et al. randomized 194 patients with moderate to severe cellulitis to 2 g intravenous cefazolin daily or 2 g intravenous ceftriaxone daily, while both groups received probenecid 1 g orally [35]. Outcomes were similar, 91·8% versus 92·7% clinical cure, with cost savings associated with the cefazolin group. However, the majority of patients were intravenous drug users with injection site infections, follow-up was not complete and patients were given a prescription for oral penicillin and cloxacillin upon enrollment. Grayson et al. randomized 116 patients who presented with moderate to severe cellulitis to 2 g intravenous cefazolin and 1 g probenecid orally or 1 g intravenous ceftriaxone and placebo [36]. Clinical cure rates were similar: 86% in the cefazolin arm versus 96% in the ceftriaxone arm ($P = 0.11$) and remained equivalent up to 1 month of follow up, 96% versus 91% ($P = 0.55$). Both studies excluded patients with penicillin allergies, septic patients requiring hospitalization, patients with evidence of osteomyelitis, and significant renal failure.

Oral antibiotics with a broad spectrum of antimicrobial activity and equivalent bioavailability to intravenous regimens offer another alternative for the outpatient management of patients with complicated skin and soft-tissue infections. In a randomized trial comparing intravenous or oral levofloxacin and intravenous ticarcillin/clavulanate alone or followed by oral amoxicillin/clavulanate, 44 of 200 patients in the levofloxacin group had oral therapy alone [25]. Forty patients (90·9%) in this subset had clinical cure, which was a similar rate to the overall responses: 84.1% in the levofloxacin group and 80.4% in the ticarcillin/clavulanate group. Although the subset receiving only oral levofloxacin was not specifically analyzed, the authors caution that it may have had less severe disease. The other fluoroquinolones, for example moxifloxacin, also with improved gram-positive activity, could be expected to be similarly effective.

There are many options for patients with more complicated cellulitis, and choice of antibiotic should be individualized based on the patient's history and any extenuating circumstances. For most patients, outpatient therapy is safe and effective. Once daily regimens such as cefazolin and probenecid provide an easy, effective, and low-cost alternative. Follow-up and clinical response should dictate changes of antibiotic therapy.

Furuncles and carbuncles

Furuncles or "boils" are infections of hair follicles usually caused by *S. aureus*. Typically lesions are painful, erythematous nodules with an overlying pustule. When several furuncles coalesce to form a larger abscess this is a carbuncle. Large furuncles and carbuncles need incision and drainage [7]. Warm compresses promote drainage and antibiotics are rarely required unless there are systemic symptoms or an extensive cellulitis [7].

Outbreaks can occur within families and individuals in close living quarters (e.g. in prisons). Sports teams, especially involving contact sports, can also experience outbreaks. Recurrent furunculosis seems to be associated with *S.aureus* nasal colonization [41]. The National Health and Nutrition Examination Survey (NHANES) demonstrated an overall colonization prevalence of *S. aureus* of 32.4% among non-institutionalized Americans, with the highest rates seen in people younger than 65 years and males [42]. Surveillance studies have demonstrated that approximately 20% of individuals are persistently colonized with one type of strain (persistent carriers), 60% carry *S. aureus* intermittently and the remainder are noncarriers [43]. Those most at risk for persistent colonization appear to express high avidity binding receptors for *S. aureus*, along with being at high risk of environmental exposure to *S. aureus* through poor living conditions due to poverty, homelessness, overcrowding, poor hygiene, hospitalization, residence in a long-term care facility, or incarceration [42,43].

Eradication with mupirocin [44] (applied to the nares for 5 days each month) or systemic treatment with low-dose clindamycin [45] (150 mg/day for 3 months) is effective in reducing recurrence rates of furunculosis.

Soft-tissue infections and MRSA infection

The majority of *S. aureus* strains still remain sensitive to cloxacillin, but MRSA strains causing infection continue to increase in prevalence, with country-specific prevalence rates as high as 50% in Japan, Eastern Europe, the Middle East and South America [46]. While MRSA infections were first reported in hospitalized patients in 1967, more recent reports have identified MRSA strains causing infection in community-dwelling individuals who have neither previous admission to hospitals nor risk factors for disease [47]. These infectious diseases syndromes have been classified as healthcare-associated (HA-MRSA) and community-associated MRSA (CA-MRSA), respectively. Currently, the most important clinical differentiating characteristics are their phenotypic susceptibility patterns, with the majority of CA-MRSA still retaining sensitivity to trimethoprim-sulfamethoxazole, tetracyclines, and clindamycin [47]. Community isolates frequently contain genes for the virulence factor Panton-Valentine leukocidin [47].

The prevalence of MRSA colonization in the USA has been estimated to be 1.5% (95% CI 1.2–1.8), with 19.7% (95% CI 12.4–28.8%) of these MRSA strains being classified as CA-MRSA [48]. There are increasing reports implicating CA-MRSA as the leading cause of emergency room visits for SSTI in certain populations, especially in the young, minorities, intravenous drug users, men who have sex with men, military personnel, and inmates of correctional facilities [47]. Clinical and epidemiologic risk factors, however, cannot reliably distinguish between MRSA and methicillin-sensitive *S. aureus* [49].

Treatment outcomes for patients with mild to moderate CA-MRSA skin and soft-tissue infections are dependent on aggressive drainage of abscesses and less so on antibiotic therapy. In one randomized controlled trial conducted on patients with MRSA skin and soft-tissue infections, there was no difference in outcomes between patients receiving antibiotics compared to placebo when appropriate incision and debridement of abscesses was completed [50]. Other studies have confirmed that abscesses caused by MRSA can be cured with drainage alone [51,52]. However, in a large retrospective analysis of 492 patients with MRSA skin and soft-tissue infections, a significant increase in treatment failures (OR 2.80, 95% CI 1.26–6.22, $P = 0.01$) was demonstrated if initial therapy was with an ineffective agent [53]. These results were confirmed in another study of empirical therapy for community *S. aureus* infections which showed that use of an effective agent was associated with greater clinical resolution (OR 5.91, 95% CI 3.14–11.13) when controlled for incision, drainage and HIV status [54]. Guidelines for the management of CA-MRSA recommend for those patients with a mild to moderate SSTI in a high-risk population for CA-MRSA, empiric therapy consist of a 5- to 10-day course of an antibiotic effective against CA-MRSA (e.g., TMP-SMX, clindamycin, or doxycycline) [55–57]. Counseling regarding the importance of good hand hygiene and wound treatment is recommended in conjunction with treatment, in order to prevent the transmission of MRSA to close contacts and the recurrence of infection [55,57].

For those patients with more severe SSTI at high risk for CA-MRSA, it is recommended that empiric therapy with parenteral systemic antibiotic therapy be initiated, along with admission to hospital with appropriate contact precautions and drainage of abscesses [57]. Empiric therapy with vancomycin is currently the first-line choice, although parenteral formulations of TMP-SMX or clindamycin are acceptable alternatives [55]. Other alternatives to vancomycin include linezolid, tigecycline, daptomycin, or quinupristin-dalfopristin [56]. These alternatives to vancomycin should only be considered after consultation with an infectious diseases specialist because of their risk profiles and cost, and lack of familiarity of use among physicians.

Treatment to eradicate MRSA colonization is not routinely recommended for individual CA-MRSA infections [55,57]. In a cluster-randomized placebo-controlled trial of mupirocin in soldiers, there was no decrease in infections (difference in infection rate between placebo and mupirocin groups 0.2%, 95% CI -1.3 to 1.7%) and new colonization was not prevented, despite eradication of CA-MRSA in colonized participants [58]. Decolonization may be considered for those patients with recurrent CA-MRSA infections or where there is evidence of ongoing transmission, but optimal regimens have not been established [57].

Necrotizing fasciitis

Case presentation 2

A previously healthy carpenter presents to the Emergency Department with fever and a painful arm. Yesterday at work he began to notice a sore right shoulder, was assessed in the Emergency Department later that evening, and diagnosed with a soft-tissue injury. Today he has pain in his shoulder and upper arm as well as fever and lethargy. On examination he is in moderate to severe distress from the pain, his temperature is 38.9°C, heart rate 122 per minute, and blood pressure of 90/60 mmHg. There is no obvious trauma or rash on his arm, but it is generally swollen and exquisitely tender to palpation and on movement of the shoulder or elbow. You begin to wonder if this man has a life-threatening infection.

Necrotizing fasciitis involves infection of the subcutaneous tissue with rapid spread and destruction of skin, subcutaneous fat, and fascia. Fortunately, it is a relatively uncommon life- and limb-threatening infection, but requires early recognition, prompt surgical intervention, and appropriate antibiotics. Many names have been used based upon clinical circumstances and pathogen, for example classic (clostridial) gas gangrene, clostridial cellulitis, non-clostridial gas gangrene, Fournier gangrene, Meleney's synergistic gangrene, necrotizing cellulitis, crepitant cellulitis, streptococcal gangrene, and, in the lay press, the term "flesh-eating bacteria" has been coined. Classification systems have also been developed based on pathogen [10] but are unhelpful clinically.

The literature on necrotizing fasciitis is predominately empiric, based on retrospective reviews and small case series. With the emergence of group A streptococcal fasciitis and associated toxic shock syndrome, more knowledge and understanding has been gained, but because of the relative rarity of cases and the complexity of the illness, randomized trials of management will be difficult to undertake.

The incidence of necrotizing fasciitis has been estimated at four cases per million [59]. A prospective cohort study monitoring the incidence of group A streptococcus in Ontario, Canada between 1991 and 1995 showed an increasing incidence from 0·85 per million to 3·5 per million during the study [60]. The CDC has estimated 500 to 1500 cases of group A streptococcus worldwide annually [61].

The presentation of necrotizing fasciitis can vary from the appearances of a simple cellulitis or soft-tissue injury to the classic hemorrhagic bullae, presence of soft-tissue gas, septic shock, and multiorgan failure. Toxic shock syndrome and multiorgan failure were also present in 47% of patients with group A streptococcus necrotizing fasciitis [60]. Most cases of necrotizing fasciitis initially present with a cellulitis but progress over hours to days with spreading erythema and edema. Hemorrhagic bullae can form as a result of skin necrosis secondary to vessel thrombosis. Pain out of proportion to clinical findings is commonly reported as an important early sign. Anesthetic skin due to destruction of nerves can be a late sign. Soft-tissue gas is a classic finding especially with clostridial infection. Estimates of the frequency of these signs and symptoms are not available.

Necrotizing fasciitis should be considered in any patient with "cellulitis" and systemic symptoms of fever and tachycardia, or rapidly spreading infection. Commonly necrotizing fasciitis starts at a pre-existing skin lesion, such as a surgical site, trauma, chronic skin problems (e.g., pressure ulcer, diabetic foot, ischemic ulcer, or psoriasis), and in children varicella infection predisposes to necrotizing fasciitis [10,59,60,62–65]. In Kaul et al. a predisposing skin lesion was present in 74% of cases of group A streptococcus necrotizing fasciitis [60]. Any underlying medical condition, such as diabetes, alcohol abuse, immunosuppressive illness or treatment, cardiac disease, peripheral vascular disease, chronic lung disease, or chronic renal failure, should increase the suspicion for necrotizing fasciitis [10,59,60,62,63,65]. In Kaul et al. one or more of these conditions were present in 71% of cases [60]. Any area of the body can be involved, but the lower extremity accounted for 53% of cases, while the upper extremity was involved 29% of the time [60].

Necrotizing fasciitis can be caused by many organisms and usually is polymicrobial with a mixture of aerobic and anaerobic bacteria. One review showed that 85% of confirmed cases of necrotizing fasciitis were polymicrobial, while *S. aureus*, *S. pyogenes*, and *Clostridium* spp. were the most commonly isolated single pathogen [66]. Usual aerobic pathogens are *S. aureus*, *S. pyogenes*, and *E. coli*, while *Clostridium* spp., *Bacteroides fragilis*, and *Peptostreptococcus* spp. are predominate anaerobes. Rarely, and usually as a co-pathogen, other gram-positive organisms such as *Streptococcus pneumoniae*, gram-negatives such as *Pseudomonas aeruginosa*, *Serratia*, *Vibrio*, *Proteus*, *Enterobacter*, *Pasteurella*, *Eikenella*, and *Neisseria* spp., and anaerobes *Fusobacterium* and *Prevotella* spp. can cause necrotizing fasciitis.

The gold standard for diagnosis is surgical exploration to determine fascial involvement and to provide material for culture and microscopic examination [10,59,62–65,67]. Surgical exploration will also indicate the need for surgical debridement. In a small retrospective study, a frozen-section biopsy with urgent histopathologic analysis reduced mortality [68]. Fine-needle aspirate is positive for bacteria or pus 80% of the time [69]. Soft-tissue gas observed clinically or with plain films is diagnostic, but not always present. Ultrasound, CT, and MRI have all been used to aid in the diagnosis of necrotizing fasciitis [69–75] but performance indicators (sensitivity and specificity) of ultrasound and CT in diagnosing necrotizing fasciitis have not been published. In two studies, totalling 25 patients, MRI had a 100% sensitivity but the specificity ranged from 75% to 100% [73,74]. Other conditions (e.g., cellulitis and abscesses) can be indistinguishable from necrotizing fasciitis [75]. Imaging should not delay definitive surgical treatment in the unstable patient. Laboratory investigations such as creatinine kinase, C-reactive protein, serum sodium, white blood cell count, serum calcium, creatinine, urea, and coagulation profiles have all been proposed to aid diagnosis, but lack sensitivity to reliably rule out necrotizing fasciitis [10,59,60,76,77].

> ## Case presentation 2 (continued)
>
> As you page the surgeon and begin resuscitating this young man, you wonder which antibiotics you could give immediately to cover the potential pathogens and whether there are other therapies that might save his life.

Immediate resuscitation, including ventilatory and inotropic support, prompt surgical debridement or amputation, and broad-spectrum parenteral antibiotics are the mainstay of management [10,11,59,60, 62–65,67]. Owing to the diversity of potential pathogens and because the majority of cases of necrotizing fasciitis are associated with polymicrobial infection, the most commonly recommended initial antibiotic is a β-lactam/β-lactamase inhibitor plus clindamycin [10,11,39,62–65,67,78]. Acceptable alternative regimens include single agents such as carbapenems, second-generation cephalosporins or fluoroquinolones with anaerobic activity and combinations with ampicillin and metronidazole or clindamycin, with either a third-generation cephalosporin, an aminoglycoside, fluoroquinolone, or aztreonam [10,11,59,62–65,78]. With animal models of group A streptococcus necrotizing fasciitis, clindamycin has been shown to have more effective killing power than penicillin, because bacteria reach the stationary growth phase rapidly and penicillin loses effectiveness in this phase [79]. Clinical data seem to support this with improved

survival in patients treated with clindamycin [60,78]. Also owing to its effect on protein synthesis inhibition and toxin production, clindamycin may improve survival in patients with group A streptococcus necrotizing fasciitis [10,60,62]. Once a pathogen(s) has been identified, antibiotics should be tailored to the pathogen(s). For group A streptococcus necrotizing fasciitis, penicillin and clindamycin is recommended [7,10,60,62]. In penicillin-allergic patients, a second- or third-generation (if *Pseudomonas* is a consideration) cephalosporin can usually be safely substituted [80,81]. If a patient has a true penicillin/cephalosporin allergy a fluoroquinolone, macrolide, or vancomycin may be alternatives.

In a case–control study intravenous immunoglobulin (IG) dosed at 2 g/kg appears to decrease mortality in patients with group A streptococcus necrotizing fasciitis [82], and in one small randomized trial mortality was 3.6 fold higher in the placebo group 4 deaths compared with the IG group 2 deaths although the results were not statistically significant [83]. All patients in these studies had toxic shock syndrome. Intravenous IG appears to modulate the superantigen response in group A streptococcus necrotizing fasciitis [60,82]. A conservative nonsurgical approach to group A streptococcus necrotizing fasciitis, using penicillin (4 million units every 6 hours), clindamycin (900 mg every 6 hours), and intravenous IG (2 g/kg) has been proposed. Seven successful cases (six with TSS) treated with this regimen have been reported [84]. Surgery was either not performed or only limited exploration was carried out. With the significant morbidity of large area debridement, this regimen potentially offers an alternative approach to group A streptococcus necrotizing fasciitis, but these preliminary data need further study, and currently an aggressive surgical approach remains an important component of management. Intravenous IG use in other forms of necrotizing fasciitis has not been studied and there is no evidence to support its use in these settings.

Hyperbaric oxygen therapy (HBO) has been used as an adjunct for necrotizing fasciitis. Multiple small, retrospective studies have been done in both clostridial and nonclostridial necrotizing fasciitis with variable results. A metaanalysis showed a significant reduction in mortality in both groups: 19% versus 45% in clostridial necrotizing fasciitis and 20·7% versus 43·5% in nonclostridial necrotizing fasciitis [85].

HBO should not delay surgical debridement and unstable patients should not be transferred, but this treatment modality should be used if available.

Mortality for necrotizing fasciitis is estimated to be around 40% [62]. Specifically group A streptococcus necrotizing fasciitis had an observed mortality of 34–43% [60,63]. Hypotension on presentation is associated with an 18-fold increase in death [60]. Age over 65, bacteremia, chronic illness, and multiorgan failure also were associated with increased mortality [60,86]. For a specific discussion of postoperative necrotizing fasciitis see Chapter 16, Infections in General Surgery.

Diabetic foot infections

Case presentation 3

A 63-year-old man with a longstanding history of type 2 diabetes, complicated by peripheral neuropathy and chronic renal insufficiency, presents with a 2-day history of increasing drainage from an ulcer on his right foot. Today redness and swelling in his foot was noted. On examination he is afebrile, with a normal heart rate and blood pressure. On his right foot, he has a 2 cm ulcer on the sole between the 1st and 2nd metatarsal heads, with swelling and erythema to the mid-foot dorsally. His blood sugar is 18 mmol/liter and his WBC count is normal. Knowing the difficult nature of diabetic foot infections, you wonder which antibiotic, oral or parenteral, outpatient or inpatient, and other therapies might help in treating this man.

Due to the triad of vascular insufficiency, peripheral neuropathy, and impaired immune function, foot ulceration and infection are common among diabetic patients. Foot infections are among the most common cause for hospital admission in such patients [86,87]. Osteomyelitis is present in an estimated 20% of complicated infections and diabetic foot infection accounts for 50% of lower extremity amputations [88–90]. In 1996, 86 000 lower extremity amputations were performed on diabetic patients in the USA [90]. Diabetic foot infections need a multidisciplinary team approach involving endocrinologist, podiatrist, wound care specialist, diabetic educators, plastic, orthopedic, and vascular surgeons, and infectious disease specialist for their care [91] but the

treatment of many patients is not in line with current guidelines [92].

Usually diabetic foot infections occur in a preexisting ulcer and prior trauma is common [93]. Peripheral neuropathy is the greatest risk factor for foot ulcers and infection [94] and patients often have no complaints of pain. Patients will usually have discharge from the ulcer, erythema, swelling, and unexplained hyperglycemia but there is no evidence a "signs-and-symptoms" checklist is a useful method of identifying infection in chronic wounds [95]. If there is no draining ulcer but the foot is erythematous and swollen, a Charcot foot (diabetic neuroarthropathy) should be considered [96].

Diabetic foot infections can be classified into two groups:
- non-limb-threatening, which have <2 cm of surrounding erythema extending from the ulcer, not a full-thickness ulcer and no systemic signs of toxicity;
- limb-threatening, which have >2 cm of surrounding erythema, full-thickness ulcer, presence of an abscess or soft-tissue gas, rapid progression, and signs of systemic toxicity [86,96].

Two-thirds of patients with limb-threatening infections have no fever, chills or elevated white blood cell count [97].

Surface cultures from wounds are not useful for identifying infection in chronic wounds [95]. Curettage of the base following debridement, or aspiration from non-necrotic tissue, may yield more dependable results to identify the infecting pathogen(s) [86,96]. In non-limb-threatening infection, S. aureus and group B streptococcus are considered the major pathogens [97–100]. Enterococcus spp., gram-negatives and anaerobes are often cultured, but it is unclear if they are colonizers or pathogens [96,101]. In moderate to severe diabetic foot infections, gram-negatives such as E. coli, Proteus spp., P. aeruginosa, Serratia spp., and Enterobacter spp., and anaerobes, such as Bacteroides and Peptostreptococcus spp., are often isolated and usually considered pathogenic [86,96–105].

For non-limb-threatening infections, initial antimicrobial therapy can be directed towards S. aureus and streptococci, and a first-generation cephalosporin, for example, cefazolin, is an appropriate choice. In a randomized, prospective trial of non-limb-threatening diabetic foot infections, 56 outpatients received 2 weeks of either oral cefalexin 500 mg four times a day or clindamycin 300 mg four times a day as an outpatient [98]. From curettage specimens, 89% yielded gram-positive organisms (42% as a sole pathogen), 36% gram-negatives and 13% anaerobes. After 2 weeks of therapy, 91% were cured or improved, while of the five failures, three went on to cure with another agent covering gram-positive organisms (clindamycin, ampicillin, or cloxacillin). One of the other treatment failures had polymicrobial growth and, despite parenteral antibiotics for 2 months, ultimately required a forefoot amputation.

For limb-threatening diabetic foot infections, broad-spectrum antibiotics are recommended and many of the trials of complicated or moderate to severe cellulitis included diabetic foot infections. Randomized trials specifically performed on diabetic foot infections included use of ampicillin/sulbactam [103,104], imipenem/cilastin [104], cefoxitin [99], ceftizoxime [105], ofloxacin [103], moxifloxacin [106], and ertapenem [107]. All the trials had similar results with clinical cure or improvement in the range of 80–90%. A systematic review concluded that the evidence was too weak to recommend any particular antimicrobial agent for foot ulcers in diabetes [108]. In certain circumstances, outpatient therapy would be appropriate depending on diabetic control, extent of infection, and availability of follow-up.

There are other interventions that can be used in the management of diabetic foot infections. The type of wound dressing is an underused tool and new technologies in skin substitutes have shown promise in chronic ulcers, but further research is required to support their use in diabetic foot infections [86,95,109]. A randomized controlled trial of negative pressure wound therapy for the treatment of diabetic foot ulcers reported greater ulcer closure with negative pressure therapy compared with moist wound dressings [110] but a systematic review that included all kinds of wounds found little evidence to support negative pressure therapy [111]. Non-weight-bearing and even rigid immobilization is often recommended, although no randomized trials have been performed [112–115]. Hyperbaric oxygenation has been shown to improve healing of chronic ulcers [116], is cost-effective when compared to standard care [117], and has been effective in several small studies in diabetic foot infections [118–120]. Urgent vascular bypass surgery can be an option if ischemia is a major contributor to a non-healing ulcer or infection. The risks of such surgery must be balanced with the expected benefit for each patient [121].

For a further discussion on the management of complicated infections and osteomyelitis in diabetic patients, refer to Chapter 3, Bone and Joint Infections.

Animal bites

Case presentation 4

A 59-year-old woman, who was trying to intervene in a fight between the family dog and a neighborhood dog, notices a 2 cm laceration over the 5th metacarpophalangeal joint after the squabble was broken up. She has a past history of angina and hypercholesterolemia and is unsure when her last tetanus booster was given. Both pets have been immunized annually. You wonder, should you close the laceration? Does she need prophylaxis and, if so, with which antibiotic? Should she receive treatment for rabies?

Animal bites are very common. The vast majority of people never seek medical attention. Dog bites account for 90% of all bites, cats (5%), humans (2%), rodents (2%), and all other animals less than 1% [122]. It is estimated than 4·5 million dog bites occur annually in the USA and 7·3–18 per 10 000 bites seek medical attention [123–125]. An estimated 10 000 hospitalizations and 20 deaths per year occur secondary to dog bites, most being in children [124,126]. Deaths are usually due to the attack itself and only rarely from secondary infectious complications. Most bites are from family pets and a minority from stray animals.

Patients with bites have a bimodal pattern of presentation. If children are bitten, if the injury is significant, or if there are concerns over the potential for infection, or for tetanus and rabies, medical attention is sought immediately. Later, patients will present with signs and symptoms of secondary infection. An estimated 3–18% of dog bites and 28–80% of cat bites become infected [127]. Most bites occur on the hand or arm, children are more likely to be bitten on the face, males are more likely to be bitten by a dog, and females more likely to be bitten by a cat [128].

Important historical information to focus on include the past medical history of the patient, especially any history of immunosuppression or significant chronic disease, status of tetanus immunization, time of and circumstances surrounding the event (provoked or unprovoked), and details concerning the animal, for example health, ownership, and location. Many patients will be reluctant to divulge information owing to concern over reprisal on the animal by local authorities. Many cities and regions have mandatory reporting of animal bites. The wound should be assessed for site and potential for nerve, tendon, bone, or joint involvement, especially on the hands and feet. Any wound over a metacarpophalangeal joint should be considered a clench fist injury (punch injury). If the patient presents with established infection, systemic signs, site and extent of infection, lymphadenopathy, and possibility of tenosynovitis, osteomyelitis and septic arthritis should be considered.

Copious irrigation, debridement of necrotic tissue, and removal of foreign bodies are essential in early management of bite wounds [126–128]. Puncture wounds should be irrigated with a needle or plastic tip catheter inserted into the wound. Infected wounds should be opened if previously sutured, eschar removed and abscesses drained, then irrigated copiously. Closure of bite wounds is controversial, as there are no randomized studies of this intervention. Wounds less than 24 hours old, with no signs of infection, on the face, trunk, or proximal extremities can probably be closed safely [127]. All wounds on hands or feet, should be left open, especially if caused by cat or human [126–128].

Talan et al. have examined the bacteriology of infected dog or cat bites [129]. They examined the pathogens responsible for 50 dog bites and 57 cat bites. There were a mean of five pathogens per wound with a range of 0–16. For dogs, the most common aerobic bacteria were *Pasteurella* spp. (50% of patients) especially *Pasteurella canis*, *Streptococcus* spp. (46%), *Staphylococcus* spp. (46%), *Neisseria* spp. (16%), and *Corynebacterium* spp. (12%), while the most frequent anaerobes were *Fusobacterium* spp. (32%), *Bacteroides* spp. (30%), *Porphyromonas* spp. (28%), and *Prevotella* spp. (28%). Cats had similar bacteria, with the exception that *Pasteurella* spp. grew in 75% of cases with *P. multocida* being the most frequent species. From these data, the authors recommended a β-lactam/

β-lactamase inhibitor or a second-generation cephalosporin with anaerobic activity. The combination of clindamycin and a fluoroquinolone was also recommended. Treatment guidelines have been published [7], however there are no prospective trials nor comparative studies of different antibiotic regimens for treating infected animal bites.

In human bites, the usual organisms are *S. aureus*, *Streptococcus* spp., and anaerobes, as well as an organism specific to the oral flora of humans, a fastidious gram-negative rod, *Eikenella corrodens*. It has an unusual sensitivity profile in that it is sensitive to penicillin and β-lactam/β-lactamase inhibitors, but relatively resistant to cloxacillin, first-generation cephalosporins, erythromycin, and clindamycin [126]. A β lactam/β-lactamase inhibitor combination is an appropriate initial choice.

The majority of patients with infected bite wounds can be managed as outpatients with oral antibiotics. Alternatively, parenteral antibiotics could be initiated with stepdown to oral therapy when the infection is resolving. This can be accomplished on an out- or inpatient basis, depending on clinical circumstances.

Antibiotic prophylaxis of animal bites is controversial. A Cochrane Library systematic review showed a favorable odds ratio for prophylaxis of cat and human bites, but not dogs, and for prophylaxis in hand wounds, but not face/neck or trunk wounds [130]. A randomized, blinded, placebo-controlled trial of 185 patients with animal bites using amoxicillin/clavulanate for prophylaxis, showed no difference in wounds less than 9 hours old, but a significant difference in those 9–24 hours old [131]. Therefore the animal, location of wound, and time to presentation all seem to affect the risk of infection and need for prophylaxis.

Animal bites can potentially transmit rabies and many patients will seek medical attention for fear of rabies infection. This is a rare occurrence in industrialized countries. In Canada, 22 rabies cases have been reported in 56 years [128]. In the USA, 32 cases over 16 years have been reported [132]. Immunized animals who are acting normally over a period of 10 days are not rabid. In certain areas, wild animals such as bats, raccoons, skunks, and foxes have been rabid. Local public health authorities can be a valuable resource in ascertaining the risk of rabies transmission in an individual case and the need for post-exposure prophylaxis.

Infections of skin and underlying soft tissue are a common problem in primary care. While most infections are managed without complication, those referred to the hospitalist/consultant are often in patients who have failed therapy, have significant comorbidity, or have a life- or limb-threatening infection. A thorough understanding of both common and unusual infectious etiologies, and local resistance patterns, are important in guiding antimicrobial choices. As well, other interventions to improve outcome can be employed and should be considered as part of the management of patients.

References

1 Darmstadt GL, Lane AT. Impetigo: an overview. Pediatr Dermatol 1994;11(4):293–303.

2 Ferrieri P, Dajani AS, Wannamaker LW, et al. Natural history of impetigo. I. Site sequence of acquisition and familial patterns of spread of cutaneous streptococci. J Clin Invest 1972;51(11):2851–62.

3 Adams B. Dermatological disorders of the athlete. Sports Med 2002;32:309–21.

4 George A, Rubin G. A systematic review and meta-analysis of treatments for impetigo. Br J Gen Pract 2003;53(491): 480–7.

5 Yun HJ, Lee SW, Yoon GM, et al. Prevalence and mechanisms of low- and high-level mupirocin resistance in staphylococci isolated from a Korean hospital. J Antimicrob Chemother 2003;51(3):619–23.

6 Koning S, Verhagen AP, van Suijlekom-Smit LW, et al. Interventions for impetigo. Cochrane Database of Syst Rev 2003 (2), CD003261, DOI 10.1002/14651858.

7 Stevens DL, Bisno AL, Chambers HF, et al. Practice guidelines for the diagnosis and management of skin and soft-tissue infections. Clin Infect Dis 2005 Nov;41(10): 1373–406.

8 Dong SL, Kelly KD, Oland RC, et al. ED management of cellulitis: a review of five urban centers. Am J Emerg Med 2001;19(7):535–40.

9 Ginsberg MB. Cellulitis: analysis of 101 cases and review of the literature. South Med J 1981;74(5):530–3.

10 Bisno AL, Stevens DL. Streptococcal infections of skin and soft tissues. N Engl J Med 1996;334(4):240–5.

11 Slaven EM, DeBlieux PM, Skin and soft-tissue infections: the common, the rare and the deadly. Emerg Med Prac 2001;3:1–24.

12 Doern GV, Jones RN, Pfaller MA, et al. Bacterial pathogens isolated from patients with skin and soft-tissue infections: frequency of occurrence and antimicrobial susceptibility patterns from the SENTRY Antimicrobial Surveillance Program (United States and Canada, 1997). SENTRY Study Group (North America). Diag Micro Infect Dis 1999;34:65–72.

13 Jorup-Ronstrom C. Epidemiological, bacteriological and complicating features of erysipelas. Scand J Infect Dis 1986;18(6):519–24.

14 Goldgeiger MH. The microbial evaluation of acute cellulitis. Cutis. 1983;31:649–56.

15 Sigurdsson AF, Gudmundsson S. The etiology of bacterial cellulitis as determined by fine-needle aspiration. Scand J Infect Dis 1989;21(5):537–42.

16 Uman SJ, Kunin CM. Needle aspiration in the diagnosis of soft tissue infections. Arch Intern Med 1975;135(7):959–61.

17 Sachs MK. The optimum use of needle aspiration in the bacteriologic diagnosis of cellulitis in adults. Arch Intern Med. 1990 Sep;150(9):1907–12.

18 Perl B, Gottehrer NP, Raveh D, et al. Cost-effectiveness of blood cultures for adult patients with cellulitis. Clin Infect Dis 1999;29(6):1483–8.

19 Powers RD. Soft tissue infections in the emergency department: the case for the use of "simple" antibiotics. South Med J 1991;84(11):1313–5.

20 Hepburn MJ, Dooley DP, Skidmore PJ, et al. Comparison of short-course (5 days) and standard (10 days) treatment for uncomplicated cellulitis. Arch Intern Med 2004;164(15):1669–74.

21 McNamara DR, Tleyjeh IM, Berbari EF, et al. A predictive model of recurrent lower extremity cellulitis in a population-based cohort. Arch Intern Med 2007;167(7):709–15.

22 Wang JH, Liu YC, Cheng DL, et al. Role of benzathine penicillin G in prophylaxis for recurrent streptococcal cellulitis of the lower legs. Clin Infect Dis 1997;25(3):685–9.

23 Kremer M, Zuckerman R, Avraham Z, et al. Long-term antimicrobial therapy in the prevention of recurrent soft-tissue infections. J Infect 1991;22(1):37–40.

24 Tan JS, Wishnow RM, Talan DA, et al. Treatment of hospitalized patients with complicated skin and skin structure infections: double-blind, randomized, multicenter study of piperacillin-tazobactam versus ticarcillin-clavulanate. The Piperacillin/Tazobactam Skin and Skin Structure Study Group. Antimicrob Agents Chemother 1993;37(8):1580–6.

25 Graham DR, Talan DA, Nichols RL, et al. Once-daily, high-dose levofloxacin versus ticarcillin-clavulanate alone or followed by amoxicillin-clavulanate for complicated skin and skin-structure infections: a randomized, open-label trial. Clin Infect Dis 2002;35(4):381–9.

26 Garau J, Blanquer J, Cobo L, et al. Prospective, randomised, multicentre study of meropenem versus imipenem/cilastatin as empiric monotherapy in severe nosocomial infections. Eur J Clin Microbiol Infect Dis 1997;16(11):789–96.

27 Gentry LO, Rodriguez-Gomez G, Zeluff BJ, et al. A comparative evaluation of oral ofloxacin versus intravenous cefotaxime therapy for serious skin and skin structure infections. Am J Med 1989;87(6C):57S–60S.

28 Gentry LO, Ramirez-Ronda CH, Rodriguez-Noriega E, et al. Oral ciprofloxacin vs parenteral cefotaxime in the treatment of difficult skin and skin structure infections. A multicenter trial. Arch Intern Med 1989;149(11):2579–83.

29 Stevens DL, Smith LG, Bruss JB, et al. Randomized comparison of linezolid (PNU-100766) versus oxacillin-dicloxacillin

for treatment of complicated skin and soft tissue infections. Antimicrob Agents Chemother 2000;44(12):3408–13.

30 Eron LJ, Park CH, Hixon DL, et al. Ceftriaxone therapy of bone and soft tissue infections in hospital and outpatient settings. Antimicrob Agents Chemother 1983;23(5):731–7.

31 Tarshis GA, Miskin BM, Jones TM, et al. Once-daily oral gatifloxacin versus oral levofloxacin in treatment of uncomplicated skin and soft tissue infections: double-blind, multicenter, randomized study. Antimicrob Agents Chemother 2001;45(8):2358–62.

32 Chirurgi VA, Edelstein H, Oster SE, et al. Randomized comparison trial of teicoplanin i.v., teicoplanin i.m., and cefazolin therapy for skin and soft tissue infections caused by gram-positive bacteria. South Med J 1994;87(9):875–80.

33 Nathwani D. The management of skin and soft tissue infections: outpatient parenteral antibiotic therapy in the United Kingdom. Chemotherapy 2001;47 Suppl 1:17–23.

34 Tice AD. Once-daily ceftriaxone outpatient therapy in adults with infections. Chemotherapy 1991;37 Suppl 3:7–10.

35 Brown G, Chamberlain R, Goulding J, et al. Ceftriaxone versus cefazolin with probenecid for severe skin and soft tissue infections. J Emerg Med 1996;14(5):547–51.

36 Grayson ML, McDonald M, Gibson K, et al. Once-daily intravenous cefazolin plus oral probenecid is equivalent to once-daily intravenous ceftriaxone plus oral placebo for the treatment of moderate-to-severe cellulitis in adults. Clin Infect Dis 2002;34(11):1440–8.

37 Falagas ME, Matthaiou DK, Vardakas KZ. Fluoroquinolones vs beta-lactams for empirical treatment of immunocompetent patients with skin and soft tissue infections: a meta-analysis of randomized controlled trials. Mayo Clin Proc 2006;81(12):1553–66.

38 Leman P, Mukherjee D. Flucloxacillin alone or combined with benzylpenicillin to treat lower limb cellulitis: a randomised controlled trial. Emerg Med J 2005;22(5):342–6.

39 Poretz DM. Treatment of skin and soft-tissue infections utilizing an outpatient parenteral drug delivery device: a multicenter trial. HIAT Study Group. Am J Med 1994;97(2A):23–7.

40 Corwin P, Toop L, McGeoch G, et al. Randomised controlled trial of intravenous antibiotic treatment for cellulitis at home compared with hospital. BMJ 2005;330(7483):129.

41 Hedstrom SA. Recurrent staphylococcal furunculosis. Bacteriological findings and epidemiology in 100 cases. Scand J Infect Dis 1981;13(2):115–19.

42 Graham PL, 3rd, Lin SX, Larson EL. A U.S. population-based survey of Staphylococcus aureus colonization. Ann Intern Med 2006;144(5):318–25.

43 Kluytmans J, van Belkum A, Verbrugh H. Nasal carriage of Staphylococcus aureus: epidemiology, underlying mechanisms, and associated risks. Clin Microbiol Rev 1997;10(3):505–20.

44 Raz R, Miron D, Colodner R, et al. A 1-year trial of nasal mupirocin in the prevention of recurrent staphylococcal nasal colonization and skin infection. Arch Intern Med 1996;156(10):1109–12.

45 Klempner MS, Styrt B. Prevention of recurrent staphylococcal skin infections with low-dose oral clindamycin therapy. JAMA 1988;260(18):2682–5.

46 Boyce JM, Cookson B, Christiansen K, et al. Methicillin-resistant Staphylococcus aureus. Lancet Infect Dis 2005;5(10):653–63.

47 Weber JT. Community-associated methicillin-resistant Staphylococcus aureus. Clin Infect Dis 2005;41 Suppl 4:S269–72.

48 Gorwitz RJ, Kruszon-Moran D, McAllister SK, et al. Changes in the prevalence of nasal colonization with Staphylococcus aureus in the United States, 2001–2004. J Infect Dis 2008;197(9):1226–34.

49 Miller LG, Perdreau-Remington F, Bayer AS, et al. Clinical and epidemiologic characteristics cannot distinguish community-associated methicillin-resistant Staphylococcus aureus infection from methicillin-susceptible S. aureus infection: a prospective investigation. Clin Infect Dis 2007;44(4):471–82.

50 Rajendran PM, Young D, Maurer T, et al. Randomized, double-blind, placebo-controlled trial of cephalexin for treatment of uncomplicated skin abscesses in a population at risk for community-acquired methicillin-resistant Staphylococcus aureus infection. Antimicrob Agents Chemother 2007;51(11):4044–8.

51 Moran GJ, Krishnadasan A, Gorwitz RJ, et al. Methicillin-resistant S. aureus infections among patients in the emergency department. N Engl J Med 2006;355(7):666–74.

52 Fridkin SK, Hageman JC, Morrison M, et al. Methicillin-resistant Staphylococcus aureus disease in three communities. N Engl J Med 2005;352(14):1436–44.

53 Ruhe JJ, Smith N, Bradsher RW, et al. Community-onset methicillin-resistant Staphylococcus aureus skin and soft-tissue infections: impact of antimicrobial therapy on outcome. Clin Infect Dis 2007;44(6):777–84.

54 Szumowski JD, Cohen DE, Kanaya F, et al. Treatment and outcomes of infections by methicillin-resistant Staphylococcus aureus at an ambulatory clinic. Antimicrob Agents Chemother 2007;51(2):423–8.

55 Barton M, Hawkes M, Moore D, et al. Guidelines for the prevention and management of community-associated methicillin-resistant Staphylococcus aureus: A perspective for Canadian health care practitioners. Can J Infect Dis Med Microbiol. 2006;17(Suppl C):4C–24C.

56 Nathwani D, Morgan M, Masterton RG, et al. Guidelines for UK practice for the diagnosis and management of methicillin-resistant Staphylococcus aureus (MRSA) infections presenting in the community. J Antimicrob Chemother 2008;61(5):976–94.

57 Dellit TM, Duchin J. Guidelines for evaluation and management of community-associated methiciclin-resistant Staphylococcus aureus skin and soft tissue infections in outpatient settings. 2007 [updated 2007; cited]; Available from: http://www.metrokc.gov/health/providers/epidemiology/MRSA-guidelines.pdf.

58 Ellis MW, Griffith ME, Dooley DP, et al. Targeted intranasal mupirocin to prevent colonization and infection by community-associated methicillin-resistant Staphylococcus aureus strains in soldiers: a cluster randomized controlled trial. Antimicrob Agents Chemother 2007;51(10):3591–8.

59 File TM, Jr., Tan JS, DiPersio JR. Group A streptococcal necrotizing fasciitis. Diagnosing and treating the "flesh-eating bacteria syndrome." Cleve Clin J Med 1998;65(5):241–9.

60 Kaul R, McGeer A, Low DE, et al. Population-based surveillance for group A streptococcal necrotizing fasciitis: Clinical features, prognostic indicators, and microbiologic analysis of seventy-seven cases. Ontario Group A Streptococcal Study. Am J Med 1997;103(1):18–24.

61 Centers for Disease Control and Prevention. Invasive group A streptococcal infections – United Kingdom, 1994. MMWR Morb Mortal Wkly Rep 1994 Jun 3;43(21):401–2.

62 Stevens DL. Streptococcal toxic-shock syndrome: spectrum of disease, pathogenesis, and new concepts in treatment. Emerg Infect Dis 1995;1(3):69–78.

63 Ward RG, Walsh MS. Necrotizing fasciitis: 10 years' experience in a district general hospital. Br J Surg 1991;78(4):488–9.

64 Bosshardt TL, Henderson VJ, Organ CH, Jr. Necrotizing soft-tissue infections. Arch Surg 1996;131(8):846–52; discussion 52–4.

65 Waldhausen JH, Holterman MJ, Sawin RS. Surgical implications of necrotizing fasciitis in children with chickenpox. J Pediatr Surg 1996;31(8):1138–41.

66 Elliott D, Kufera JA, Myers RA. The microbiology of necrotizing soft tissue infections. Am J Surg 2000;179(5):361–6.

67 File TM, Jr., Tan JS. Treatment of skin and soft-tissue infections. Am J Surg 1995;169(5A Suppl):27S–33S.

68 Stamenkovic I, Lew PD. Early recognition of potentially fatal necrotizing fasciitis. The use of frozen-section biopsy. N Engl J Med 1984;310(26):1689–93.

69 Lille ST, Sato TT, Engrav LH, et al. Necrotizing soft tissue infections: obstacles in diagnosis. J Am Coll Surg 1996;182(1):7–11.

70 Kaplan DM, Fliss DM, Shulman H, et al. Computed tomographic detection of necrotizing soft tissue infection of dental origin. Ann Otol Rhinol Laryngol 1995;104(2):164–6.

71 Kane CJ, Nash P, McAninch JW. Ultrasonographic appearance of necrotizing gangrene: aid in early diagnosis. Urology 1996;48(1):142–4.

72 Struk DW, Munk PL, Lee MJ, et al. Imaging of soft tissue infections. Radiol Clin North Am 2001;39(2):277–303.

73 Schmid MR, Kossmann T, Duewell S. Differentiation of necrotizing fasciitis and cellulitis using MR imaging. AJR Am J Roentgenol 1998;170(3):615–20.

74 Brothers TE, Tagge DU, Stutley JE, et al. Magnetic resonance imaging differentiates between necrotizing and non-necrotizing fasciitis of the lower extremity. J Am Coll Surg 1998;187(4):416–21.

75 Loh NN, Ch'en IY, Cheung LP, et al. Deep fascial hyperintensity in soft-tissue abnormalities as revealed by T2-weighted MR imaging. AJR Am J Roentgenol 1997;168(5):1301–4.

76 Wall DB, Klein SR, Black S, et al. A simple model to help distinguish necrotizing fasciitis from nonnecrotizing soft tissue infection. J Am Coll Surg 2000;191(3):227–31.

77 Simonart T, Simonart JM, Derdelinckx I, et al. Value of standard laboratory tests for the early recognition of group A beta-hemolytic streptococcal necrotizing fasciitis. Clin Infect Dis 2001;32(1):E9–12.

78 Zimbelman J, Palmer A, Todd J. Improved outcome of clindamycin compared with beta-lactam antibiotic treatment for invasive Streptococcus pyogenes infection. Pediatr Infect Dis J 1999;18(12):1096–100.

79 Stevens DL, Gibbons AE, Bergstrom R, et al. The Eagle effect revisited: efficacy of clindamycin, erythromycin, and penicillin in the treatment of streptococcal myositis. J Infect Dis 1988;158(1):23–8.

80 Levine BB. Antigenicity and cross-reactivity of penicillins and cephalosporins. J Infect Dis 1973;128:Suppl: S364–6.

81 Anne S, Reisman RE. Risk of administering cephalosporin antibiotics to patients with histories of penicillin allergy. Ann Allergy Asthma Immunol 1995;74(2):167–70.

82 Kaul R, McGeer A, Norrby-Teglund A, et al. Intravenous immunoglobulin therapy for streptococcal toxic shock syndrome – a comparative observational study. The Canadian Streptococcal Study Group. Clin Infect Dis 1999;28(4):800–7.

83 Darenberg J, Ihendyane N, Sjolin J, et al. Intravenous immunoglobulin G therapy in streptococcal toxic shock syndrome: a European randomized, double-blind, placebo-controlled trial. Clin Infect Dis 2003;37(3):333–40.

84 Norrby-Teglund A, Muller MP, McGeer A, et al. Successful management of severe group A streptococcal soft tissue infections using an aggressive medical regimen including intravenous polyspecific immunoglobulin together with a conservative surgical approach. Scand J Infect Dis 2005;37(3):166–72.

85 Clark LA, Moon RE. Hyperbaric oxygen in the treatment of life-threatening soft-tissue infections. Respir Care Clin N Am 1999;5(2):203–19.

86 Calhoun JH, Overgaard KA, Stevens MC. Diabetic foot ulcers and infections: current concepts. Adv Skin Wound Care 2002;15:31–42.

87 Thomson FJ, Veves A, Ashe H, et al. A team approach to diabetic foot care: the Manchester experience. Foot 1995;2:75–82.

88 Reiber GE, Pecoraro RE, Koepsell TD. Risk factors for amputation in patients with diabetes mellitus. A case-control study. Ann Intern Med 1992;117(2):97–105.

89 Armstrong DG, Lavery LA, Quebedeaux TL, et al. Surgical morbidity and the risk of amputation due to infected puncture wounds in diabetic versus nondiabetic adults. South Med J 1997;90(4):384–9.

90 Centers for Disease Control and Prevention. Diabetes Surveillance Report. 1999 [updated 1999; cited]; Available from: http://www.cdc.gov/diabetes/statistics/survl99/chap1/contents.htm.

91 Association AD. Standards of medical care in diabetes – 2008. Diabetes Care 2008;31 Suppl 1:S12–54.

92 Prompers L, Huijberts M, Apelqvist J, et al. Delivery of care to diabetic patients with foot ulcers in daily practice: results of the Eurodiale Study, a prospective cohort study. Diabet Med 2008;25(6):700–7.

93 Lavery LA, Armstrong DG, Wunderlich RP, et al. Risk factors for foot infections in individuals with diabetes. Diabetes Care 2006;29(6):1288–93.

94 Rith-Najarian SJ, Stolusky T, Gohdes DM. Identifying diabetic patients at high risk for lower-extremity amputation in a primary health care setting. A prospective evaluation of simple screening criteria. Diabetes Care 1992;15(10):1386–9.

95 Nelson EA, O'Meara S, Craig D, et al. A series of systematic reviews to inform a decision analysis for sampling and treating infected diabetic foot ulcers. Health Technol Assess 2006;10(12):iii–iv, ix–x, 1–221.

96 Caputo GM, Joshi N, Weitekamp MR. Foot infections in patients with diabetes. Am Fam Physician 1997; 56(1):195–202.

97 Gibbons GW, Eliopoulos GM. Infection of the diabetic foot. In: Kozak GP, Hoar CS, Rowbotham JL, et al., editors. Management of diabetic foot problems. Philadelphia: Saunders; 1984.

98 Lipsky BA, Pecoraro RE, Larson SA, et al. Outpatient management of uncomplicated lower-extremity infections in diabetic patients. Arch Intern Med 1990;150(4):790–7.

99 Sapico FL, Witte JL, Canawati HN, et al. The infected foot of the diabetic patient: quantitative microbiology and analysis of clinical features. Rev Infect Dis 1984;6 Suppl 1:S171–6.

100 Jones EW, Edwards R, Finch R, et al. A microbiological study of diabetic foot lesions. Diabet Med 1985; 2(3):213–15.

101 Wheat LJ, Allen SD, Henry M, et al. Diabetic foot infections. Bacteriologic analysis. Arch Intern Med 1986; 146(10):1935–40.

102 Citron DM, Goldstein EJ, Merriam CV, et al. Bacteriology of moderate-to-severe diabetic foot infections and in vitro activity of antimicrobial agents. J Clin Microbiol 2007;45(9):2819–28.

103 Lipsky BA, Baker PD, Landon GC, et al. Antibiotic therapy for diabetic foot infections: comparison of two parenteral-to-oral regimens. Clin Infect Dis 1997;24(4):643–8.

104 Grayson ML, Gibbons GW, Habershaw GM, et al. Use of ampicillin/sulbactam versus imipenem/cilastatin in the treatment of limb-threatening foot infections in diabetic patients. Clin Infect Dis 1994;18(5):683–93.

105 Hughes CE, Johnson CC, Bamberger DM, et al. Treatment and long-term follow-up of foot infections in patients with diabetes or ischemia: a randomized, prospective, double-blind comparison of cefoxitin and ceftizoxime. Clin Ther 1987;10 Suppl A:36–49.

106 Lipsky BA, Giordano P, Choudhri S, et al. Treating diabetic foot infections with sequential intravenous to oral moxifloxacin compared with piperacillin-tazobactam/amoxicillin-clavulanate. J Antimicrob Chemother 2007; 60(2):370–6.

107 Lipsky BA, Armstrong DG, Citron DM, et al. Ertapenem versus piperacillin/tazobactam for diabetic foot infections (SIDESTEP): prospective, randomised, controlled, double-blinded, multicentre trial. Lancet 2005;366(9498): 1695–703.

108 Nelson EA, O'Meara S, Golder S, et al. Systematic review of antimicrobial treatments for diabetic foot ulcers. Diabet Med 2006;23(4):348–59.

109 Veves A, Sheehan P, Pham HT. A randomized, controlled trial of Promogran (a collagen/oxidized regenerated cellulose dressing) vs standard treatment in the management of diabetic foot ulcers. Arch Surg 2002;137(7):822–7.

110 Blume PA, Walters J, Payne W, et al. Comparison of negative pressure wound therapy using vacuum-assisted closure with advanced moist wound therapy in the treatment of diabetic foot ulcers: a multicenter randomized controlled trial. Diabetes Care 2008;31(4):631–6.

111 Ubbink DT, Westerbos SJ, Nelson EA, et al. A systematic review of topical negative pressure therapy for acute and chronic wounds. Br J Surg 2008;95(6):685–92.

112 Sinacore DR. Total contact casting for diabetic neuropathic ulcers. Phys Ther 1996;76(3):296–301.

113 Helm PA, Walker SC, Pullium G. Total contact casting in diabetic patients with neuropathic foot ulcerations. Arch Phys Med Rehabil 1984;65(11):691–3.

114 Caputo GM, Ulbrecht JS, Cavanagh PR. The total contact cast: a method for treating neuropathic diabetic ulcers. Am Fam Physician 1997;55(2):605–11, 15–16.

115 Nabuurs-Franssen MH, Sleegers R, Huijberts MS, et al. Total contact casting of the diabetic foot in daily practice: a prospective follow-up study. Diabetes Care 2005;28(2):243–7.

116 Hammalund C, Sundberg T. Hyperbaric oxygen reduced size of chronic leg ulcers: a randomized double-blind study. Plast Reconstr Surg 1994;93:829–33.

117 Hailey D. Adjunctive hyperbaric oxygen therapy for diabetic foot ulcer: An economic analysis technology report: Canadian Agency for Drugs and Technologies in Health 2007 Mar Contract No.: Document Number.

118 Davis JC. The use of adjuvant hyperbaric oxygen in treatment of the diabetic foot. Clin Podiatr Med Surg 1987;4(2):429–37.

119 Oriani G, Meazza D, Favales F, et al. Hyperbaric oxygen therapy in the diabetic gangrene. J Hyperb Med 1990;5:171–5.

120 Wattel E, Mathieu DM, Fassati P, et al. Hyperbaric oxygen in the treatment of diabetic foot lesions. J Hyperb Med 1991;6:263–8.

121 Gibbons GW. Vascular evaluation and long-term results of distal bypass surgery in patients with diabetes. Clin Podiatr Med Surg 1995;12(1):129–40.

122 Callaham ML. Human and animal bites. Top Emerg Med 1982;4:1–15.

123 Thompson PG. The public health impact of dog attacks in a major Australian city. Med J Aust 1997;167(3): 129–32.

124 Weiss HB, Friedman DI, Coben JH. Incidence of dog bite injuries treated in emergency departments. JAMA 1998;279(1):51–3.

125 Sacks JJ, Kresnow M, Houston B. Dog bites: how big a problem? Inj Prev 1996;2(1):52–4.

126 Fleisher GR. The management of bite wounds. N Engl J Med 1999;340(2):138–40.

127 Goldstein EJ. Bite wounds and infection. Clin Infect Dis 1992;14(3):633–8.

128 Tannenbaum DW, Goldstein EJC, Rupprecht CE, et al. Management of animal bites. Patient Care 2002;13:54–69.

129 Talan DA, Citron DM, Abrahamian FM, et al. Bacteriologic analysis of infected dog and cat bites. Emergency Medicine Animal Bite Infection Study Group. N Engl J Med 1999;340(2):85–92.

130 Medeiros I, Saconato H. Antibiotic prophylaxis for mammalian bites. Cochrane Database Syst Rev 2001 (2), CD001738, DOI 10.1002/14651858.

131 Brakenbury PH, Muwanga C. A comparative double blind study of amoxycillin/clavulanate vs placebo in the prevention of infection after animal bites. Arch Emerg Med 1989;6(4):251–6.

132 Noah DL, Drenzek CL, Smith JS, et al. Epidemiology of human rabies in the United States, 1980 to 1996. Ann Intern Med 1998;128(11):922–30.

CHAPTER 3
Bone and joint infections

William J. Gillespie

Introduction

The evidence base for diagnosis and management of musculoskeletal infections has become stronger in the last 5 years with the publication of a number of systematic reviews and meta-analyses, and a substantial number of new primary trials. The use of likelihood ratios (LR) and diagnostic odds ratios (DOR) derived from meta-analysis of diagnostic studies should prove helpful in clinical practice. However meta-analysis of diagnostic studies is an emerging technique, subject to bias and variation in the included studies [1], and it is likely that there will be considerable refinement of the current methods in the next few years. Two important points should be kept in mind for the present. First, the performance of diagnostic tests which measure host inflammatory response may be misleading when their performance characteristics are applied to people with other disorders, particularly inflammatory polyarthritis. Second, the results of a sequence of tests using LRs derived in different contexts may also be misleading, particularly if the tests are not truly independent of each other [2]. This chapter considers three important examples of musculoskeletal infection: infectious arthritis in adults, prosthetic joint infection, and osteomyelitis in the diabetic foot.

Evidence-Based Infectious Diseases, 2nd edition. Edited by Mark Loeb, Fiona Smaill and Marek Smieja. © 2009 Wiley-Blackwell Publishing, ISBN: 978-1-4051-7026-0

Infectious arthritis

Case presentation 1

A 76-year-old woman presents to her family practitioner with a 72-hour history of increasing pain in the left knee associated with fever and malaise. She has been unable to walk for 12 hours prior to presentation. She has a 5-year history of osteoarthritis progressively affecting both knees for which she had taken a number of different non-steroidal anti-inflammatory agents, until 4 months ago when her medication was changed to paracetamol 2 g daily on account of medication-associated gastrointestinal discomfort. She has had no surgery to the knee. There is no history of gout, injury, or other recent illness. Physical examination reveals a temperature of 39°C. The left knee is held in 30 degrees of flexion; any movement from that position is extremely uncomfortable. There is a tense and tender effusion in the knee, which is warm to the touch. The right knee is cool to the touch, without a palpable effusion. Examination of cardio-respiratory, gastrointestinal, and neurological systems is normal. Blood pressure is 140/95 mmHg. Initial laboratory tests have shown hemoglobin of 10.9 mg/dL, WCC of 15 000/μL with 85% PMN and an ESR of 86 mm per hour. Radiographic examination of the knee confirms the presence of osteoarthritis. Urinalysis is negative for sugar and protein. She is admitted to hospital for investigation of acute inflammatory arthritis of the left knee.

Background

Incidence/prevalence estimates for infectious arthritis have varied [3,4], depending on case definition and case mix. The incidence in people with rheumatoid arthritis is around ten times that in the general population [3]. *Staphylococcus aureus* and streptococci remain the most frequent isolates in most reports. Other organisms may assume some importance in particular groups (e.g., tuberculous infection in immigrants from the developing world, and in people with HIV infection). The natural history of the untreated case is destruction of the infected joint. In adults, the case fatality rate may exceed 10% overall, and 25% in older people with rheumatoid arthritis [4].

Diagnosis of infectious arthritis

Clinical signs and laboratory studies

A recent systematic review [5] summarized current evidence for the predictive value of clinical signs, blood and synovial fluid analyses in the investigation of possible infectious arthritis. It found that:

1. Reported prevalence of infectious arthritis amongst patients presenting with acute monoarthritis to a specialist clinic is 8–27%.
2. Although the reference standard for confirming a diagnosis of infectious arthritis is a positive culture and Gram stain from examination of synovial fluid or tissue obtained by percutaneous needle aspiration, biopsy, or arthroscopy, the reference standard itself is imperfect. Therefore, the review included studies which had used positive Gram stain, positive aspirate or blood cultures, or response to antibiotics as a proxy reference standard.
3. A limitation of the current evidence is the lack of high-quality data in the included studies.
4. Clinical findings which characterize acute peripheral monoarticular arthritis do not predict infectious arthritis. The only clinical findings which occur in more than 50% of patients with infectious arthritis are joint pain (sensitivity 0.85; 95% CI 0.78–0.9), a history of joint swelling (sensitivity 0.78; 95% CI 0.71–0.85), and fever (sensitivity 0.57; 95% CI 0.52–0.62). Sweats (sensitivity, 0.27; 95% CI 0.20–0.34) and rigors (sensitivity, 0.19; 95% CI 0.15–0.24) are less common findings in infectious arthritis.
5. An abnormal peripheral WBC count (LR+ 1.4; 95% CI 1.1–1.8), ESR (LR+ 1.3; 95% CI 1.1–1.8), and CRP (LR+ 1.6; 95% CI 1.1–2.5) have poor diagnostic power for changing the pretest probability of

infectious arthritis, mostly due to their low specificity. Nevertheless, blood culture may occasionally identify an organism even when culture of the aspirate fails.
6. In examination of a joint aspirate, WCC greater than 100 000 cells/μL has strong diagnostic power for infectious arthritis (LR+ 28.0, 95% CI 12.0–66.0; LR– 0.71, 95% CI 0.64–0.79); WCC greater than 50 000 cells/μL has moderate diagnostic power (LR+ 7.7, 95% CI 5.7–11.0; LR– 0.42, 95% CI 0.34–0.51). Differential WCC of greater than 90% PMN carries LR+ of 3.4 (95% CI 2.8–4.2) and LR– of 0.34 (95% CI 0.25–0.47).
7. Other synovial fluid evaluations (low glucose, protein >3 g/dL, and LDH >250 U/L) predict infection weakly or not at all.

Imaging

MRI has limited diagnostic power in diagnosing infectious arthritis in adults. Two studies, both with methodologic limitations, have reported the sensitivity and specificity of MRI signs in infectious arthritis [6,7]. For individual signs (95% confidence intervals unavailable), LR+ was 4.14 and LR– 0.08 for synovial enhancement [8]; LR+ 1.96 and LR– 0.42 for periarticular bone marrow edema; and LR+ 2.11 and LR– 0.34 for bone erosion [9]. These likelihood ratios may not be valid in people with inflammatory polyarthritis, as the same signs are characteristic of rheumatoid arthritis [10].

Microbial culture

Attempts to increase the yield of positive cultures in aspirates by better techniques of sampling and transport have been made. Immediate incubation of the aspirate in blood culture bottles appears to increase the rate of successful culture [11,12]. One study (54 participants) [13], using microbiologic culture as the reference standard, found that synovial biopsy (sensitivity 0.69; specificity 1.0) had better diagnostic performance characteristics than simple aspirate (sensitivity 0.31; specificity 0.97).

There is insufficient current evidence to confirm advantage of using the polymerase chain reaction (PCR) with broad-range bacterial primers in the diagnosis of inflammatory monoarthritis in the usual diagnostic laboratory setting [8,9,14].

Case presentation 1 (continued)

Initial results from the laboratory found WCC of 15 000/μL with 85% PMN and ESR of 86 mm per hour. Synovial fluid analysis indicates WCC of 65 000/μL, with 92% PMN. No organisms were identified on Gram stain.

The prevalence of infectious arthritis amongst all the cases of inflammatory monoarthritis seen in your unit in the last 5 years is 26%, providing a prior probability of infectious arthritis of 0.26, equivalent to pre-test odds of 0.35. Using the likelihood ratios from [5], Table 3.1 shows what happens to the probability of infection as the diagnostic information builds up.

Management

There is general agreement based on cumulative experience that the treatment of infectious arthritis requires both antimicrobial therapy and the removal by joint puncture and lavage, on a number of occasions if necessary, of the inflammatory exudate from the joint [4].

Antimicrobial therapy

Provisional (empiric) therapy should begin as soon as the results of synovial fluid microscopy are available, if these support the diagnosis. Until the results of culture become available (and if no culture becomes available) a "best guess" choice should be based on local prescribing guidelines, the patient's history and findings, the known local pattern of infecting organisms, and their likely sensitivity to antimicrobial agents.

Definitive choice of antimicrobial agent is determined by the sensitivity of the etiologic microorganism. Optimal duration of therapy is not known. A consensus benchmark for RCTs evaluating new antimicrobial agents was 2–3 weeks [15]. Initially in the acutely febrile patient, intravenous therapy has usually been preferred until the temperature has returned to normal, but there is no RCT evidence to support practice.

Aspiration and lavage

Both open joint drainage and arthroscopic drainage [16] appear effective. RCT evidence for the best method of joint aspiration/lavage is unavailable. Open drainage of the hip has been traditionally advised, but arthroscopic drainage/lavage techniques are becoming established for the hip also [17].

Corticosteroid therapy

A third proposed component of therapy [4], the administration of a short course of systemic corticosteroids, improved outcomes in an experimental model [18]. In a subsequent RCT in childhood infectious

Table 3.1 Diagnostic sequence for infectious arthritis

	Pre-test probability of sepsis	Pretest odds	Point likelihood ratio from test [5]	Post-test odds	Post-test probability of sepsis
Patient has acute monoarthritis					0.26
History: prior osteoarthritis; no other obvious risk factor	0.26	0.35	1	0.35	0.26
Physical examination: fever	0.26	0.35	0.67	0.24	0.19
Blood white cell count: >15 000 cells/μL	0.19	0.24	1.40	0.33	0.25
ESR: 85 mm/h	0.25	0.33	1.30	0.43	0.30
Synovial fluid WCC: 65 000 cells/μL	0.30	0.43	7.70	3.30	0.77
Synovial fluid PMN: 92%	0.77	3.30	3.40	11.22	0.92

Note that it is the likelihood ratios from synovial fluid analysis which raise the probability of infectious arthritis from a low figure based on the frequency of infectious arthritis amongst cases of acute monoarthritis, to a level of probability which supports beginning presumptive therapy for infectious arthritis. A sensitivity analysis using the less favorable confidence limits from reference [5] raises the probability to 0.74; using the more favorable (upper) confidence limit, the probability of infectious arthritis is 0.98.

arthritis [19] a short course of dexamethasone was associated with reduced residual joint dysfunction and shortened the duration of symptoms. However its use in adults has not been reported. Given the increased risk of developing infectious arthritis associated with corticosteroid therapy of polyarthritis [20], caution is understandable at this point.

Implications for practice

In diagnosing infection in adults presenting with acute monoarthritis:

- Clinical findings and blood tests have poor diagnostic power.
- MRI has limited diagnostic power in diagnosing infectious arthritis in adults. It can distinguish anatomic and pathologic detail with great accuracy, but the signs in infection are also found in other inflammatory arthropathies.
- WCC greater than 100000 cells/μL has strong diagnostic power, WCC greater than 50000 cells/μL has moderate diagnostic power, and differential count of greater than 90% PMN has weak diagnostic power.

Implications for research

- The performance of diagnostic tests for infection which measure host inflammatory response should be evaluated in cohorts of people with suspected infection and inflammatory polyarthritis.
- The use of corticosteroids in adult septic arthritis, already used in some clinics, should be examined in carefully designed RCTs before wider adoption.

Prosthetic joint infection

Case presentation 2

A 67-year-old woman with a 14-year history of rheumatoid arthritis presents with a 1-year history of increasing discomfort in the right hip. Three years previously she had developed an acute postoperative infection following a primary elective right total hip replacement for which she had been treated by debridement, suction drainage and irrigation, and antimicrobial therapy. Recently, although she has been generally well with satisfactory control of her rheumatoid arthritis, pain in the right hip has recurred and radiographs show loosening of the implant.

Background

Although the incidence is low, prosthetic joint infections (PJI) result in substantial patient morbidity, loss of function, reduced quality of life, and societal costs. Clinical presentations range from an acute illness with local and systemic symptoms (characteristic in early postoperative and hematogenous infections), to low-grade infection leading to insidious prosthetic loosening and pain. PJI is hard to eradicate due to formation of surface biofilms on implant materials [21–23].

The incidence of infection after primary hip arthroplasty has decreased since the late 1960s, when infection rates were as high as 10% [24]. The introduction of antimicrobial prophylaxis and the development of techniques to reduce the burden of airborne bacteria in the operating room led to infection rates under 2% by the 1990s [25,26]. The increasing incidence of MRSA has raised the question of whether antibiotic prophylaxis should now include a glycopeptide, but there is insufficient current evidence to determine a threshold prevalence of MRSA at which switching to glycopeptide prophylaxis might be cost-effective [27].

Estimates of incidence of PJI derived from case series, surveillance programs, and national arthroplasty registers are susceptible to bias, due to differing diagnostic criteria for infection and operative risk case mix. Accepting that limitation, in the decade 1998–2007 [28–34] the incidence of any surgical site infection occurring within 1 year appears, overall, under 2%. Less than half of incident infections occur by 3 months. The ratio of superficial to deep SSIs in the first 3 months is approximately 3:1. By 2 years, up to 0.5% of primary total hip replacements will have had a reoperation for deep infection.

Diagnosis of prosthetic joint infection

The reference standard

There is no "gold standard" definition of prosthetic infection. Most investigators have identified a proportion of cases (10–15%) with convincing clinical evidence of infection from which it has not been possible to culture an organism. As a result, some reliance on assessing the host inflammatory response, a surrogate for infection, has been adopted in clinical practice. This is somewhat problematic for diagnosing infection in people with inflammatory polyarthritis. Neutrophils are prominent in the histology and cytology of rheumatoid arthritis [35,36]. Investigators have frequently excluded patients with inflammatory polyarthritis from studies of blood indicators, aspiration specimens, and histologic findings suggestive of inflammation. Where they have been included, subgroup information has rarely been provided.

In clinical practice, the Mayo Clinic definition [25] or a modification of it [37] has been used as a working definition. It requires the presence of at least one of four criteria – growth of the same microorganism in two or more cultures from preoperative aspirates or from intraoperative specimens; purulence of synovial fluid from an aspirate or at the implant site; presence of granulocytes on histopathologic examination of periprosthetic tissue; or presence of a sinus tract communicating with the device.

Preoperative tests

Blood investigations
In studies in people without inflammatory polyarthritis, three inexpensive blood tests have good predictive capability for supporting or ruling out a suspected PJI. Each pair of LRs (positive and negative), based on a single study only, are: ESR >30 mm/h [38] (LR+ 5.47, LR− 0.18); CRP >10 mg/L [38] (LR+ 12.0, LR− 0.08); and IL-6 >10 ng/L [39] (LR+ 20, LR+ 0.05).

Imaging
In a metaanalysis of anti-granulocyte scintigraphy [40], LR+ was 3.99 (95% CI 3.13–5.09) and LR− was 0.22 (95% CI 0.15–0.34) The data on FDG PET, although scanty, suggest that it may be a more powerful examination. One metaanalysis [41] calculated LR+ of 9.58 and LR− of 0.08. More recent data from a single center [42] indicated LR+ of 13.6 and LR− of 0.05.

Aspiration of the hip
No systematic review of the diagnostic performance of preoperative aspiration and culture has been identified. In reports from single units since the early 1990s, sensitivity has ranged from 0.12 to 0.86, and specificity from 0.81 to 1.00. A recent report [43] includes a short narrative review.

Intraoperative tests

Histology
Histologic examination may be unreliable in patients with inflammatory joint disease [44]. Variation in the quantitative criteria for making an intraoperative frozen section diagnosis of infection from histologic examination is reflected in the wide range of reports of sensitivity (0.18 to 1.00) and specificity (0.64 to 1.00) [45–55]. No systematic review of these reports is currently available. While a positive Gram stain in a tissue sample does predict infection, it has poor sensitivity (0.06) compared with a positive culture result from the same sample used as the reference standard [44,56]. Its sensitivity compared with a positive histology result as reference standard is also poor (0.12).

Microbial culture of fluid or tissue specimens
Isolation of the same organism from three or more of at least five independent tissue specimens is highly predictive of infection (LR+ 169) [44]. A single positive culture is less convincing (LR+ 4.3).

Laboratory culture of material from a possible prosthetic infection should include a careful search for small colony variants (SCVs) which contribute to the resistance to treatment of biofilm-associated infections [22,23].

Sonication of removed prostheses
Submission of the explanted implant to the laboratory, under a strict protocol, for low-energy ultrasonication appears promising. One study [57] found that sonicate fluid culture had significantly better sensitivity (0.78) than two or more positive periprosthetic-tissue cultures (0.60). Specificities for both were 0.99.

Molecular diagnosis using polymerase chain reaction
Three studies have compared the performance characteristics of polymerase chain reaction (PCR) compared with culture in PJI [58–61] and others have included material from PJI which is not reported separately. The place of PCR in the diagnosis of PJI is currently unclear.

Case presentation 2 (continued)

Recurrence of surgically acquired infection is clearly possible. The implant is no longer stable, and the condition of the soft tissues at the operative site is categorized as showing evidence of moderate damage, not surprising given the past history of two procedures, the second of which had required extensive debridement.

Following discussion she expresses her wish to consider two-stage revision arthroplasty, and asks what diagnostic tests would help to support or exclude a diagnosis of persisting infection.

The fact that she has rheumatoid arthritis means that the majority of tests in the diagnostic sequence which would normally be undertaken during preoperative evaluation to firm up a diagnosis of recurrent infection may be of limited value since the published likelihood ratios will not necessarily be reliable. Intraoperative culture will be the pivotal Investigation in her case. The circumstances in this case led to advice that operative cover with intravenous (IV) vancomycin should be commenced during surgery as soon as the tissue specimens for the laboratory had been secured.

Treatment and outcomes

Programs for cure or remission of infection, and restoration of good function after PJI have developed empirically, almost completely without support of evidence from RCTs. A management algorithm which reflects most contemporary practice illustrates how the choice of management program for individual patients may be made [62].

For a small number of people with PJI, restoration of good function may not be achievable. They may be offered removal of the prosthesis alone, or long-term suppressive antimicrobial therapy.

For the great majority, one of three approaches to the management of PJI offer odds of better than 4 to 1 of an acceptable functional outcome without recurrence of infection.

People in whom infection occurs early after implantation, or who have a late hematogenous infection, may be offered debridement of soft tissues involved in the infection, with retention of the implant and a period of antimicrobial therapy of at least 3 months [37]. Criteria for implant retention are: (1) a stable implant; (2) a pathogen with susceptibility to antimicrobial agents active against surface-adhering

microorganisms; (3) absence of a sinus tract or an abscess; and (4) duration of symptoms of infection of less than 3 weeks. Debridement and retention applied using these patient selection criteria achieved greater than 80% recurrence-free function at 2 years. A preferred antimicrobial therapy regimen for debridement/retention in hip PJI caused by methicillin-susceptible *S. aureus*, based on the results of one RCT [63], has used intravenous rifampin plus (flu)cloxacillin for 2 weeks, followed by rifampin plus ciprofloxacin or levofloxacin for 3 months.

People with PJI who do not meet these criteria are likely to be offered a further operative procedure which aims to remove the infected prosthesis, eradicate infection, and insert a new prosthesis by either one-stage or two-stage exchange arthroplasty. Delivery of antimicrobial agents, an essential component of each option, may be achieved parenterally, orally, or by the use of antibiotic-loaded bone cement (ALBC).

A comprehensive narrative review [64] of data from 1641 patients treated for PJI from 29 centers in a number of countries confirmed that two-stage exchange was associated with successful outcome with (93%) or without (86%) the use of ALBC. One-stage exchange had similar success if ALBC was used, but poorer outcome (59% success rate) if it was not. A recent report of two-stage exchange procedure with ALBC, but without the use of a prolonged course of antibiotic therapy, achieved minimum recurrence-free period of 2 years in 85% of patients [65].

Case presentation 2 (continued)

This patient agreed to advice that a two-stage exchange arthroplasty was indicated. At surgery, no fluid collection was found, and seven tissue specimens were submitted for intraoperative histology and culture. Sonication of the prosthesis was unavailable. The first stage of a two-stage arthroplasty was completed and irrigation and suction drainage initiated. After 5 days of incubation, four of seven submitted periprosthetic tissue specimens grew a small colony variant of *S. aureus*, resistant to methicillin and ciprofloxacin, and sensitive to vancomycin, rifampin, fusidic acid, and cotrimoxazole. At that point IV rifampin was added to vancomycin, and continued until day 14, when IV therapy was discontinued and oral rifampin/

continued

Case presentation 2 (continued)

cotrimoxazole therapy administered until the second stage of the two-stage exchange arthroplasty was carried out, 8 weeks following the first stage. Over the procedure, IV vancomycin was administered as surgical prophylaxis and oral rifampin/cotrimoxazole was continued for a further 3 months.

Implications for practice

In the prevention, diagnosis, and management of PJI:

- There is insufficient current evidence to determine a threshold prevalence of MRSA at which switching to glycopeptide antibiotic prophylaxis for prosthetic joint surgery might be cost-effective.
- Preoperative blood tests (ESR, CRP, IL-6) appear to be good and inexpensive screening tests in people who do not have inflammatory polyarthritis. Their diagnostic performance characteristics in people with inflammatory polyarthritis are unclear.
- Anti-granulocyte scintigraphy using monoclonal antibodies and FDG PET have good diagnostic performance characteristics in people who do not have inflammatory polyarthritis.
- Identification of PMN in preoperative aspirates or in operative tissue specimens has good diagnostic performance characteristics in people with suspected PJI who do not have inflammatory polyarthritis.
- The isolation of the same organism from culture of three or more independent operative tissue specimens in people with suspected PJI is highly predictive of infection.
- The diagnostic performance characteristics of molecular methods when compared with culture from operative tissue specimens in PJI remain unclear. Current reports show considerable heterogeneity.

Implications for research

- Further primary studies and metaanalyses of the performance of diagnostic tests used in suspected PJI should be conducted, particularly in people who have inflammatory polyarthritis.
- Although PJI affects only a small proportion of people who have undergone joint arthroplasty, and effective methods of management are available, innovative management regimens should in future be examined in large multicenter randomized trials.

Osteomyelitis in the diabetic foot

Case presentation 3

A 62-year-old man presents to his family practitioner with an infection in his left forefoot. He gives a history of type 2 diabetes mellitus of 8 years' duration, managed with oral hypoglycemic agents and diet. He is a non-(never) smoker, with a daily alcohol intake of 1–2 units. He appears systemically well; his metabolic control is adequate. Clinical examination of the foot demonstrates ulceration on the plantar surface of the foot under the 4th and 5th metatarsal heads, with a purulent discharge. Tendon, and possibly bone, are visible in the base of the ulcer. Cellulitis extends proximally above the ankle. His family practitioner refers him for further evaluation to the local multidisciplinary diabetes clinic.

Background

Incidence and prevalence

Foot ulceration is the major predisposing factor in diabetic foot infections. Approximately 15% of over 150 million people worldwide with diabetes mellitus will develop foot ulceration at some time in their life [66]. Estimates of incidence derived from cohort studies have varied depending on case mix, from 11 to 65 per 1000 person-years [67–71]. Over 50% of foot ulcers may become infected [70]. Annual incidence of infection in a clinic population with foot ulcers has been estimated at 5–9% [70,71].

Pathology and microbiology

Although a penetrating injury may implant pathogens directly into bone, contiguous soft-tissue infection preceded by skin ulceration accounts for most cases of osteomyelitis in the feet of diabetic patients. Devascularization of areas of bone may create a favorable environment for the establishment of biofilm-associated infection [21–23] with its associated resistance to antimicrobial therapy. Thus, surgical debridement of the infected bone remains an essential component of successful control of osteomyelitis in most cases.

Aerobic gram-positive cocci (particularly *S. aureus,* but also coagulase negative staphylococci and group B streptococci) are found in the majority of cases of osteomyelitis in the diabetic foot. Many isolates are methicillin-resistant [72]. Polymicrobial infections are more common in chronic ulcers, and in people who have recently received antimicrobial therapy [73].

Classification schemes for diabetic foot ulcers have evolved over the last 25 years. The widely used Wagner Scale [74] is based on clinical impression of the pathologic anatomy. The University of Texas (UT) Classification [75,76] (Table 3.2) may be a better predictor of clinical outcome, as it takes into account the presence of both infection and ischemia. The International Working Group on the Diabetic Foot (IWGDF) diabetic foot risk classification, based on both anatomic and physiologic features, initially validated in 2001, is predictive of the risk of both ulceration and of amputation [77]. An update has recently been proposed [78].

Risk factors for infection and amputation in the presence of ulceration

Factors in the clinical presentation of a diabetic foot ulcer which are significantly associated with infection have been evaluated in a large cohort study [79], using multivariate analysis. These factors, with risk ratios (RR), were:

- wound depth to bone RR 6.7 (2.3–19.9)
- wound duration ≥ 30 days RR 4.7 (1.6–13.4)
- recurrent foot wound RR 2.4 (1.3–4.5)
- traumatic wound etiology RR 2.4 (1.1–5.0)
- peripheral vascular disease RR 1.9 (1.0–3.6).

The Infectious Diseases Society of America (IDSA) and IWGDF have collaborated in developing a classification scheme for infection severity which predicts the likelihood of amputation in the presence of a foot ulcer

in a patient with diabetes (see Table 3.3). Validation of this classification was reported in 2007 [80].

Case presentation 3 (continued)

Physical examination at the diabetic foot clinic provides further information. He has mild retinopathy. Both popliteal pulses are palpable. No pulses are palpable in either leg below the knee. Blunt probing of the ulcer contacts bone. Both feet show intrinsic (hammer toe) deformities and are insensitive to the 5·07 Semmes–Weinstein filament test. Plain radiographs demonstrate soft-tissue swelling and loss of definition of tissue planes, and zonal osteopenia in the heads of both 4th and 5th metatarsals. These appearances are consistent with osteomyelitis.

This patient's history and findings appear consistent with a moderate infection (UT B3, IDSA/IWGDF grade 3). Further investigations are begun to establish the extent of the infection in his foot, and in particular to gain anatomic detail of the apparent involvement of the 4th and 5th metatarsals.

Principles of diagnosis and management

The principles of diagnosis and management of diabetic foot infections are set out in an evidence-based guideline [81] published in 2004. Although the evidence base for some of its recommendations has been strengthened by the subsequent publication of metaanalyses, and by some new primary studies, they continue to represent best practice.

Table 3.2 University of Texas Foot Ulcer Classification [75]

Wound grade	Stage 0	Stage 1	Stage 2	Stage 3
A Clean wounds	Pre- or post-ulcerative site that has healed	Superficial wound not involving tendon, capsule, or bone	Wound penetrating to tendon or capsule	Wound penetrating bone or joint
B Non-ischemic infected wounds	Pre- or post-ulcerative site that has healed	Superficial wound not involving tendon, capsule, or bone	Wound penetrating to tendon or capsule	Wound penetrating bone or joint
C Ischemic non-infected wounds	Pre- or post-ulcerative site that has healed	Superficial wound not involving tendon, capsule, or bone	Wound penetrating to tendon or capsule	Wound penetrating bone or joint
D Ischemic infected wounds	Pre- or post-ulcerative site that has healed	Superficial wound not involving tendon, capsule, or bone	Wound penetrating to tendon or capsule	Wound penetrating bone or joint

Table 3.3 Diabetic foot infection classification schemes [80]

Clinical findings	Infectious Diseases Society of America Classification	International Working Group on the Diabetic Foot Classification
Wound without purulence or any manifestations of inflammation	Uninfected	Grade 1
Manifestations of inflammation (purulence or erythema, pain, tenderness, warmth, or induration); any cellulitis or erythema extends ≤2 cm around ulcer, and infection is limited to skin or superficial subcutaneous tissues; no local complications or systemic illness	Mild infection	Grade 2
Infection in a patient who is systemically well and metabolically stable but has more than one of the following – cellulitis extending ≥2 cm; lymphangitis; spread beneath fascia; deep tissue abscess; gangrene; muscle, tendon, joint, or bone involvement	Moderate Infection	Grade 3
Infection in a patient with systemic toxicity or metabolic instability (e.g., fever, chills, tachycardia, hypotension, confusion, vomiting, leukocytosis, acidosis, hyperglycemia, or azotemia)	Severe infection	Grade 4

Diagnosis of osteomyelitis

As in the diagnosis of prosthetic joint infections, establishing a single clinically useful diagnostic reference standard for osteomyelitis in the diabetic foot is somewhat problematic. The interpretation of microbial culture results may be complex or misleading due to prior antimicrobial therapy, polymicrobial infection, and superficial wound contamination. For these reasons, positive culture or positive histology from a bone biopsy is generally accepted as the reference standard for evaluating diagnostic tests.

Clinical findings

A positive probe-to-bone test provides moderate diagnostic evidence of osteomyelitis. One systematic review [82] (21 included studies, 403 participants) found summary LR+ 6.4 (95% CI 3.6–11.0). A negative test has a summary LR of 0.39 (95% CI 0.20–0.76).

Physician's assessment of the ulcer as Wagner Grade >2 provides moderate diagnostic evidence of osteomyelitis [82]. More evidence is required, as this finding is derived from two small studies (total of 43 participants) which reported LR+ of 3.9 (95% CI 0.96–16) [83] and 13 (95% CI 0.82–203) [84].

One study (35 participants) [85] reported that physician's "clinical judgment" predicted LR + of 9.2 (0.57–147) and LR- of 0.70 (0.53–0.92).

Blood investigations

An ESR above 70 mm/h in the context of a diabetic ulcer supports a diagnosis of osteomyelitis. An ESR of less than 70 mm/h does not rule it out. One systematic review [82] presented data from two studies (64 participants) [85,86]. ESR ≥70 mm/h had summary LR+ of 11.0 (95% CI 1.6–79) and LR− of 0.34 (95% CI 0.06–1.9).

The sensitivity of an elevated white blood cell count for a diagnosis of osteomyelitis was evaluated in one small study [87], which found poor sensitivity regardless of the cut-off used [82], and provided no data to calculate specificity.

Microbiological investigations

Superficial swabs from an ulcer or curettage from its edges and base are poor predictors of osteomyelitis, and of the microbial isolates from bone biopsy. One study with 16 participants [88], found that culture of soft tissue obtained by curettage of the edges and base of an ulcer was a poor predictor of osteomyelitis confirmed by histological examination of a debridement bone specimen (LR+ 1.0, 95% CI 0.65–1.5; LR− 1.0, 95% CI 0.08–13).

Four studies [89–92] compared the microbiologic isolate from a superficial swab with the isolate from a deep tissue biopsy. All used slightly different methods which are summarized in Table 3.4.

Table 3.4 Studies comparing sampling techniques for diagnosis of diabetic foot osteomyelitis

Study	n	Index test	Reference Standard	Diagnostic performance of index test
Bill 2001 [89]	38	Superficial swab	Punch biopsy ulcer base, immediately following swab	Sensitivity 0.79, specificity 0.6, LR+ 1.96, LR− 0.36
Slater 2004 [90]	60	Superficial swab	Deep soft-tissue or bone sample at the junction of nonviable and viable tissue at debridement immediately following swab	Sensitivity 0.62*
Senneville 2006 [91]	69	Superficial swab	Percutaneous bone biopsy within 72h of swab	Sensitivity 0.17*
Kessler 2006 [92]	21	Superficial swab	Percutaneous needle to bone surface immediately after swab	Sensitivity 0.19*

*Sensitivity calculated using number of superficial swab isolates identical to deep tissue isolates.

Preliminary data on the use of miniaturized oligo-nucleotide arrays [93] to differentiate colonized from infected wounds in <1 day found that genes for both virulence and resistance factors were present significantly more often in clinically infected wounds. The implications of this new technique in clinical practice remain to be established.

Plain radiographs

Plain radiographs have weak predictive value in the diagnosis of lower extremity osteomyelitis in people with diabetes. Nevertheless, they are inexpensive, easily obtained in most healthcare facilities, and provide useful clinical and anatomic information. One systematic review [82] reported a metaanalysis (7 studies; 217 participants). Summary LR+ was 2.3 (95% CI 1.56–3.3) and LR− was 0.63 (95% CI 0.51–0.78).

Limited specificity may be explained, first, by the observation that the bone changes of established osteomyelitis may also be seen in neuropathic bone and joint disease without infection. Contributing to limited sensitivity is the delay between onset of osteomyelitis and the onset of radiologic signs, typically 7–14 days.

Magnetic resonance imaging

Magnetic resonance imaging (MRI) has moderate predictive value in the diagnosis of foot osteomyelitis, but if changes indicating osteomyelitis have been seen on plain radiographs, it may not always be necessary [94]. Eleven of 16 studies in one systematic review [95] included predominantly diabetic patients, and in six, all participants had ulceration. Summary LR+ was 3.8 (95% CI 2.5–5.8) and LR− 0.14 (95% CI 0.08–0.26). A particular advantage of MRI is the excellent anatomic detail of the extent of infection in bone, which facilitates surgical planning.

Nuclear imaging

The diagnostic accuracy of ^{99m}Tc bone scanning, indium scanning, and WBC imaging techniques is inferior to that of MRI in head-to-head comparison. One systematic review [95] found that MRI was markedly superior (DOR 149.9; 95% CI 54.6–411.3) compared with bone scan (DOR 3.6; 95% CI 1.0–13.3) At the 90% sensitivity cut point, the specificity for MRI was 0.98 compared with 0.29 for technetium. In 9 studies that compared plain radiography with MRI, MRI outperformed plain radiography (DOR 81.5; 95% CI 14.2–466.1 compared with DOR 3.3; 95% CI 2.2–5.0). In three studies comparing MRI with white blood cell (WBC) labeling, DOR for MRI was 120.3 (95% CI 61.8–234.3) compared with 3.4 (95% CI 0.2–62.2) for WBC studies. Another systematic review [96] found that ^{99m}Tc bone scanning, indium scanning, and WBC imaging techniques lacked useful specificity (range 0.62–0.89) in the diagnosis of infection in the diabetic foot.

Three studies [97–99] have compared MRI and FDG PET in people with diabetic foot disorders. FDG PET appears to distinguish between neuropathic osteoarticular changes and osteomyelitis, but a clear picture of the cost-effectiveness of FDG PET compared with MRI awaits further comparative data.

Clinical presentation 3 (continued)

The clinical and radiologic evidence so far indicates that there is an open ulcer, a cellulitis, and a probable osteomyelitis, based on the positive probe-to-bone test and the plain radiographs. MRI shows reduced marrow signal intensity in T1-weighted sequences, and increased signal on fat-suppressed T2-weighted sequences in both 4th and 5th metatarsals, confined to the metatarsal heads and the distal third of each shaft. Soft tissue edema surrounds both 4th and 5th metatarsal heads, and cortical destruction is present on the plantar aspect of the shaft of the 4th metatarsal. Image-guided percutaneous biopsy from a dorsal approach using a 10 gauge Craig needle sampled both metatarsal heads.

As local community-acquired MRSA prevalence has been low, and the patient had no obvious MRSA risk factors, empiric antimicrobial therapy with cefalexin was commenced immediately after biopsy, and a formal surgical debridement planned for 72 hours later.

Although this patient had not been considered at high risk for MRSA, both samples grew a pure culture of MRSA susceptible to vancomycin, linezolid, daptomycin, doxycycline ($MIC_{90} \leq 2\,\mu g/mL$), trimethoprim-sulfamethoxazole ($MIC_{90} \leq 0.5/9.5\,\mu g/mL$) but resistant to clindamycin ($MIC_{90} > 8\,\mu g/mL$). No anaerobes were identified. The histologic appearances were those of osteomyelitis. Antimicrobial therapy was changed to vancomycin and trimethoprim-sulfamethoxazole when the cultures were received.

Treatment and outcomes

Surgical management

Based on long collective experience, but no RCTs, surgery continues to be a normal component of the management of osteomyelitis in the diabetic foot. Accordingly, surgical management follows the general principles of surgical management of osteomyelitis – resection of necrotic bone and soft tissue, management of the post-resection defect, and wound closure. The use of flaps to manage defects after forefoot surgery may be indicated in younger patients. In older patients, most surgeons have felt it appropriate to avoid primary skin closure, even where it seems technically possible, preferring delayed primary or secondary closure.

A review of the outcome of predominantly medical therapy for foot osteomyelitis (11 case series, 546 patients) [100] found remission rates of 25% to 91%. In a recent retrospective report of nonsurgical management from nine diabetes clinics (50 patients) [101], the remission rate was 64%. These reports raise the hypothesis that there may be a subset of diabetics with foot osteomyelitis who can be effectively managed in this way.

Choice of antimicrobial agent

A systematic review of primary studies published up to November 2002 found 23 RCTs evaluating the effectiveness or cost-effectiveness of antimicrobial agents in the treatment of diabetic foot infections [102]. Eight of these studies were double blind. The review, unsurprisingly in view of the heterogeneity of study participants, agents, pathogens, and outcome measures, found no evidence of the superiority of any particular intravenous or oral antibiotic regimen over any other. Metaanalysis was not conducted.

The clinical relevance of a systematic review with such a broad scope is limited; a more appropriate scope might be antibiotic X versus antibiotic Y in the treatment of infection with isolate pattern Z. But that presupposes that all primary studies also ask clinically useful questions formulated in this manner. However, the reviewers made some very pertinent observations. The quality of many of the trials was poor, particularly in respect of allocation concealment and blinding. The authors found little agreement on what is the key outcome measure for assessing the effectiveness of an antimicrobial in the management of diabetic foot ulcers. No trials reported the impact of interventions on health-related quality of life or on the development of antibiotic resistance. These are challenges for the pharmaceutical industry and the research community to consider.

Empiric preliminary antimicrobial therapy should be based on the likely microbial etiology and the current local antimicrobial prescribing policy. If an infection is severe (IDSA/IWGDF grade 4) current guidelines [81] recommend the use of broad-spectrum agents, but in mild to moderate infection, therapy against gram-positive cocci may be sufficient. Isolation of MRSA from community-acquired infections appears to be increasing [73] and antimicrobial prescribing policies may need to take that into account.

Duration of antimicrobial therapy

Optimum duration of antimicrobial therapy has not been established using RCTs. Recommended duration of antibacterial therapy [81] ranges from 1 to 4 weeks for soft tissue infection, to >6 weeks if the complete resection of the infected bone is not achieved. If resection is complete (e.g., amputation of a toe with infection involving the middle phalanx and distal interphalangeal joint), and wound healing is proceeding satisfactorily, a shorter period is often sufficient.

General supportive management

The fundamentals of good diabetic foot care continue to apply during treatment of a diabetic foot infection, and the search for optimum wound dressing constitutes an area of active research. Both are beyond the scope of this chapter.

Adjuvant therapy: G-CSF

A recent systematic review [103] concluded that administration of G-CSF therapy does not appear to hasten the clinical resolution of diabetic foot infection or ulceration but is associated with a reduced rate of amputation and other surgical procedures. However, neither of the two included RCTs which recruited mainly participants with osteomyelitis [104,105] had power to demonstrate any significant effect for these outcomes.

Adjuvant therapy: hyperbaric oxygen therapy

One systematic review [106] included four small trials (147 participants with foot ulcers due to diabetes). Data from these studies indicated that hyperbaric oxygen therapy (HBOT) significantly reduced the risk of major amputation and may have improved the rate of healing at 1 year. However, the authors of the review warned that in view of the small size, methodologic shortcomings, and poor reporting of the studies, this finding should be interpreted cautiously. One subsequent small RCT (28 participants) [107] found that ulcer diameter decreased significantly more in the treatment group by 15 days.

In view of the doubt about its effectiveness, and the substantial costs associated with its use, the introduction of HBOT for diabetic foot infections, including osteomyelitis, does not appear justified at present.

Implications for practice

In the diagnosis and management of osteomyelitis in the diabetic foot:

- An ESR above 70 mm/h supports a diagnosis of osteomyelitis.
- Superficial swabs from an ulcer or curettage from its edges and base are poor predictors of osteomyelitis, and of the microbial isolates from bone biopsy.
- Plain radiographs have weak predictive value in the diagnosis of osteomyelitis.
- MRI has moderate predictive value in the diagnosis of osteomyelitis.
- The diagnostic accuracy of ^{99m}Tc bone scanning, indium scanning, and anti-granulocyte scintigraphy is inferior to that of MRI in head-to-head comparison.
- The role of FDG PET in the diagnosis of osteomyelitis remains unclear.
- Empirical antimicrobial therapy pending culture and sensitivity data should be based on the severity of the infection and the expected susceptibility of the likely etiologic agent(s).
- Antimicrobial therapy for osteomyelitis generally should last 4–6 weeks, but a shorter duration is sufficient if the entire infected bone is removed, and probably a longer duration is needed if infected bone remains.
- The effectiveness of adjuvant therapy with G-CSF is unclear.
- The effectiveness of HBOT is unclear.

Implications for research

- More data are needed to establish confident estimates of the predictive value of clinical and laboratory tests and imaging studies used in diagnosis of infection.
- Multicenter studies should be considered comparing nonoperative with operative management of foot osteomyelitis in some situations (e.g., perhaps UT B3 IDSA moderate infections).
- To have clinical relevance, RCTs and systematic reviews of antimicrobial therapy should more

precisely define the inclusion criteria for participants and the indication to use a particular agent.

Conclusion

The evidence base for treating bone and joint infections is improving, but much remains to be done. Greater interdisciplinarity, a focus on research questions about whose importance there is consensus, collaboration between multiple centers, and good study design remain challenges for the research community.

References

1 Whiting P, Rutjes AW, Reitsma JB, et al. Sources of variation and bias in studies of diagnostic accuracy: a systematic review. Ann Intern Med 2004;140:189–202.

2 ter Riet G, Kessels AG, Bachmann LM. Systematic reviews of evaluations of diagnostic and screening tests. Two issues were simplified. BMJ 2001;323(7322):1188.

3 Kaandorp CJE, Dinant HJ, van de Laar MAFJ, et al. Incidence and sources of native and prosthetic joint infection: a community based prospective survey. Ann Rheum Dis 1997;56:470–5.

4 Tarkowski A. Infection and musculoskeletal conditions: Infectious arthritis. Best Prac Res Clin Rheumatol 2006; 20:1029–4.

5 Margaretten ME, Kohlwes J, Moore D, Bent S. Does this adult patient have septic arthritis? JAMA. 2007;297:1478–88.

6 Karchevsky M, Schweitzer ME, Morrison WB, et al. MRI findings of septic arthritis and associated osteomyelitis in adults. AJR Am J Roentgenol 2004;182:119–22.

7 Graif M, Schweitzer ME, Deely D, et al. The septic versus nonseptic inflamed joint: MRI characteristics. Skeletal Radiol 1999;28:616–20.

8 Fihman V, Hannouche D, Bousson V, et al. Improved diagnosis specificity in bone and joint infections using molecular techniques. J Infect 2007;55:510–17.

9 Yang S, Ramachandran P, Hardick A, et al. Rapid PCR-based diagnosis of septic arthritis by early gram-type classification and pathogen identification. J Clin Microbiol 2008;46(4):1386–90.

10 Jimenez-Boj E, Nöbauer-Huhmann I, Hanslik-Schnabel B, et al. Bone erosions and bone marrow edema as defined by magnetic resonance imaging reflect true bone marrow inflammation in rheumatoid arthritis. Arthritis Rheum 2007;56:1118–24.

11 Von Essen R. Culture of joint specimens in bacterial arthritis. Impact of blood culture bottle utilization. Scand J Rheumatol 1997;26:293–300.

12 Yagupsky P, Press J. Use of the isolator 1.5 microbial tube for culture of synovial fluid from patients with septic arthritis. J Clin Microbiol 1997;35:2410–12.

13 Piriou P, Garreau DL, Wattincourt L, et al. Simple punction versus notch needle-biopsy for bacteriological diagnosis of osteoarticular infection. A prospective study on 54 cases. [French] Rev Chir Orthop Reparatrice Appar Mot 1998;84:685–8.

14 Jalava J, Skurnik M, Toivanen A, et al. Bacterial PCR in the diagnosis of joint infection. Ann Rheum Dis 2001;60:287–9.

15 Norden C, Nelson JD, Mader JT, et al. Evaluation of new anti-infective drugs for the treatment of infectious arthritis in adults. Clin Infect Dis 1992;15(Suppl.1):S167–S171.

16 Stutz G, Kuster MS, Kleinstuck F, et al. Arthroscopic management of septic arthritis: stages of infection and results. Knee Surg Sports Traumatol Arthrosc 2000;8:270–4.

17 Nusem I, Jabur MK, Playford EG. Arthroscopic treatment of septic arthritis of the hip. Arthroscopy 2006;22:902.e1–3.

18 Sakiniene E, Bremell T, Tarkowski A. Corticosteroids ameliorate the course of experimental superantigen-triggered *Staphylococcus aureus* arthritis. Arthritis Rheum 1996;39:1596–605.

19 Odio CM, Ramirez T, Pharmd GA, et al. Double blind, randomized, placebo-controlled study of dexamethasone therapy for hematogenous septic arthritis in children. Pediatr Infect Dis J 2003;22:883–8.

20 Edwards CJ, Cooper C, Fisher D, et al. The importance of the disease process and disease-modifying antirheumatic drug treatment in the development of septic arthritis in patients with rheumatoid arthritis. Arthritis Rheum 2007;57:1151–7.

21 Costerton JW, Stewart PS, Greenberg EP. Bacterial biofilms: a common cause of persistent infections. Science 1999;284:1318–22.

22 von Eiff C. *Staphylococcus aureus* small colony variants: a challenge to microbiologists and clinicians. Int J Antimicrob Agents 2008;31(6):507–10.

23 Neut D, van der Mei HC, Bulstra S, et al. The role of small-colony variants in failure to diagnose and treat biofilm infections in orthopedics. Acta Orthop 2007;78:299–308.

24 Lidgren L. Joint prosthetic infections: A success story. Acta Orthop Scand 2001;72:553–6.

25 Berbari EF, Hanssen AD, Duffy MC, et al. Risk factors for prosthetic joint infection: Case–control study. Clin Infect Dis 1998;27:1247–54.

26 Peersman G, Laskin R, Davis J, et al. The Insall award paper: Infection in total knee replacement: A retrospective review of 6489 total knee replacements. Clin Orthop 2001;392:15–23.

27 Cranny G, Elliott R, Weatherly H, et al. A systematic review and economic model of switching from non-glycopeptide to glycopeptide antibiotic prophylaxis for surgery. Health Technol Assess 2008;12:1–168.

28 Barnes S, Salemi C, Fithian D, et al. An enhanced benchmark for prosthetic joint replacement infection rates. Am J Infect Control 2006;34:669–72.

29 The Swedish Hip Arthroplasty Register. Annual Report 2005. at http://www.jru.orthop.gu.se/

30 New Zealand Orthopaedic Association National Joint Registry. Eight year report. January 1999 to December 2006. www.cdhb.govt.nz/njr/

31 Thomas C, Cadwallader HL, Riley TV. Surgical-site infections after orthopaedic surgery: statewide surveillance using linked administrative databases. J Hosp Infect 2004;57:25–30.

32 Health Protection Agency. Second Report of the Mandatory Surveillance of Surgical Site Infection in Orthopaedic Surgery. April 2004 to March 2006. London: Health Protection Agency, January 2007. Available from: www.hpa.org.uk

33 National Nosocomial Infections Surveillance (NNIS) System Report, data summary from January 1992 through June 2004, issued October 2004. Am J Infect Control 2004;32:470–85.

34 Horan TC, Gaynes RE, Martone WJ, et al. CDC definitions of nosocomial surgical site infections, 1992: a modification of CDC definitions of surgical wound infections. Infect Control Hosp Epidemiol 1992;13:606–8.

37 Zimmerli W. Infection and musculoskeletal conditions: Prosthetic-joint-associated infections. Best Pract Res Clin Rheumatol 2006;20:1045–63.

35 Weissmann G. Pathogenesis of rheumatoid arthritis. J Clin Rheumatol 2004;10(3 Suppl):S26–31.

36 Niki Y, Matsumoto H, Otani T, et al. Five types of inflammatory arthritis following total knee arthroplasty. J Biomed Mater Res A 2007;81:1005–10.

38 Austin MS, Ghanem E, Joshi A, et al. A simple, cost-effective screening protocol to rule out periprosthetic infection. J Arthroplasty 2008;23:65–8.

39 Di Cesare PE, Chang E, Preston CF, et al. Serum interleukin-6 as a marker of periprosthetic infection following total hip and knee arthroplasty. J Bone Joint Surg Am 2005;87:1921–7.

40 Pakos EE, Trikalinos TA, Fotopoulos AD, et al. Prosthesis infection: diagnosis after total joint arthroplasty with anti-granulocyte scintigraphy with 99mTc-labeled monoclonal antibodies – a meta-analysis. Radiology 2007;242:101–8.

41 Crymes WB Jr, Demos H, Gordon L. Detection of musculoskeletal infection with 18F-FDG PET: review of the current literature. J Nucl Med Technol 2004;32:12–15.

42 Pill SG, Parvizi J, Tang PH, et al. Comparison of fluorodeoxyglucose positron emission tomography and (111)indium-white blood cell imaging in the diagnosis of periprosthetic infection of the hip. J Arthroplasty 2006; 21(6 Suppl 2):91–7.

43 Ali F, Wilkinson JM, Cooper JR, et al. Accuracy of joint aspiration for the preoperative diagnosis of infection in total hip arthroplasty. J Arthroplasty 2006;21:221–6.

44 Atkins BL, Athanasou N, Deeks JJ, et al. Prospective evaluation of criteria for microbiological diagnosis of prosthetic-joint infection at revision arthroplasty. The OSIRIS Collaborative Study Group. J Clin Microbiol 1998;36:2932–9.

45 Banit DM, Kaufer H, Hartford JM. Intraoperative frozen section analysis in revision total joint arthroplasty. Clin Orthop Relat Res 2002;401:230–8.

46 Bori G, Soriano A, García S, et al. Usefulness of histological analysis for predicting the presence of microorganisms at the time of reimplantation after hip resection arthroplasty for the treatment of infection. J Bone Joint Surg Am 2007;89:1232–7.

47 Della Valle CJ, Bogner E, Desai P, et al. Analysis of frozen sections of intraoperative specimens obtained at the time of reoperation after hip or knee resection arthroplasty for the treatment of infection. J Bone Joint Surg Am 1999; 81:684–9.

48 Feldman DS, Lonner JH, Desai P, et al. The role of intraoperative frozen sections in revision total joint arthroplasty. J Bone Joint Surg Am 1995;77:1807–13.

49 Fehring TK, McAlister JA Jr. Frozen histologic section as a guide to sepsis in revision joint arthroplasty. Clin Orthop Relat Res 1994;304:229–37.

50 Francés Borrego A, Martínez FM, Cebrian Parra JL, et al. Diagnosis of infection in hip and knee revision surgery: intraoperative frozen section analysis. Int Orthop 2007; 31:33–7.

51 Lonner JH, Desai P, Dicesare PE, et al. The reliability of analysis of intraoperative frozen sections for identifying active infection during revision hip or knee arthroplasty. J Bone Joint Surg Am 1996;78:1553–8.

52 Musso AD, Mohanty K, Spencer-Jones R. Role of frozen section histology in diagnosis of infection during revision arthroplasty. Postgrad Med J 2003;79:590–3.

53 Nuñez LV, Buttaro MA, Morandi A, et al. Frozen sections of samples taken intraoperatively for diagnosis of infection in revision hip surgery. Acta Orthop 2007;78:226–30.

54 Pace TB, Jeray KJ, Latham JT Jr. Synovial tissue examination by frozen section as an indicator of infection in hip and knee arthroplasty in community hospitals. J Arthroplasty 1997;12:64–9.

55 Pandey R, Drakoulakis E, Athanasou NA. An assessment of the histological criteria used to diagnose infection in hip revision arthroplasty tissues. J Clin Pathol 1999;52: 118–23.

56 Spangehl MJ, Masri BA, O'Connell JX, et al. Prospective analysis of preoperative and intraoperative investigations for the diagnosis of infection at the sites of two hundred and two revision total hip arthroplasties. J Bone Joint Surg Am 1999;81:672–83.

57 Trampuz A, Piper KE, Jacobson MJ, et al. Sonication of removed hip and knee prostheses for diagnosis of infection. N Engl J Med 2007;357:654–63.

58 Panousis K, Grigoris P, Butcher I, et al. Poor predictive value of broad-range PCR for the detection of arthroplasty infection in 92 cases. Acta Orthop 2005;76:341–6.

59 Kordelle J, Hossain H, Stahl U, et al. [Usefulness of 16S rDNA polymerase-chain-reaction (PCR) in the intraoperative detection of infection in revision of failed arthroplasties] Z Orthop Ihre Grenzgeb 2004;142:571–6.

60 Gallo J, Sauer P, Dendis M, et al. [Molecular diagnostics for the detection of prosthetic joint infection] Acta Chir Orthop Traumatol Cech 2006;73:85–91.

61 Tarkin IS, Henry TJ, Fey PI, et al. PCR rapidly detects methicillin-resistant staphylococci in periprosthetic infection. Clin Orthop Relat Res 2003;(414):89–94.

62 Giulieri SG, Graber P, Ochsner PE, et al. Management of infection associated with total hip arthroplasty according to a treatment algorithm. Infection 2004;32:222–8.

63 Zimmerli W, Widmer AF, Blatter M, et al. Role of rifampin for treatment of orthopaedic implant-related staphylococcal infections: a randomized controlled trial. Foreign-Body Infection (FBI) Study Group. JAMA 1998;279:1537–41.

64 Langlais F. Can we improve the results of revision arthroplasty for infected total hip replacement? J Bone Joint Surg Br 2003;85:637–40.

65 Stockley I, Mockford BJ, Hoad-Reddick A, et al. The use of two-stage exchange arthroplasty with depot antibiotics in the absence of long-term antibiotic therapy in infected total hip replacement. J Bone Joint Surg Br 2008;90:145–8.

66 Boulton AJ. The diabetic foot: a global view. Diab Metab Res Rev 2000;16(Suppl. 1):S2–S5.

67 Muller IS, de Grauw WJ, van Gerwen WH, et al. Foot ulceration and lower limb amputation in type 2 diabetic patients in Dutch primary health care. Diab Care 2002;25:570–4.

68 Eneroth M, Larsson J, Apelqvist J. Deep foot infections in patients with diabetes and foot ulcer: an entity with different characteristics, treatments, and prognosis. J Diab Complic 1999;13:254–63.

69 Boyko EJ, Ahroni JH, Stensel V, et al. A prospective study of risk factors for diabetic foot ulcer. The Seattle Diabetic Foot Study. Diab Care 1999;22:1036–42.

70 Ramsey SD, Newton K, Blough D, et al. Incidence, outcomes, and cost of foot ulcers in patients with diabetes. Diabetes Care 1999;22:382–7.

71 Lavery LA, Armstrong DG, Wunderlich RP, et al. Diabetic foot syndrome: evaluating the prevalence and incidence of foot pathology in Mexican Americans and non-Hispanic whites from a diabetes disease management cohort. Diabetes Care 2003;26:1435–8.

72 Dang C, Prasad Y, Bouton A, et al. Methicillin-resistant Staphylococcus aureus in the diabetic foot clinic: a worsening problem. Diabet Med 2003;20:159–61.

73 Cavanagh PR, Lipsky BA, Bradbury AW, et al. Treatment for diabetic foot ulcers. Lancet 2005;366(9498):1725–35.

74 Wagner FW . The diabetic foot. Orthopedics 1987;10:163–7.

75 Lavery LA, Armstrong DG, Harkless LB. Classification of diabetic foot wounds. J Foot Ankle Surg 1996;35:528–31.

76 Oyibo SO, Jude EB, Tarawneh I, et al. A comparison of two diabetic foot ulcer classification systems: the Wagner and the University of Texas wound classification systems. Diabetes Care 2001;24:84–8.

77 Peters EJ, Lavery LA. Effectiveness of the diabetic foot risk classification system of the International Working Group on the Diabetic Foot. Diab Care 2001;24:1442–7.

78 Lavery LA, Peters EJ, Williams JR, et al. Re-evaluating the way we classify the diabetic foot: restructuring the diabetic foot risk classification system of the International Working Group on the Diabetic Foot. Diabetes Care 2008;31:154–6.

79 Lavery LA, Armstrong DG, Wunderlich RP, et al. Risk factors for foot infections in individuals with diabetes. Diabetes Care 2006;29:1288–93.

80 Lavery LA, Armstrong DG, Murdoch DP, et al. Validation of the Infectious Diseases Society of America's diabetic foot infection classification system. Clin Infect Dis 2007;44:562–5.

81 Lipsky BA, Berendt AR, Deery HG, et al. Infectious Diseases Society of America. Diagnosis and treatment of diabetic foot infections. Clin Infect Dis 2004;39:885–910.

82 Butalia S, Palda VA, Sargeant RJ, et al. Does this patient with diabetes have osteomyelitis of the lower extremity? JAMA 2008;299:806–13.

83 Enderle MD, Coerper S, Schweizer HP, et al. Correlation of imaging techniques to histopathology in patients with diabetic foot syndrome and clinical suspicion of chronic osteomyelitis. The role of high-resolution ultrasound. Diabetes Care 1999;22:294–9.

84 Vesco L, Boulahdour H, Hamissa S, et al. The value of combined radionuclide and magnetic resonance imaging in the diagnosis and conservative management of minimal or localized osteomyelitis of the foot in diabetic patients. Metabolism 1999;48:922–7.

85 Newman LG, Waller J, Palestro CJ, et al. Unsuspected osteomyelitis in diabetic foot ulcers. Diagnosis and monitoring by leukocyte scanning with indium in 111 oxyquinoline. JAMA 1991;266:1246–51.

86 Kaleta JL, Fleischli JW, Reilly CH. The diagnosis of osteomyelitis in diabetes using erythrocyte sedimentation rate: a pilot study. J Am Podiatr Med Assoc 2001;91:445–50.

87 Armstrong DG, Lavery LA, Sariaya M, et al. Leukocytosis is a poor indicator of acute osteomyelitis of the foot in diabetes mellitus. J Foot Ankle Surg 1996;35:280–3.

88 Oyen WJ, Netten PM, Lemmens JA, et al. Evaluation of infectious diabetic foot complications with indium-111-labeled human nonspecific immunoglobulin G. J Nucl Med 1992;33:1330–6.

89 Bill TJ, Ratliff CR, Donovan AM, et al. Quantitative swab culture versus tissue biopsy: a comparison in chronic wounds. Ostomy Wound Manage 2001;47:34–7.

90 Slater RA, Lazarovitch T, Boldur I, et al. Swab cultures accurately identify bacterial pathogens in diabetic foot wounds not involving bone. Diabet Med 2004;21:705–9.

91 Senneville E, Melliez H, Beltrand E, et al. Culture of percutaneous bone biopsy specimens for diagnosis of diabetic foot osteomyelitis: concordance with ulcer swab cultures. Clin Infect Dis 2006;42:57–62.

92 Kessler L, Piemont Y, Ortega F, et al. Comparison of microbiological results of needle puncture vs. superficial swab in infected diabetic foot ulcer with osteomyelitis. Diabet Med 2006;23:99–102.

93 Sotto A, Richard JL, Jourdan N, et al. Miniaturized oligonucleotide arrays: a new tool for discriminating colonization from infection due to Staphylococcus aureus in diabetic foot ulcers. Diabetes Care 2007;30:2051–6.

94 Leibovici L. Review: magnetic resonance imaging is an accurate test for diagnosing foot osteomyelitis. ACP J Club 2007;147:20.

95 Kapoor A, Page S, Lavalley M, et al. Magnetic resonance imaging for diagnosing foot osteomyelitis: a meta-analysis. Arch Intern Med 2007;167:125–32.

96 Capriotti G, Chianelli M, Signore A. Nuclear medicine imaging of diabetic foot infection: results of meta-analysis. Nucl Med Commun 2006;27:757–64.

97 Höpfner S, Krolak C, Kessler S, et al. Preoperative imaging of Charcot neuroarthropathy in diabetic patients: comparison of ring PET, hybrid PET, and magnetic resonance imaging. Foot Ankle Int 2004;25:890–5.

98 Basu S, Chryssikos T, Houseni M, et al. Potential role of FDG PET in the setting of diabetic neuro-osteoarthropathy: can it differentiate uncomplicated Charcot's neuroarthropathy from osteomyelitis and soft-tissue infection? Nucl Med Commun 2007;28:465–72.

99 Schwegler B, Stumpe KD, Weishaupt D, et al. Unsuspected osteomyelitis is frequent in persistent diabetic foot ulcer and better diagnosed by MRI than by 18F-FDG PET or 99mTc-MOAB. Intern Med 2008;263:99–106.

100 Jeffcoate WJ, Lipsky BA. Controversies in diagnosing and managing osteomyelitis of the foot in diabetes. Clin Infect Dis 2004;39 Suppl 2:S115–22.

101 Senneville E, Lombart A, Beltrand E, et al. Outcome of diabetic foot osteomyelitis treated non-surgically: a retrospective cohort study. Diabetes Care 2008;31(4):637–42.

102 Nelson EA, O'Meara S, Golder S, et al. Systematic review of antimicrobial treatments for diabetic foot ulcers. Diabet Med 2006;23:348–59.

103 Cruciani M, Lipsky BA, Mengoli C, et al. Are granulocyte colony-stimulating factors beneficial in treating diabetic foot infections?: A meta-analysis. Diabetes Care 2005;28:454–60.

104 de Lalla F, Pellizzer G, Strazzabosco M, et al. Randomized prospective controlled trial of recombinant granulocyte colony-stimulating factor as adjunctive therapy for limb-threatening diabetic foot infection. Antimicrob Agents Chemother 2001;45:1094–8.

105 Gough A, Clapperton M, Rolando N, et al. Randomised placebo-controlled trial of granulocyte-colony stimulating factor in diabetic foot infection. Lancet 1997;350(9081):855–9.

106 Kranke P, Bennett M, Roeckl-Wiedmann I, et al. Hyperbaric oxygen therapy for chronic wounds. Cochrane Database Syst Rev 2004 (2), CD004123, DOI: 10.1002/14651858.

107 Kessler L, Bilbault P, Ortéga F, et al. Hyperbaric oxygenation accelerates the healing rate of nonischemic chronic diabetic foot ulcers: a prospective randomized study. Diabetes Care 2003;26:2378–82.

CHAPTER 4

Infective endocarditis

Scott D. Halpern, Elias Abrutyn & Brian L. Strom

Case presentation

A 47-year-old man presents to the emergency room with a 1-week history of fever, malaise, and back pain. The patient's symptoms began insidiously, but have been severe enough to keep him home from work for the past 2 days. The patient was previously healthy, but reports having been told he had a heart murmur caused by mitral valve prolapse. He has no significant family history of medical illness. Further questioning reveals that the patient had a tooth extracted 5 weeks prior to presentation. He does not recall having taken antibiotics prior to the extraction (or at any time during the past 2 months). He denies having ever used intravenous drugs.

Physical examination reveals a temperature of 38.3°C (101.8°F), pulse of 90 per minute, and blood pressure of 120/80 mmHg. Diffuse petechiae are seen on the sublingual oral mucosa, and a grade III/VI holosystolic regurgitant murmur is most audible at the apex. Initial lab results are significant for a hemoglobin of 115 g/L (11.5 mg/dL) and an erythrocyte sedimentation rate of 70 mm/h. Urinalysis shows microscopic hematuria. An ELISA for antibodies to HIV is negative.

You admit the patient with a presumptive diagnosis of infective endocarditis, and arrange for three sets of blood cultures to be obtained, spaced so that 12 hours may pass between drawing the first and last set. You wonder whether this patient should be further examined by transthoracic or transesophageal echocardiography.

Diagnosis

Epidemiology

There are generally five steps to determining whether a particular patient has infective endocarditis (IE). First, the clinician should consider, prior to obtaining any information from diagnostic studies, the probability that any patient with similar demographic and clinical characteristics would develop the disease (i.e., the prior probability of disease). Because IE is an incident disease, it is best to consider probabilities expressed as incidence, rather than prevalence, so as to gauge a patient's risk of developing IE over time.

Reported incidence rates of IE range from 1.6 to 11.6 cases per 100 000 person-years [1–7]. Much of the variation is attributable to the proportion of people who have prosthetic valves, the proportion who use intravenous drugs, and the population's age distribution (older patients having higher incidences of IE [3,6]; Fig. 4.1).

For this patient, the most applicable estimate to consider – that specific to cases of community-acquired, native-valve IE – is 3.56 to 4.81 cases per 100 000 person-years [5]. Though this chapter focuses on suspected cases of community-acquired, native-valve endocarditis, it is important to note that the risk for IE is higher among patients with prosthetic valves, those who use intravenous drugs [8], and those at risk for nosocomial infections. These differences in the prior probability of IE may influence decisions regarding the appropriate use of diagnostic criteria and tests in these populations.

Clinical presentation

The second step in diagnosing IE involves both a careful physical examination, with special evaluation for the common cardiac, neurologic, vascular, and immunologic manifestations of the disease (many of which

Evidence-Based Infectious Diseases, 2nd edition. Edited by Mark Loeb, Fiona Smaill and Marek Smieja. © 2009 Wiley-Blackwell Publishing, ISBN: 978-1-4051-7026-0

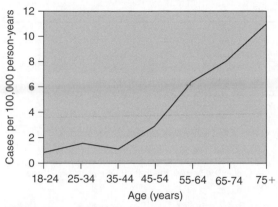

Figure 4.1 Age-specific person-years of community native valve non-IVDU cases residing in six contiguous counties (Philadelphia, Delaware, Montgomery, Bucks, and Chester Counties, PA, and Camden County, NJ) during a 27-month (August, 1988–October, 1990) recruitment period. Person-years of follow-up were calculated by multiplying the population in each age-stratum by 27 months/12 = 2.25 years of case accrual. Data from reference [5]: Berlin JA, Abrutyn E, Strom BL, et al. Incidence of infective endocarditis in the Delaware Valley, 1988–1990. Am J Cardiol 1995;76:933–6.

are listed in Table 4.1), and a medical history focused on whether the patient has any known risk factors for developing IE. With regard to this patient, it is known that patients with mitral valve prolapse (MVP) are 8 to 19 times more likely to develop IE than patients without MVP [9,10]. By contrast, it is useful to know that this patient was HIV-negative, as patients infected with HIV are approximately five times more likely to develop IE (independent of intravenous drug use) [8], with the precise risk being related to the level of immunodeficiency [11]. Other risk factors for IE that have been documented in case–control studies include congenital heart disease [9], prior cardiac valvular surgery [9], rheumatic fever [9], heart murmur without other known cardiac abnormalities [9], previous episodes of IE [9], severe kidney disease [12], diabetes mellitus [12], and prior skin infections [12] or wounds [13].

Blood culture

Third, clinicians should arrange for blood cultures to be obtained prior to the initiation of empiric antimicrobial treatment. Proper timing and technique of blood cultures remain the keys to accurate diagnosis; unfortunately, errors remain common [14]. Multiple blood cultures should be obtained over time so as to demonstrate persistent bacteremia if culturable organisms are present. Valid utilization of the Duke criteria (see below) requires that three independent sets of blood cultures (independent venipunctures) be obtained, with at least 12 hours separating the first and last [15]. More than 99% of cases of true bacteremia or fungemia can be detected with three venipunctures [16,17]. Ideally, each venipuncture should yield at least 15 mL of blood [17], though some culture systems may have different requirements. Organisms commonly associated with community-acquired, native-valve IE are listed in Table 4.2.

Echocardiography

The fourth diagnostic step to be considered is echocardiography. Many studies evaluating patients with confirmed or rejected IE based on pathologic specimens or long-term follow-up have firmly established that transesophageal echocardiography (TEE) has better operating characteristics than transthoracic echocardiography (TTE). For example, in two case series, the sensitivity of TEE for diagnosing IE (in the absence of other clinical information) was 94–100%, and the specificity was 100% [18,19]. By contrast, the sensitivity of TTE in these two series was 44–50%, and the specificity was 93–98%, when the same echocardiographic findings were required for diagnosis [18,19].

TEE is also superior for detecting specific lesions, such as vegetations, perivalvular abscesses, valvular aneurysms, and valvular perforations, that are commonly associated with both the presence of IE and the patient's prognosis [20–29]. In addition, despite early concerns about safety, the procedure carries a very low risk of complication [30].

Despite the superiority of TEE, there are two reasons why it should not be routinely used as a first-line diagnostic test for every patient suspected of having IE. First, among patients with very high or very low probabilities of IE based on history and physical examination, TTE and TEE yield highly concordant diagnostic classifications [31]. Though incorporating the results of TEE improves the sensitivity of the Duke criteria (see below) for diagnosing both culture-positive [32] and culture-negative [33] endocarditis

Table 4.1 The Duke criteria* for diagnosis of infective endocarditis

Major criteria

I Positive blood culture for infective endocarditis

A   Typical microorganism for IE from 2 separate blood cultures
   1   Viridans streptococci (including nutritionally variant strains), *Streptococcus bovis*, HACEK[†] group, or
   2   Community-acquired *Staphylococcus aureus* or enterococci, in the absence of a primary focus, or

B   Persistently positive blood culture, defined as recovery of a microorganism consistent with IE from:
   1   Blood cultures drawn more than 12 hours apart, or
   2   All of 3 or a majority of 4 or more separate blood cultures, with first and last drawn at least 1 hour apart

II Evidence of endocardial involvement

A   Positive echocardiogram for IE
   1   Oscillating intracardiac mass, on valve or supporting structures, or in the path of regurgitant jets, or on implanted
       material, in the absence of an alternative anatomic explanation, or
   2   Abscess, or
   3   New partial dehiscence of prosthetic valve, or

B   New valvular regurgitation (increase or change in preexisting murmur not sufficient)

Minor criteria

I Predisposition: predisposing heart condition or intravenous drug use

II Fever: ≥38.0°C (100.4°F)

III Vascular phenomena: major arterial emboli, septic pulmonary infarcts, mycotic aneurysm, intracranial hemorrhage,
       conjunctival hemorrhages, Janeway lesions

IV Immunologic phenomena: glomerulonephritis, Osler nodes, Roth spots, rheumatoid factor

V Microbiologic evidence: positive blood culture but not meeting major criterion as noted previously,[‡] or serologic evidence
      of active infection with organism consistent with IE

VI Echocardiogram: consistent with IE but not meeting major criterion as note previously

---

*Adapted from reference [15]. The diagnosis of "definite endocarditis" is made on pathologic grounds when appropriate pathologic specimens from surgery or autopsy reveal positive histology and/or culture. The diagnosis of "definite endocarditis" is made on clinical grounds when 2 major criteria, 1 major and 3 minor criteria, or 5 minor criteria are met. The diagnosis of "possible endocarditis" is given when patients present with findings consistent with IE, but falling short of the requirements for definite endocarditis. The diagnosis of endocarditis is "rejected" if there is a firm alternative diagnosis to explain the clinical manifestations, if there is resolution of the manifestations suggesting IE with ≤4 days of antibiotic therapy, or if no pathologic evidence of IE is found at surgery or autopsy, in patients who received ≤4 days of antibiotic therapy.
†*Haemophilus* spp., *Actinobacillus actinomycetemcomitans*, *Cardiobacterium hominis*, *Eikenella* spp., and *Kingella kingae*.
‡Excluding single positive cultures for coagulase-negative staphyloccoci and organisms that do not cause IE.

compared to classifications based on TTE results, this improvement is largely confined to (1) patients with intermediate probabilities of IE on clinical grounds, and (2) patients with prosthetic valves [31,32].

The second reason to limit the use of TEE is that it is only cost-effective as a first-line test in these same two groups of patients [34]. Indeed, a detailed decision analysis suggests that among patients with very low (e.g., <2%) probabilities of IE, short-term treatment of bacteremia in the absence of echocardiography is warranted, whereas among patients with high probabilities of disease (e.g., >60%, as might be observed among patients with persistently positive bacteremia without another known cause) it is most cost-effective to treat empirically for endocarditis, regardless of echocardiographic results [34]. This analysis recommends the use of TEE as a first-line test for patients with intermediate probabilities of disease, though initial use of TTE, followed by TEE in the event of negative or inconclusive results, remains a recommended strategy [35].

Regardless of the probability of IE, echocardiography retains an important role in the identification of patients who have complications of IE, such as perivalvular abscess, aneurysm, and valvular perforation. Because TEE is clearly superior to TTE in identifying such complications, it ought to be used whenever complications are suspected, or whenever there is a need to rule them out [21,27]. TEE is also indicated for defining underlying structural abnormalities in that predispose patients to future IE [35].

Table 4.2 Common etiologic agents of community-acquired, native-valve endocarditis*

Organism	Proportion of cases (%)
Streptococcus species	50
Viridans, alpha-hemolytic	35
S. bovis	12
Other streptococci	< 5
Staphylococcus species	30
S. aureus	25
Coagulase-negative	5
Enterococcus species	7
HACEK[†] group	< 5
Gram-negative bacilli	< 5
Other bacteria/polymicrobial	< 5
Fungi	< 5
Culture-negative	5

*These proportions are approximations based on data from a large number of series. Observed proportions may vary considerably based on features of the local population, including the proportion of intravenous drug users, patients with prosthetic valves, and age distribution.

[†]*Haemophilus* spp., *Actinobacillus actinomycetemcomitans*, *Cardiobacterium hominis*, *Eikenella* spp., and *Kingella kingae*.

Diagnostic criteria

Another reason to use echocardiography is that it enables formal diagnosis of "definite," "possible," or "rejected" IE using the well-established Duke criteria (Table 4.1) [15]. Incorporating clinical, laboratory, and echocardiographic information, the Duke criteria – the fifth diagnostic step in making a diagnosis of endocarditis – have been shown repeatedly [36–40] to have more favorable operating characteristics than the earlier Beth Israel criteria [41]. A retrospective evaluation of 410 patients also showed that the Duke criteria had good agreement (72–90%) with expert clinical judgment [42].

The operating characteristics of the Duke Criteria are best determined using studies, or subgroups within studies, for which the diagnosis of endocarditis was eventually proven or rejected by surgery, autopsy, and/or long-term follow-up. Considering only such studies, and grouping "definite" *and* "possible" categorizations as positive tests, the sensitivity of the Duke criteria is 98–100% [15,36,38–40,43] and the specificity is 93% [44]. If only a "definite" categorization on the Duke criteria is considered as a positive test, the sensitivity drops to 72–80%

[15,38,39,43] (69% in elderly patients) [40], while the specificity rises to 99% [44].

The Duke criteria are also valid for diagnosing culture-negative endocarditis, with one study of 49 patients with pathologically proven or rejected IE showing a sensitivity of 72%, and specificity of 100% when serial blood cultures are negative [33]. In light of this reduced sensitivity with retained specificity, several authors have recently proposed modifications to the Duke criteria [43,45,46]. However, we cannot recommend the routine use of any of these proposed modifications until further investigation of their comparative value is available. For example, these studies are uniform in suggesting that the sensitivity of the Duke criteria might be improved, without sacrificing specificity, by adding the serologic diagnosis of Q fever (caused by *Coxiella burnetii*) as a major criterion [45–47]. However, the incremental value of such modifications may only be realized in geographic areas where Q fever accounts for an important proportion of IE cases.

These estimates of sensitivity and specificity are more robust than corresponding estimates of positive and negative predictive values because the latter are strongly influenced by the underlying prevalence of disease in a given population. Nonetheless, predictive values answer the more clinically relevant question of whether a patient with a positive (or negative) categorization using the Duke criteria does (or does not) have IE. One study of the negative predictive value of the Duke criteria suggested it was at least 92% when both "definite" and "possible" categorizations are considered positive tests [48]. Presently, the positive predictive value of the Duke criteria can only be estimated by jointly considering the results of several small, independent samples of patients with pathologically confirmed diagnoses. On the basis of these reports on heterogeneous patient samples, the positive predictive value appears to be ≥85% for diagnosing both culture-positive and culture-negative IE in patients with native or prosthetic valves [32,33,36].

Proper diagnosis of the presented patient should therefore be based on the Duke criteria, incorporating information obtained from a thorough history and physical examination, three sets of blood cultures, and TEE. If the blood cultures are negative, and the patient is classified as "possible IE" according to the Duke criteria, further diagnostic tests, reviewed elsewhere [33,49–53], may be warranted.

Case presentation (continued)

After overnight incubation, Gram stains of blood culture specimens obtained at 2 of the three separate venipunctures reveal Gram-positive cocci in chains. The following day, these cultures grow viridans *Streptococcus*, and are found to be highly susceptible to penicillin (MIC ≤ 0.1 μg/mL) on day 3. Transesophageal echocardiography reveals a moderate-sized, mobile mass attached to the atrial surface of the anterior leaflet of a prolapsed mitral valve, and color Doppler study shows mitral regurgitation with no evidence of extension of the intracardiac lesion. The patient appears hemodynamically stable, and has no evidence of renal dysfunction. Evaluation for signs of congestive heart failure reveals only 1+ edema in the lower extremities. No rales are appreciated, no S3 is audible, and the jugular veins are not distended. A chest radiograph is clear. While deciding upon the most appropriate course of antibiotics, you wonder whether evaluation for mitral valve replacement is warranted.

Antimicrobial management

This patient meets two major criteria in the Duke classification – isolation of a typical organism for IE, and echocardiographic detection of an oscillating mass attached to a valvular leaflet – and is thus classified as having "definite endocarditis." Determination of the most appropriate antibiotic regimen requires consideration of the appropriate agent(s), their dose, route of administration, duration of treatment, and whether such treatment requires prolonged hospitalization.

A working group of the American Heart Association has provided thorough treatment recommendations for IE caused by both typical [54] and atypical [49] organisms. Few randomized trials of these regimens have been conducted because the disease itself is rare, and specific etiologies are rarer still. Recruiting sufficient numbers of patients with IE caused by specific bacteria is therefore difficult. Furthermore, the excellent efficacy of known regimens that would be used in control subjects makes type II errors likely in all but extremely large trials. We will limit our discussion to reviewing the best available evidence on regimens for treating the most common causes of native-valve IE in non-drug users, viridans streptococci and *Streptococcus bovis*.

With few trials to guide treatment recommendations, decisions must be guided by case series documenting the efficacy of various regimens against streptococcal species. The viridans streptococci include several species, such as *S. mutans*, *S. sanguis*, *S oralis* (*mitis*), and *S. salivarius*. The treatment of penicillin-susceptible *S. bovis*, a nonenterococcal, group D streptococcus, is similar, and is often grouped with viridans species in these series.

Four weeks of antimicrobial treatment is traditionally recommended for IE caused by penicillin-sensitive streptococci [54]. Typical regimens include parenteral penicillin, either alone or in tandem with an aminoglycoside. More recently, a single daily dose of intravenous or intramuscular ceftriaxone (2 g/day) for 4 weeks has been shown to be effective in treating endocarditis caused by sensitive strains of streptococci [55–57]. One small randomized trial showed that both this 4-week regimen, as well as a modified regimen of 2 weeks of parenteral ceftriaxone followed by 2 weeks of oral amoxicillin, were curative in all 15 patients receiving each regimen (one possible relapse was noted among the group receiving 4 weeks of ceftriaxone [55]. However, this trial was not adequately powered to determine whether clinically important differences exist in the efficacy of these regimens.

The efficacy of shorter-course (2-week) antimicrobial therapy (typically for patients without longstanding symptoms) has been suggested by uncontrolled studies for 50 years [58,59]. Penicillin alone was initially used in sensitive isolates [58], although more recent series have shown lower relapse rates when an aminoglycoside was added [59,60]. This is attributable to synergistic bactericidal activity between the agents.

Single daily doses of ceftriaxone (2 g/day IV) plus netilmicin (4 mg/kg/day IV) for 2 weeks have recently been shown to be effective, achieving clinical cure in 89% of patients, and microbiologic cure in 100% of patients with documented streptococcal endocarditis [61]. In a randomized trial of 51 evaluable patients, Sexton et al. showed that a 2-week regimen of single daily doses of ceftriaxone (2 g/day IV) plus gentamicin (3 mg/kg/day IV) produced the same 96% cure rate as a 4-week regimen of ceftriaxone alone [57].

Despite these promising results with 2-week therapy, and the tremendous benefits they afford in reducing length of stay in the hospital, several important considerations may limit their widespread use. First, more extensive evaluation of the efficacy of single daily doses of aminoglycosides is needed. Second, clinicians may be reluctant to add an aminoglycoside for patients at high risk for nephrotoxicity or ototoxicity. Lastly, although isolates of penicillin-tolerant viridans streptococci and *S. bovis* remain uncommon, they have been noted in several recent series [62]. Four weeks of treatment is a prudent option in such cases [62]. A Cochrane Library meta-analysis evaluating the addition of aminoglycosides to standard therapy for endocarditis found greater nephrotoxicity without evidence of definite clinical benefit [63].

Case series suggest that for selected patients with susceptible isolates of viridans streptococci, no evidence of hemodynamic instability, and no other complications of IE, several of these regimens can be safely administered on an outpatient basis [55,56]. However, there have been no published trials directly comparing inpatient and outpatient antimicrobial therapy for IE. Such trials seem unlikely because they would need to be extremely large to detect small, but clinically important differences in the rates of treatment failure. In the absence of such comparative evidence, physicians must weigh, for each individual patient, the risks and costs of remaining in the hospital versus the risks for having IE complications unattended to in the outpatient setting [63].

In summary, there are several viable options for treating patients with penicillin-susceptible, viridans streptococcus or *S. bovis* IE on native valves. These are listed in Table 4.3. If the isolates show relative penicillin resistance ($0.1\,\mu g/mL$ < MIC < $0.5\,\mu g/mL$), 4 weeks of penicillin (18 million units per 24 hours IV) should be combined with gentamicin (1 mg/kg IM or IV every 8 hours) for at least the first 2 weeks [54,65]. For patients allergic to β-lactam antibiotics, vancomycin hydrochloride (30 mg/kg per 24 hours IV in two equally divided doses) should be used for 4 weeks [54].

Case presentation (continued)

You start the patient on IV penicillin (18 million units per 24 hours), plus IV gentamicin 1 mg/kg every 8 hours. You planned treatment for 2 weeks, but after 2 days, the patient becomes progressively dyspneic at rest. Pulse oximetry reveals an oxygen saturation of 89% on room air. Jugular venous distension is evident at 8 cm above the sternal notch, and rales are auscultated bilaterally. A second chest radiograph reveals patchy infiltrates in the lower lung fields bilaterally.

Surgical intervention

Indications for cardiac surgery

Traditional indications for cardiac surgery in IE include: moderate to severe heart failure, severe valvular dysfunction, perivalvular abscesses, multiple embolic events, prosthetic valve endocarditis, fungal infection, persistent bacteremia despite theoretically adequate antibiotic treatment, and, possibly, the

Table 4.3 Suggested therapeutic regimens for the treatment of native-valve endocarditis due to penicillin-susceptible (MIC < 0.1 mg/mL) viridans streptococci and *S. bovis*

Antibiotic regimen	Dosage and route	Duration
Aqueous crystalline penicillin G sodium	12–18 million units per 24 h IV, continuously or in 6 equally divided doses	4 weeks
Ceftriaxone sodium	2 g once daily IV or IM	4 weeks
Aqueous crystalline penicillin G sodium	12–18 million units per 24 h IV, continuously or in 6 equally divided doses	2 weeks
with gentamicin sulfate	1 mg/kg IM or IV every 8 hours	
Ceftriaxone sodium	2 g once daily IV or IM	
with netilmicin	4 mg/kg daily IV	2 weeks

Modified from reference [5].

echocardiographic detection of large, mobile vegetations [66]. Although 35 years of clinical experience supports the adherence to these indications, the lack of controlled studies makes it difficult to determine the validity or relative strengths of each. In deciding whether to proceed to surgery for an individual patient, careful (and perhaps separate) evaluation of hemodynamic and infectious disease considerations is warranted.

Timing of surgical intervention

Whether proceeding to surgery early (i.e., during the active stage of IE) [67] confers an additional risk for recurrence or mortality remains controversial. There are no randomized trials of the timing of surgical intervention, although one such trial of early surgical intervention compared with medical therapy is ongoing [68]. Clinicians should therefore be mindful that the results of the available cohort studies may be biased if patients with more severe disease, and hence poorer prognosis, were preferentially selected for earlier surgical intervention.

Aranki and colleagues reported that among patients with mitral valve IE, proceeding to surgery before sterilizing the diseased valve with antimicrobial therapy was not associated with a poorer postoperative prognosis [69]. By contrast, among patients with aortic valve IE, delaying operation until the initial IE had healed was associated with more favorable outcomes [70]. Other series show no association between surgery in active IE and poorer prognosis, regardless of the valve involved [71,72].

Several retrospective cohort studies indicate that early surgical intervention may improve short- and/or long-term outcomes in patients with *Staphylococcus aureus* IE [67,73–75] and in any patient with IE complicated by CHF [75,76]. There remains no evidence indicating a benefit to early surgical intervention in patients with uncomplicated streptococcal IE. However, a prospective, randomized trial of medical versus early surgical intervention among patients with uncomplicated IE would be needed to overcome the selection biases that likely influence the foregoing conclusions. Unfortunately, such a trial would still be limited by the inability to blind patients to their received treatment.

Decisions to proceed to surgery must therefore be tailored to the individual patient, and should be based on consideration of at least three groups of factors. First, physicians should consider the patient's risks for operative mortality. Second, physicians should consider the patient's risks for postsurgical complications such as relapse (resumption of the clinical picture of endocarditis, including isolation of the same microorganism, within 6 months of initial treatment), recurrence (development of a new clinical picture also consistent with endocarditis, but with a different microorganism or occurring more than 6 months after the initial episode), embolic events, worsening heart failure, need for subsequent valve replacement, and death. Finally, physicians should consider the short- and long-term prognoses of patients managed surgically versus those managed medically. Several case series have evaluated these prognostic issues.

Prognosis

Relapse and recurrence

Long-term (≥10 years) follow-up of inception cohorts of non-intravenous drug users diagnosed with IE suggest that 0–3% of patients will have relapsing IE, and 6–12% will have recurrent IE [29,72,77]. Series of surgically managed patients show a higher (20–25%) incidence of recurrence [78] though, again, the severity of disease may be higher among such patients. Recurrence is more likely in patients with initial IE on a prosthetic valve, those with positive valve cultures at the time of surgery, and in those with persistent fever more than 7 days postoperatively [78]. To monitor for relapses, which typically manifest within 4 weeks of the cessation of treatment, it is recommended that at least one set of blood cultures be obtained in the 8 weeks following completion of antimicrobial treatment [54]. However, the costs and benefits of different strategies have not been evaluated.

The need for subsequent valvular surgery

Several large case series indicate that approximately 10–20% of patients initially operated on for IE will need another valve replacement [77,79,80]. Patients at higher risk for requiring late valve replacement include those with recurrent IE [77], those with initial endocarditis on a prosthetic valve [77], those with initial involvement of the aortic valve [72],) and those with positive cultures of valvular material obtained intraoperatively [80].

Embolic events

Embolic events, typically caused by the fragmentation and dislodging of valvular vegetations, have been reported to occur in 9–44% of patients after being diagnosed with IE [81–83]; many others will have already experienced embolic complications by the time of presentation [83,84]. The variability among these retrospective cohort studies is attributable to differing frequencies of early surgical intervention, heterogeneity in the underlying severity of disease among cohorts, and to whether or not computed tomography was used to detect silent emboli. Once appropriate antimicrobial therapy is initiated, the risk of embolic events decreases precipitously, particularly after the first week of therapy [81,85]. The most common sites for embolization are the central nervous system, spleen, lungs, kidneys, peripheral arteries, retinal artery, and coronary vessels [81–83].

Because of the frequency and substantial morbidity associated with embolic events in IE, and the (untested) premise that early surgical intervention could prevent many embolic events, several investigators have conducted retrospective cohort studies to determine whether patients' risks for embolism could be predicted by echocardiography [81–83,86–89]. The results of these studies have been mixed, depending on the size of study samples, whether TTE or TEE was used, and whether or not computed tomography was used to detect silent emboli. The larger studies using TEE to evaluate vegetations have consistently found that vegetation size (>10 mm) and mobility are each associated with an elevated risk for embolism [83, 87,89]. However, the fact that embolism also occurs in many patients without detectable vegetations raises doubts as to the clinical utility of routinely screening patients for embolism risk using TEE [90].

Congestive heart failure

Symptoms of congestive heart failure (CHF) are found at presentation in more than half of patients with IE. Other patients will experience incident CHF or worsening CHF after the initial infection has healed with appropriate treatment. Patients with native valve endocarditis are more likely to present with CHF symptoms than are those with prosthetic valve endocarditis [28]. Though severe CHF is an indication for early surgery, intractable pulmonary edema and impaired left ventricular systolic function are independent predictors of operative mortality [79].

Early and late mortality

Advances in the diagnosis and management of IE have had substantial impact on overall mortality, though it remains discouragingly high. Recent case series of consecutive patients with IE report survival rates of approximately 75% at 1 year, dropping to approximately 70% at 10 years [29]. Survival is significantly better among patients with initial native valve endocarditis than among those with prosthetic valve endocarditis [29,91].

Among all patients with IE, risk factors for early mortality (typically defined as within 6 weeks of diagnosis) include older age [29] a variety of cardiac complications [29,79,92] and neurologic complications [84,93]. Among patients managed surgically, early postoperative mortality (typically defined as occurring within 30 days of surgery or prior to discharge from the hospital, whichever comes second) occurs in 8–16%, depending on the preoperative clinical severity of the cohort [28,71,79,91]. Risk factors for early operative mortality include older age, S. aureus infection, perivalvular abscess with fistulization, worse preoperative heart failure, and preoperative renal failure [28,71,79,94].

Late mortality appears to be greater among men [77], older patients [28,77], patients with S. aureus infection [28], perivalvular abscess [27,76,95], and those with initial IE on a prosthetic valve [69].

Case presentation (continued)

Based on this patient's worsening CHF and risk for embolism, mitral valve replacement is performed on the seventh day of admission. Six days later, the patient is stable and discharged to home, where arrangements have been made for him to complete his antibiotic course. Before leaving, the patient inquires as to whether he could have prevented this episode of endocarditis. He also asks what he should do in the future to prevent recurrence.

Antibiotic prophylaxis against infective mendocarditis is no longer recommended for high-risk patients, including those who, like this patient, have MVP and regurgitation, before they undergo many dental, genitourinary, and gastrointestinal procedures [96]. While this was previously the recommendation, the value of this recommendation has been repeatedly questioned [9,97–99], and there is evidence that many physicians do not follow it [14,100]. In the 2008 update of the American College of Cardiology/American Heart Association guidelines on infective endocarditis, prophylaxis is now recommended *only* for patients at highest risk of poor outcome should they contract endocarditis (prosthetic valves, congenital heart disease, cardiac transplant patients with valve regurgitation) [96].

The low incidence of infective endocarditis makes it unlikely that a randomized, controlled trial of prophylactic efficacy will be undertaken to resolve this question definitively. As a result, several groups have used alternate methods to provide insights into the potential utility of prophylaxis.

Three case–control studies have directly evaluated the efficacy of antibiotic prophylaxis [13,101,102]. The first reported that prophylaxis provides clinically and statistically significant protection against IE [101]. However, this analysis was based on only 8 patients who developed IE and 24 controls, and misclassification of just one of the cases would nullify the results entirely [101]. Furthermore, selective recall of having taken antibiotic prophylaxis among patients with cardiac lesions who did not develop IE may have inflated the observed efficacy. The second and third studies of efficacy, both of which were larger, found no significant benefit of prophylaxis [13,102].

Another approach to quantifying the potential value of prophylaxis is to determine whether procedures known to induce transient bacteremia occur more commonly among patients who develop endocarditis than among those who do not. One hospital-based case–control study [13] and one population-based case–control study [9] have evaluated these risk factors. Both studies found that dental treatments were not associated with an increased risk for IE [9,13], even among patients with known cardiac lesions [9]. Because such patients represent those for whom prophylaxis is recommended [96], the lack of an association between dental treatments and IE in this group suggests that even strict adherence to these recommendations would yield little benefit.

Finally, investigators have conducted formal decision analyses considering both the incidence of IE

in patients with mitral valve prolapse who undergo dental procedures, and the incidence of adverse drug reactions following prophylaxis [103,104]. These analyses indicate that prophylaxis is extremely unlikely to produce a net health benefit, and that it could not plausibly provide such a benefit at a cost that society might consider reasonable.

These findings are, perhaps, to be expected considering that only 10.6% of patients who develop IE would have been targets of prophylaxis by virtue of having both a preexisting cardiac lesion and a dental procedure [9]. Therefore, not only does there exist no good evidence supporting the efficacy of known prophylactic regimens, but there is substantial evidence to suggest that prophylaxis could not prevent a sizeable number of IE cases, even if a uniformly effective regimen were developed.

This patient should therefore be told that his episode of IE was an unfortunate occurrence that could not have (reasonably) been prevented with known interventions. Maintaining good oral hygiene with regular flossing may be beneficial [12]. The patient should also be told that his risk for IE is now markedly increased due to both his having had IE in the past, and his having a prosthetic mitral valve [9]. Formal evaluation of the costs and benefits of prophylaxis in such a high-risk population is needed to guide the patient in preventing future episodes.

References

1 Smith RH, Radford DJ, Clark RA, Julian DJ. Infective endocarditis: a survey of cases in the South-East region of Scotland. Thorax 1976;31:373–9.

2 Hickey AJ, MacMahon SW, Wilcken DEL. Mitral valve prolapse and bacterial endocarditis: when is antibiotic prophylaxis necessary? Am Heart J 1985;109:431–5.

3 Griffin MR, Wilson WR, Edwards WD, O'Fallon WM, Kurland LT. Infective endocarditis, Olmsted County, Minnesota, 1950 through 1981. JAMA 1985;254:1199–202.

4 King JW, Nguyen VQ, Conrad SA. Results of a prospective statewide reporting system for infective endocarditis. Amer J Med Sci 1988;295:517–27.

5 Berlin JA, Abrutyn E, Strom BL, et al. Incidence of infective endocarditis in the Delaware Valley, 1988–1990. Am J Cardiol 1995;76:933–6.

6 Hogevick H, Olaison L, Andersson R, Lindeberg J, Alestig K. Epidemiologic aspects of infective endocarditis in an urban population: a 5-year prospective study. Medicine (Baltimore) 1995;74:324–39.

7 Bouza E, Menasalvas A, Munoz P, Vasallo FJ, Del Mar Moreno M, Fernandez MAG. Infective endocarditis – A propospective study at the end of the twentieth century. Medicine (Baltimore) 2001;80:298–307.

8 Spijkerman IJB, van Ameijden EJC, Mientjes GHC, Coutinho RA, van den Hoek A. Human immunodeficiency virus infection and other risk factors for skin abscesses and endocarditis among injection drug users. J Clin Epidemiol 1996;49:1149–54.

9 Strom BL, Abrutyn E, Berlin JA, et al. Dental and cardiac risk factors for infective endocarditis: a population-based case-control study. Ann Intern Med 1998;129:761–9.

10 Clemens J, Horwitz R, Jaffe C, Feinstein A, Stanton B. A controlled evaluation of the risk of bacterial endocarditis in persons with mitral-valve prolapse. N Engl J Med 1982;307:776–81.

11 Manoff SB, Vlahov D, Herskowitz A, et al. Human immunodeficiency virus infection and infective endocarditis among injecting drug users. Epidemiology 1996;7:566–70.

12 Strom BL, Abrutyn E, Berlin JA, et al. Risk factors for infective endocarditis: Oral hygiene and nondental exposures. Circulation 2000;102:2842–8.

13 Lacassin F, Hoen B, Leport C, et al. Procedures associated with infective endocarditis in adults. A case control study. Eur Heart J 1995;16:1968–74.

14 Delahaye F, Rial M-O, de Gevigney G, Ecochard R, Delaye J. A critical appraisal of the quality of the management of infective endocarditis. J Am Coll Cardiol 1999;33:788–93.

15 Durack DT, Lukes AS, Bright DK. New criteria for diagnosis of infective endocarditis: utilization of specific echocardiographics findings. Am J Med 1994;96:200–9.

16 Washington JA, II. Blood cultures: principles and techniques. Mayo Clin Proc 1975;50:91–8.

17 Weinstein M, Reller L, Murphy J, Lichtenstein K. Clinical significance of positive blood cultures: a comprehensive analysis of 500 episodes of bacteremia and fungemia in adults. I. Laboratory and epidemiologic observations. Rev Infect Dis 1983;5:35–53.

18 Pedersen WE, Walker M, Olsen JD, et al. Value of transesophageal echocardiography as an adjunct to transthoracic echocardiography, in evaluation of native and prosthetic valve endocarditis. Chest 1991;100:351–6.

19 Shively BK, Gurule FT, Roldan CA, Leggett JH, Schiller NB. Diagnostic value of transesophageal echocardiography compared with transthoracic echocardiography in infective endocarditis. J Am Coll Cardiol 1991;18:391–7.

20 Birmingham GD, Rahko PS, Ballantyne F. Improved detection of infective endocarditis with transesophageal echocardiography. Am Heart J 1992;123:774–81.

21 De Castro S, d'Amati G, Cartoni D, et al. Valvular perforation in left-sided infective endocarditis: a prospective echocardiographic evaluation and clinical outcome. Am Heart J 1997;134:656–64.

22 Daniel WG, Mugge A, Martin RP, et al. Improvement in the diagnosis of abscesses associated with endocarditis by transesophageal echocardiography. N Engl J Med 1991;324:795–800.

23 Daniel WG, Schroeder E, Nonnast-Daniel B, Lichtlen PR. Conventional and transesophageal echocardiography in the diagnosis of infective endocarditis. Eur Heart J 1987;8(suppl J):303–6.

24 Erbel R, Rohmann S, Drexler M, et al. Improved diagnostic value of echocardiography in patients with infective endocarditis by transesophageal approach: a prospective study. Eur Heart J 1988;9:43–53.

25 Taems MA, Gussenhoven EJ, Bos E, et al. Enhanced morphological diagnosis in infective endocarditis by transesophageal echocardiography. Br Heart J 1990;63:109–13.

26 Shapiro SM, Young E, De Guzman S, et al. Transesophageal echocardiography in diagnosis of infective endocarditis. Chest 1994;105:377–82.

27 Blumberg EA, Karalis DA, Chandrasekaran K, et al. Endocarditis-associated paravalvular abscesses: do clinical parameters predict the presence of abscess? Chest 1995;107:898–903.

28 Choussat R, Thomas D, Isnard R, et al. Perivalvular abscesses associated with endocarditis: clinical features and prognostic factors of overall survival in a series of 233 cases: Perivalvular Abscess French Multicentre Study. Eur Heart J 1999;20:232–41.

29 Castillo JC, Anguita MP, Ramirez A, et al. Long term outcome of infective endocarditis in patients who were not drug addicts: a 10 year study. Heart 2000;83:525–30.

30 Daniel WG, Erbel R, Kaspar W, et al. Safety of transesophageal echocardiography, a multicenter survey of 10,419 examinations. Circulation 1993;83:817–21.

31 Lindner JR, Case RA, Dent JM, Abbott RD, Scheld WM, Kaul S. Diagnostic value of echocardiography in suspected endocarditis: an evaluation based on the pretest probability of disease. Circulation 1996;93:730–6.

32 Roe MT, Abramson MA, Li J, et al. Clinical information determines the impact of transesophageal echocardiography on the diagnosis of infective endocarditis by the Duke Criteria. Am Heart J 2000;139:945–51.

33 Kupferwasser LI, Darius H, Muller AM, et al. Diagnosis of culture-negative endocarditis: the role of the Duke criteria and the impact of transesophageal echocardiography. Am Heart J 2001;142:146–52.

34 Heidenreich PA, Masoudi FA, Maini B, et al. Echocardiography in patients with suspected endocarditis: a cost-effectiveness analysis. Am J Med 1999;107:198–208.

35 Cheitlin MD, Alpert JS, Armstrong WF, et al. ACC/AHA Guidelines for the Clinical Application of Echocardiography: A Report of the American College of Cardiology/American Heart Association Task Force on Practice Guidelines (Committee on Clinical Application of Echocardiography) Developed in Collaboration With the American Society of Echocardiography. Circulation 1997;95:1686–744.

36 Bayer AS, Ward JI, Ginzton LE, Shapiro SM. Evaluation of new clinical criteria for the diagnosis of infective endocarditis. Am J Med 1994;96:211–19.

37 Hoen B, Selton-Suty C, Danchin N, et al. Evaluation of the Duke Criteria versus the Beth Israel Criteria for the

diagnosis of infective endocarditis. Clin Infect Dis 1995; 21:905–9.

38 Cecchi E, Parrini A, Chinaglia F, et al. New diagnostic criteria for infective endocarditis. Eur Heart J 1997;18:1149–56.

39 Heiro M, Nikoskelainen J, Hartiala JJ, Saraste MK, Kotilainen PK. Diagnosis of infective endocarditis. Sensitivity of the Duke vs. von Reyn criteria. Arch Intern Med 1998;158:18–24.

40 Gagliardi JP, Nettles RE, McCarthy DE, Sanders LL, Corey GR, Sexton DJ. Native valve infective endocarditis in elderly and younger adult patients: comparison of clinical features and outcomes with use of Duke Criteria and the Duke Endocarditis Database. Clin Infect Dis 1998; 26:1165–8.

41 von Reyn CF, Levy BS, Arbeit RD, Friedland G, Crumpacker CS. Infective endocarditis: an analysis based on strict case definitions. Ann Intern Med 1981;94:505–17.

42 Sekeres MA, Abrutyn E, Berlin JA, et al. An assessment of the usefulness of the Duke criteria for diagnosing active infective endocarditis. Clin Infect Dis 1997;24:1185–90.

43 Lamas CC, Eykyn SE. Suggested modifications to the Duke criteria for the clinical diagnosis of native valve and prosthetic valve endocarditis: analysis of 118 pathologically proven cases. Clin Infect Dis 1997;25:713–19.

44 Hoen B, Beguinot I, Rabaud C, et al. The Duke criteria for diagnosing infective endocarditis are specific: analysis of 100 patients with acute fever of unknown origin. Clin Infect Dis 1996;23:298–302.

45 Fournier P-E, Casalta J-P, Habib G, Messana T, Raoult D. Modification of the diagnostic criteria proposed by the Duke Endocarditis Service to permit improved diagnosis of Q Fever endocarditis. Am J Med 1996;100:629–33.

46 Li JS, Sexton DJ, Mick N, et al. Proposed modifications to the Duke criteria for the diagnosis of infective endocarditis. Clin Infect Dis 2000;30:633–8.

47 Habib G, Derumeaux G, Avierinos J-F, et al. Value and limitations of the duke criteria for the diagnosis of infective endocarditis. J Am Coll Cardiol 1999;33:2023–9.

48 Dodds GAI, Sexton DJ, Durack DT, et al. Negative predictive value of the Duke Criteria for infective endocarditis. Am J Cardiol 1996;77:403–7.

49 Bayer AS, Bolger AF, Taubert KA, et al. Diagnosis and management of infective endocarditis and its complications. Circulation 1998;98:2936–48.

50 Mylonakis E, Calderwood SB. Infective endocarditis in adults. N Engl J Med 2001;345:1318–30.

51 Hoen B, Selton-Suty C, Lacassin F, et al. Infective endocarditis in patients with negative blood cutltures: analysis of 88 cases from a one-year nationwide survey in France. Clin Infect Dis 1995;20:501–6.

52 Fournier PF, Raoult D. Non-culture laboratory methods for diagnosis of infective endocarditis. Curr Infect Dis Rep 1999;1:136–41.

53 Brouqi P, Raoult D. Endocarditis due to rare and fastidious bacteria. Clin Microbiol Rev 2001;14:177–207.

54 Wilson WR, Karchmer AW, Dajani AS, et al. Antibiotic treatment of adults with infective endocarditis due to Streptococci, Enterococci, Staphylococci, and HACEK microorganisms. JAMA 1995;274:1706–13.

55 Stamboulian D, Bonvehi P, Arevalo C, et al. Antibiotic management of outpatients with endocarditis due to penicillin-susceptible streptococci. Rev Infect Dis 1991;13:S160–3.

56 Francioli PF, Etienne J, Hoigne R, Thys J, Gerber A. Treatment of streptococcal endocarditis with a single daily dose of ceftriaxone sodium for 4 weeks. Efficacy and outpatient treatment feasibility. JAMA 1992;267:264–7.

57 Sexton DJ, Tenenbaum MJ, Wilson WR, et al. Ceftriaxone once daily for four weeks compared with ceftriaxone plus gentamicin once daily for two weeks for treatment of endocarditis due to penicillin-susceptible streptococci. Clin Infect Dis 1998;27:1470–4.

58 Hamburger M, Stein L. Streptococcus viridans subacute bacterial endocarditis. Two week treatment schedule with penicillin. JAMA 1952;149:542–5.

59 Tan JS, Kaplan S, Terhune CA, Jr., Hamburger M. Successful two-week treatment schedule for penicillin-susceptible streptococcus viridans endocarditis. Lancet 1971;2:1340–3.

60 Wilson WR, Thompson RL, Wilkowske CJ, et al. Short-term therapy for streptococcal infective endocarditis: combined intramuscular administration of penicillin and streptomycin. JAMA 1981;245:360–3.

61 Francioli PF, Ruch W, Stamboulian D, and the International Infective Endocarditis Study Group. Treatment of streptococcal endocarditis with a single dose of ceftriaxone and netilmicin for 14 days: A prospective multicenter study. Clin Infect Dis 1995;21:1406–10.

62 Hoen B. Special issues in the management of infective endocarditis caused by gram-positive cocci. Infect Dis Clin North Am 2002;16(2):437–52,xi.

63 Falagas ME, Matthaiou DK, Bliziotis IA. The role of aminoglycosides in combination with a beta-lactam for the treatment of bacterial endocarditis: a meta-analysis of comparative trials. J Antimicrob Chemother 2006;57:639–47.

64 Andrews M-M, von Reyn CF. Patient selection criteria and management guidelines for outpatient parenteral antibiotic therapy for native valve infective endocarditis. Clin Infect Dis 2001;33:203–9.

65 Working Party of the British Society for Antimicrobial Therapy. Antibiotic treatment of Streptococcal, Enterococcal, and Staphylococcal endocarditis. Heart 1998;79:207–10.

66 Olaison L, Pettersson G. Current best practices and guidelines: indications for surgical intervention in infective endocarditis. Infect Dis Clin North Am 2002;16(2):453–75,xi.

67 Bishara J, Leibovici L, Gartman-Israel D, et al. Long-term outcome of infective endocarditis: the impact of early surgical intervention. Clin Infect Dis 2001;33:1636–43.

68 San Roman JA, Lopez J, Revilla A, et al. Rationale, design and methods for the early surgery in infective endocarditis study (ENDOVAL 1): a multicenter, prospective, randomized trial comparing the state-of-the-art therapeutic strategy versus early surgery strategy in infective endocarditis. Am Heart J 2008;156:431–6.

69 Aranki SF, Adams DH, Rizzo RJ, et al. Determinants of early mortality and late survival in mitral valve endocarditis. Circulation 1995;92(9 Suppl):II143–9.

70 Aranki SF, Santini F, Adams DH, et al. Aortic valve endocarditis. Determinants of early survival and late morbidity. Circulation 1994;90:II175–82.

71 Jault F, Gandjbakhch I, Rama A, et al. Active native valve endocarditis: determinants of operative death and late mortality. Ann Thorac Surg 1997;63:1737–41.

72 Tornos MP, Permanyer-Miralda G, Olona M, et al. Long-term complications of native valve infective endocarditis in non-addicts. Ann Intern Med 1992;117: 567–72.

73 Malquarti V, Saradarian W, Etienne J, et al. Prognosis of native valve infective endocarditis: a review of 253 cases. Eur Heart J 1984;5(Suppl C):11–20.

74 Delahaye F, Ecochard R, de Gevigney G, et al. The long-term prognosis of infective endocarditis. Eur Heart J 1995;16(Suppl B):48–53.

75 Richardson JV, Karp RB, Kirklin JW, Dismukes WE. Treatment of infective endocarditis: a 10-year comparative analysis. Circulation 1978;58:589–97.

76 Croft CH, Woodward W, Elliott A, Commerford PJ, Barnard CN, Beck W. Analysis of surgical versus medical therapy in active complicated native valve infective endocarditis. Am J Cardiol 1983;51:1650–5.

77 Mansur AJ, Dal Bo CMR, Fukushima JT, Issa VS, Grinberg M, Pomerantzeff PMA. Relapses, recurrences, valve replacements, and mortality during the long-term follow-up after infective endocarditis. Am Heart J 2001;141: 78–86.

78 Renzulli A, Carozza A, Romano G, et al. Recurrent infective endocarditis: a multivariate analysis of 21 years of experience. Ann Thorac Surg 2001;72:39–43.

79 Alexiou C, Langley SM, Stafford H, Lowes JA, Livesey SA, Monro JL. Surgery for active culture-positive endocarditis: determinants of early and late outcome. Ann Thorac Surg 2000;69:1448–54.

80 Renzulli A, Carozza A, Marra C, et al. Are blood and valve cultures predictive for long-term outcome following surgery for infective endocarditis? Eur J Cardiothorac Surg 2000;17:228–33.

81 Steckelberg JM, Murphy JG, Ballard D, et al. Emboli in infective endocarditis: the prognostic value of echocardiography. Ann Intern Med 1991;114:635–40.

82 De Castro S, Magni G, Beni S, et al. Role of transthoracic and transesophageal echocardiography in predicting embolic events in patients with active infective endocarditis involving native cardiac valves. Am J Cardiol 1997;80: 1030–4.

83 Di Salvo G, Habib G, Pergola V, et al. Echocardiography predicts embolic events in infective endocarditis. J Am Coll Cardiol 2001;37:1069–76.

84 Heiro M, Nikoskelainen J, Engblom E, Marttila R, Kotilainen P. Neurologic manifestations o finfective endocarditis: a 17-year experience in a teaching hospital in Finland. Arch Intern Med 2000;160:2781–7.

85 Alestig K, Hogevick H, Olaison L. Infective endocarditis: a diagnostic and therapeutic challenge for the new millenium. Scand J Infect Dis 2000;32:343–56.

86 Heinle S, Wilderman N, Harrison K, et al. Value of transthoracic echocardiography in predicting embolic events in active infective endocarditis. Am J Cardiol 1994;74: 799–801.

87 Mugge A, Daniel WG, Frank G, Lichtlen PR. Echocardiography in infective endocarditis: reassessment of the prognostic implications of vegetation size determined by the transthoracic and the transesophageal approach. J Am Coll Cardiol 1989;14:631–8.

88 Sanfilippo AJ, Picard MH, Newell JB, et al. Echocardiographic assessment of patients with infectious endocarditis: prediction of risk for complications. J Am Coll Cardiol 1991;18:1191–9.

89 Rohmann S, Erbel R, Gorge G, et al. Clinical relevance of vegetation localization by transoesophageal echocardiography in infective endocarditis. Eur Heart J 1992;13: 446–52.

90 Shapiro S, Kupferwasser LI. Echocardiography predicts embolic events in infective endocarditis. J Am Coll Cardiol 2001;37:1077–9.

91 Delay D, Pellerin M, Carrier M, et al. Immediate and long-term results of valve replacement for native and prosthetic valve endocarditis. Ann Thorac Surg 2000;70:1219–23.

92 Meine TJ, Nettles RE, Anderson DJ, et al. Cardiac conduction abnormalities in endocarditis defined by the Duke Criteria. Am Heart J 2001;142:280–5.

93 Roder BL, Wandall DA, Espersen F, Frimodt-Moller N, Skinhoj P, Rosdahl VT. Neurologic manifestations in *Staphylococcus aureus* endocarditis: a review of 260 bacteremic cases in nondrug addicts. Am J Med 1997;102: 379–86.

94 Bauernschmitt R, Jakob HG, Vahl C-F, Lange R, Hagl S. Operation for infective endocarditis: Results after implantation of mechanical valves. Ann Thorac Surg 1998;65:359–64.

95 Aguado JM, Gonzalez-Vilchez F, Martin-Duran R, Arjona R, Vazquez de Prada JA. Perivalvular abscesses associated with endocarditis. Clinical features and diagnostic accuracy of two-dimensional echocardiography. Chest 1993;104: 88–93.

96 Nishimura RA, Carabella BA, Faxon DP, et al. ACC/AHA 2008 guideline update on valvular heart disease: focused update on infective endocarditis. Circulation 2008;118:887–96.

97 Durack DT, Kaplan EL, Bisno AL. Apparent failures of endocarditis prophylaxis: analysis of 52 cases submitted to a national registry. JAMA 1983;250:2318–22.

98 Levison ME, Abrutyn E. Infective endocarditis: current guidelines on prophylaxis. Curr Infect Dis Rep 1999; 1:119–25.

99 Roberts GJ. Dentists are innocent! "Everyday" bacteremia is the real culprit: a review and assessment of the evidence that dental surgical procedures are a principal cause of bacterial endocarditis in children. Pediatr Cardiol 1999;20:317–35.

100 Seto TB, Kwiat D, Taira DA, Douglas PS, Manning WJ. Physicians' recommendations to patients for use of antibiotic prophylaxis to prevent endocarditis. JAMA 2000;284:68–71.

101 Imperiale TF, Horwitz RI. Does prophylaxis prevent post-dental infective endocarditis? A controlled evaluation of protective efficacy. Am J Med 1990;88:131–6.

102 van der Meer JTM, van Wijk W, Thompson J, Vandenbroucke JP, Valkenburg HA, Michel MF. Efficacy of anitbiotic prophylaxis for prevention of native-valve endocarditis. Lancet 1992;339:135–9.

103 Bor DH, Himmelstein DU. Endocarditis prophylaxis for patients with mitral valve prolapse. Am J Med 1984;76:711–17.

104 Clemens J, Ransohoff DF. A quantitative assessment of pre-dental antibiotic prophylaxis for patients with mitral-valve prolapse. J Chronic Dis 1984;37:531–44.

CHAPTER 5

Meningitis and encephalitis

Kara B. Mascitti & Ebbing Lautenbach

Meningitis

Case presentation 1

A 30-year-old male presents to the emergency department with a 24-hour history of fever and headache. The patient's symptoms began abruptly and have worsened steadily over the last day. His wife reports that in the last 6 hours he has become somewhat confused. He has no significant past medical or surgical history. He takes no medications and denies alcohol, tobacco, or drug use. His family history is likewise non-contributory. Physical examination reveals a temperature of 38.5°C, a pulse of 110 beats per minute, and a blood pressure of 130/70 mmHg. He does not demonstrate photophobia or neck stiffness. His neurologic examination is non-focal but he is orientated only to person. Initial laboratory evaluation is remarkable for a white blood cell count of 21.4 × 10^9/L. You admit the patient with the presumptive diagnosis of meningitis, order two sets of blood cultures, and plan to perform a lumbar puncture (LP). You wonder whether to order a computed tomography (CT) scan prior to the LP to rule out an intracranial mass lesion, as well as whether antibiotics can be withheld until after the CT and LP have been performed.

Diagnosis

Epidemiology

The acute meningitis syndrome may be caused by a wide variety of infectious pathogens as well as by

noninfectious diseases and syndromes (Box 5.1) [1–5]. Given its frequency and clinical impact, this chapter will focus specifically on acute bacterial meningitis. The annual incidence of bacterial meningitis varies by geographic region, from between

Box 5.1 Differential diagnosis of acute meningitis

Bacteria
- *Streptococcus pneumoniae*
- *Neisseria meningitidis*
- *Listeria monocytogenes*
- *Hemophilus influenzae*
- *Streptococcus agalactiae*
- *Escherichia coli*
- *Klebsiella pneumoniae*
- *Pseudomonas aeruginosa*
- *Salmonella* spp.
- *Nocardia* spp.
- *Mycobacterium tuberculosis*

Rickettsiae
- *Rickettsia rickettsii*
- *Rickettsia conorii*
- *Rickettsia prowazekii*
- *Rickettsiae typhi*
- *Ehrlichia* and *Anaplasma* spp.

Spirochetes
- *Treponema pallidum*
- *Borrelia burgdorferi*
- *Leptospira* spp.

Protozoa and helminths
- *Naegleria fowleri*

Continued

Evidence-Based Infectious Diseases, 2nd edition. Edited by Mark Loeb, Fiona Smaill and Marek Smieja. © 2009 Wiley-Blackwell Publishing, ISBN: 978-1-4051-7026-0

Box 5.1   (continued)

- *Angiostrongylus cantonensis*
- *Balisascaris procyonis*
- *Strongyloides stercoralis*
- *Toxoplasma gondii*
- *Plasmodium falciparum*

Viruses
- Nonpolio enteroviruses (Echoviruses, Coxsackieviruses)
- Mumps virus
- Arboviruses
- Herpesviruses
- Lymphocytic choriomeningitis virus
- Human immunodeficiency virus
- Adenovirus
- Parainfluenza viruses type 3
- Influenza virus
- Measles virus

Fungi
- *Cryptococcus neoformans*
- *Coccidioides immitis*
- *Histoplasma capsulatum*
- *Blastomyces dermatitidis*
- *Paracoccidioides brasiliensis*
- *Candida* spp.
- *Aspergillus* spp.
- *Sporothrix schenckii*

Neoplastic diseases
- Lymphomatous meningitis
- Carcinomatous meningitis
- Leukemia

Intracranial tumors and cysts
- Craniopharyngioma
- Dermoid/epidermoid cyst
- Teratoma

Medications
- Antimicrobial agents*
- Non-steroidal anti-inflammatory agents
- OKT3
- Azathioprine
- Cytosine arabinoside
- Immune globulin
- Ranitidine

Systemic illnesses
- Systemic lupus erythematosus
- Vogt–Koyanagi–Harada syndrome
- Sarcoidosis
- Behçet disease
- Rheumatoid arthritis
- Polymyositis
- Wegener granulomatosis
- Familial Mediterranean fever
- Kawasaki syndrome

Miscellaneous
- Seizures
- Migraine
- Serum sickness
- Heavy metal poisoning

Adapted from references [1–5].
*Trimethoprim, sulfamethoxazole, ciprofloxacin, penicillin, cephalosporins, metronidazole, isoniazid, pyrazinamide.

4 and 6 cases per 100 000 adults in developed countries, to up to 10 times higher in less developed nations [6–9].

The incidence of bacterial meningitis has been profoundly affected by the introduction of the *Hemophilus influenzae* type B vaccine in 1987 and the *Streptococcus pneumoniae* conjugate vaccine in 2000. Rates of *H. influenzae* type B disease in children have declined by more than 95% [10], and rates of pneumococcal meningitis in children have declined by almost 70% [11,12]. More recently in 2005, the *Neisseria meningitidis* conjugate vaccine was introduced and, in addition to existing recommendations for use in groups at high-risk of infection, it is now routinely recommended in the US for adolescents before high school entry, which should further reduce the incidence of bacterial meningitis in this age group [13].

The net result of these vaccines and routine immunization programs in developed nations has not only been a reduction in the overall incidence of bacterial meningitis, but also a change in the age distribution of these infections [6]. The median age of persons with bacterial meningitis increased from 15 months in 1986 to 39 years currently [14], such that bacterial meningitis in the US in now predominantly a disease of adults. Unfortunately, epidemics of bacterial meningitis, especially due to *N. meningitidis*, continue to occur in developing nations, often affecting a large number of adolescents and adults [15]. This chapter thus focuses on bacterial meningitis in the adult population.

Etiology of bacterial meningitis

In an extensive surveillance project of 13 974 cases of bacterial meningitis in the US, 80% of cases were accounted for by *S. pneumoniae*, *N. meningitidis*, and *H. influenzae* [6]. These data were confirmed by several smaller case series of adult bacterial meningitis, which taken together suggest the prevalence of specific organisms to be: *S. pneumoniae* (20–53%), *N. meningitidis* (3–56%), *Listeria monocytogenes* (6–13%), and *H. influenzae* (<8%) [6,8,16–18]. The most likely causative organism depends on several factors including age, immunocompromise, preceding head trauma, recent neurosurgery, and site of acquisition (community-acquired vs. healthcare-acquired) (Table 5.1) [19,20].

While this chapter will focus on community-acquired meningitis, healthcare-acquired meningitis is also a significant problem. The National Nosocomial Infection Surveillance System (NNIS) noted an incidence of 5.6 nonsurgical, healthcare-acquired infections of the central nervous system (CNS) for every 100 000 patients discharged from the hospital between 1986 and 1993, with meningitis accounting for 91% of cases [21]. Unlike community-acquired meningitis, the most common pathogens in healthcare-acquired meningitis are gram-negative bacilli and staphylococci [16,20].

Clinical presentation

Given the documented association between early institution of antimicrobial therapy and both reduced mortality as well as improved neurologic outcomes [22–26], rapid recognition and diagnosis of meningitis is imperative. The relative sensitivity of any given sign or symptom has varied across selected studies published within the past 15 years (Table 5.2) [8,16–18, 27]. Fever is arguably the most common finding, and is often accompanied by other signs or symptoms [19]. Rash, particularly petechiae or purpura, are most common in meningococcal meningitis, but may also be observed in patients with meningitis caused by *S. pneumoniae*, *H. influenzae*, and *L. monocytogenes* [8,16].

The classic clinical presentation of acute meningitis consists of the triad of fever, neck stiffness, and an

Table 5.1 Empiric treatment of bacterial meningitis

Patient population	Likely pathogens	Antimicrobial	Dosage and route	Duration[§]
Immunocompetent Age 18–50 years	*S. pneumoniae* *N. meningitidis*	Vancomycin[†] Cefotaxime Ceftriaxone	15 mg/kg IV every 6 hours[¶], *plus* 2 g IV every 6 hours, or 2 g IV every 12 hours,	10–14 days
Immunocompetent Age >50 years	*S. pneumoniae* *N. meningitidis* Gram-negative bacilli *L. monocytogenes*	Vancomycin[†] Cefotaxime Ceftriaxone Ampicillin	15 mg/kg IV every 6 hours[¶], *plus* 2 g IV every 6 hours, or 2 g IV every 12 hours, *plus* 2 g IV every 4 hours	14–21 days
Impaired cellular immunity	*L. monocytogenes* Gram-negative bacilli	Ampicillin Ceftazidime	2 g IV every 4 hours, *plus* 50–100 mg/kg IV every 8 hours[‡]	14–21 days
Head trauma, neurosurgery, cerebrospinal shunt	Staphylococci *S. pneumoniae* Gram-negative bacilli	Vancomycin[†] Ceftazidime	15 mg/kg IV every 6 hour[¶], *plus* 50–100 mg/kg IV every 8 hours[‡]	≥21 days

Modified from references [19,20].
[†] Vancomycin provides additional coverage for penicillin-resistant *S. pneumoniae*.
[¶] Up to a total of 2 g per day.
[‡] Up to a total of 2 g every 8 hours.
[§] Suggested duration of therapy for specific pathogens: *H. influenzae* (7 days), *N. meningitidis* (7 days), *S. pneumoniae* (10–14 days), *L. monocytogenes* (≥21 days), gram-negative bacilli and staphylococci (21 days).

Table 5.2 Symptoms and signs associated with bacterial meningitis in adults

Author/Year [ref]	N*	Fever (%)	Neck stiffness (%)	Altered MS (%)	Head-ache (%)	Nausea/ vomiting (%)	Focal neuro signs (%)	Rash (%)
Durand 1993 [16]	259	95	88	78	NR	NR	29	11
Sigurdardottir 1997 [18]	127	97	82	66	NR	NR	10	52
Andersen 1997 [27]†	174	99	99	8	NR	52	NR	74
Hussein 2000 [17]	100	97	87	56	66	55	23	10
Van de Beek 2004 [8]	671	77	83	83	87	74	33	26

* Number of patients: 279 cases in 259 patients [16]; 132 cases in 127 patients [18], 103 cases in 100 patients [17]; 696 cases in 671 patients [8].
MS, mental status.
† Limited to cases of *N. meningitidis*.

altered mental status [9]. Recent reviews have found that only 44–67% of patients with bacterial meningitis present with this classic triad [8,16–18]; however, 99–100% of patients will have at least one of these findings [16,18]. It has thus been suggested that the diagnosis of bacterial meningitis may be effectively eliminated in a patient who presents without any of these findings [28].

Cerebrospinal fluid culture

If the diagnosis of bacterial meningitis is a consideration, a lumbar puncture (LP) should be performed promptly [9]. Routine morphologic and chemical analysis of the cerebrospinal fluid (CSF) in suspected bacterial meningitis should include a cell count, white blood cell differential count, glucose concentration, protein concentration, Gram stain, and bacterial culture [4]. The appearance of the CSF in bacterial meningitis is typically turbid and/or discolored with an opening pressure in the range 200–500 mmH$_2$O (Table 5.3) [4,16–18]. The white blood cell count usually ranges from 1000 to 5000 cells $\times$ 10^6/L (1000 to 5000/mm^3) with greater than 80% neutrophils [4,16–18]. Protein and glucose concentrations are usually 0.1–0.5 g/L (100–500 mg/dL) and <2.2 mol/L (40 mg/dL), respectively [4,16–18]. Recent large series of adult meningitis have noted that between 48% and 60% of CSF Gram stains from adults with bacterial meningitis were positive while CSF culture was positive in 65–80% of patients (Table 5.3) [16–18].

Patients partially treated with antibiotics may be less likely to have a positive CSF culture or Gram stain result, but such therapy has minimal effect on CSF indices such as leukocyte count [29]. Even after institution of appropriate antibiotics for meningitis, the CSF picture usually remains abnormal for at least 48–72 hours [30]. On the other hand, CSF pleocytosis, low CSF glucose, and elevated CSF protein may be found even in the absence of infection. Finally, the Gram stain of CSF from patients with gram-negative bacillary or post-neurosurgery meningitis is less often as positive as for pneumococcal and meningococcal meningitis [31].

Blood culture

Blood cultures should also be made in the evaluation of a patient with suspected bacterial meningitis, particularly if a CSF sample cannot be obtained prior to initiation of antibiotics (for example, when neuroimaging is planned prior to LP) [9]. Blood cultures in bacterial meningitis have been noted to be positive in 19–77% of patients [8,18,22,27].

Other diagnostic modalities

Rapid bacterial antigen testing

The use of rapid bacterial antigen testing, or latex agglutination testing, remains controversial. Reviews have noted that only 0.3–3% of all CSF bacterial antigen tests were positive [32–34]. However, the false-positive rate exceeded the true positive rate, and therapy was not altered on the basis of any of the true-positive rapid antigen results [32–34]. The false-positive results led to additional cost, prolonged hospitalization, and some clinical complications. Furthermore, all true-positive CSF samples showed the causative microorganisms by Gram stain [32–34]. In light of these findings, it has been suggested that rapid antigen testing

Table 5.3 Cerebrospinal fluid analysis in bacterial meningitis in adults

Author/Year [ref]	N*	Opening pressure >300 mm H$_2$O (%)	Leukocyte count >1000/mm^3 (%)	Percent neutrophils ≥80% (%)	Protein >0.2 g/L (%)	Glucose ≤2.8 mol/L (%)	Gram stain positive (%)	CSF culture positive (%)
Durand 1993 [16]	259	39	28 (>5000/mm^3)	79	56	50 (>2.2 mol/L)	46	83
Sigurdardottir 1997 [18]	127	48	20	88	85 (>0.5 mol/L)	89 (<0.5 mol/L)	57	80
Hussein 2000 [17]	100	NR	56	74	67	72	48	65

* Number of patients: 279 cases in 259 patients [16]; 132 cases in 127 patients [18], 103 cases in 100 patients [17].

should not be used routinely for the determination of the bacterial etiology of meningitis [20]. It may, however, be useful for patients with suspected bacterial meningitis with a negative CSF Gram stain result, or those who have been pretreated with antimicrobial therapy and have negative Gram stain and CSF culture results, although this requires further study [20].

Polymerase chain reaction

Polymerase chain reaction (PCR) of CSF has been used to detect microbial DNA in the CSF of patients with suspected bacterial meningitis. Primers have been developed that permit the simultaneous detection of the most common organisms, including *N. meningitidis*, *S. pneumoniae*, and *H. influenzae* [3]. Several studies have evaluated diagnostic performance of PCR in cases of bacterial meningitis caused by a range of organisms as compared to the gold standard of culture. Reported sensitivities ranged from 94% to 100% and specificity ranged from 91% to 98% [35], suggesting that PCR targeting a broad range of bacterial pathogens might be useful for excluding the diagnosis of bacterial meningitis, although this requires further study [20]. Furthermore, PCR may also have a role in improving diagnosis of bacterial meningitis in patients with negative CSF cultures, but further refinements are needed before PCR can be routinely recommended [20].

Another important role of PCR is in the detection of viral (specifically enteroviral) meningitis. In a multicenter study, 476 CSF specimens were collected from patients with suspected aseptic meningitis [36]: 68 samples were positive for enterovirus by PCR (14.4%), whereas 49 samples were positive by

culture (10.4%). The sensitivity and specificity of the enterovirus PCR test (using viral culture as the "gold standard") were 85.7% and 93.9%, respectively. Rapid PCR-based detection of enteroviral meningitis would facilitate early decision-making regarding discontinuation of empiric antibacterial therapy as well as shortened hospitalization.

Neuroimaging

There exists controversy regarding the need to perform neuroimaging prior to the performance of the LP. Despite no evidence, clinicians frequently perform computed tomography (CT) imaging prior to LP in order to rule out intracranial abnormalities which might increase the risk of brain herniation resulting from removal of cerebrospinal fluid during LP [37]. In a survey of 201 physicians who had ordered a CT prior to LP, stated reasons for this practice included suspicion that a focal brain abnormality was present (59%), belief that this practice was standard of care (34%), and a fear of litigation (5%) [38].

The risk of routine CT scanning prior to LP in patients with meningitis is that this practice is associated with a delay in performing LP and initiation of antimicrobial therapy [38]. This delay in initiation of antimicrobial therapy in turn increases the risk of a poor clinical outcome [22–26].

In a study of 235 patients who underwent head CT prior to LP, clinical features associated with an abnormal finding on CT were age >60 years, immunocompromise, history of CNS disease, history of seizure within 1 week before presentation, as well as the following neurologic abnormalities: abnormal level of consciousness, inability to answer two consecutive questions correctly or to follow two consecutive commands, gaze palsy, abnormal visual fields, facial palsy, arm drift, leg drift, and abnormal language [38]. Of the 96 patients in whom none of these features was present, 93 had a normal CT scan. Although the negative predictive value of the approach was not 100%, the three patients who were misclassified underwent LP without subsequent brain herniation [38]. While these results should be validated in future studies, they suggest that a routine CT scan can safely be avoided in favor of careful evaluation of the clinical findings of patients with suspected meningitis [20,39].

Possible indications for CT or magnetic resonance imaging (MRI) following initiation of therapy include persistent focal neurologic findings, persistently positive CSF cultures despite appropriate antimicrobial therapy, and persistent elevation of CSF polymorphonuclear leukocyte percentage after more than 10 days of therapy [40]. Neuroimaging is also indicated in patients with recurrent meningitis.

Therapy

Case presentation 1 (continued)

The patient undergoes LP without prior CT scanning. CSF reveals an opening pressure of 250 mmH$_2$O, and the patient is started on vancomycin 15 mg/kg IV every 6 hours and ceftriaxone 2 g IV every 12 hours. Subsequently, the CSF demonstrates a leukocyte count of 2400 × 10^6/L (2400/mm^3) with 70% neutrophils, protein concentration of 0.32 g/L (320 mg/dL), and a glucose concentration of 3.4 mol/L (62 mg/dL). The Gram stain reveals gram-positive cocci in pairs and chains.

Antimicrobials

Early initiation of antimicrobial therapy is essential in the approach to bacterial meningitis [9]. Early diagnosis and therapy reduce morbidity and mortality, particularly if antimicrobial therapy is initiated before meningitis progresses to a high severity level [8,16,22]. If neuroimaging prior to LP is considered, antibiotics should not be delayed until neuroimaging is complete [9]. In this situation, blood cultures should be obtained and antibiotics then administered [20]. The choice of empiric antibiotic depends on which organisms are most likely causative, which in turn depends on several factors including age, immunocompromise, recent surgery or instrumentation, and local antimicrobial resistance patterns (Table 5.1) [9,20]. Due to the high prevalence of penicillin-resistant S. pneumoniae, vancomycin is routinely recommended as part of the initial empiric antibiotic regimen pending culture and susceptibility results [20].

Corticosteroids

Adjunctive corticosteroid therapy for bacterial meningitis remains controversial. Animal studies of meningitis have shown that bacterial lysis resulting from antimicrobial therapy leads to inflammation in the subarachnoid space which in turn may contribute to poor outcomes [41,42]. These studies have also demonstrated that adjunctive corticosteroid therapy reduces cerebrospinal fluid inflammation and subsequent neurologic sequelae [41,42]. A number of randomized controlled trials have examined the possible role of corticosteroid therapy in pediatric meningitis but have come to differing conclusions. A metaanalysis of these trials showed a beneficial effect of adjunctive dexamethasone therapy in reducing severe hearing loss in children with H. influenzae type B meningitis and further suggested a similar benefit in reducing hearing loss in those children with pneumococcal meningitis [43].

In adults, early published trials were limited by methodologic flaws and inconclusive results [44–47]. More recently, however, in a multicenter trial of 301 adults with bacterial meningitis randomized to adjuvant dexamethasone vs placebo, administration of dexamethasone (10 mg) at 15 to 20 minutes before or with the first dose of antibiotic (and continued every 6 hours for 4 days) resulted in a statistically significant reduction in the risk of an unfavorable outcome (assessed with the Glasgow Outcome Scale) [48]. Dexamethasone therapy was also associated with a statistically significant reduction in mortality, most pronounced for the subgroup of patients with meningitis due to S. pneumoniae. However, there was no significant beneficial effect of dexamethasone therapy on neurologic sequelae, including hearing loss [48]. A recent metaanalysis confirmed these results, showing that adjuvant corticosteroid therapy reduced mortality from 22% to 12% and reduced neurologic sequelae from 22% to 14% [49].

More recently published studies on the use of dexamethasone as adjuvant therapy for bacterial meningitis in developing countries showed variable results. In areas such as Vietnam where mortality from bacterial meningitis is low, dexamethasone (when given with ceftriaxone) significantly decreased rates of death and disability in cases of proven bacterial infection [50]. However, in Africa, where both HIV prevalence and death rates from bacterial meningitis are high, adjuvant dexamethasone therapy seemed to offer no benefit in terms of mortality or rates of disability [51]. Thus, the debate about the value of corticosteroids in acute bacterial meningitis in developing countries will likely continue [52].

Currently, for patients in the US, routine adjunctive dexamethasone therapy is recommended in the initial treatment of those patients with suspected *S. pneumoniae* meningitis [20,53], but should only be continued if the CSF Gram stain reveals gram-positive diplococci or if blood or CSF cultures are positive to *S. pneumoniae* [20]. The ultimate role of dexamethasone in the treatment of other types of bacterial meningitis, however, needs to be clarified in future studies. In particular, future studies should focus on the possible reduction by corticosteroids of penetration of certain antibiotics (especially vancomycin) into the CNS [54]. Dexamethasone reduces blood–brain barrier permeability and may impede the penetration of vancomycin into the subarachnoid space [54]. This issue is especially relevant as the use of vancomycin for suspected bacterial meningitis increases because of concern regarding the continued emergence of penicillin-resistant *S. pneumoniae* [20]. Of note, while treatment with dexamethasone did not reduce vancomycin levels in the CSF in children with bacterial meningitis [55], treatment failures have been reported in adults who received standard doses of vancomycin and adjunctive dexamethasone [56].

Preventive therapy

Hemophilus influenzae

Currently available *H. influenzae* type B conjugate vaccines are highly immunogenic with more than 95% of infants developing protective antibody concentrations after a primary series of two or three doses. Use of this vaccine has been extremely effective at reducing the incidence of *H. influenzae* meningitis worldwide, often by more than 90% [57,58]. The American Academy of Pediatrics recommends that all infants should receive a primary series of *H. influenzae* vaccine beginning at 2 months of age [59].

Streptococcus. pneumoniae

Use of the 23-valent pneumococcal vaccine to prevent bacteremic pneumococcal disease is recommended in certain high-risk groups [60]. The efficacy of this vaccine against meningitis due to *S. pneumoniae* has never been specifically proven, but has been suggested to be approximately 50% [61,62]. The more recently developed heptavalent pneumococcal conjugate vaccine (PCV-7) has been demonstrated to have excellent efficacy in the prevention of invasive pneumococcal disease in infants and children [63], and its use is now recommended in all infants under 2 years of age [64]. Use of the conjugate vaccine is not, however, currently recommended in adults owing to limited experience in this population. Reductions in invasive pneumococcal disease rates due to the heptavalent vaccine have recently leveled off due to increases (albeit relatively small) in infections caused by non-PCV7 serotypes. Expanded-valency conjugate vaccines for children are currently in clinical trials [65].

Neisseria meningiditis

Routine meningococcal vaccination is currently recommended for certain high-risk groups which include [66]:

- college freshmen living in dormitories
- microbiologists who are routinely exposed to isolates of *N. meningitidis*
- military recruits
- persons who travel to or reside in countries in which *N. meningitidis* is hyperendemic or epidemic, particularly if contact with the local population will be prolonged
- persons who have terminal complement component deficiencies
- persons who have anatomic or functional asplenia.

There are currently two available meningococcal vaccines which both cover serotypes A, C, Y, and

W-135. The polysaccharide vaccine is recommended among eligible children age 2–10 and adults >55 [66]. A more recently approved conjugate vaccine is preferred among eligible people ages 11–55 [66]. The polysaccharide vaccine is not recommended for use in children age <2 due to poor immunogenicity and relatively short duration of protection [66]. The conjugate vaccine has not been studied in this group.

In addition to these high-risk groups, it also recommended that all children age 11–12 be routinely vaccinated with the conjugate vaccine due to the high risk of meningococcal disease among adolescents and college students [66].

In addition to routine vaccination, both vaccine types are also recommended for use in control of meningococcal outbreaks. While sufficient experience exists to recommend vaccination in controlling outbreaks due to serogroup C meningococcal disease only, use of either vaccine may be applicable to control of outbreaks due to other vaccine preventable serogroups (A, Y, and W-135). [66] The conjugate vaccine is preferred over the polysaccharide vaccine if the population targeted for vaccination includes people ages 11–55 [66].

Prognosis

Case presentation 1 (continued)

The patient's CSF culture subsequently demonstrates growth of *S. pneumoniae*, which is resistant to penicillin but susceptible to ceftriaxone. Vancomycin therapy is thus discontinued. The patient's fever, headache, and confusion resolve by day 3 of therapy, although the patient now complains of mild ataxia. He completes 14 days of therapy with ceftriaxone and his ataxia has resolved by the time of his hospital discharge.

While almost uniformly fatal in the pre-antibiotic era, the impact of bacterial meningitis remains great today. Mortality rates in meningitis in recent series have ranged from 19% to 37% [3,8,16–18].

Several factors have been associated with increased mortality in patients with bacterial meningitis including advanced age [8,16,18,22], obtunded mental state [8,16,22], seizures [8,16,22], hypotension [8,22], and platelet count of less than 100×10^6/L (100 000/mm^3)

[27]. A recently published prediction model found that six variables routinely available within 1 hour of admission (age, heart rate, Glasgow Coma Scale score, presence of cranial nerve palsies, CSF leukocyte count, presence of gram-positive cocci on CSF Gram stain) reliably predicted unfavorable outcome in adults with bacterial meningitis [67]. Increased fatality has also been associated with absence of typical symptoms and signs, presumably due to a delay in diagnosis [68]. Indeed, despite the recognized association between delay in administration of antibiotics and mortality [22–26], recent evidence notes that the median duration from initial presentation to administration of antibiotics was 4 hours, with 30% of patients waiting longer than 1 hour between performance of an LP and administration of antibiotics [22]. Mortality rates also vary substantially across infecting organisms: *S. pneumoniae* (26–28%); *N. meningitidis* (10–16%), *L. monocytogenes* (32–38%), *H. influenzae* (11–17%), and culture negative (9–10%) [16,18].

CNS sequelae occur in up to 50% of previously healthy patients following meningitis, and include dizziness, tiredness, mild memory deficiencies, gait ataxia, aphasia, seizures, cerebral edema, intracerebral hemorrhage, and hydrocephalus [8,69,70]. In one prospective study, persistent cognitive impairment was detected in 27% of adults despite good recovery from pneumococcal meningitis [71]. Systemic complications of bacterial meningitis may include septic shock, acute respiratory distress syndrome, and disseminated intravascular coagulation [8,70].

Encephalitis

Case presentation 2

A 64-year-old woman is brought to the emergency department by her daughter after a new-onset seizure. The patient had been well until 48 hours prior when she had the abrupt onset of fever and headache. Over the next 2 days, she developed confusion and exhibited bizarre behavior, and subsequently had a seizure. She has no significant past medical history. She takes no medications and does not use alcohol, tobacco, or drugs. The season is spring. The patient is retired and spends most of her time indoors and has not traveled recently. Her daughter recalls no exposure to animals. On physical examination, she has a temperature of 38.9°C, a pulse of 100 beats per minute, and a blood pressure of 140/64 mmHg. She is minimally responsive, without nuchal rigidity or focal neurologic findings. Her Glasgow Coma Scale score is 8. A serum white blood cell count is normal. A CT scan of the head reveals no intracranial mass lesions. Evaluation of CSF demonstrates a leukocyte count of 500 × 10^6/L (500 cells/mm^3) with lymphocyte predominance, an elevated protein concentration of 0.98 g/L (980 mg/dL), and a normal glucose. You admit the patient with a diagnosis of acute encephalitis and institute intravenous acyclovir for the possibility of herpes simplex virus-1 encephalitis. You wonder what other diagnostic testing should be done.

Box 5.2   Diseases that may mimic viral encephalitis

- Abscess or subdural empyema
    bacterial
    listerial
    fungal
    mycoplasmal
- Tuberculosis
- Cryptococcosis
- Rickettsial infection
- Toxoplasmosis
- Mucormycosis
- Meningococcal meningitis
- Tumor
- Subdural hematoma
- Systemic lupus erythematosus
- Adrenal leukodystrophy
- Toxic encephalopathy
- Reye syndrome
- Vascular disease

Adapted from reference [75].

Diagnosis

Epidemiology

Encephalitis indicates inflammation of the brain, and is distinguished from meningitis by the presence of abnormal brain function, which may manifest as altered mental status, motor or sensory deficits, or movement disorders [72]. The incidence of acute encephalitis varies according to geographical location but has been estimated at between 5 and 10 cases per 100 000 patient-years (highest in the young and elderly) [72], with approximately 20 000 cases of encephalitis occurring annually in the US [73].

While almost 100 agents have been associated with encephalitis, viruses are by far the most common cause, with the most life-threatening being herpes simplex virus (HSV) and arboviruses [74]. It is important to rule out other potentially treatable conditions that may mimic viral encephalitis (Box 5.2) [75].

Since clinical syndromes and routine laboratory tests are often nonspecific, the diagnosis of viral encephalitis may be difficult. To aid in the diagnosis, certain epidemiologic features should be elicited, including: time of year, location and prevalent disease in the area, recent travel, occupational exposures, recreational activities (e.g., caving or hiking), and animal contacts (e.g., insect or animal bites) [72,73,76]. This chapter will focus primarily on viral encephalitis in adults in the US.

Etiology of viral encephalitis

Encephalitis resulting from viral infection can manifest as two distinct disease entities:

- Acute viral encephalitis – results from direct invasion of neurons by the virus, with subsequent inflammation and neuronal destruction.
- Postinfectious encephalomyelitis – may occur following a variety of viral infections, usually of the respiratory tract; perivascular inflammation and demyelination of the white matter are prominent.

The most common viruses causing acute encephalitis in the US are enteroviruses, followed by HSV and arboviruses (Box 5.3) [35,77]. Less common viral etiologies include other herpes viruses, adenoviruses, measles, mumps, and the human immunodeficiency virus (HIV). Rare causes of encephalitis such as rabies would be suspected based on exposure and occupational information.

Enteroviral infections (including coxsackieviruses, echoviruses, and polioviruses) peak in the summer and fall, and children and young adults are most commonly affected (Table 5.4) [73].

HSV type 1 is the most common cause of severe nonepidemic viral encephalitis in the US, accounting

Box 5.3 Causative agents for acute viral encephalitis in the United States

Arboviruses

- La Crosse virus
- Eastern equine encephalitis virus
- Western equine encephalitis virus
- St Louis encephalitis virus
- West Nile virus
- Venezuelan equine encephalitis virus
- Powassan virus
- Snowshoe Hare virus
- Jamestown Canyon virus

Enteroviruses

- Coxsackievirus A and B
- Echoviruses
- Poliovirus

Herpesviruses

- Herpes simplex virus type 1
- Herpes simplex virus type 2
- Cytomegalovirus
- Epstein–Barr virus
- Varicella zoster virus
- Human herpesvirus 6
- Simian herpes B virus

Other viruses

- Measles virus
- Mumps virus
- Adenovirus
- Human immunodeficiency virus
- Influenza
- Rabies virus
- JC virus
- Lymphocytic choriomeningitis virus

Adapted from reference [77].

Table 5.4 Seasonal preferences of selected viruses causing encephalitis

Time of year	Virus
Summer/fall	Enteroviruses
	West Nile virus
	La Crosse virus
	Eastern equine encephalitis virus
	Western equine encephalitis virus
	St Louis encephalitis
Winter/spring	Measles virus
	Mumps virus
	Varicella zoster virus
Any season	Herpes simplex virus type 1
	Human immunodeficiency virus
	Rabies virus

Adapted from reference [73].

in the US and peak in late summer and early fall when exposure to vectors is highest. First documented in the US in 1999, West Nile virus (WNV) is now the most common cause of epidemic viral encephalitis [35,79,80]. The next most common arboviruses causing encephalitis are the California encephalitis (CE) group (La Crosse virus) and the togaviruses: western equine encephalitis (WEE), eastern equine encephalitis (EEE), and St Louis encephalitis (SLE) [35, 81,82]. Venezuelan equine encephalitis (VEE) has also caused small epidemics in Florida, Louisiana, and Texas [83,84] and Powassan virus, which is transmitted by ticks, has caused rare cases in New England [85].

Epidemiologic features may help narrow the diagnosis in arboviral infections, including:

- age of the patient
- location where the infection was acquired
- incidences of other cases of arboviral infections in the area (Table 5.5) [75,86].

Two paramyxoviruses, measles and mumps, are rarely seen now because of effective childhood vaccines, but were significant causes of encephalitis in the pre-vaccine era [73]. In recent years, however, multistate outbreaks of mumps in the US suggest this virus may still be important to consider [87,88]. These infections usually occur in the winter and spring. A postinfectious encephalitis develops in approximately 1 in 1000 cases of measles [89] and

for about 10% of all cases of encephalitis [73,78]. It has a bimodal distribution, with most cases occurring in patients under 20 and over 50 years of age [75,78]. The virus has no seasonal predilection, occurring at any time of the year.

Arthropod-borne viruses (arboviruses) are a heterogeneous group of viruses transmitted by the bite of arthropod vectors (mosquitoes and ticks). They are a common cause of sporadic and epidemic encephalitis

Table 5.5 Epidemiologic features of encephalitis caused by arboviruses in the United States

Virus	Geographical distribution	Age of typical patients	Mortality rate (%)
West Nile	East, mid-west, Gulf coast, southern USA	Adults, esp. elderly	20
La Crosse	Central, eastern USA	<15 years	1
Eastern equine	East, Gulf coast, southern USA	Young children and >50 years	>30
Western equine	West, mid west USA	Infants and >50 years	2–3
St Louis	Central, western, southern USA	>50 years	10–20
Powassan	New England	Any age	50

Adapted from references [75,86].

typically 4–8 days after the rash, during convalescence [81]. Subacute sclerosing panencephalitis (SSPE) is a chronic degenerative disease that presents insidiously with myoclonus and seizure activity an average of 7 years after acute measles infections [86]. CNS disease from mumps, including encephalitis, complicates about 1% of infections [86] and usually occurs in older children or adults. It may occur before, during, or up to 2 weeks after parotid gland swelling or in the absence of parotitis.

Seroconversion to HIV infection and primary HIV disease has been associated with acute, self-limited encephalitis syndromes [81]. Patients with the acquired immunodeficiency syndrome (AIDS) can develop CNS disease from a number of unusual organisms, such as toxoplasmosis, pneumocystis, *Cryptococcus*, cytomegalovirus, and JC polyoma virus (progressive multifocal leukoencephalopathy) [90].

Rabies is transmitted by the bite of an infected animal and is a rare cause of encephalitis in the US. Most human disease in the US is due to bat transmission, although a history of bat bite is uncommon [91]. Other animals that are most often infected include foxes, skunks, and racoons.

Postinfectious encephalomyelitis is an acute inflammatory demyelinating disease that accounts for approximately 10–15% of cases of acute encephalitis in the US [76,92]. It most commonly develops after an infection of the respiratory tract (particularly influenza [93]), a viral exanthema such as measles or varicella, or, in the past, immunization with the vaccinia virus [76,92]. Worldwide, measles is the most common etiologic agent [73]. The pathogenesis is thought to be an autoimmune response triggered by the viral infection, with activation of lymphocytes against myelin [76,92].

Clinical presentation

The triad of fever, headache, and altered level of consciousness is the clinical hallmark of acute viral encephalitis [72,75]. Additional clinical findings often include disorientation, disturbance in behavior and speech, and focal or diffuse neurologic abnormalities such as hemiparesis and seizures [72].

Herpes simplex type 1

The onset of HSV-1 encephalitis (HSE) is usually abrupt, although a subacute prodrome of frontal headache and malaise may occur less commonly. Fever is present in 90% of cases, headache is prominent early in the course of the disease, and the majority of patients have signs suggesting a localized lesion involving one or both temporal lobes [78,94]. These findings often include dramatic personality changes, which may be the first clinical manifestation. Following these behavioral changes, patients may develop aphasia, anosmia, temporal lobe seizures, and hemiparesis. Unlike with HSV-2 meningitis, mucocutaneous herpetic lesions are rarely seen with HSV-1 encephalitis [86].

Arboviruses

The clinical spectrum of illness due to arboviruses is broad, ranging from a mild febrile illness to aseptic meningitis to fatal encephalitis [82,95]. The onset of encephalitis may be abrupt or subacute, and begins with nonspecific symptoms of fever, headache, nausea, and vomiting. CNS symptoms usually begin on day 2 or 3, and symptoms can range widely from only mild deficits to coma [82,96]. Focal abnormalities much as hemiparesis, tremors, seizures, and cranial nerve palsies can occur [82,86,96]. EEE is the most virulent of the arboviral encephalitides and produces symptomatic disease with a high frequency in all age groups and a mortality of 30% [97,98].

In most people, infection with WNV is subclinical or causes a self-limited febrile illness [80,99,100]. Only about 1 in 150 infections results in severe neurologic disease, and advanced age (50 years of age and older) is by far the greatest risk factor for this complication [99]. Encephalitis is more common than meningitis, and symptoms of severe muscle weakness or flaccid paralysis suggestive of Guillain–Barre syndrome may provide a clue to the diagnosis of WNV.

Enteroviruses

While most enteroviral encephalitides are mild, patients with agammaglobulinemia may develop a chronic, lethal form of enteroviral encephalitis [101].

Other herpesviruses

Cytomegalovirus and Epstein–Barr virus can cause acute encephalitis syndromes [78,102,103]. Varicella zoster virus (VZV) infections may also be complicated by encephalitis, which usually develops a week after the exanthema begins [102,104,105]. Acute cerebellar ataxia is the most common complication of chickenpox [73,86,106]. An eruption of herpes zoster may be complicated by encephalomyelitis and granulomatous arteritis, the latter of which has been associated with zoster ophthalmicus [73].

Rabies

The common presentation of rabies is one of agitation, delirium, and hydrophobia, which ultimately progresses to coma and death [107]. The incubation period usually ranges from days to months but may be as long as a year.

Postinfectious encephalomyelitis

The clinical presentation of postinfectious encephalomyelitis resembles that of an acute viral encephalitis, except that there is usually a history of an exanthema or nonspecific respiratory or gastrointestinal illness about 5 days to 3 weeks prior to the onset of CNS disease [86,92].

Laboratory findings

Peripheral white blood cell counts are rarely helpful because they may be normal, slightly elevated, or slightly low [108]. Evaluation of CSF in viral encephalitis reflects the inflammatory nature of the disease, typically demonstrating a mononuclear pleocytosis, ranging from 10 to 2000 $\times$ 10^6/L (10 to 2000 cells/mm^3), an elevated protein level, and a normal or slightly low glucose. Polymorphonuclear cells may be present early in the disease, so it may be useful to repeat the lumbar puncture in 24 hours [109]. CSF PCR to detect viral nucleic acids is the superior diagnostic test in most cases of viral encephalitis; culture of CSF for isolation of viruses has only a sensitivity of 14–24% compared with PCR [35].

In HSE, CSF may be normal in 3–5% of patients [94]. The presence of red blood cells in the absence of a traumatic lumbar puncture is suggestive, but not diagnostic, of necrotizing HSV-1 infection [86]. The availability of CSF PCR techniques to detect HSV DNA has revolutionized the diagnosis of HSE, allowing for rapid, sensitive, and specific diagnosis [35]. In several series, PCR was found to have a sensitivity of greater than 95% with a specificity of 94% to 100%, and it can be positive as early as one day after disease onset [35]. Studies have found no effect on PCR yield during the first week of antiviral therapy, although the sensitivity of the test declines during the second week of treatment [35].

Antibody titers in the CSF or serum are not helpful in establishing an early diagnosis of HSE, and viral cultures are insensitive [35]. HSV antigen is detected later than HSV DNA and has a sensitivity of only 33% [35]. The historical gold standard for diagnosis has been brain biopsy with demonstration of HSV in the brain tissue; however, the sensitivity has been reported to be only 60–70%, possibly because of sampling error or improper specimen handling [35]. For this reason, as well as the less invasive nature of lumbar puncture, PCR has largely replaced the need for brain biopsy [35].

The diagnosis of arboviral infections is usually obtained by serologic assays for virus-specific IgM antibodies on serum and/or CSF. Both acute and convalescent (4 weeks) titers should be measured to confirm acute infection [75]. Viral cultures and PCR testing of CSF, blood, or tissue samples are generally of low yield, except in the case of VEE where blood and throat cultures are frequently positive [86].

A limitation of serologic tests is the possibility of cross-reactivity because of close antigenic relationships among the flaviviruses; for example, patients with WNV may test positive if they had recent infection with SLE or dengue, or vaccination for yellow fever or Japanese encephalitis [99]. A positive IgM test for WNV can be confirmed (eliminate positives caused by cross-reaction) by a WNV plaque-reduction neutralization antibody test (PRNT) titer of greater than 20 [35].

A case of WNV can be confirmed by any one of the following criteria:

• a 4-fold rise in serum antibody titer
• isolation of virus, genomic sequences, or antigen from tissue, blood, CSF, or other body fluid
• specific IgM antibodies in CSF or serum by EIA, confirmed by PRNT [110].

When WNV infection is suspected, CSF should be obtained for PCR or IgM confirmed with PRNT, and PCR should be performed on peripheral blood if CSF is not available [35].

The best diagnostic method for confirmation of rabies is detection of rabies virus RNA in saliva by reverse-transcriptase PCR [75]. Diagnosis may also be made by direct fluorescence antibody staining of viral antigens from a nuchal skin biopsy or brain tissue, isolation of rabies virus in a cell cultures from CSF, saliva, or brain tissue, or a rabies-neutralizing antibody titer of 5 in the CSF or serum in an unvaccinated person [111].

The recommended laboratory tests for viral causes of encephalitis are listed in Table 5.6 [35,77,86].

Other diagnostic modalities

Magnetic resonance imaging (MRI)

MRI with enhancement is superior to CT in detecting early lesions in cases of viral encephalitis, although early in disease both imaging modalities may be unremarkable [112–114]. In HSE, MRI images tend to show lesions in the orbital-frontal and temporal lobes [112,113]. In WNV encephalitis, MR imaging findings can be normal, although abnormal T2-weighted signal can be seen in lobar gray and white matter [114]. MRI is the most helpful test in distinguishing postinfectious encephalomyelitis from viral encephalitis since there is usually pronounced enhancement of multifocal white matter lesions [74].

Electroencephalogram (EEG)

EEG is of value in diagnosing encephalitis, particularly in patients with HSE. Periodic high-voltage spike wave activity and slow-wave complexes emanating

Table 5.6 Recommended laboratory tests in the diagnosis of viral encephalitis

Etiology	Diagnostic tests recommended
Herpes simplex virus type 1	PCR and cell culture of CSF and tissue
West Nile virus	PCR testing of CSF, IgM antibody of CSF and serum (with confirmation by neutralization antibody test)
Other arboviruses[†]	IgM and IgG antibody of serum and CSF, antigen detection and PCR (brain tissue) available for some viruses
Enterovirus	PCR and cell culture of CSF
Varicella zoster virus	PCR and cell culture of CSF and tissue
Cytomegalovirus	PCR and cell culture of CSF and tissue
Epstein–Barr virus	PCR of CSF and tissue, serum antibody (often inconclusive)
Rabies virus	PCR of saliva or tissue, antigen testing of skin biopsy, brain tissue, or corneal impressions
JC polyoma virus (agent of progressive multifocal leukoencephalopathy)	PCR of CSF, PCR or in situ hybridization of brain tissue
Colorado tick fever virus	Antibody (serum)
Human immunodeficiency virus	Laboratory tests not specific for central nervous system involvement
Herpes B virus	Cell culture or PCR of lesion (special biocontainment laboratory required)
Post-infectious encephalitis[‡]	Document recent infection at primary site outside CSF

Adapted from references [35,77,86].
PCR, polymerase chain reaction; CSF, cerebrospinal fluid; IgM, immunoglobulin M; IgG, immunoglobulin G.
[†] Includes common arboviruses in North America including St Louis encephalitis, La Crosse encephalitis, eastern equine encephalitis, and western equine encephalitis.
[‡] Post-infectious encephalitis usually caused by measles virus, varicella zoster virus, influenza virus, and vaccinia (pox) virus.

from the temporal lobes at 2- to 3-second intervals are highly suggestive of HSE [75]. However, these findings are not specific for HSE [115].

Therapy

> ### Case presentation 2 (continued)
>
> You order PCR testing of the CSF for HSV. An MRI of the brain reveals enhancing lesions in both temporal lobes. An EEG shows diffuse slowing as well as bilateral periodic discharges in the temporal regions, suggestive of HSE.

Proven antiviral therapy is currently limited to HSV. In two separate trials comparing vidarabine to acyclovir in HSE, acyclovir was found to be superior [116,117]. The recommended dose is 10 mg/kg [4] intravenously every 8 hours for 10–14 days [118]. The dose should be adjusted in patients with renal insufficiency. Both mortality and later sequelae can be substantially reduced if therapy is instituted before there is a major alteration in consciousness [117]. Therefore, early treatment is essential and should be initiated as soon as the diagnosis is suspected. Although several new antiviral drugs with activity against HSV are available in oral formulations with good bioavailability, none has been studied for HSV infections of the CNS. Currently under investigation is the approach of repeat CSF examination after completion of intravenous acyclovir therapy and continuing high-dose oral valacyclovir for 3 months if HSV is still detected by PCR [72].

Treatment of arboviral encephalitis is primarily supportive, as there are no proven therapies. Ribavirin and interferon-2b have been shown to have activity against WNV in vitro, but no controlled trials have been done evaluating these agents [119]. Pooled immunoglobulin from populations previously exposed to WNV offer protection in a mouse model of encephalitis [120] and human studies are currently under way.

Treatment of enteroviral meningitis with pleconaril, an anti-picornaviral agent, has been studied in two clinical trials (one adult, one pediatric) [121]. While no benefit was shown for the primary endpoint of complete resolution of headache, a subgroup analysis showed accelerated headache resolution in patients with moderate to severe disease [121].

No FDA approval for this drug has been pursued at this time.

Treatment of postinfectious encephalomyelitis is largely supportive. The use of corticosteroids is often advocated, but no controlled trails have evaluated their efficacy and safety [92]. There is no established treatment of rabies, short of supportive therapy, once symptoms have begun.

Preventive therapy

There is currently no vaccine available to prevent HSV infection, although several are in preclinical and clinical development [122]. A number of vaccines are also being developed for WNV infection, but none are currently available for human use [79]. A live, attenuated Japanese encephalitis vaccine is available and has been used successfully to reduce the risk of infection in children in China and India [95,123]. Prevention of arboviral infections, however, rests largely on mosquito control and avoidance measures. The live attenuated measles and mumps vaccines are extremely effective in preventing these infections. Recognition of potential exposure to an animal infected with rabies should prompt prophylactic treatment with rabies vaccine and immunoglobulin [124].

Prognosis

> ### Case presentation 2 (continued)
>
> The patient's CSF PCR for HSV is positive and she completes a 14-day course of intravenous acyclovir. She has a slow recovery over several weeks with no clinical evidence of relapse and is transferred to a rehabilitation facility. Six months after the encephalitis, she is living independently but functioning at a lower level than previously and has short-term memory impairment and anosmia.

In the absence of therapy, mortality for HSV-1 encephalitis exceeds 70%, with only 2.5% of patients regaining normal function [75]. Even with acyclovir therapy, morbidity and mortality remain high, with a mortality of 19% and 28% at 6 months and 18 months after therapy, respectively [117]. Poorer outcome was associated with older age, a Glasgow Coma Scale score of <6 at presentation, and the presence of encephalitis for >4 days prior to initiation of therapy [117].

Many patients who survive are left with severe, debilitating sequelae, including aphasia, anosmia, problems with cognitive function, and motor and sensory deficits [125]. Clinical relapses may also occur after completion of therapy in a small percentage (4–7%) of patients [116,117,126], due to either reactivation of viral infection or proinflammatory immunologic responses [127,128]. Although some authors advocate a longer course of acyclovir therapy (14–21 days) to prevent relapse [126], no definitive evidence exists that a longer duration of therapy is associated with a decreased rate of relapse.

In cases of arbovirus encephalitis, mortality rates and the presence of neurologic sequelae depend on the specific organism and age of the patient, with the extremes of age having worse outcome [75]. The case fatality rate among hospitalized patients with WNV encephalitis is approximately 20%, with advanced age and diabetes identified as risk factors for mortality [99]. Finally, rabies is uniformly fatal in nonimmunized patients [86,107].

References

1 Fitch MT, Abrahamian FM, Moran GJ, Talan DA. Emergency department management of meningitis and encephalitis. Infect Dis Clin North Am 2008;22(1):33–52, v–vi.

2 Moris G, Garcia-Monco JC. The challenge of drug-induced aseptic meningitis. Arch Intern Med 1999;159(11):1185–94.

3 Tunkel A. Bacterial Meningitis. Philadelphia: Lippincott Williams & Wilkins, 2001.

4 Tunkel A, Scheld W. Acute meningitis. In: Mandell G, Bennett J, Dolin R, eds. Principles and Practice of Infectious Diseases. Sixth ed. Philadelphia: Churchill Livingstone, 2005.

5 Lee BE, Davies HD. Aseptic meningitis. Curr Opin Infect Dis 2007;20(3):272–7.

6 Schuchat A, Robinson K, Wenger JD, et al. Bacterial meningitis in the United States in 1995. Active Surveillance Team. N Engl J Med 1997;337(14):970–6.

7 Schut ES, de Gans J, van de Beek D. Community-acquired bacterial meningitis in adults. Pract Neurol 2008;8(1):8–23.

8 van de Beek D, de Gans J, Spanjaard L, Weisfelt M, Reitsma JB, Vermeulen M. Clinical features and prognostic factors in adults with bacterial meningitis. N Engl J Med 2004;351(18):1849–59.

9 van de Beek D, de Gans J, Tunkel AR, Wijdicks EF. Community-acquired bacterial meningitis in adults. N Engl J Med 2006;354(1):44–53.

10 Bisgard KM, Kao A, Leake J, Strebel PM, Perkins BA, Wharton M. Haemophilus influenzae invasive disease in the United States, 1994–1995: near disappearance of a vaccine-preventable childhood disease. Emerg Infect Dis 1998;4(2):229–37.

11 Kyaw MH, Lynfield R, Schaffner W, et al. Effect of introduction of the pneumococcal conjugate vaccine on drug-resistant Streptococcus pneumoniae. N Engl J Med 2006;354(14):1455–63.

12 Whitney CG, Farley MM, Hadler J, et al. Decline in invasive pneumococcal disease after the introduction of protein-polysaccharide conjugate vaccine. N Engl J Med 2003;348(18):1737–46.

13 Bilukha OO, Rosenstein N. Prevention and control of meningococcal disease. Recommendations of the Advisory Committee on Immunization Practices (ACIP). MMWR Morb Mortal Wkly Rep 2005;54(RR-7):1–21.

14 Dery M, Hasbun R. Changing epidemiology of bacterial meningitis. Curr Infect Dis Rep 2007;9(4):301–7.

15 Stephens DS, Greenwood B, Brandtzaeg P. Epidemic meningitis, meningococcaemia, and Neisseria meningitidis. Lancet 2007;369(9580):2196–210.

16 Durand ML, Calderwood SB, Weber DJ, et al. Acute bacterial meningitis in adults. A review of 493 episodes. N Engl J Med 1993;328(1):21–8.

17 Hussein AS, Shafran SD. Acute bacterial meningitis in adults. A 12-year review. Medicine (Baltimore) 2000;79(6):360–8.

18 Sigurdardottir B, Bjornsson OM, Jonsdottir KE, Erlendsdottir H, Gudmundsson S. Acute bacterial meningitis in adults. A 20-year overview. Arch Intern Med 1997;157(4):425–30.

19 Fitch MT, van de Beek D. Emergency diagnosis and treatment of adult meningitis. Lancet Infect Dis 2007;7(3):191–200.

20 Tunkel AR, Hartman BJ, Kaplan SL, et al. Practice guidelines for the management of bacterial meningitis. Clin Infect Dis 2004;39(9):1267–84.

21 Farr B, Scheld W. Nosocomial meningitis. Ochner Clin Rep 1998;10:1–7.

22 Aronin SI, Peduzzi P, Quagliarello VJ. Community-acquired bacterial meningitis: risk stratification for adverse clinical outcome and effect of antibiotic timing. Ann Intern Med 1998;129(11):862–9.

23 Lu CH, Huang CR, Chang WN, et al. Community-acquired bacterial meningitis in adults: the epidemiology, timing of appropriate antimicrobial therapy, and prognostic factors. Clin Neurol Neurosurg 2002;104(4):352–8.

24 Miner JR, Heegaard W, Mapes A, Biros M. Presentation, time to antibiotics, and mortality of patients with bacterial meningitis at an urban county medical center. J Emerg Med 2001;21(4):387–92.

25 Proulx N, Frechette D, Toye B, Chan J, Kravcik S. Delays in the administration of antibiotics are associated with mortality from adult acute bacterial meningitis. Q J Med 2005;98(4):291–8.

26 Short WR, Tunkel AR. Timing of Administration of Antimicrobial Therapy in Bacterial Meningitis. Curr Infect Dis Rep 2001;3(4):360–4.

27 Andersen J, Backer V, Voldsgaard P, Skinhoj P, Wandall JH. Acute meningococcal meningitis: analysis of features of the disease according to the age of 255 patients. Copenhagen Meningitis Study Group. J Infect 1997;34(3):227–35.

28 Attia J, Hatala R, Cook DJ, Wong JG. The rational clinical examination. Does this adult patient have acute meningitis? JAMA 1999;282(2):175–81.

29 Conly JM, Ronald AR. Cerebrospinal fluid as a diagnostic body fluid. Am J Med 1983;75(1B):102–8.

30 Blazer S, Berant M, Alon U. Bacterial meningitis. Effect of antibiotic treatment on cerebrospinal fluid. Am J Clin Pathol 1983;80(3):386–7.

31 Mancebo J, Domingo P, Blanch L, Coll P, Net A, Nolla J. Post-neurosurgical and spontaneous gram-negative bacillary meningitis in adults. Scand J Infect Dis 1986;18(6):533–8.

32 Finlay FO, Witherow H, Rudd PT. Latex agglutination testing in bacterial meningitis. Arch Dis Child 1995;73(2):160–1.

33 Maxson S, Lewno MJ, Schutze GE. Clinical usefulness of cerebrospinal fluid bacterial antigen studies. J Pediatr 1994;125(2):235–8.

34 Perkins MD, Mirrett S, Reller LB. Rapid bacterial antigen detection is not clinically useful. J Clin Microbiol 1995;33(6):1486–91.

35 Thomson RB, Jr., Bertram H. Laboratory diagnosis of central nervous system infections. Infect Dis Clin North Am 2001;15(4):1047–71.

36 van Vliet KE, Glimaker M, Lebon P, et al. Multicenter evaluation of the Amplicor Enterovirus PCR test with cerebrospinal fluid from patients with aseptic meningitis. The European Union Concerted Action on Viral Meningitis and Encephalitis. J Clin Microbiol 1998;36(9):2652–7.

37 Archer BD. Computed tomography before lumbar puncture in acute meningitis: a review of the risks and benefits. Cmaj 1993;148(6):961–5.

38 Hasbun R, Abrahams J, Jekel J, Quagliarello VJ. Computed tomography of the head before lumbar puncture in adults with suspected meningitis. N Engl J Med 2001;345(24):1727–33.

39 Steigbigel NH. Computed tomography of the head before a lumbar puncture in suspected meningitis – is it helpful? N Engl J Med 2001;345(24):1768–70.

40 Kline MW, Kaplan SL. Computed tomography in bacterial meningitis of childhood. Pediatr Infect Dis J 1988;7(12):855–7.

41 Scheld WM, Dacey RG, Winn HR, Welsh JE, Jane JA, Sande MA. Cerebrospinal fluid outflow resistance in rabbits with experimental meningitis. Alterations with penicillin and methylprednisolone. J Clin Invest 1980;66(2):243–53.

42 Tauber MG, Khayam-Bashi H, Sande MA. Effects of ampicillin and corticosteroids on brain water content, cerebrospinal fluid pressure, and cerebrospinal fluid lactate levels in experimental pneumococcal meningitis. J Infect Dis 1985;151(3):528–34.

43 McIntyre PB, Berkey CS, King SM, et al. Dexamethasone as adjunctive therapy in bacterial meningitis. A meta-analysis of randomized clinical trials since 1988. JAMA 1997;278(11):925–31.

44 Ahsan T, Shahid M, Mahmood T, et al. Role of dexamethasone in acute bacterial meningitis in adults. J Pak Med Assoc 2002;52(6):233–9.

45 Gijwani D, Kumhar MR, Singh VB, et al. Dexamethasone therapy for bacterial meningitis in adults: a double blind placebo control study. Neurol India 2002;50(1):63–7.

46 Girgis NI, Farid Z, Mikhail IA, Farrag I, Sultan Y, Kilpatrick ME. Dexamethasone treatment for bacterial meningitis in children and adults. Pediatr Infect Dis J 198;8(12):848–51.

47 Thomas R, Le Tulzo Y, Bouget J, et al. Trial of dexamethasone treatment for severe bacterial meningitis in adults. Adult Meningitis Steroid Group. Intensive Care Med 1999;25(5):475–80.

48 de Gans J, van de Beek D. Dexamethasone in adults with bacterial meningitis. N Engl J Med 2002;347(20):1549–56.

49 van de Beek D, de Gans J, McIntyre P, Prasad K. Steroids in adults with acute bacterial meningitis: a systematic review. Lancet Infect Dis 2004;4(3):139–43.

50 Nguyen TH, Tran TH, Thwaites G, et al. Dexamethasone in Vietnamese adolescents and adults with bacterial meningitis. N Engl J Med 2007;357(24):2431–40.

51 Scarborough M, Gordon SB, Whitty CJ, et al. Corticosteroids for bacterial meningitis in adults in sub-Saharan Africa. N Engl J Med 2007;357(24):2441–50.

52 Greenwood BM. Corticosteroids for acute bacterial meningitis. N Engl J Med 2007;357(24):2507–9.

53 Tunkel AR, Scheld WM. Corticosteroids for everyone with meningitis? N Engl J Med 2002;347(20):1613–5.

54 Coyle PK. Glucocorticoids in central nervous system bacterial infection. Arch Neurol 1999;56(7):796–801.

55 Klugman KP, Friedland IR, Bradley JS. Bactericidal activity against cephalosporin-resistant Streptococcus pneumoniae in cerebrospinal fluid of children with acute bacterial meningitis. Antimicrob Agents Chemother 1995;39(9):1988–92.

56 Viladrich PF, Gudiol F, Linares J, et al. Evaluation of vancomycin for therapy of adult pneumococcal meningitis. Antimicrob Agents Chemother 1991;35(12):2467–72.

57 Peltola H. Worldwide Haemophilus influenzae type b disease at the beginning of the 21st century: global analysis of the disease burden 25 years after the use of the polysaccharide vaccine and a decade after the advent of conjugates. Clin Microbiol Rev 2000;13(2):302–17.

58 Prasad K, Karlupia N. Prevention of bacterial meningitis: an overview of Cochrane systematic reviews. Respir Med 2007;101(10):2037–43.

59 Recommended immunization schedules for children and adolescents – United States, 2008. Pediatrics 2008;121(1):219–20.

60 Prevention CfDCa. Recommended Adult Immunization Schedule – United States, October 2007 – September 2008. MMWR Morb Mortal Wkly Rep 2008;56:Q1-Q4.

61 Bolan G, Broome CV, Facklam RR, Plikaytis BD, Fraser DW, Schlech WF, 3rd. Pneumococcal vaccine efficacy in selected populations in the United States. Ann Intern Med 1986;104(1):1–6.

62 Butler JC, Breiman RF, Campbell JF, Lipman HB, Broome CV, Facklam RR. Pneumococcal polysaccharide vaccine efficacy. An evaluation of current recommendations. JAMA 1993;270(15):1826–31.

63 Black S, Shinefield H, Fireman B, et al. Efficacy, safety and immunogenicity of heptavalent pneumococcal conjugate vaccine in children. Northern California Kaiser Permanente Vaccine Study Center Group. Pediatr Infect Dis J 2000;19(3):187–95.

64 Prevention CfDCa. Recommended Immunization Schedules for Persons Aged 0–18 Years – United States, 2008. MMWR Morb Mortal Wkly Rep 2008;57:Q1–Q4.

65 CDC. Invasive pneumococcal disease in children 5 years after conjugate vaccine introduction – eight states, 1998–2005. MMWR Morb Mortal Wkly Rep 2008;57(6):144–8.

66 Prevention. CfDCa. Prevention and Control of Meningococcal Disease Recommendations of the Advisory Committee on Immunization Practices (ACIP). MMWR Morb Mortal Wkly Rep 2005;54(RR-7):1–21.

67 Weisfelt M, van de Beek D, Spanjaard L, Reitsma JB, de Gans J. A risk score for unfavorable outcome in adults with bacterial meningitis. Ann Neurol 2008;63(1):90–7.

68 Rasmussen HH, Sorensen HT, Moller-Petersen J, Mortensen FV, Nielsen B. Bacterial meningitis in elderly patients: clinical picture and course. Age Ageing 1992;21(3):216–20.

69 Bohr V, Paulson OB, Rasmussen N. Pneumococcal meningitis. Late neurologic sequelae and features of prognostic impact. Arch Neurol 1984;41(10):1045–9.

70 Pfister HW, Feiden W, Einhaupl KM. Spectrum of complications during bacterial meningitis in adults. Results of a prospective clinical study. Arch Neurol 1993;50(6):575–81.

71 van de Beek D, Schmand B, de Gans J, et al. Cognitive impairment in adults with good recovery after bacterial meningitis. J Infect Dis 2002;186(7):1047–52.

72 Solomon T, Hart IJ, Beeching NJ. Viral encephalitis: a clinician's guide. Pract Neurol 2007 Oct;7(5):288–305.

73 Whitley RJ. Viral encephalitis. N Engl J Med 1990;323(4):242–50.

74 Davies NW, Sharief MK, Howard RS. Infection-associated encephalopathies: their investigation, diagnosis, and treatment. J Neurol 2006;253(7):833–45.

75 Whitley RJ, Gnann JW. Viral encephalitis: familiar infections and emerging pathogens. Lancet 2002;359(9305):507–13.

76 Kennedy PG. Viral encephalitis. J Neurol 2005;252(3):268–72.

77 Redington JJ, Tyler KL. Viral infections of the nervous system, 2002: update on diagnosis and treatment. Arch Neurol 2002;59(5):712–18.

78 Whitley RJ. Herpes simplex encephalitis: adolescents and adults. Antiviral Res 2006;71(2–3):141–8.

79 Gubler DJ. The continuing spread of West Nile virus in the western hemisphere. Clin Infect Dis 2007;45(8):1039–46.

80 Petersen LR, Marfin AA, Gubler DJ. West Nile virus. JAMA 2003;290(4):524–8.

81 Johnson RT. Acute encephalitis. Clin Infect Dis 1996;23(2):219–24; quiz 25–6.

82 Solomon T. Flavivirus encephalitis. N Engl J Med 2004;351(4):370–8.

83 Ventura AK, Buff EE, Ehrenkranz NJ. Human Venezuelan equine encephalitis virus infection in Florida. Am J Trop Med Hyg 1974;23(3):507–12.

84 Zehmer RB, Dean PB, Sudia WD, Calisher CH, Sather GE, Parker RL. Venezuelan equine encephalitis epidemic in Texas, 1971. Health Serv Rep 1974;89(3):278–82.

85 Embil JA, Camfield P, Artsob H, Chase DP. Powassan virus encephalitis resembling herpes simplex encephalitis. Arch Intern Med 1983;143(2):341–3.

86 Gluckman S, DiNuble M. Infections of the central nervous system: acute viral infections. In: Weiner W, Shulman L, eds. Emergent and Urgent Neurology. Philadelphia: Lippincott WIlliams & Wilkins, 1999.

87 CDC. Update: multistate outbreak of mumps – United States, January 1–May 2, 2006. MMWR Morb Mortal Wkly Rep 2006;55(20):559–63.

88 Bloom S, Wharton M. Mumps outbreak among young adults in UK. BMJ 2005;331(7508):E363–4.

89 Johnson RT, Griffin DE, Hirsch RL, et al. Measles encephalomyelitis – clinical and immunologic studies. N Engl J Med 1984;310(3):137–41.

90 Simpson DM, Tagliati M. Neurologic manifestations of HIV infection. Ann Intern Med 1994;121(10):769–85.

91 CDC. Human rabies – Alberta, Canada, 2007. MMWR Morb Mortal Wkly Rep 2008;57(8):197–200.

92 Kennedy PG. Viral encephalitis: causes, differential diagnosis, and management. J Neurol Neurosurg Psychiatry 2004;75 Suppl 1:i10–15.

93 Morishima T, Togashi T, Yokota S, et al. Encephalitis and encephalopathy associated with an influenza epidemic in Japan. Clin Infect Dis 2002;35(5):512–7.

94 Whitley RJ, Soong SJ, Linneman C, Jr., Liu C, Pazin G, Alford CA. Herpes simplex encephalitis. Clinical Assessment. JAMA 198215;247(3):317–20.

95 Gould EA, Solomon T. Pathogenic flaviviruses. Lancet 2008;371(9611):500–9.

96 Haglund M, Gunther G. Tick-borne encephalitis – pathogenesis, clinical course and long-term follow-up. Vaccine 2003;21 Suppl 1:S11–8.

97 Przelomski MM, O'Rourke E, Grady GF, Berardi VP, Markley HG. Eastern equine encephalitis in Massachusetts: a report of 16 cases, 1970–1984. Neurology 1988;38(5):736–9.

98 Tsai TF. Arboviral infections in the United States. Infect Dis Clin North Am 1991;5(1):73–102.

99 Petersen LR, Marfin AA. West Nile virus: a primer for the clinician. Ann Intern Med 2002;137(3):173–9.

100 Petersen LR, Roehrig JT, Hughes JM. West Nile virus encephalitis. N Engl J Med 2002;347(16):1225–6.

101 McKinney RE, Jr., Katz SL, Wilfert CM. Chronic enteroviral meningoencephalitis in agammaglobulinemic patients. Rev Infect Dis 1987;9(2):334–56.

102 Whitley RJ, Cobbs CG, Alford CA, Jr., et al. Diseases that mimic herpes simplex encephalitis. Diagnosis, presentation, and outcome. NIAD Collaborative Antiviral Study Group. JAMA 1989;262(2):234–9.

103 Arribas JR, Storch GA, Clifford DB, Tselis AC. Cytomegalovirus encephalitis. Ann Intern Med 1996;125(7):577–87.

104 Koskiniemi M, Piiparinen H, Rantalaiho T, et al. Acute central nervous system complications in varicella zoster virus infections. J Clin Virol 2002;25(3):293–301.

105 Gilden DH, Kleinschmidt-DeMasters BK, LaGuardia JJ, Mahalingam R, Cohrs RJ. Neurologic complications of the reactivation of varicella-zoster virus. N Engl J Med 2000;342(9):635–45.

106 Cameron JC, Allan G, Johnston F, Finn A, Heath PT, Booy R. Severe complications of chickenpox in hospitalised children in the UK and Ireland. Arch Dis Child 2007;92(12):1062–6.

107 Fishbein DB, Robinson LE. Rabies. N Engl J Med 1993;329(22):1632–8.

108 Griffin D. Encephaltis, Myelitis, and Neuritis. In: Mandell G, Bennett J, Dolin R, eds. PRinciples and practice of infectious diseases. Philadelphia: Chruchill Livingstone, 2005.

109 Feigin RD, Shackelford PG. Value of repeat lumbar puncture in the differential diagnosis of meningitis. N Engl J Med 1973;289(11):571–4.

110 CDC. Case definitions for infectious conditions under public health surveillance. Centers for Disease Control and Prevention. MMWR Morb Mortal Wkly Rep 1997; 46(RR-10):1–55.

111 CDC. Summary of notifiable diseases, United States, 1999 MMWR Morb Mortal Wkly Rep 1999;48(53).

112 McCabe K, Tyler K, Tanabe J. Diffusion-weighted MRI abnormalities as a clue to the diagnosis of herpes simplex encephalitis. Neurology 2003;61(7):1015–6.

113 Tien RD, Felsberg GJ, Osumi AK. Herpesvirus infections of the CNS: MR findings. AJR Am J Roentgenol 1993;161(1):167–76.

114 Foerster BR, Thurnher MM, Malani PN, Petrou M, Carets-Zumelzu F, Sundgren PC. Intracranial infections: clinical and imaging characteristics. Acta Radiol 2007;48(8):875–93.

115 Brick JF, Brick JE, Morgan JJ, Gutierrez AR. EEG and pathologic findings in patients undergoing brain biopsy for suspected encephalitis. Electroencephalogr Clin Neurophysiol 1990;76(1):86–9.

116 Skoldenberg B, Forsgren M, Alestig K, et al. Acyclovir versus vidarabine in herpes simplex encephalitis. Randomised multicentre study in consecutive Swedish patients. Lancet 1984;2(8405):707–11.

117 Whitley RJ, Alford CA, Hirsch MS, et al. Vidarabine versus acyclovir therapy in herpes simplex encephalitis. N Engl J Med 1986;314(3):144–9.

118 Whitley RJ, Lakeman F. Herpes simplex virus infections of the central nervous system: therapeutic and diagnostic considerations. Clin Infect Dis 1995;20(2):414–20.

119 Anderson JF, Rahal JJ. Efficacy of interferon alpha-2b and ribavirin against West Nile virus in vitro. Emerg Infect Dis 2002;8(1):107–8.

120 Ben-Nathan D, Lustig S, Tam G, Robinzon S, Segal S, Rager-Zisman B. Prophylactic and therapeutic efficacy of human intravenous immunoglobulin in treating West Nile virus infection in mice. J Infect Dis 2003;188(1):5–12.

121 Desmond RA, Accortt NA, Talley L, Villano SA, Soong SJ, Whitley RJ. Enteroviral meningitis: natural history and outcome of pleconaril therapy. Antimicrob Agents Chemother 2006;50(7):2409–14.

122 Whitley RJ, Roizman B. Herpes simplex viruses: is a vaccine tenable? J Clin Invest 2002;110(2):145–51.

123 Marfin AA, Eidex RS, Kozarsky PE, Cetron MS. Yellow fever and Japanese encephalitis vaccines: indications and complications. Infect Dis Clin North Am 2005;19(1):151–68, ix.

124 Rupprecht CE, Gibbons RV. Clinical practice. Prophylaxis against rabies. N Engl J Med 2004;351(25):2626–35.

125 McGrath N, Anderson NE, Croxson MC, Powell KF. Herpes simplex encephalitis treated with acyclovir: diagnosis and long term outcome. J Neurol Neurosurg Psychiatry 1997;63(3):321–6.

126 VanLandingham KE, Marsteller HB, Ross GW, Hayden FG. Relapse of herpes simplex encephalitis after conventional acyclovir therapy. JAMA 1988;259(7):1051–3.

127 Skoldenberg B, Aurelius E, Hjalmarsson A, et al. Incidence and pathogenesis of clinical relapse after herpes simplex encephalitis in adults. J Neurol 2006;253(2):163–70.

128 Yamada S, Kameyama T, Nagaya S, Hashizume Y, Yoshida M. Relapsing herpes simplex encephalitis: pathological confirmation of viral reactivation. J Neurol Neurosurg Psychiatry 2003;74(2):262–4.

CHAPTER 6

Management of community-acquired pneumonia

David C. Rhew

Case presentation 1

A 63-year-old man presents to your office with fever and a productive cough. His symptoms began 3 days ago. He has hypertension and is being treated with an angiotensin-converting enzyme inhibitor. He does not smoke and has had no recent travel or ill contacts. Does this patient have pneumonia, where antibiotic treatment is warranted, or does the patient have a viral upper respiratory infection, in which case antibiotic treatment may be withheld?

Burden of illness/relevance to clinical practice

Treating patients using an evidence-based approach may ultimately improve care and reduce costs [1–3]. The objective of this chapter is to review the clinical evidence for the management of patients with community-acquired pneumonia (CAP) and to report the highest level of evidence as it pertains to management issues.

MEDLINE, EMBASE, Best Evidence, and Cochrane Systematic Review databases were searched from January 1966 through July 2007 using search terms for the following topics: diagnosis (history and physical examination, chest x-ray, sputum Gram's stain or culture, blood cultures, serology (*M. pneumoniae*, *C. pneumoniae*, *Legionella*, urine legionella antigen), admission decision, empiric antibiotic choice, treatment duration,

and prevention (pneumococcal vaccine, influenza vaccine). The American College of Physicians (ACP) Journal Club and the 2007 BMJ *Clinical Evidence* textbook were handsearched to identify additional references. Articles were excluded if they were of non-English language, addressed primarily hospital- or nursing-home acquired pneumonia, focused on pediatrics, or were nonhuman or in vitro studies. Articles in the following order were preferred: metaanalyses of randomized controlled trials (RCTs), systematic reviews of RCTs with no metaanalysis, > RCTs > metaanalyses of non-RCTs, systematic reviews of non-RCTs, non-randomized or observational studies [4,5].

Case presentation 1 (continued)

Upon physical examination, the patient has a temperature of 38°C (100.4°F), respiratory rate of 32 breaths per minute, pulse of 100 beats per minute, and systolic blood pressure of 145 mmHg and diastolic pressure of 90 mmHg. The examination of the chest is normal. Based on the history, you suspect CAP. However, the chest examination demonstrates no abnormalities. Does a normal chest examination rule out CAP? How confident are you that he has CAP based on the history alone? Should you order a chest radiograph?

Clinical history and physical examination

This type of case is a common scenario for clinicians who practice in ambulatory settings. An important question is the diagnostic accuracy of the history and

Evidence-Based Infectious Diseases, 2nd edition. Edited by Mark Loeb, Fiona Smaill and Marek Smieja. © 2009 Wiley-Blackwell Publishing, ISBN: 978-1-4051-7026-0

physical examination in making the diagnosis of CAP. A 1997 review [6] identified four prospective studies [7–10] that applied an independent, blind comparison with a reference standard to address this question. The conclusion was that no individual element of the history or physical examination possesses a likelihood ratio high or low enough to rule CAP in or out. This conclusion was also supported by a 2003 systematic review of testing strategies for CAP [11].

The question that follows is whether a *combination* of findings from the history and physical examination can help establish the diagnosis of CAP. Several prospective studies have examined this issue. Diehr et al. [7] assigned points based on the presence of each of the following findings: rhinorrhea (−2 points), sore throat (−1 point), night sweats (+1 point), myalgias (+1 point), sputum production (+1 point), respiratory rate >25 breaths per minute (+2 points), and temperature ≥37.8°C (100°F) (+2 points). Patients who had a score of −1 or greater were considered to have pneumonia. A threshold score of −1 was associated with a positive likelihood ratio (+LR) of 1.5 and a negative likelihood ratio (−LR) of 0.22. A threshold score of +1 was associated with a +LR of 5.0 and a −LR of 0.47, while a threshold score of +3 had a +LR of 14.0 and a −LR of 0.82.

Singal et al. [9] estimated the probability of CAP based on the following formula: $1/(1 + e^{-Y})$, where $Y = -3.095 + (1.214,$ if cough present) $+ (1.007,$ if fever present) $+ (0.823,$ if crackles present).

Heckerling et al. [10] estimated the probability of pneumonia by first determining how many of the following five findings were present: (1) absence of asthma, (2) temperature >37.8°C (100°F), (3) decreased breath sounds, (4) crackles, and (5) heart rate >100 beats per minute. The number of findings in combination with the prevalence (i.e., pretest probability) of pneumonia could then be applied to a nomogram to determine the post-test probability of pneumonia. The prediction rule had good discriminative ability, with a receiver operating characteristic (ROC) area of 0.82 in the derivation cohort and ROC areas of 0.82 and 0.76 in the two validation cohorts.

In another study, Gennis et al. [8] proposed that chest radiographs be obtained for one or more of the following: respiratory rate >30 breaths per minute, heart rate >100 beats per minute, and temperature ≥37.8°C (100°F). The presence of any these vital sign abnormalities was associated with a +LR of 1.2. The absence of all of these vital sign abnormalities was associated with a −LR of 0.18 for diagnosing pneumonia.

According to a national survey, 5% of patients with cough have pneumonia [12]. Assuming this pretest probability, and applying the above prediction rules to our patient, the Diehr rule [7] would predict a probability of CAP of 42%, the Singal rule [9] a probability of 29%, the Heckerling rule [10] a probability of 3%, and the Gennis rule a probability of 6%. This wide variability illustrates the difficulty in estimating the "true" probability for CAP by applying prediction rules. Moreover, a prospective observational study by Emerman et al. [13] has found that physician judgment is more sensitive (86%) in predicting CAP than any of the four prediction rules (Diehr, Singal, Heckerling, and Gennis).

Chest radiograph

The gold standard for confirming pneumonia remains the chest radiograph (CXR) [11]. However, do findings from the CXR influence care? A prospective randomized study of patients with acute cough (lasting less than 1 month) found that physicians may miss pneumonia based on clinical findings alone and that the increased use of CXR may result in more frequent appropriate treatment [14]. One observational study of patients with suspected pneumonia showed that CXR findings influence medical management in 69% of cases [15]. Finally, it should be noted that a negative CXR in a patient with presumed pneumonia does not necessarily warrant discontinuation of antibiotics. Some patients hospitalized with presumed pneumonia but who have a negative CXR have been shown to have serious lower respiratory tract infections resulting in bacteremia and death [16]. For these patients, continuation of antibiotic treatment would be justified.

Case presentation 1 (continued)

You decide to order a CXR, and the CXR demonstrates the presence of a left lower lung infiltrate without pleural effusion. Should you admit the patient to the hospital? Do you need to order any other tests to help you make this decision?

Admission decision

The decision to admit the patient to hospital or treat in the ambulatory setting may be facilitated by applying a prediction rule. In this case, the prediction rule provides the clinician with the probability that a specific adverse outcome (e.g., death) is likely to occur, based on the presence or absence of patient-specific factors at the time of presentation. The rationale is that patients deemed to be at low risk for adverse outcomes may be safely treated in the ambulatory setting, while those considered to be at higher risk may require hospitalization. However, there are no randomized controlled trials that directly demonstrate the benefit of such prediction rules.

The modified British Thoracic Society prediction rule [17] has been derived and validated in the largest cohort ($n = 1068$) of CAP patients outside of the US. The modified British Thoracic Society rule assigns 1 point for each of the following findings at the time of initial assessment: (a) confusion; (b) urea >7 mmol/L; (c) respiratory rate ≥30/min; (d) low systolic (<90 mmHg) or low diastolic (≤60 mmHg) blood pressure; and (e) age ≥65 years. Patients who receive a score of 0–1 (group 1) have a 30-day mortality rate of 1.5% and are considered appropriate candidates for ambulatory management. Patients who receive a score of 2 (group 2) have a 30-day mortality rate of 9.2% and may be eligible for brief hospitalization or supervised ambulatory care. Patients with a score of 3–5 (group 3) have a 30-day risk of death of 22% and should be treated in the hospital.

The prediction rule that has been most extensively validated is the rule developed by Fine and colleagues [18]. This prediction rule (sometimes referred to as the Pneumonia Severity Index [PSI] or Fine Prediction rule) and the corresponding score (sometimes referred to as the Patient Outcomes Research Team [PORT] score) was retrospectively derived from a cohort of 14 199 patients with CAP from the 1989 MedisGroups comparative hospital database and prospectively validated in a cohort of 38 039 patients with CAP from the 1991 Pennsylvania MedisGroups database. According to the PSI [18], risk factors for worse outcomes are associated with a point score. Age is often the most important risk factor, with one point given for each year of age (with 10 points subtracted for women). Other risk factors receive individual scores that range from 10 to 30 points. These include patient demographics,

comorbid conditions, physical examination findings, and laboratory results. Patients who receive a score ≤70 (class I or II) have an attributable risk of death within 30 days of <1% and are considered appropriate candidates for ambulatory management. Patients who receive a score of 71–90 (class III) have an associated 30-day mortality rate of up to 2.8% and may be eligible for brief hospitalization, or alternatively, ambulatory management with close follow-up [19,20]. However, in one retrospective study [21] ($n = 1889$), one-third of patients who fulfilled low-risk criteria (class I–III) had one or more contraindications to ambulatory care, and for this group of patients, inpatient care was still warranted. This demonstrates that such prediction rules do need to be superseded by clinical judgment. Patients with scores 91–130 (class IV) have a 30-day risk of death of between 8.2% and 9.3%, and patients with score >130 (class V) have a 30-day risk of death between 27.0% and 31.1%. It is recommended that class IV and V patients be treated in the hospital [18].

Case presentation 1 (continued)

The complete blood count and serum chemistries are all within normal limits. You calculate that the patient has a PSI score of 83 (class III) and contemplate admitting him to the hospital. If you admit the patient, what diagnostic tests should you order? What is the value of ordering a sputum Gram stain and culture? What about blood cultures? Should you order tests to detect the presence of 'atypical' pathogens (*Mycoplasma*, *Chlamydia*, *Legionella*)?

Diagnostic tests

Sputum Gram stain and culture

To decide whether or not to order a diagnostic test, it is first necessary to understand the test's diagnostic characteristics (e.g., sensitivity, specificity, positive and negative likelihood ratios, receiver operating characteristic [ROC] curves) [22]. A 1996 metaanalysis evaluated the sensitivity and specificity of sputum Gram stain in community-acquired pneumococcal pneumonia [23]. Inclusion criteria included: confirmed diagnosis of pneumococcal CAP, comparison to an independent reference standard, and all patients being properly accounted for (i.e., enough data provided to construct a 2 × 2 table of true positives, true negatives, false positives, and false negatives). Three blinded reviewers assessed the quality of the studies to determine eligibility for this review. A total of 12 studies published between 1966 and 1993 met inclusion criteria. These 12 studies enrolled a total of 1322 patients and evaluated 17 test characteristics. The results demonstrated that the sensitivity of sputum Gram stain ranged between 15% to 100%, and the specificity ranged between 11% and 100%. In 10 of the 17 estimations, sputum culture was the reference standard. The authors noted a trend ($P = 0.07$) for increased interpreter training and greater diagnostic accuracy. The conclusion of this study was that no single estimate of sensitivity and specificity could be determined for sputum Gram stain in pneumococcal CAP, and that the results of sputum Gram staining could be misleading, especially if the interpreter was not well trained.

Clinical studies have demonstrated conflicting results as to whether sputum Gram stain and culture provide useful information in the management of patients hospitalized with CAP. In one prospective study [24] ($n = 533$), sputum samples of good quality were obtained from only 39% (210 of 533) of hospitalized patients. In another prospective study [25] ($n = 74$), sputum Gram stain was unable to identify the pathogen affecting any of 74 hospitalized adult patients with nonsevere CAP. This study also showed that sputum cultures identified pathogens in only 4 (5%) patients. A retrospective study [26] ($n = 108$) analyzed the diagnostic effectiveness of sputum cultures and sputum Gram stains among inpatients with bacteremic pneumococcal pneumonia. The authors concluded that sputum Gram stains had some diagnostic value when moderate or abundant gram-positive diplococci were evident but that the overall results of sputum cultures had limited impact on the diagnosis of pneumococcal pneumonia. Another retrospective study [27] ($n = 184$) examined the value of initial microbiologic studies (MBSs) in adults who were admitted for CAP and managed according to the 1993 ATS guidelines [28]. In this study, 14 patients with severe CAP had their antibiotic regimens changed due to a nonresponse to their initial regimen. Three of these patients had their antibiotic regimens changed based on MBSs, while 11 had empiric antibiotic regimen changes. The mortality rate for patients whose antibiotics were changed based on MBSs was no different from that for patients who had antibiotics changed empirically (67% versus 64%, respectively; P-value not reported). The authors concluded that initial MBSs were not warranted except in high-risk patients who were more likely to harbor resistant organisms.

Blood cultures

Clinical studies have demonstrated that the incidence of positive blood cultures in adult patients hospitalized with CAP ranges from 0% to 26.8% [25,27,29–53]. One prospective study ($n = 209$) has shown that the yield from blood cultures increases with worsening severity of illness (PSI class I: 5.3%, II: 10.2%, III: 10.3%, IV: 16.1%, V: 26.7%) [48], while another prospective study ($n = 760$) has not shown this to be the case (PSI class I and II: 8%, III: 6.2%, IV: 4.6%, V: 5.2%) [54]. A retrospective study has found that the yield from patients who have received antibiotics prior to blood cultures is significantly lower than that from patients who have not (0% [0/23] vs 16.6% [5/30] patients, respectively; $P < 0.05$) [55]. The incidence of positive blood cultures in the ambulatory setting is considerably lower than that seen in inpatients. According to a study of 1350 ambulatory patients with a variety of infections including CAP the incidence of positive blood cultures is 1.8% [56], while a study of 204 patients with severe CAP (i.e., requiring ICU) has shown a yield from blood cultures of 21.1% [29]. In summary, these data suggest that blood cultures may provide information on the etiology of pneumonia for patients with CAP, especially for those who are hospitalized and sicker (e.g., requiring ICU care).

An important question is whether blood culture results change clinical management and improve outcomes for patients with CAP. A 1996 metaanalysis [57] demonstrated that bacteremia is associated with an increased risk for death (OR 2.8, 95% CI 2.3–3.6), and a large retrospective study ($n = 14069$) has found an association between drawing blood cultures prior to antibiotics and lower 30-day mortality rate (adjusted OR 0.92, 95% CI 0.82–1.02; $P = 0.10$) [58]. Also, several studies have specifically addressed whether drawing blood cultures has an impact on clinical management. A large retrospective analysis of a database ($n = 10275$) [59] found that positive blood cultures for penicillin-susceptible

S. *pneumoniae* in hospitalized patients does not have an impact on fluoroquinolone use. One small retrospective study has shown that the results of blood cultures do not lead to a change in the initial empiric antibiotic regimen [55]. Other studies suggest that the results of positive blood cultures may occasionally change the management of patients with CAP [27,29–35,37–53,60] but do not lower mortality [48].

Serologies

Various types of serologic tests exist for atypical pathogens. For *M. pneumoniae* these include enzyme-linked immunosorbent assay (ELISA), complement fixation, and cold agglutinins; for *C.pneumoniae* microimmunofluorescence is used; and for *Legionella* species immunofluorescence assay [61]. However, results from serologic tests to diagnose "atypical" pathogens often return after the patient has been discharged and do not impact the treatment plan [62].

Urine legionella antigen

The urine legionella antigen test identifies *Legionella pneumophila* serogroup I, which is the most common serogroup causing illness. The sensitivity of the test is 70% and specificity is 100%, with a quick turnaround time [63]. Use of the urine legionella antigen test has been demonstrated to expedite the time to diagnosis of legionella by 5 days [64].

Case presentation 1 (continued)

What empiric antibiotics should you order if you decide to treat your patient in the ambulatory setting? What about the inpatient setting? If a patient is admitted and started on intravenous (IV) antibiotics, when would the patient be stable enough to be switched from IV to oral antibiotics and sent home?

Antibiotic treatment

Ambulatory treatment

There are no RCTs that have compared multiple antibiotic regimens to determine which is the most suitable for ambulatory patients with CAP. A 2005

metaanalysis [65] showed that there was no difference in treatment failure between patients with non-severe CAP who received a β-lactam antibiotic alone versus those who received a regimen that included an antibiotic with activity against "atypical" pathogens. Furthermore, one prospective observational study [66] ($n = 864$) showed that ambulatory CAP patients who received antibiotics in accordance with 1993 ATS guidelines [28] experienced no difference in outcomes (mortality, subsequent hospitalization, medical complications, symptom resolution, return to work and usual activities, health-related quality of life, and antimicrobial costs) as compared to those who received other antibiotics. In summary, the evidence indicates that ambulatory patients with CAP may be successfully treated with either a β-lactam antibiotic or an antibiotic with activity against "atypical" pathogens.

Inpatient treatment

While many clinical trials have compared individual empiric antibiotic regimens, fewer studies have compared multiple different empiric regimens. One metaanalysis suggested that empiric antibiotic treatment with either azithromycin or a respiratory fluoroquinolone was superior to comparator agents in the treatment of CAP. One 2002 metaanalysis [67] showed that azithromycin reduced clinical failures by one-third (random effects odds ratio 0.63, 95% CI 0.41–0.95) as compared with other antibiotics in the treatment of CAP. Another 2002 metaanalysis [68] demonstrated that respiratory fluoroquinolones reduced the incidence of therapeutic failures as compared with macrolides, β-lactam antibiotics, and doxycycline for patients with CAP. However, a more recent metaanalysis [69] found no difference in mortality between empiric antibiotic regimens that covered for "atypical" pathogens versus those that did not cover for "atypical" pathogens in hospitalized patients with CAP.

Some of the largest evaluations of the relationship between the initial choice of antibiotics and clinical outcomes have involved use of administrative databases. A retrospective study [70] ($n = 44\,814$) of hospitalized CAP patients showed that dual therapy with a macrolide plus either ceftriaxone, another cephalosporin, penicillin, or quinolone was associated with a lower 30-day mortality rate and shorter length of stay than monotherapy with the non-macrolide agent. A retrospective study [71] ($n = 10\,069$) of Medicare patients hospitalized in 10 Western US states during 1993, 1995, and 1997 demonstrated an association between lower 30-day mortality and the initial empiric antibiotic regimens including either a macrolide or fluoroquinolone. Another retrospective study [72] ($n = 12\,945$) used a non-pseudomonal third-generation cephalosporin as a referent and demonstrated that three antibiotic regimens were associated with significantly lower 30-day mortality rates compared to the referent: second-generation cephalosporin plus macrolide, third-generation cephalosporin (non-pseudomonal) plus macrolide, respiratory fluoroquinolone alone. Results from these large retrospective analyses suggest that coverage for "atypical" pathogens with either a macrolide or an anti-pneumococcal quinolone is important in the treatment of inpatients with CAP.

In summary, data are conflicting as to which antibiotic or class of antibiotic is most appropriate for the inpatient treatment of CAP patients. Findings from a 2005 metaanalysis [69] of RCTs suggest that coverage for "atypical" pathogens does not reduce mortality. On the other hand, findings from large observational studies suggest that coverage for "atypical" pathogens is associated with lower 30-day mortality rates for patients hospitalized with CAP. It should also be noted that a 2004 metaanalysis [73] of RCTs has shown that patients hospitalized with CAP can be safely and effectively treated with oral antibiotic therapy.

Duration of treatment

RCTs have compared shorter versus longer courses of antibiotic treatment of patients with CAP.

In these studies, duration of shorter course therapy can be as few as 1 to 7 days [74–93], with rates of clinical resolution not significantly different between the shorter and longer courses of therapy. These data indicate that patients with mild to moderate disease (e.g., PSI I–III) can potentially be treated with antibiotic regimens as short as 1–3 days. Often the antibiotic of choice is azithromycin because of its long half-life [78–80,83–85,92,93]. However, one RCT by el Moussaoui [90] shows that 3 days of oral amoxicillin was just as effective as 10 days of oral amoxicillin for patients with CAP with a PSI score ⩽110

(i.e., class I–III). Patients with more severe disease (e.g., PSI class IV) may potentially be treated with 5–7 days of antibiotics [77,91].

Prevention

Vaccines

Several metaanalyses [94–101] have evaluated the pneumococcal vaccine in adults. Data from the most recent 2007 [96] and 2004 [94] metaanalyses indicate that the polysaccharide pneumococcal vaccine reduces the incidence of invasive pneumococcal disease in adults and the immunocompetent elderly (55 years and older), but does not reduce the incidence of pneumonia or death in adults with or without chronic illness or in the elderly (55 years and older).

Several systematic reviews and metaanalyses have evaluated the efficacy of the influenza vaccine in elderly persons [102–105], healthy adults [106], and healthcare workers [107–109].

Data from the most recent 2006 metaanalysis by Rivetti and colleagues [104] of RCTs and non-RCTs demonstrates that for the elderly when the influenza vaccine is well matched against the circulating strain of virus, the influenza vaccine is 46% (95% CI 30–58%) effective in preventing pneumonia, 45% (95% CI 16–64%) effective in preventing hospital admission, and 42% (95% CI 17–59%) effective in preventing death due to influenza or pneumonia for elderly patients residing in long-term care facilities (note: vaccine effectiveness = 1 – odds ratio). For elderly patients living in the community, the vaccine is 26% (95% CI 12–38%) effective in preventing hospital admission for influenza or pneumonia and 42% (95% CI 24–55%) effective in preventing all-cause death. Data from the most recent 2007 metaanalysis by Demicheli and colleagues [106] of randomized and non-randomized trials shows that for healthy adults the influenza vaccine is 30% effective (95% CI 17–41%) against influenza-like illness. In cases of laboratory-confirmed influenza infection, when the influenza vaccine matched the circulating strain, the influenza vaccine is 80% (95% CI 56–91%) effective. This decreases to 50% (95% CI 27–65%) when the vaccine does not match with the circulating strain.

Data from the most recent 2006 metaanalyses by Thomas and colleagues [108,109] of RCTs and non-RCTs show that vaccination of healthcare workers who treat elderly (60 years or older) patients residing in a long-term care facility results in lower incidence of influenza-related illness, but only when the patients are also vaccinated; the results are not significant when only the healthcare worker is vaccinated.

In summary, data from recent metaanalyses indicate that the pneumococcal vaccine reduces the incidence of invasive pneumococcal disease in adults (including the elderly), but does not reduce the incidence of pneumococcal pneumonia or death. Recent metaanalyses on the influenza vaccine demonstrate that the influenza vaccine is effective in preventing death due to influenza or pneumonia for elderly patients residing in long-term care facilities, especially when the healthcare worker is also vaccinated. The influenza vaccine is also effective in preventing influenza in healthy adults.

References

1 Weingarten S. Translating practice guidelines into patient care: guidelines at the bedside. [Review] Chest 2000;118:4S–7S.

2 Grimshaw JM, Russell IT. Effect of clinical guidelines on medical practice: a systematic review of rigorous evaluations. [see comments]. Lancet 1993;342:1317–22.

3 Bahtsevani C, Uden G, Willman A. Outcomes of evidence-based clinical practice guidelines: a systematic review. Int J Technol Assess Health Care 2004;20:427–33.

4 BMJ Publishing Group. Clinical Evidence, vol.6. London: BMJ Publishing Group, 2001.

5 Rhew DC, Goetz MB, Shekelle PG. Evaluating quality indicators for patients with community-acquired pneumonia. J Comm J Qual Improv 2001;27:575–90.

6 Metlay JP, Kapoor WN, Fine MJ. Does this patient have community-acquired pneumonia? Diagnosing pneumonia by history and physical examination. JAMA 1997;278:1440–5.

7 Diehr P, Wood RW, Bushyhead J, et al. Prediction of pneumonia in outpatients with acute cough – a statistical approach. Journal of Chronic Diseases 1984;7:215–25.

8 Gennis P, Gallagher J, Falvo C, et al. Clinical criteria for the detection of pneumonia in adults: guidelines for ordering chest roentgenograms in the emergency department. Journal of Emergency Medicine 1989;7:263–8.

9 Singal BM, Hedges JR, Radack KL. Decision rules and clinical prediction of pneumonia: evaluation of low-yield criteria. Annals of Emergency Medicine 1989;18:13–20.

10 Heckerling PS, Tape TG, Wigton RS, et al. Clinical prediction rule for pulmonary infiltrates. [see comments]. Ann Intern Med 1990;113:664–70.

11 Metlay JP, Fine MJ. Testing strategies in the initial management of patients with community-acquired pneumonia. [Review] Annals of Internal Medicine 2003;138:109–18.

12 Metlay JP, Stafford RS, Singer DE. National trends in the management of acute cough by primary care physicians. J Gen Intern Med 1997;12(suppl), 77.

13 Emerman CL, Dawson N, Speroff T, et al. Comparison of physician judgment and decision aids for ordering chest radiographs for pneumonia in outpatients. Ann Emerg Med 1991;20:1215–19.

14 Bushyhead JB, Wood RW, Tompkins RK, et al. The effect of chest radiographs on the management and clinical course of patients with acute cough. Medical Care 1983;21:661–73.

15 Speets AM, Hoes AW, van der Graaf Y, et al. Chest radiography and pneumonia in primary care: diagnostic yield and consequences for patient management. Eur Respir J 2006;28:933–8.

16 Basi SK, Marrie TJ, Huang JQ, et al. Patients admitted to hospital with suspected pneumonia and normal chest radiographs: epidemiology, microbiology, and outcomes. Am J Med 2004;117:305–11.

17 Lim WS, van der Eerden MM, Laing R, et al. Defining community-acquired pneumonia severity on presentation to hospital: an international derivation and validation study. Thorax 2003;58:377–82.

18 Fine MJ, Auble TE, Yealy DM, et al. A prediction rule to identify low-risk patients with community-acquired pneumonia [see comments]. N Engl J Med 1997;336:243–50.

19 Atlas SJ, Benzer TI, Borowsky LH, et al. Safely increasing the proportion of patients with community-acquired pneumonia treated as outpatients: an interventional trial. Arch Intern Med 1998;158:1350–6.

20 Carratala J, Fernandez-Sabe N, Ortega L, et al. Outpatient care compared with hospitalization for community-acquired pneumonia: a randomized trial in low-risk patients. Ann Intern Med 2005;142:165–72.

21 Labarere J, Stone RA, Scott OD, et al. Factors associated with the hospitalization of low-risk patients with community-acquired pneumonia in a cluster-randomized trial. J Gen Intern Med 2006;21:745–52.

22 Jaeschke R, Guyatt GH, Sackett DL. Users' guides to the medical literature. III. How to use an article about a diagnostic test. B. What are the results and will they help me in caring for my patients? The Evidence-Based Medicine Working Group. JAMA 1994;271:703–7.

23 Reed WW, Byrd GS, Gates RHJ, et al. Sputum gram's stain in community-acquired pneumococcal pneumonia. A meta-analysis. Western Journal of Medicine 1996;165: 197–204.

24 Roson B, Carratala J, Verdaguer R, et al. Prospective study of the usefulness of sputum Gram stain in the initial approach to community-acquired pneumonia requiring hospitalization. Clin Infect Dis 2000;31:869–74.

25 Theerthakarai R, El Halees W, Ismail M, et al. Nonvalue of the initial microbiological studies in the management of nonsevere community-acquired pneumonia. [see comments]. Chest 2001;119:181–4.

26 Watanakunakorn C, Bailey TA. Adult bacteremic pneumococcal pneumonia in a community teaching hospital, 1992–1996. A detailed analysis of 108 cases. Arch Intern Med 1997;157:1965–71.

27 Sanyal S, Smith PR, Saha AC, et al. Initial microbiologic studies did not affect outcome in adults hospitalized with community-acquired pneumonia. Am J Respir Crit Care Med 1999;160:346–8.

28 Niederman MS, Bass JBJ, Campbell GD, et al. Guidelines for the initial management of adults with community-acquired pneumonia: diagnosis, assessment of severity, and initial antimicrobial therapy. American Thoracic Society. Medical Section of the American Lung Association. Am Rev Respir Dis 1993;148:1418–26.

29 Rello J, Bodi M, Mariscal D, et al. Microbiological testing and outcome of patients with severe community-acquired pneumonia. Chest 2003;123:174–80.

30 Lehtomaki K, Leinonen M, Takala A, et al. (1988) Etiological diagnosis of pneumonia in military conscripts by combined use of bacterial culture and serological methods. Eur J Clin Microbiol Infect Dis 1988;7:348–54.

31 McNabb WR, Shanson DC, Williams TD, et al. Adult community-acquired pneumonia in central London. J Roy Soc Med 1984;77:550–5.

32 Ishida T, Hashimoto T, Arita M, et al. Etiology of community-acquired pneumonia in hospitalized patients: a 3-year prospective study in Japan. [see comments]. Chest 1998;114:1588–93.

33 Ostergaard L, Andersen PL. Etiology of community-acquired pneumonia. Evaluation by transtracheal aspiration, blood culture, or serology. Chest 1993;104:1400–7.

34 Marrie TJ. Bacteremic community-acquired pneumonia due to viridans group streptococci. Clin Invest Med – Medecine Clinique et Experimentale 1993;16:38–44.

35 Fang GD, Fine M, Orloff J, et al. New and emerging etiologies for community-acquired pneumonia with implications for therapy. A prospective multicenter study of 359 cases. Medicine 1990;69:307–16.

36 British Thoracic Society PHLS. Community-acquired pneumonia in adults in British hospitals in 1982–1983: a survey of aetiology, mortality, prognostic factors and outcome. Q J Med 1987;62:195–220.

37 Venkatesan P, Gladman J, MacFarlane JT, et al. A hospital study of community acquired pneumonia in the elderly. Thorax 1990;45:254–8.

38 Marrie TJ, Durant H, Yates L. Community-acquired pneumonia requiring hospitalization: 5-year prospective study. Rev Infect Dis 1989;11:586–99.

39 Porath A, Schlaeffer F, Lieberman D. The epidemiology of community-acquired pneumonia among hospitalized adults. J Infect 1997;34:41–8.

40 Marston BJ, Plouffe JF, File TMJ, et al. Incidence of community-acquired pneumonia requiring hospitalization. Results of a population-based active surveillance Study in Ohio. The Community-Based Pneumonia Incidence Study Group. Arch Int Med 1997;157:1709–18.

41 Rello J, Quintana E, Ausina V, et al. A three-year study of severe community-acquired pneumonia with emphasis on outcome. Chest 1993;103:232–5.

42 Socan M, Marinic-Fiser N, Kraigher A, et al. Microbial aetiology of community-acquired pneumonia in hospitalised patients. Eur J Clin Microbiol Infect Dis 1999;18: 777–82.

43 Woodhead MA, Arrowsmith J, Chamberlain-Webber R, et al. The value of routine microbial investigation in community-acquired pneumonia. [see comments]. Respiratory Medicine 1991;85:313–17.

44 Bartlett JG, Mundy LM. Community-acquired pneumonia. [see comments]. [Review] [48 refs]. N Engl J Med 1995;333:1618–24.

45 Levy M, Dromer F, Brion N, et al. Community-acquired pneumonia. Importance of initial noninvasive bacteriologic and radiographic investigations. Chest 1988;93:43–8.

46 Lim I, Shaw DR, Stanley DP, et al. A prospective hospital study of the aetiology of community-acquired pneumonia. Med J Australia 1989;151:87–91.

47 Ruiz M, Ewig S, Marcos MA, et al. Etiology of community-acquired pneumonia: impact of age, comorbidity, and severity. Am J Respir Crit Care Med 1999;160:397–405.

48 Waterer GW, Wunderink RG. The influence of the severity of community-acquired pneumonia on the usefulness of blood cultures. Respir Med 2001;95:78–82.

49 MacFarlane JT, Finch RG, Ward MJ, et al. Hospital study of adult community-acquired pneumonia. Lancet 1982;2:255–8.

50 Ewig S, Bauer T, Hasper E, et al. Value of routine microbial investigation in community-acquired pneumonia treated in a tertiary care center. Respiration 1996;63:164–9.

51 Mundy LM, Auwaerter PG, Oldach D, et al. Community-acquired pneumonia: impact of immune status. Am J Respir Crit Care Med 1995;152:1309–15.

52 Leroy O, Santre C, Beuscart C, et al. A five-year study of severe community-acquired pneumonia with emphasis on prognosis in patients admitted to an intensive care unit. Intens Care Med 1995;21:24–31.

53 Moine P, Vercken JB, Chevret S, et al. Severe community-acquired pneumococcal pneumonia. The French Study Group of Community-Acquired Pneumonia in ICU. Scand J Infect Dis 1995;27:201–6.

54 Campbell SG, Marrie TJ, Anstey R, et al. The contribution of blood cultures to the clinical management of adult patients admitted to the hospital with community-acquired pneumonia: a prospective observational study.[comment]. Chest 2003;123:1142–50.

55 Glerant JC, Hellmuth D, Schmit JL, et al. Utility of blood cultures in community-acquired pneumonia requiring hospitalization: influence of antibiotic treatment before admission. Respir Med 1999;93:208–12.

56 Sturmann KM, Bopp J, Molinari D, et al. Blood cultures in adult patients released from an urban emergency department: a 15-month experience. Acad Emerg Med 1996;3:768–75.

57 Fine MJ, Smith MA, Carson CA, et al. Prognosis and outcomes of patients with community-acquired pneumonia. A meta-analysis. JAMA 1996;275:134–41.

58 Meehan TP, Fine MJ, Krumholz HM, et al. Quality of care, process, and outcomes in elderly patients with pneumonia [see comments]. JAMA 1997;278:2080–4.

59 Chang NN, Murray CK, Houck PM, et al. Blood culture and susceptibility results and allergy history do not influence fluoroquinolone use in the treatment of community-acquired pneumonia. Pharmacotherapy 2005;25:59–66.

60 British Thoracic Society. Community-acquired pneumonia in adults in British hospitals in 1982–1983: a survey of aetiology, mortality, prognostic factors and outcome. The British Thoracic Society and the Public Health Laboratory Service. Q J Med 1987;62:195–220.

61 Bartlett J, Dowell S, Mandell L, et al. Practice guidelines for the management of community-acquired pneumonia in adults: guidelines from the Infectious Disease Society of America. Clin Infect Dis 2000;31:347–82.

62 Mundy LM, Oldach D, Auwaerter PG, et al. Implications for macrolide treatment in community-acquired pneumonia. Hopkins CAP Team. [see comments]. Chest 1998;113:1201–6.

63 Stout JE, Yu VL. Legionellosis. [see comments]. [Review]. N Engl J Med 1997;337:682–7.

64 Formica N, Yates M, Beers M, et al. The impact of diagnosis by legionella antigen test on the epidemiology and outcomes of legionnaires' disease. Epidemiol Infect 2001;127:275–80.

65 Mills GD, Oehley MR, Arrol B. Effectiveness of beta lactam antibiotics compared with antibiotics active against atypical pathogens in non-severe community acquired pneumonia: meta-analysis. BMJ 2005;330:456.

66 Gleason PP, Kapoor WN, Stone RA, et al. Medical outcomes and antimicrobial costs with the use of the American Thoracic Society guidelines for outpatients with community-acquired pneumonia. JAMA 1997;278:32–9.

67 Contopoulos-Ioannidis DG, Ioannidis JP, Chew P, et al. Meta-analysis of randomized controlled trials on the comparative efficacy and safety of azithromycin against other antibiotics for lower respiratory tract infections. J Antimicrob Chemother 2001;48:691–703.

68 Salkind AR, Cuddy PG, Foxworth JW. Fluoroquinolone treatment of community-acquired pneumonia: a meta-analysis. Ann Pharmacother 2002;36:1938–43.

69 Robenshtok E, Shefet D, Gafter-Gvili A, Paul M, Vidal L, Leibovici L. Empiric antibiotic coverage of atypical pathogens for community acquired pneumonia in hospitalized adults. Cochrane Database Syst Rev 2008 (1), CD004418, DOI: 10.1002/14651858. pub3.

70 Brown RB, Iannini P, Gross P, et al. Impact of initial antibiotic choice on clinical outcomes in community-acquired pneumonia: analysis of a hospital claims-made database. [comment]. Chest 2003;123:1503–11.

71 Houck PM, MacLehose RF, Niederman MS, et al. (2001) Empiric antibiotic therapy and mortality among medicare pneumonia inpatients in 10 western states: 1993, 1995, and 1997. Chest 2001;119:1420–6.

72 Gleason PP, Meehan TP, Fine JM, et al. Associations between initial antimicrobial therapy and medical outcomes for hospitalized elderly patients with pneumonia [see comments]. Arch Intern Med 1999;159:2562–2572.

73 Marras TK, Nopmaneejumruslers C, Chan CK. Efficacy of exclusively oral antibiotic therapy in patients hospitalized with nonsevere community-acquired pneumonia: a retrospective study and meta-analysis. Am J Med 2004;116:385–93.

74 Tellier G, Chang JR, Asche CV, et al. Comparison of hospitalization rates in patients with community-acquired pneumonia treated with telithromycin for 5 or 7 days or clarithromycin for 10 days. Curr Med Res Opin 2004;20:739–47.

75 Tellier G, Niederman MS, Nusrat R, et al. Clinical and bacteriological efficacy and safety of 5- and 7-day regimens of telithromycin once daily compared with a 10-day regimen of clarithromycin twice daily in patients with mild to moderate community-acquired pneumonia. J Antimicrob Chemother 2004;54:515–23.

76 Siegel RE, Alicea M, Lee A, et al. Comparison of 7 versus 10 days of antibiotic therapy for hospitalized patients with uncomplicated community-acquired pneumonia: a prospective, randomized, double-blind study. Am J Ther 1999;6:217–22.

77 Shorr AF, Zadeikis N, Xiang JX, et al. A multicenter, randomized, double-blind, retrospective comparison of 5- and 10-day regimens of levofloxacin in a subgroup of patients aged > or = 65 years with community-acquired pneumonia. Clin Ther 2005;27:1251–9.

78 Schonwald S, Kuzman I, Oreskovic K, et al. Azithromycin: single 1.5 g dose in the treatment of patients with atypical pneumonia syndrome – a randomized study. Infection 1999;27:198–202.

79 Schonwald S, Barsic B, Klinar I, et al. Three-day azithromycin compared with ten-day roxithromycin treatment of atypical pneumonia. Scand J Infect Dis 1994;26:706–10.

80 Schonwald S, Skerk V, Petricevic I, et al. Comparison of three-day and five-day courses of azithromycin in the treatment of atypical pneumonia. Eur J Clin Microbiol Infect Dis 1991;10:877–80.

81 Schonwald S, Gunjaca M, Kolacny-Babic L, et al. Comparison of azithromycin and erythromycin in the treatment of atypical pneumonias. J Antimicrob Chemother 1990;25 Suppl A:123–6.

82 Rovira E, Martinez-Moragon E, Belda A, et al. Treatment of community-acquired pneumonia in outpatients: randomized study of clarithromycin alone versus clarithromycin and cefuroxime. Respiration 1999;66:413–18.

83 Rizzato G, Montemurro L, Fraioli P, et al. Efficacy of a three-day course of azithromycin in moderately severe community-acquired pneumonia. Eur Respir J 1995;8:398–402.

84 Rahav G, Fidel J, Gibor Y, et al. Azithromycin versus comparative therapy for the treatment of community acquired pneumonia. Int J Antimicrob Agents 2004;24:181–4.

85 O'Doherty B, Muller O. Randomized, multicentre study of the efficacy and tolerance of azithromycin versus clarithromycin in the treatment of adults with mild to moderate community-acquired pneumonia. Azithromycin Study Group. Eur J Clin Microbiol Infect Dis 1998;17:828–33.

86 Niederman MS, Chang JR, Stewart J, et al. Hospitalization rates among patients with community-acquired pneumonia

treated with telithromycin vs clarithromycin: results from two randomized, double-blind, clinical trials. Curr Med Res Opin 2004;20:969–80.

87 Leophonte P, File T, Feldman C. Gemifloxacin once daily for 7 days compared to amoxicillin/clavulanic acid thrice daily for 10 days for the treatment of community-acquired pneumonia of suspected pneumococcal origin. Respir Med 2004;98:708–20.

88 Kuzman I, kovic-Rode O, Oremus M, et al. Clinical efficacy and safety of a short regimen of azithromycin sequential therapy vs standard cefuroxime sequential therapy in the treatment of community-acquired pneumonia: an international, randomized, open-label study. J Chemother 2005;17:636–42.

89 Kinasewitz G, Wood RG. Azithromycin versus cefaclor in the treatment of acute bacterial pneumonia. Eur J Clin Microbiol Infect Dis 1991;10:872–7.

90 el Moussaoui R, de Borgie CA, van den Broek P, et al. Effectiveness of discontinuing antibiotic treatment after three days versus eight days in mild to moderate-severe community acquired pneumonia: randomised, double blind study. BMJ 2006;332:1355.

91 Dunbar LM, Wunderink RG, Habib MP, et al. High-dose, short-course levofloxacin for community-acquired pneumonia: a new treatment paradigm. Clin Infect Dis 2003;37:752–60.

92 Drehobl MA, De Salvo MC, Lewis DE, et al. Single-dose azithromycin microspheres vs clarithromycin extended release for the treatment of mild-to-moderate community-acquired pneumonia in adults. Chest 2005;128:2230–7.

93 D'Ignazio J, Camere MA, Lewis DE, et al. Novel, single-dose microsphere formulation of azithromycin versus 7-day levofloxacin therapy for treatment of mild to moderate community-acquired Pneumonia in adults. Antimicrob Agents Chemother 2005;49:4035–41.

94 Conaty S, Watson L, Dinnes J, et al. The effectiveness of pneumococcal polysaccharide vaccines in adults: a systematic review of observational studies and comparison with results from randomised controlled trials. Vaccine 2004;22:3214–24.

95 Cornu C, Yzebe D, Leophonte P, et al. Efficacy of pneumococcal polysaccharide vaccine in immunocompetent adults: a meta-analysis of randomized trials. Vaccine 2001; 19:4780–90.

96 Moberley S, Holden J, Tatham DP, Andrews RM. Vaccines for preventing pneumococcal infection in adults. Cochrane Database Syst Rev 2008 (1), CD000422, DOI: 10.1002/14651858. pub2.

97 Fedson DS, Liss C. Precise answers to the wrong question: prospective clinical trials and the meta-analyses of pneumococcal vaccine in elderly and high-risk adults. Vaccine 2004;22:927–46.

98 Fine MJ, Smith MA, Carson CA, et al. Efficacy of pneumococcal vaccination in adults. A meta-analysis of randomized controlled trials. Arch Int Med 1994;154: 2666–77.

99 Hutchison BG, Oxman AD, Shannon HS, et al. Clinical effectiveness of pneumococcal vaccine. Meta-analysis. [see comments]. Can Fam Phys 1999;45:2381–93.

100 Moore RA, Wiffen PJ, Lipsky BA. Are the pneumococcal polysaccharide vaccines effective? Meta-analysis of the prospective trials. BMC Fam Pract 2000;1:1.

101 Watson L, Wilson BJ, Waugh N. Pneumococcal polysaccharide vaccine: a systematic review of clinical effectiveness in adults. Vaccine 2002;20:2166–73.

102 Gross PA, Hermogenes AW, Sacks HS, et al. The efficacy of influenza vaccine in elderly persons. A meta-analysis and review of the literature. Ann Int Med 1995;123: 518–27.

103 Jefferson T, Rivetti D, Rivetti A, et al. Efficacy and effectiveness of influenza vaccines in elderly people: a systematic review. Lancet 2005;366:1165–74.

104 Rivetti D, Jefferson T, Thomas R, et al. Vaccines for preventing influenza in the elderly. Cochrane Database Syst Rev 2006 (3), CD004876, DOI: 10.1002/14651858.

105 Vu T, Farish S, Jenkins M, et al. A meta-analysis of effectiveness of influenza vaccine in persons aged 65 years and over living in the community. Vaccine 2002;20:1831–6.

106 Demicheli V, Di Pietrantonj C, Jefferson TO, Rivetti A, Rivetti D. Vaccines for preventing influenza in healthy adults. Cochrane Database Syst Rev 2007 (2), CD001269, DOI: 10.1002/14651858. pub3.

107 Burls A, Jordan R, Barton P, et al. Vaccinating healthcare workers against influenza to protect the vulnerable – is it a good use of healthcare resources? A systematic review of the evidence and an economic evaluation. Vaccine 2006;24:4212–21.

108 Thomas RE, Jefferson TO, Demicheli V, et al. Influenza vaccination for health-care workers who work with elderly people in institutions: a systematic review. Lancet Infect Dis 2006;6:273–9.

109 Thomas RE, Jefferson T, Demicheli V, Rivetti D. Influenza vaccination for healthcare workers who work with the elderly. Cochrane Database Syst Rev 2006 (3), CD005187, DOI: 10.1002/14651858.

CHAPTER 7

Tuberculosis

Peter Daley & Marek Smieja

Case presentation 1

A 40-year-old man, who emigrated from India to Canada 2 years previously, presents with irregular fever and cough for several weeks. He is coughing up thick clear coin-like bits of sputum, sometimes streaked with blood. He had hemoptysis on one occasion. His fever is more marked in the evenings and he has cold sweats at night. He also has marked loss of appetite, and has lost some 10 kg of weight in the past 2 months. He smokes cigarettes but denies drinking alcohol. He works in the construction industry, but has been unable to work for a month.

On examination, the patient is thin, almost to the point of emaciation; the ribs stand out prominently, and the trachea is deviated to the right side. There is a hollow beneath the right clavicle. The skin feels hot and dry to the touch although there is no actual fever. There is dullness to percussion over the apex of the lung. Auscultation reveals moist crepitations and bronchial breathing over the same regions.

A chest radiograph reveals a dense opacity in the right apical region with a small cavity in the middle of the opacity. You admit him to hospital into a negative pressure, aerosol isolation room, and order sputum examination for acid-fast bacilli (AFB) and mycobacterial culture. To your surprise, his first sputum examination is negative for AFB. You wonder whether polymerase chain reaction (PCR) for *Mycobacterium tuberculosis* would help to rapidly diagnose this man's suspected pulmonary tuberculosis.

Evidence-Based Infectious Diseases, 2nd edition. Edited by Mark Loeb, Fiona Smaill and Marek Smieja. © 2009 Wiley-Blackwell Publishing, ISBN: 978-1-4051-7026-0

Epidemiology

Tuberculosis (TB) is an infectious disease caused by the bacterium *Mycobacterium tuberculosis*, and remains a major cause of morbidity and mortality throughout the world. An estimated 1.7 billion people, or nearly one-third of the world's population, have been infected, and every year there are an estimated 8.8 million new cases and 1.6 million deaths [1]. Global TB incidence was stable in 2005, but prevalence continued to rise [1]. TB was the eighth leading cause of death worldwide in 2002, and is projected to drop to twenty-third by 2030 [2]. TB is second only to HIV as a single cause of infectious disease-related mortality. TB was responsible for the loss of 14.3 million disability-adjusted life-years in 2005 [3]. About 95% of the total burden of TB is in resource-poor countries, especially in southeast Asia and sub-Saharan Africa [4].

Targets set by the World Health Organization (WHO) to achieve 70% case detection and 85% treatment success by 2005 were not met. Global case detection in 2006 was 60% (52–69%) and treatment success was 84% [1]. Interventions to meet the targets set by the Global Plan to Stop TB would cost an additional US$1.1 billion in 2007 [1]. In resource-poor nations, and particularly in sub-Saharan Africa, the HIV epidemic, poverty, displacement of populations caused by war or famine, and lack of comprehensive treatment and control programs have contributed to a resurgence of TB, prompting the World Health Organization to declare a Global Health Emergency in 1993. No country with a severe HIV epidemic has been able to successfully control TB.

In India, which alone accounts for 2 million active TB cases and 0.5 millions deaths per year, a large-scale effort to improve laboratory services, drug supplies and standardized regimens, directly-observed therapy, and improved reporting methods resulted in a major improvement in the proportion of patients completing therapy. It is estimated that the Revised National TB Control Program in India has prevented more than 1 million TB deaths since 1997 [1].

In contrast with high TB burden resource-poor nations, with annual TB incidence rates of between 60 and 641 cases per 100000 [1], the USA, Canada, and most industrialized countries have witnessed a steady decline in TB incidence through much of the 20th century. However, between 1985 and 1992, an unexpected increased incidence was observed. This has been attributed in part to the HIV epidemic, to an increased number of refugees from endemic countries, and to delayed recognition and control of inner-city outbreaks by underfunded public health departments [5]. With renewed government commitment, incidence has been declining since 1992, to 4.6 per 100000 in the year 2006, with a 46% decline observed between 1992 and 2006 [6]. In the year 2006, 26 of 50 American states reported an incidence of 3.5 cases per 100000 or fewer, the interim goal for the new millennium set out in 1989 by the Advisory Council for the Elimination of Tuberculosis strategic plan of the Centers for Disease Control and Prevention (CDC) [7]. These states, representing over one-quarter of the American population, are classified as "low-incidence states" and targeted for TB elimination. The Advisory Council for Elimination of Tuberculosis defined "eradication" as a level of less than 0.1 cases per 100000 per year [8].

Risk factors for infection and disease

The principal mode of transmission for *M. tuberculosis* is by airborne droplets, and consequently the primary focus is in the lungs. Infection generally does not manifest as disease, and progression to disease depends on a number of contributing factors. The risk factors for developing TB can be divided into factors that increase the probability of exposure to infection and factors that increase the probability of disease among those who become infected.

Given the low incidence of TB in industrialized countries, the major risk factor for exposure is previous habitation in endemic areas. Refugees and immigrants from TB-endemic areas of the world are at high risk of developing TB because of previous exposure, particularly in their first 5–10 years after arrival [9,10]. Initially, their TB incidence is similar to their country of origin, and after 5 years or more approaches that of their adopted country. Other groups at risk of TB exposure are household or institutional contacts of active TB cases, aboriginals, the homeless, injection drug users, and people in long-term care institutions [5,11–14]. Many of the elderly were exposed to TB in their childhood, particularly if born outside of the USA and Canada, as TB was epidemic throughout Europe and most of the world at that time. The elderly with previous infection are at risk for reactivation, particularly if they have an abnormal chest X-ray film and have never received "preventive treatment" [14], now termed treatment of latent TB infection (LTBI) [15].

Among those previously or concurrently exposed to *M. tuberculosis* infection, a number of risk factors have been shown to predispose to developing active disease. The strongest risk factors are concurrent HIV infection, associated with 50–200-fold increases in TB incidence [16,17]. The Centers for Disease Control and Prevention (CDC) recommend HIV testing in all patients diagnosed with TB [16]. Other risk factors include increasing age, malignancy, silicosis, liver or kidney disease, transplantation and other immunosuppression, chronic use of corticosteroids, alcoholism, malnutrition, gastrectomy, jejunoileal bypass, and diabetes mellitus [15,18]. New drugs such as tumor necrosis factor-alpha blockers, used for patients with severe rheumatoid arthritis, have been found to increase reactivation of TB [19]. In Mexico, indoor air pollution from traditional wood stoves was found to be strongly associated with developing TB (adjusted OR of 2·4) [20]. Smoking is a newly recognized but extremely prevalent risk factor for TB infection [21–25]. One metaanalysis of 16 studies published between 1956 and 2002 found increased pulmonary and extrapulmonary TB among smokers and their children [24] and a further metaanalysis of 33 studies showed a significantly increased risk of latent TB infection, a significantly increased risk of clinical TB and positive associations of smoking with TB mortality and passive smoking with TB [26].

Among new tuberculin skin test converters, 5% develop active TB within 2 years, and a further 5% are estimated to develop TB life-long [27]. These estimates are derived from studies in the 1950s and 1960s, when TB prevalence in the community was markedly higher than at present. Whether exposure to infection still carries the same risk today is unclear. Among patients with untreated HIV, the risk following exposure to *M. tuberculosis* may be as high as 8% per year, or a cumulative 50% or higher risk of developing active TB [17].

Diagnosis

Clinical presentation

The classic clinical features of active pulmonary TB include chronic cough, hemoptysis, expectoration of thick sputum, and constitutional symptoms such as fatigue or night sweats, anorexia, and weight loss. Although many case series exist, there are few population-based studies that describe symptoms of TB. In a population-based study set in Los Angeles County, in which 12% of patients had HIV, the incidence of cough was 48%, fever 29%, weight loss 45%, and hemoptysis 21% [28]. Cough for 2 weeks or more was only present in 52% of patients with pulmonary TB, while fever of over 2 weeks' duration was present in only 29%. The other population-based study was from the Ivory Coast, where 44% of patients had HIV [29]. In this study, cough was present in 80%, fever in 69%, and weight loss in 74%. Other studies have shown variable results. In one case series from Chicago of 110 patients, where 44 patients had pulmonary TB, only one patient with TB did not have either an abnormal chest radiograph, 2 or more weeks of cough, sputum production, or weight loss [30]. Predictive models have been developed to help better predict who requires hospital isolation in patients with suspected TB [31]. However, although these models were more sensitive than the existing respiratory isolation policy (91% and 82% for two retrospective groups vs 71% for isolation policy), the results are limited to smear-positive patients.

Chest radiograph

The diagnosis of pulmonary TB requires compatible changes on chest radiograph, accompanied by culture or other evidence of infection with *M. tuberculosis*. Radiographic changes depend on how recent the infection is, concomitant medical conditions (such as HIV or diabetes), and host reaction (fibrosis,

calcification). Pulmonary TB can be primary or post-primary. Primary TB commonly occurs in the lower lung since the droplet is preferentially inhaled into this region, but may involve any lobe. In about 5% of cases, the primary lesion results in clinical pneumonia, which is seen as a lobar or segmental infiltrate with ipsilateral lymphadenopathy. Multiple lobes may also be involved with gross mediastinal lymph node enlargement with or without pleural effusion. Primary TB is increasingly found in adults with acute TB in outbreaks in Canada and other industrialized countries, as many people have had no prior exposure to TB [32]. The areas of consolidation in primary TB may undergo cavitation, referred to as "progressive primary disease." Occasionally, a completely normal X-ray film may be seen in patients with small parenchymal or endobronchial lesions.

The predictive value and reproducibility of a radiograph system for screening of active TB was assessed in one study [33]. Inter-reader agreement using five broad categories was moderate (kappa values of 0·44–0·56). The adjusted odds of active TB, relative to normal or minor findings or granulomas, was 10·2 (95% CI 3.2–33) for fibronodular changes, 46·1 (95% CI 18–117) for parenchymal infiltrates, and 11.6 (95% CI 3·6–37) for pleural effusion.

Diabetic, compared with nondiabetic patients, more commonly had lower lobe disease and were more likely to have cavitation [34]. HIV-positive patients were more likely to have a primary pneumonia, pleural effusions, and multilobe disease. The X-ray film was altered by immune status: among 135 HIV/TB coinfected patients, CD4 T-lymphocyte count of <200 cells/L were more likely than those with counts >200 cells/L to have hilar adenopathy, and less likely to have cavitation [35].

Chest radiograph may be unable to distinguish active from inactive disease, or to exclude concomitant disease such as lung cancer. In such cases, high resolution CT or gallium scanning may be helpful. In a small case series, CT had 93% sensitivity and 100% specificity for detecting active pulmonary TB; gallium scanning had 100% sensitivity and 82% specificity [36].

Immunologic testing

The tuberculin skin test, and gamma-interferon release by lymphocytes stimulated with mycobacterial antigen, can detect infection with *M. tuberculosis*. Both tests are discussed extensively later in this chapter, under the heading of prevention of TB. For the diagnosis of active TB, the tuberculin skin test is often positive ($>5\,mm$ in HIV or close contact to known active case, otherwise $>10\,mm$). However, due to false positives (from previous BCG vaccination or other mycobacteria) and false negatives (anergy from malnutrition, HIV, or other immune compromise), the skin test is only helpful if unequivocally positive ($>20\,mm$). Even in such cases, lung disease may be due to other causes. At least 25% of patients with acute TB will have false-negative skin tests, although these may convert to positive as the patient is recovering.

The interferon gamma release assay (IGRA) has been shown to be more specific than the tuberculin skin test, correlate better with TB exposure, and be less confounded by BCG vaccination and nontuberculous mycobacterial infection [37]. IGRA cannot distinguish active from latent TB. For the diagnosis of latent TB infection, IGRA and tuberculin skin test have similar sensitivity, but IGRA has greater specificity (Elispot 97.7% and Quantiferon 92.5%) [38]. Discordance between skin test and IGRA is unexplained, as are conversions and reversions of results with serial testing.

The role of IGRA for the diagnosis of active TB in high TB burden countries has been assessed [9]. Among HIV-infected adults, sensitivity is 81–90% but specificity is poor due to indeterminate results. IGRA: CD_4 cell ratio may be helpful for diagnosis. Among HIV-negative adults, current IGRA have no role in the diagnosis of active TB. IGRA do not have prognostic or predictive capacity in active TB. The diagnosis of active TB should generally require the isolation of organism.

Microbiologic testing

Confirmatory diagnosis of active TB requires demonstration of the pathogen in appropriately stained smears together with culture of the organism or amplification of specific RNA or DNA. Although TB can affect any part of the body, the lungs are by far the most commonly affected. Hence sputum, and in the case of children, gastric lavage, is the most commonly examined specimen. Early morning specimens are best. The diagnostic yield of the third sputum specimen is only 2–5%, and so two specimens may be adequate, especially when a second clinic visit can be avoided [40]. Bronchoscopy may be indicated if the patient cannot cough up sputum, although most such patients can be identified by inducing sputum production with hypertonic saline [41]. Bronchial washings, brushings, and biopsy specimens may be obtained, and sputum that is collected immediately after bronchoscopy is frequently positive. A variety of other specimens such as urine, cerebrospinal fluid, pleural fluid, pus, or tissue biopsy specimens can be collected in suspected cases of extrapulmonary TB, but the yield of smear is low. Histopathologic examination may reveal granulomatous inflammation. Fresh or frozen tissue can be cultured for mycobacteria. Formalin-fixed tissue, while inappropriate for culture, may still be subjected to AFB stains followed by PCR.

During specimen collection, patients produce an aerosol that may be hazardous to the healthcare worker or others in close proximity to the patient. For this reason, the workers should use protective masks while collecting the specimens. The specimens must be collected in an isolated, well-ventilated area. Sputum induction is particularly prone to generating aerosols that infect staff and other patients.

Smear examination

Mycobacteria are acid-fast bacteria, which can be demonstrated in appropriately prepared specimens by Ziehl–Neelsen (ZN) or related stains. At least 100 fields, which examine only 1% of the entire smear, must be examined under the oil immersion objective before a specimen is declared negative. To find one acid-fast bacillus per field, there must be a minimum of 10^6 bacilli/mL of sputum; hence if there are 5000 bacilli/mL, there is only a 50% chance of finding the bacillus [42]. Thus the sensitivity of the smear examination is low. In surveys, the smear detects only about 50% of all culture-positive cases. Sensitivity is increased using fluorescent stains as compared to conventional Ziehl-Neelsen method, with similar specificity [43]. For laboratories doing high volume work, fluorescent microscopy has the further advantage of allowing more rapid specimen screening, although specialized instruments and skilled laboratory staff are required [42]. Using newer inexpensive, long-lasting light-emitting diode bulbs can allow conversion of conventional light microscopes to fluorescent capacity. Pretreatment of sputum by physical or chemical means is associated with an increase in smear sensitivity as compared to direct smearing [44].

Whereas a positive AFB smear may be diagnostic in an endemic country, fewer than 50% of AFB-positive sputa in industrialized countries may be due to *M. tuberculosis*. The remainder are due to nontuberculous mycobacteria, including *M. kansasii*, *M. avium intercellulare* complex, and *M. xenopii*. Thus, a positive AFB smear requires confirmation by culture, and, where available, by PCR.

Mycobacterial culture

As sputum AFB stain is insensitive, culture for mycobacteria will markedly improve detection of pulmonary TB. Results of culture by the conventional solid egg media take 2–8 weeks, whereas culture using the BACTEC radiometric system or other liquid media gives results in 4–14 days. Only sputum smear examination and PCR are available rapidly enough to influence the management of the acutely sick patient. Culture is estimated to be 80–85% sensitive, and 98–99% specific. Culture has an analytic sensitivity many times greater than sputum examination, and can detect as few as 10–100 bacilli/mL. However, suboptimal specimen collection or overly aggressive laboratory decontamination may result in false-negative cultures. Newer rapid liquid culture techniques such as MODS are more rapid, sensitive, and less costly than conventional culture [45]. After the colonies grow, they are identified by biochemical tests or, more rapidly, by nucleic acid hybridization. Newer identification tests based on detection of TB-specific antigens show improved performance over biochemical tests, and are very inexpensive [46,47].

Drug susceptibility testing is conventionally performed once an organism has been grown, and takes one more week. With current liquid broth methods, detection and drug susceptibility testing results are often available within 3–4 weeks. Newer colorimetric redox indicator methods are rapid and simple and have 89–100% sensitivity and specificity for rifampin and isoniazid results [48]. Molecular approaches to detection of resistance mutations offer single-day results that are comparable to conventional methods [49].

Nucleic acid amplification tests

Nucleic acid amplification tests (NAAT), whether in-house or commercially produced, are increasingly used to rapidly diagnose TB. They can be used for confirmation of smear-positive sputa, or applied directly for detection from sputum, fluids, or tissue. In low-prevalence countries, AFB-positive smears often represent nontuberculous mycobacteria. PCR is able in such cases to rapidly exclude *M. tuberculosis*, with implications for treatment and infection control. PCR would not be cost-effective in high-prevalence areas, since AFB-positive smears in such settings are virtually diagnostic. In either setting, PCR does not currently replace culture since the latter remains more sensitive, and a cultured organism is required to determine drug susceptibilities and for molecular fingerprinting.

Commercial NAAT applied to respiratory specimens has 96% sensitivity and 85% specificity in smear-positive specimens and 66% sensitivity and 98% specificity in smear-negative [50] but these estimates are suspect as studies are heterogeneous [51]. In-house NAAT applied to respiratory specimens show widely variable performance with high heterogeneity between studies, making summary estimates meaningless [52].

Commercial NAAT applied to pleural fluid demonstrates 62% sensitivity and 98% specificity, but in-house NAAT is highly heterogeneous [53]. Similarly commercial NAAT applied to cerebrospinal fluid gave 56% sensitivity and 98% specificity with variable results from in-house assays [54]. NAAT from tissue taken from suspected TB lymphadenitis showed highly variable performance [55].

Generally, studies reporting diagnostic performance of new tests for TB suffer from methodologic deficiencies, with poor blinding, inappropriate reference standard, no description of selection criteria, and use of discrepant analysis [56]. Guidelines on diagnostic testing have been published and future evaluations should comply with these in order to make results interpretable [57,58].

Since PCR detects virtually all AFB-positive specimens, and a proportion of AFB-negatives, it is being investigated for routine initial specimen examination. However, as *M. tuberculosis* may present in only some 1% of specimens submitted to a laboratory in a low-prevalence country the routine use of PCR is not cost-effective. However, if there is high clinical suspicion of TB, PCR is recommended despite AFB-negative smears [59].

Serological tests

Commercial antibody tests from blood demonstrate inadequate and variable performance for the diagnosis of TB, and are not recommended despite their widespread use in TB-endemic countries [60–62]. In contrast, adenosine deaminase testing of sterile fluids has excellent performance for the diagnosis of extrapulmonary TB, whether used for pleural fluid [63], pericarditis [64] or peritonitis [65].

Phage-based tests

Mycobacteriophage-based assays have been proposed for detection of TB and detection of drug resistance. Few studies have reported direct application to sputum specimens, but several studies show high sensitivity but low specificity for drug resistance detection [66,67]. Further large-scale work on phage assays has been stopped due to inadequate diagnostic performance.

Molecular fingerprinting

In industrialized countries with a low prevalence of TB, reactivation of latent TB disease accounts for the majority of clinical cases of TB. The uniqueness of cultured isolates can be demonstrated by molecular fingerprinting methods such as IS6110 or spoligotyping [68–71]. The finding of clustered isolates strongly suggests recent transmission, and has been shown in several settings to be much more sensitive than conventional public health contact tracing for identifying community outbreaks. Thus, in an outbreak in Baltimore, only 30% of clustered isolates had been detected by contact tracing. National and international databases are being set up to look for temporal and spatial clustering of *M. tuberculosis* isolates, and will be particularly important in low-prevalence countries for identifying otherwise undetected outbreaks. The worldwide occurrence of a multidrug-resistant "Beijing/W" strain was shown using molecular epidemiologic methods to be present not only in Asia, but as far as New York, Cuba, and Estonia [72].

Case presentation 1 (continued)

Your patient's second and third sputum samples are acid-fast positive for small numbers of characteristic bacilli. A nucleic acid amplification test confirms *M. tuberculosis* and you start him on isoniazid (INH), rifampicin (rifampin), pyrazinamide, and ethambutol. He consents to HIV antibody testing and tests negative. Two weeks later his culture confirms *M. tuberculosis*. One week later, his isolate is found to be fully susceptible to all first-line antituberculous drugs, and you discontinue his ethambutol. You plan to treat him with three drugs for a total of 2 months, followed by a further 4 months of isoniazid and rifampicin. You warn him about potential drug side effects, and prescribe vitamin B6 to minimize his chance of neuropathy. You notify the local public health department to arrange contact tracing. You ask the department about the availability of directly observed therapy (DOT), and wonder about the need for DOT in this man.

Treatment

The aim of treatment is to cure patients, prevent relapses, and avert deaths. The treatment of pulmonary TB has been subjected to numerous randomized clinical trials, primarily in developing and high-prevalence countries, although no systematic review of such trials was identified. A number of studies conducted by the British Medical Research Council in Singapore, Hong Kong, India, and East Africa compared various durations and regimens [73], and found that a combination of INH, rifampicin, and pyrazinamide for 2 months, followed by INH and rifampicin for a further 4 months, resulted in high (>96%) cure rates. The CDC recommends these three drugs, together with ethambutol, for initial treatment of TB [74].

For sputum-negative, culture-positive disease, randomized trials have demonstrated that 4 months or longer of therapy yielded very low relapse rates of 1–4% (depending on initial drug susceptibility) [75]. Inclusion of sputum-negative, culture-negative patients with compatible chest radiographs in these trials, however, suggests that these may have fallen more in the category of treatment of "latent TB infection" rather than necessarily representing active TB. Longer regimens result in higher success rates, but at a cost of lower adherence rates. There is not adequate evidence reporting relapse rate or mortality to compare short and long regimens [76].

There is no evidence to suggest that fluoroquinolones should be included in first-line regimens, and ciprofloxacin substitution has shown higher relapse and adverse event rates [77]. Rifabutin was not superior to rifampin in five trials [78].

In addition to examining the duration of therapy, randomized clinical trials have examined the efficacy of twice-weekly INH and rifampin in the continuation phase versus daily therapy. A Cochrane Library systematic review found that there was insufficient evidence to state that intermittent therapy was as effective as daily therapy [79]. Of 399 patients, intermittent therapy cured 99.5% versus 100% in the daily treatment arm. Relapses were 2.5% and 0%, respectively. However, as only a single trial was identified, the authors conclude that larger studies are required to more precisely estimate long-term cure. Intermittent regimens may be particularly attractive as part of supervised programs in which all doses are administered and witnessed by medical personnel (directly observed therapy, "DOT").

The effect of DOT remains unclear. There are cohort and before-and-after data to demonstrate the effectiveness of WHO's DOTS program, which utilizes DOT and short-course (6-month) therapy [6,80]. However, the program also emphasizes a number of other effective aspects of TB treatment including:

- appropriate laboratory facilities and training for microscopic diagnosis
- providing drugs and establishing conveniently located clinics
- appropriate record-keeping and follow-up.

While this program, properly implemented, has clearly worked in areas such as India [6], it remains unclear to what extent the direct supervision of pill-taking was responsible for the improvements.

In a metaanalysis of six randomized controlled trials of DOT or usual care, Volmink and Garner found no effect of DOT [81]. They note, however, that many of the DOT programs examined had poorly motivated staff and were inconvenient for patients to access. In one RCT of DOT in which patients were given a choice of treatment site, adherence was improved. The authors note that DOT is often more expensive than standard therapy, and requires a paternalistic model of medical care at variance with most other therapies. The authors note that an emphasis on incentives and enablers is probably as important as DOT. In many industrialized countries, DOT is used quite selectively for patients with multidrug-resistant (MDR)-TB, or among homeless people, injection drug users, or other groups at high risk of poor adherence.

Even with DOT, high adherence rates are not assured. Clinical trials of health education, monetary incentives, and reminders have found that monetary incentives were very effective at improving adherence to clinic visits among injection drug users on TB treatment [82]. In one randomized trial, a $5 incentive improved compliance two-fold compared with no intervention or education alone [83].

Adjunctive therapies for TB that have been studied include corticosteroids and immunotherapy, with a large RCT demonstrating more rapid symptom control [84]. A metaanalysis of corticosteroid use concluded that, compared with placebo, steroids were associated with more rapid resolution of pulmonary infiltrates, and did not affect sputum conversion [85]. There is insufficient evidence to recommend steroid treatment for TB pericarditis [86] or pleuritis [87], but it is indicated to reduce death and neurologic deficit in TB meningitis among HIV-negative patients [88].

Immunotherapy with *Mycobacterium vaccae* has been studied in seven trials, and summarized in a systematic review [89]. Immunotherapy was ineffective in altering mortality (OR 1.09; 95% CI 0.79–1.49), or in altering the proportion of study subjects with negative sputum smears or cultures. Immunotherapy was associated with increased local side effects including ulceration and scarring. The authors conclude that immunotherapy does not benefit TB patients.

The treatment of TB in the setting of HIV consists of standard therapies. Duration of treatment is not clear. HIV-coinfected patients tend to do equally well clinically and microbiologically, but they have an increased case fatality and TB recurrence rate, due to HIV effects. Timing of initiation of cotherapy is controversial as mortality is high, but immune reconstitution inflammatory syndrome (IRIS) may cause treatment discontinuation. Early ART is favored [90] and guidelines suggest a delay of only 2–8 weeks in those with CD4+ T-lymphocytes of fewer than 200×10^6/L (200 cells/mL) [91].

Three further interventions have demonstrated effectiveness. First, as TB is an AIDS-defining illness, all coinfected patients should be offered appropriate highly active antiretroviral therapy (HAART). This has not been studied specifically in an RCT, but can be extrapolated from cohort studies indicating high death rates in TB/HIV-coinfected patients in the pre-HAART era, and low mortality among AIDS patients taking appropriate antiretroviral medications (see Chapter 11). Second, secondary prevention with INH given to HIV/TB-coinfected patients was more effective than placebo in preventing recurrent TB [92]. This study was undertaken in Haiti, and its results are probably generalizable to other developing nations with high prevalence of TB. However, secondary prevention is unlikely to be useful in low-prevalence settings, since reinfection rather than relapse was probably responsible for recurrent TB [93]. Third, HIV/TB-coinfected patients have been shown to benefit from trimethoprim/sulfamethoxazole (TMP/SMX). In an RCT, TMP/SMX was more effective than placebo in preventing death and repeat hospitalization among coinfected patients [94]. However, CD4+ T-lymphocyte counts were not available in that study, and are most likely a better method for stratifying risk among HIV/TB-coinfected patients and for assessing the need for prophylaxis of opportunistic infections.

Drug-resistant TB

The World Health Organization reported in 2008 a global population-weighted proportion of drug resistance among new cases of 17.0% (any resistance) and 2.9% (isoniazid and rifampin resistant or "MDR"). Among previously treated cases, 35.0% had any resistance and 15.3% had MDR. MDR-TB is at critical levels in specific regions of the world, including Estonia, Latvia, the Oblasts of Ivanovo and Tomsk in Russia, and the provinces of Henan and Zhejiang in China. MDR-TB has been associated with poorer response to therapy, higher mortality, and higher treatment costs [95–98]. While no randomized clinical trials of therapy are available to guide optimal management strategies, guidelines suggest at least four drugs to which the organism is known or presumed to be susceptible, with at least 18 months duration of treatment [99]. For pulmonary MDR-TB not responding to multiple chemotherapy, surgical resection has been demonstrated to be effective in a number of case series [100,101].

In 2006, the first reports of extensively drug-resistant TB (XDR) emerged, from South Africa [102]. This strain is resistant to isoniazid and rifampin as well as at least one quinolone and one injectable agent [103]. The mortality in the first report was 100%, with a median survival time of 16 days among 44 patients, all of whom had HIV infection. The strain was clonal and probably nosocomially spread. Since then XDR has been reported from every country with the capacity to detect it [104]. Forty-five countries have at least one XDR case, and the proportion of MDR cases that meet the XDR definition range from 0 to 30% [105]. XDR cases have a significantly worse clinical outcome than MDR [106,107].

Case presentation 1 (continued)

You treat your patient for a total of 6 months. At 1 and 2 months, his sputum smears and culture are negative, and he is unable to produce sputum thereafter. You see him monthly to assess symptoms and adherence. At 4 weeks, his transaminase levels rise to 3 times baseline. As he is asymptomatic, you continue his therapy and these normalize by week 8. He completes therapy and is asked to present 1 year later for X-ray film follow-up. Contact tracing reveals no immediate family or fellow workers with symptoms or a positive TB skin test. You reassure him and his wife that the chances of a future recurrence are very low, and quite treatable if recurrence does occur.

Prevention of TB

Case presentation 2

You are asked to see a 25-year-old asymptomatic woman who recently immigrated to Canada from the Philippines. Her screening intracutaneous 5-unit PPD test is positive at 13 mm of induration. She does not recall any previous skin testing. She received BCG vaccine as a young child and has had no known exposure to active TB among family, friends, or occupational contacts. She denies respiratory symptoms, has an unremarkable clinical examination, and has a normal chest radiograph. You diagnose latent TB infection (LTBI) and recommend INH treatment for 9 months. You measure baseline liver enzymes, and counsel her regarding potential side effects. You wonder whether the BCG vaccine is responsible for her TB skin test reactivity. You have read about a new blood test for TB and wonder if this would provide firmer evidence for *M. tuberculosis* exposure. Finally, you wonder whether a 6-month or 9-month regimen of INH is preferred.

BCG vaccination

Prevention of active TB has focused on two strategies: vaccination of children with BCG (bacille

Calmette–Guérin), and tuberculin skin testing followed by treatment of LTBI. Childhood immunization with BCG has been studied in three separate metaanalyses, which pooled both randomized controlled trials and case–control studies [108–110]. BCG was shown to reduce miliary and meningeal TB by 75–86%, and pulmonary TB in children by 50%. However, great variation in efficacy was seen in different trials, and explained in part by distance from the equator [111]. The disadvantages of routine BCG vaccination include false-positive tuberculin skin tests (see below), which compromises contact tracing and initiation of INH treatment of LTBI; cutaneous abscesses; and occasional disseminated BCG.

The tuberculin skin test

The tuberculin skin test consists of injecting 5 units of purified protein derivative "S" (PPD-S) intracutaneously into the volar aspect of the forearm, and measuring the millimeters of induration in the transverse diameter 48–72 hours later. The tuberculin skin test is a well-validated measure of infection with *M. tuberculosis*. It is not, however, an optimal test for the diagnosis of active disease.

The test measures delayed-type hypersensitivity to mycobacterial antigen. Conversion of the skin test may take 3 months after exposure to infection, and a change of 10 mm or more identifies patients who are at high risk for developing active TB (estimated at 5% in the next 2 years, and a further 5% lifelong) [27].

In the immunocompetent individual without acute symptoms of TB, the test approaches 100% sensitivity [11]. Among patients with acute TB, false negatives of 25% have been reported. Such anergy may be specific for *M. tuberculosis*, or there may be a general anergy to multiple antigens. Anergy is more common among HIV-positive and other immunocompromised patients, or among the malnourished. Although individuals anergic to multiple antigens can be identified by testing intracutaneous responses to candida, tetanus, mumps, or other common antigens, these tests have poor reproducibility and are no longer recommended [112].

False-positive tuberculin skin tests may result from previous BCG vaccination or from exposure to other mycobacteria. A metaanalysis has shown that, while BCG vaccination is associated with skin test positivity, the skin test is rarely >15 mm, and the effects

rarely persist beyond 15 years [113]. Other endemic mycobacteria may also cause false-positive tuberculin skin tests, and the cut-off for "positivity" in such areas may need to be >12 mm or >15 mm of induration.

Various cut-off values for interpreting tuberculin skin test positivity have been recommended [114,115]. In India and many areas with high TB prevalence, >12 mm is used as a cut-off for positivity. In the USA, the use of three different cut-off points has been recommended. For patients with HIV, recent contact with a patient with active TB, or signs of previous TB on chest radiograph, a skin test of >5 mm identifies infection. For patients with other risk factors for infection, >10 mm is used as a cut-off. These include immigrants from endemic countries and patients with silicosis, liver or kidney disease, gastrectomy or ileal bypass, the homeless, or aboriginals. In patients at low risk of infection or disease, >15 mm is used. However, testing low-risk individuals with tuberculin skin tests are no longer generally recommended [15]. A fourth criterion for positivity is a change in induration by 5 mm between serial tests. For individuals undergoing screening prior to employment, a baseline tuberculin test may stimulate remote immunity due to previous BCG or *M. tuberculosis* infection. Such "boosting" of immunity is identified by the two-step tuberculin test, in which the skin test is repeated 1 week or more after the initial test. Detection of the boosted response prevents ascribing the boosted response to recent exposure, should the person be retested in the future [116].

Tuberculin testing is recommended to aid diagnosis (see previous discussion) and to identify asymptomatic infected individuals who may be candidates for treatment of LTBI. When contacts of an active case are investigated, a skin test of >5 mm indicates recent exposure and >5% risk of active TB. Such patients have been shown to benefit from monotherapy with INH.

Interferon gamma release assays

Given the difficulties in interpreting the tuberculin skin test, and the need for the patient to return for a second visit, other tests for detecting immune responses to *M. tuberculosis* have been developed [117–120]. Interferon gamma release assays detect interferon produced by an in vitro memory immune response to antigens specific to *M. tuberculosis* such as ESAT-6, CFP-10, and TB 7.7. This test has been shown to correlate well with skin testing [121], and is approved by the Food and Drug Administration (FDA) in the USA. It is recommended to be used in the USA in place of tuberculin skin test in all testing situations [122]. This test is less influenced by BCG vaccination, correlates better with TB exposure, and is more specific than the tuberculin skin test [37].

Treatment of LTBI

Treatment of latent TB infection is the strategy of treating asymptomatic infected patients to prevent future active TB [11]. INH monotherapy for 6–12 months, rifampicin for 4 months, or rifampicin/pyrazinamide for 2 months, have all been studied in randomized clinical trials of LTBI. The comparator in these trials was either placebo, or INH.

Three metaanalyses for treatment of LTBI were identified. For non-HIV patients, Cochrane reviewers identified 11 randomized trials of INH versus placebo, which enrolled 73 375 people between 1952 and 1994 [123]. They calculated an overall efficacy for INH versus placebo to be a relative risk of 0.40 (95% CI 0·31–0.52, a relative risk reduction of 60%). INH also reduced extrapulmonary TB and TB deaths, whereas all-cause mortality was unchanged (RR 1.10; 95% CI 0.94, 1.28). Durations of less than 6 months were no more effective than placebo. Both 6- and 12-month regimens were more effective than placebo, with relative risks of 0.44 (95% CI 0.27–0.73) and 0.38 (95% CI 0.28–0.50), respectively. Direct comparison of the efficacies of these two regimens is misleading, however, as heterogeneous study populations were randomized in the various studies. In the only direct randomized comparison of 6 versus 12 months [124], relative efficacy was a 65% and 75% reduction, respectively (RR 1.4; 95% CI 0.8–2.4). The difference was not statistically significant. In subgroup analyses, those who took 80% or more of their drug had efficacy of 93% with 12 months' treatment, versus 69% with the 6-month regimen. On the basis of this study, and a reinterpretation of the Alaskan US Public Health Service study [125], the CDC has recommended 9 months of treatment for latent TB infection [11].

In HIV-positive people, two metaanalyses have been published [126,127]. Any prophylaxis regimen was more effective than placebo with a relative risk of active TB of 0.64 (95% CI 0·51–0·81). Those with a positivie tuberculin skin test had more benefit (RR 0.38; 95% CI: 0.25–0.57) than those with a negative tuberculin skin test (RR 0.83; 95% CI: 0.58–1.18). In spite of the reduction in subsequent active TB with preventive therapy, all-cause mortality was not reduced (RR 0·95; 95% CI: 0.85–1.06), although a beneficial estimate.

Other effective regimens studied in randomized trials include rifampicin alone for 4 months, or rifampicin with pyrazinamide for 2 months. The combination of rifampicin with pyrazinamide has been studied in three RCTs, and shown to be at least as effective as INH with similar tolerability [128–130]. Subsequently, a case series reported a number of individuals with hepatotoxicity, including a number of deaths, secondary to the combination of rifampicin with pyrazinamide [131]. The CDC now recommends caution with this regimen [132], and does not recommend this regimen for pregnant women.

Current ATS/CDC recommendations for treatment of LTBI are: 9 (preferred) or 6 months of INH, or 4 months of rifampicin. The 2-month regimen of rifampicin and pyrazinamide should only be considered if the risks justify the benefits. For latent MDR-TB infection, two drugs are recommended to which susceptibility has been demonstrated in the index case. These would usually include pyrazinamide and a quinolone, although one case series demonstrated that this combination is poorly tolerated [133].

In cases exposed to known MDR-TB, the role of prophylaxis is unclear and individual decisions should be made based on risks and benefits [134,135].

Case presentation 2 (continued)

Your patient is treated with daily INH and vitamin B6. She increasingly complains of tiredness and headaches, and difficulty concentrating on her university studies. After 5 months, she has decided that she will not continue with treatment. You convince her to complete 6 months of therapy, which you know to be an acceptable alternative to the full 9 months recommended by the CDC, and she agrees to this. You emphasize to her that treatment for latent TB infection is imperfect and that a small chance of future TB remains. You recommend that, should she ever develop symptoms compatible with TB, she will need to be investigated for this. You estimate that her baseline lifetime risk of TB reactivation was up to 5%, and following treatment, you have reduced this risk to 2% or less.

References

1 Global tuberculosis control: surveillance, planning, financing. WHO report 2007. Geneva: World Health Organization; 2007. Report No.: WHO/HTM/TB/2007.376.

2 Mathers CD, Loncar D. Projections of global mortality and burden of disease from 2002 to 2030. PLoS Med 2006;3(11): e442.

3 Projections of Mortality and Burden of Disease 2006. Geneva: World Health Organization; 2006.

4 Kochi A. The global tuberculosis situation and the new control strategy of the WHO. Tubercle 1991;72:1–6.

5 Control of tuberculosis in the United States. Joint Statement of the American Thoracic Society, the Centers for Disease Control, and the Infectious Disease Society of America. Respir Care 1993;38:929–39.

6 Khatri GR, Frieden TR. Controlling tuberculosis in India. N Engl J Med 2002;347:1420–5.

7 CDC. Reported Tuberculosis in the United States, 2006. Atlanta, Georgia: US Department of Health and Human Services, CDC; 2007.

8 CDC. A strategic plan for the elimination of tuberculosis in the United States. MMWR 1989;38(S-3).

9 Cowie RL, Sharpe JW. Tuberculosis among immigrants: interval from arrival in Canada to diagnosis. A 5-year study in southern Alberta. CMAJ 1998;158:599–602.

10 Marks GB, Bai J, Simpson SE, Sullivan EA, Stewart GJ. Incidence of tuberculosis among a cohort of tuberculin-positive refugees in Australia: reappraising the estimates of risk. Am J Respir Crit Care Med 2000;162:1851–4.

11 Revised treatment and testing guidelines for latent tuberculosis infection. Rep Med Guidel Outcomes Res 2000;11:9–10.

12 Prevention and control of tuberculosis among homeless persons. Recommendations of the Advisory Council for the Elimination of Tuberculosis. MMWR Recomm Rep 1992;41(RR-5):13–23.

13 Prevention and control of tuberculosis in US communities with at-risk minority populations. Recommendations of the Advisory Council for the Elimination of Tuberculosis. MMWR Recomm Rep 1992;41(RR-5):1–11.

14 Prevention and control of tuberculosis in facilities providing long-term care to the elderly. Recommendations of the Advisory Committee for Elimination of Tuberculosis. MMWR Recomm Rep 1990;39(RR-10):7–13.

15 Centers for Disease Control and Prevention. Targeted tuberculin testing and treatment of latent tuberculosis infection. MMWR 2000;49(RR-6):1–51.

16 Rose VL. CDC calls for tuberculosis screening and treatment for all patients with HIV infection. Am Fam Physician 1999;59:1682,1687.

17 Selwyn PA, Hartel D, Lewis VA, et al. A prospective study of the risk of tuberculosis among intravenous drug users with human immunodeficiency virus infection. N Engl J Med 1989;320:545–50.

18 Thulstrup AM, Molle I, Svendsen N, Sorensen HT. Incidence and prognosis of tuberculosis in patients with cirrhosis of the liver. A Danish nationwide population based study. Epidemiol Infect 2000;124:221–5.

19 Long R, Gardam M. Tumor necrosis factor-alpha inhibitors and the reactivation of latent tuberculosis infection. CMAJ 2003;168:1153–6.

20 Perez-Padilla R, Perez-Guzman C, Baez-Saldana R, Torres-Cruz A. Cooking with biomass stoves and tuberculosis: a case control study. Int J Tuberc Lung Dis 2001;5:441–7.

21 Yach D. Partnering for better lung health: improving tobacco and tuberculosis control. Int J Tuberc Lung Dis 2000;4:693–7.

22 Gajalakshmi V, Peto R, Kanaka TS, Jha P. Smoking and mortality from tuberculosis and other diseases in India: retrospective study of 43 000 adult male deaths and 35 000 controls. Lancet 2003;362:507–15.

23 Kolappan C, Gopi PG. Tobacco smoking and pulmonary tuberculosis. Thorax 2002;57:964–6.

24 Maurya V, Vijayan VK, Shah A. Smoking and tuberculosis: an association overlooked. Int J Tuberc Lung Dis 2002;6:942–51.

25 Tekkel M, Rahu M, Loit HM, Baburin A. Risk factors for pulmonary tuberculosis in Estonia. Int J Tuberc Lung Dis 2002;6:887–94.

26 Lin HH, Ezzati M, Murray M. Tobacco smoke, indoor air pollution and tuberculosis: a systematic review and meta-analysis. PLoS Med 2007;4(1):e20.

27 Ferebee SH. Controlled chemoprophylaxis trials in tuberculosis: a general review. Bibl Tuberc 1970;26: 28–106.

28 Miller AG, Asch SM, Yu EI, et al. A population-based survey of tuberculosis symptoms: how atypical are atypical presentations? Clin Infect Dis 2000;293–9.

29 Gnaore E, Sassan-Morokro M, Kassim S, et al. A comparison of clinical features in tuberculosis associated with infection with human immunodeficiency viruses 1 and 2. Trans Royal Soc Trop Med Hyg 1993;87:57–9.

30 Cohen R, Muzaffar S, Capellan J, Azar H, Chinikamwala M. The validity of classic symptoms and chest radiograph configuration in predicting pulmonary tuberculosis. Chest 1996;109:420–3.

31 Tattevin P, Casalino E, Fleury L, et al. The validity of medical history, classic symptoms, and chest radiographs in predicting pulmonary tuberculosis. Chest 1996;115:1248–53.

32 Long R, Cowie R. Tuberculosis: 4. Pulmonary disease. CMAJ 1999;160:1344–8.

33 Graham S, Das GK, Hidvegi RJ, et al. Chest radiograph abnormalities associated with tuberculosis: reproducibility and yield of active cases. Int J Tuberc Lung Dis 2002;137–42.

34 Perez-Guzman C, Torres-Cruz A, Villarreal-Velarde H, Salazar-Lezama MA, Vargas MH. Atypical radiological images of pulmonary tuberculosis in 192 diabetic patients: a comparative study. Int J Tuberc Lung Dis 2001;5:455–61.

35 Perlman DC, el Sadr WM, Nelson ET, et al. Variation of chest radiographic patterns in pulmonary tuberculosis by degree of human immunodeficiency virus-related immunosuppression. The Terry Beirn Community Programs for Clinical Research on AIDS (CPCRA). The AIDS Clinical Trials Group (ACTG). Clin Infect Dis 1997;25:242–6.

36 Lai FM, Liam CK, Paramsothy M, George J. The role of 67gallium scintigraphy and high resolution computed tomography as predictors of disease activity in sputum smear-negative pulmonary tuberculosis. Int J Tuberc Lung Dis 1997;1:563–9.

37 Pai M, Riley LW, Colford JM, Jr. Interferon-gamma assays in the immunodiagnosis of tuberculosis: a systematic review. Lancet Infect Dis 2004;4(12):761–76.

38 Menzies D, Pai M, Comstock G. Meta-analysis: new tests for the diagnosis of latent tuberculosis infection: areas of uncertainty and recommendations for research. Ann Intern Med 2007;146(5):340–54.

39 Daley P, Chordia P. What is the clinical utility of interferon-γ release assays for the diagnosis of TB in high-TB-burden countries? Future Medicine 2008;5(3).

40 Mase SR, Ramsay A, Ng V, et al. Yield of serial sputum specimen examinations in the diagnosis of pulmonary tuberculosis: a systematic review. Int J Tuberc Lung Dis 2007;11(5):485–95.

41 Anderson C, Inhaber N, Menzies D. Comparison of sputum induction with fiber-optic bronchoscopy in the diagnosis of tuberculosis. Am J Respir Crit Care Med 1995;152 (Pt 1):1570–4.

42 Laszlo A. Tuberculosis: 7. Laboratory aspects of diagnosis. CMAJ 1999;160:1725–9.

43 Steingart KR, Henry M, Ng V, et al. Fluorescence versus conventional sputum smear microscopy for tuberculosis: a systematic review. Lancet Infect Dis 2006;6(9):570–81.

44 Steingart KR, Ng V, Henry M, et al. Sputum processing methods to improve the sensitivity of smear microscopy for tuberculosis: a systematic review. Lancet Infect Dis 2006;6(10):664–74.

45 Moore DA, Evans CA, Gilman RH, et al. Microscopic-observation drug-susceptibility assay for the diagnosis of TB. N Engl J Med 2006;355(15):1539–50.

46 Hirano K, Aono A, Takahashi M, Abe C. Mutations including IS6110 insertion in the gene encoding the MPB64 protein of Capilia TB-negative Mycobacterium tuberculosis isolates. J Clin Microbiol 2004;42(1):390–2.

47 Hillemann D, Rusch-Gerdes S, Richter E. Application of the Capilia TB assay for culture confirmation of Mycobacterium tuberculosis complex isolates. Int J Tuberc Lung Dis 2005;9(12):1409–11.

48 Martin A, Portaels F, Palomino JC. Colorimetric redox-indicator methods for the rapid detection of multidrug resistance in Mycobacterium tuberculosis: a systematic review and meta-analysis. J Antimicrob Chemother 2007;59(2):175–83.

49 Barnard M, Albert H, Coetzee G, O'Brien R, Bosman ME. Rapid molecular screening for multidrug-resistant tuberculosis in a high-volume public health laboratory in South Africa. Am J Respir Crit Care Med 2008;177(7):787–92.

50 Greco S, Girardi E, Navarra A, Saltini C. Current evidence on diagnostic accuracy of commercially based nucleic acid amplification tests for the diagnosis of pulmonary tuberculosis. Thorax 2006;61(9):783–90.

51 Ling DI, Flores LL, Riley LW, Pai M. Commercial nucleic-acid amplification tests for diagnosis of pulmonary tuberculosis in respiratory specimens: meta-analysis and meta-regression. PLoS ONE 2008;3(2):e1536.

52 Flores LL, Pai M, Colford JM, Jr., Riley LW. In-house nucleic acid amplification tests for the detection of Mycobacterium tuberculosis in sputum specimens: meta-analysis and meta-regression. BMC Microbiol 2005;5:55.

53 Pai M, Flores LL, Hubbard A, Riley LW, Colford JM, Jr. Nucleic acid amplification tests in the diagnosis of tuberculous pleuritis: a systematic review and meta-analysis. BMC Infect Dis 2004;4:6.

54 Pai M, Flores LL, Pai N, Hubbard A, Riley LW, Colford JM, Jr. Diagnostic accuracy of nucleic acid amplification tests for tuberculous meningitis: a systematic review and meta-analysis. Lancet Infect Dis 2003;3(10):633–43.

55 Daley P, Thomas S, Pai M. Nucleic acid amplification tests for the diagnosis of tuberculous lymphadenitis: a systematic review. Int J Tuberc Lung Dis 2007;11(11):1166–76.

56 Pai M, O'Brien R. Tuberculosis diagnostics trials: do they lack methodological rigor? Expert Rev Mol Diagn 2006; 6(4):509–14.

57 Bossuyt PM, Reitsma JB, Bruns DE, et al. Towards complete and accurate reporting of studies of diagnostic accuracy: the STARD initiative. Ann Clin Biochem 2003;40(Pt 4): 357–63.

58 Whiting PF, Weswood ME, Rutjes AW, Reitsma JB, Bossuyt PN, Kleijnen J. Evaluation of QUADAS, a tool for the quality assessment of diagnostic accuracy studies. BMC Med Res Methodol 2006;6:9.

59 Sarmiento OL, Weigle KA, Alexander J, Weber DJ, Miller WC. Assessment by meta-analysis of PCR for diagnosis of smear-negative pulmonary tuberculosis. J Clin Microbiol 2003;41:3233–40.

60 Steingart KR, Henry M, Laal S, et al. A systematic review of commercial serological antibody detection tests for the diagnosis of extrapulmonary tuberculosis. Postgrad Med J 2007;83(985):705–12.

61 Steingart KR, Henry M, Laal S, et al. A systematic review of commercial serological antibody detection tests for the diagnosis of extrapulmonary tuberculosis. Thorax 2007;62(10):911–8.

62 Steingart KR, Henry M, Laal S, et al. Commercial serological antibody detection tests for the diagnosis of pulmonary tuberculosis: a systematic review. PLoS Med 2007;4(6):e202.

63 Goto M, Noguchi Y, Koyama H, Hira K, Shimbo T, Fukui T. Diagnostic value of adenosine deaminase in tuberculous pleural effusion: a meta-analysis. Ann Clin Biochem 2003;40(Pt 4):374–81.

64 Tuon FF, Silva VI, Almeida GM, Antonangelo L, Ho YL. The usefulness of adenosine deaminase in the diagnosis of tuberculous pericarditis. Rev Inst Med Trop Sao Paulo 2007;49(3):165–70.

65 Riquelme A, Calvo M, Salech F, et al. Value of adenosine deaminase (ADA) in ascitic fluid for the diagnosis of tuberculous peritonitis: a meta-analysis. J Clin Gastroenterol 2006;40(8):705–10.

66 Kalantri S, Pai M, Pascopella L, Riley L, Reingold A. Bacteriophage-based tests for the detection of Mycobacterium

tuberculosis in clinical specimens: a systematic review and meta- analysis. BMC Infect Dis 2005;5(1):59.

67 Pai M, Kalantri S, Pascopella L, Riley LW, Reingold AL. Bacteriophage-based assays for the rapid detection of rifampicin resistance in *Mycobacterium tuberculosis*: a meta-analysis. J Infect 2005;51(3):175–87.

68 Hernandez-Garduno E, Kunimoto D, et al. Predictors of clustering of tuberculosis in Greater Vancouver: a molecular epidemiologic study. CMAJ 2002;167:349–52.

69 Kulaga S, Behr M, Musana K, et al. Molecular epidemiology of tuberculosis in Montreal. CMAJ 2002; 167:353–4.

70 Kulaga S, Behr MA, Schwartzman K. Genetic fingerprinting in the study of tuberculosis transmission. CMAJ 1999;161:1165–9.

71 Murray MB. Molecular epidemiology and the dynamics of tuberculosis transmission among foreign-born people. CMAJ 2002;167:355–6.

72 Glynn JR, Whiteley J, Bifani PJ, Kremer K, van Soolingen D. Worldwide occurrence of Beijing/W strains of *Mycobacterium tuberculosis*: a systematic review. Emerg Infect Dis 2002;8:843–9.

73 Fox W, Ellard GA, Mitchison DA. Studies on the treatment of tuberculosis undertaken by the British Medical Research Council tuberculosis units, 1946–1986, with relevant subsequent publications. Int J Tuberc Lung Dis 1999;3(Suppl.2): S231–S279.

74 From the Centers for Disease Control and Prevention. Initial therapy for tuberculosis in the era of multidrug resistance: recommendations of the Advisory Council for the Elimination of Tuberculosis. JAMA 1993;270: 694–8.

75 A controlled trial of 3-month, 4-month, and 6-month regimens of chemotherapy for sputum-smear-negative pulmonary tuberculosis. Results at 5 years. Hong Kong Chest Service/Tuberculosis Research Center, Madras/ British Medical Research Council. Am Rev Respir Dis 1989;139:871–6.

76 Gelband H. Regimens of less than six months for treating tuberculosis. Cochrane Database Syst Rev 1999 (4), CD001362, DOI 10.1002/14651858.

77 Ziganshina LE, Squire SB. Fluoroquinolones for treating tuberculosis. Cochrane Database Syst Rev 2008 (1), CD004795, DOI 10.1002/14651858.

78 Davies G, Cerri S, Richeldi L. Rifabutin for treating pulmonary tuberculosis. Cochrane Database Syst Rev 2007 (4), CD005159, DOI 10.1002/14651858.

79 Mwandumba HC, Squire SB. Fully intermittent dosing with drugs for treating tuberculosis in adults (Cochrane Review). Chichester, UK: John Wiley & Sons, Ltd. The Cochrane Library, Issue 4, 2003.

80 Olle-Goig JE, Alvarez J. Treatment of tuberculosis in a rural area of Haiti: directly observed and non-observed regimens. The experience of Hospital Albert Schweitzer. Int J Tuberc Lung Dis 2001;5:137–41.

81 Volmink J, Garner P. Directly observed therapy for treating tuberculosis (Cochrane Review). Chichester, UK: John Wiley & Sons, Ltd. The Cochrane Library, Issue 4, 2003.

82 Volmink J, Garner P. Systematic review of randomized controlled trials of strategies to promote adherence to tuberculosis treatment. BMJ 1997;315:1403–6.

83 Tulsky JP, Pilot L, Hahn JA, et al. Adherence to isoniazid prophylaxis in the homeless: a randomized controlled trial. Arch Intern Med 2000;160:697–702.

84 Lee CH, Wang WJ, Lan RS, Tsai YH, Chiang YC. Corticosteroids in the treatment of tuberculous pleurisy. A double-blind, placebo-controlled, randomized study. Chest 1988;94:1256–9.

85 Smego RA, Ahmed N. A systematic review of the adjunctive use of systemic corticosteroids for pulmonary tuberculosis. Int J Tuberc Lung Dis 2003;7:208–13.

86 Mayosi BM, Ntsekhe M, Volmink JA, Commerford PJ. Interventions for treating tuberculous pericarditis. Cochrane Database Syst Rev 2002 (4), CD000526, DOI 10.1002/14651858.

87 Engel ME, Matchaba PT, Volmink J. Corticosteroids for tuberculous pleurisy. Cochrane Database Syst Rev 2007 (4), CD001876, DOI 10.1002/14651858.

88 Prasad K, Singh MB. Corticosteroids for managing tuberculous meningitis. Cochrane Database Syst Rev 2008 (1), CD002244, DOI 10.1002/14651858.

89 de Bruyn G, Garner P. *Mycobacterium vaccae* immunotherapy for treating tuberculosis (Cochrane Review). Chichester, UK: John Wiley & Sons, Ltd. The Cochrane Library, Issue 4, 2003.

90 Schiffer JT, Sterling TR. Timing of antiretroviral therapy initiation in tuberculosis patients with AIDS: a decision analysis. J Acquir Immune Defic Syndr 2007;44(2):229–34.

91 Antiretroviral therapy for HIV infection in adults and adolescents in resource-limited settings: Towards universal access. Recommendations for a public health approach. Geneva: World Health Organization; 2006.

92 Fitzgerald DW, Desvarieux M, Severe P, et al. Effect of posttreatment isoniazid on prevention of recurrent tuberculosis in HIV-1 infected individuals: a randomized trial. Lancet 2000;356:1470–4.

93 van Rie A, Warren R, Richardson M, et al. Exogenous reinfection as a cause of recurrent tuberculosis after curative treatment. N Engl J Med 1999;341:1174–9.

94 Wiktor SZ, Sassan-Morokro M, Grant AD, et al. Efficacy of trimethoprim-sulphamethoxazole prophylaxis to decrease morbidity and mortality in HIV-1 infected patients with tuberculosis in Abidjan, Cote d'Ivoire: a randomized controlled trial. Lancet 1999;353:1469–75.

95 Geerligs WA, Van Altena R, De Lange WCM, van Soolingen D, Van Der Werf TS. Multidrug-resistant tuberculosis: long-term treatment outcome in the Netherlands. Int J Tuberc Lung Dis 2000;4:758–64.

96 Flament-Saillour M, Robert J, Jarlier V, Grosset J. Outcome of multi-drug-resistant tuberculosis in France: a nation-wide case-control study. Am J Respir Crit Care Med 1999;160:587–93.

97 Singla R, Al Sharif N, Al Sayegh MO, Osman MM, Shaikh MA. Influence of anti-tuberculosis drug resistance on the treatment outcome of pulmonary tuberculosis patients

receiving DOTS in Riyadh, Saudi Arabia. Int J Tuberc Lung Dis 2002;6:585–91.

98 Subhash HS, Ashwin I, Jesudason MV, et al. Clinical characteristics and treatment response among patients with multidrug-resistant tuberculosis: a retrospective study. Indian J Chest Dis Allied Sci 2003;45:97–103.

99 Hopewell PC, Pai M, Maher D, Uplekar M, Raviglione MC. International standards for tuberculosis care. Lancet Infect Dis 2006;6(11):710–25.

100 Chiang CY, Yu MC, Bai KJ, et al. Pulmonary resection in the treatment of patients with pulmonary multidrugresistant tuberculosis in Taiwan. Int J Tuberc Lung Dis 2001;5:272–7.

101 Sung SW, Kang CH, Kim YT, et al. Surgery increased the chance of cure in multi-drug resistant pulmonary tuberculosis. Eur J Cardiothorac Surg 1999;16:187–93.

102 Gandhi NR, Moll A, Sturm AW, et al. Extensively drug-resistant tuberculosis as a cause of death in patients co-infected with tuberculosis and HIV in a rural area of South Africa. Lancet 2006;368(9547):1575–80.

103 Case definition for extensively drug-resistant tuberculosis. Wkly Epidemiol Rec 2006;81(42):408.

104 Matteelli A, Migliori GB, Cirillo D, Centis R, Girard E, Raviglion M. Multidrug-resistant and extensively drug-resistant *Mycobacterium tuberculosis*: epidemiology and control. Expert Rev Anti Infect Ther 2007;5(5):857–71.

105 Anti-tuberculosis drug resistance in the world. Fourth global report. Geneva: World Health Organization; 2008. Report No.: WHO/HTM/TB/2008.394.

106 Migliori GB, Besozzi G, Girardi E, et al. Clinical and operational value of the extensively drug-resistant tuberculosis definition. Eur Respir J 2007;30(4):623–6.

107 Migliori GB, Lange C, Girardi E, et al. Extensively drug-resistant tuberculosis is worse than multidrug-resistant tuberculosis: different methodology and settings, same results. Clin Infect Dis 2008;46(6):958–9.

108 Colditz GA, Brewer TF, Berkey CS, et al. Efficacy of BCG vaccine in the prevention of tuberculosis. Meta-analysis of the published literature. JAMA 1994;271:698–702.

109 Colditz GA, Berkey CS, Mosteller F, et al. The efficacy of bacillus Calmette-Guerin vaccination of newborns and infants in the prevention of tuberculosis: meta-analyses of the published literature. Pediatrics 1995;96(Pt 1):29–35.

110 Brewer TF. Preventing tuberculosis with bacillus Calmette-Guerin vaccine: a meta-analysis of the literature. Clin Infect Dis 2000;31(Suppl.3):S64–S67.

111 Wilson ME, Fineberg HV, Colditz GA. Geographic latitude and the efficacy of bacillus Calmette-Guerin vaccine. Clin Infect Dis 1995;20:982–91.

112 Anergy skin testing and tuberculosis [corrected] preventive therapy for HIV-infected persons: revised recommendations. Centers for Disease Control and Prevention. MMWR Recomm Rep 1997;46(RR-15):1–10.

113 Wang L, Turner MO, Elwood RK, Schulzer M, FitzGerald JM. A meta-analysis of the effect of Bacille Calmette Guerin vaccination on tuberculin skin test measurements. Thorax 2002;57:804–9.

114 Targeted tuberculin testing and treatment of latent tuberculosis infection. American Thoracic Society. MMWR Recomm Rep 2000;49(RR-6):1–51.

115 Duchin JS, Jereb JA, Nolan CM, Smith P, Onorato IM. Comparison of sensitivities to two commercially available tuberculin skin test reagents in persons with recent tuberculosis. Clin Infect Dis 1997;25:661–3.

116 Sepkowitz KA, Feldman J, Louther J, et al. Benefit of two step PPD testing of new employees at a New York City hospital. Am J Infect Control 1997;25:283–6.

117 Stuart RL, Olden D, Johnson PD, et al. Effect of anti-tuberculosis treatment on the tuberculin interferongamma response in tuberculin skin test (TST) positive health care workers and patients with tuberculosis. Int J Tuberc Lung Dis 2000;4:555–61.

118 Arend SM, Engelhard AC, Groot G, et al. Tuberculin skin testing compared with T-cell responses to *Mycobacterium tuberculosis*-specific and non-specific antigens for detection of latent infection in persons with recent tuberculosis contact. Clin Diagn Lab Immunol 2001;8:1089–96.

119 Boras Z, Juretic A, Rudolf M, Uzarevic B, Trescec A. Cellular and humoral immunity to purified protein derivative (PPD) in PPD skin reactive and nonreactive patients with pulmonary tuberculosis: comparative analysis of antigen-specific lymphocyte proliferation and IgG antibodies. Croat Med J 2002;43:301–5.

120 Mazurek GH, Villarino ME. Guidelines for using the QuantiFERON-TB test for diagnosing latent *Mycobacterium tuberculosis* infection. Centers for Disease Control and Prevention. MMWR Recomm Rep 2003;52(RR-2):15–18.

121 Mazurek GH, LoBue PA, Daley CL, et al. Comparison of a whole-blood interferon-gamma assay with tuberculin skin testing for detecting latent *Mycobacterium tuberculosis* infections. JAMA 2001;286:1740–7.

122 Guidelines for using the Quantiferon-TB Gold test for detecting *Mycobacterium tuberculosis* infection, United States. Atlanta; 2005.

123 Smieja MJ, Marchetti CA, Cook DJ, Smaill FM. Isoniazid for preventing tuberculosis in non-HIV infected persons (Cochrane Review). Chichester, UK: John Wiley & Sons, Ltd. The Cochrane Library, Issue 4, 2003.

124 Efficacy of various durations of isoniazid preventive therapy for tuberculosis: five years of follow up in the IUAT trial. International Union Against Tuberculosis Committee on Prophylaxis. Bull World Health Organ 1982;60:555–64.

125 Comstock GW. How much isoniazid is needed for prevention of tuberculosis among immunocompetent adults? Int J Tuberc Lung Dis 1999;3:847–50.

126 Bucher HC, Griffith LE, Guyatt GH, et al. Isoniazid prophylaxis for tuberculosis in HIV infection: a metaanalysis of randomized controlled trials. AIDS 1999;13:501–7.

127 Woldehanna S, Volmink J. Treatment of latent tuberculosis infection in HIV infected persons. Cochrane Database Syst Rev 2004 (1), CD000171, DOI 10.1002/14651858.

128 Halsey NA, Coberly JS, Desormeaux J, et al. Randomized trial of isoniazid versus rifampicin and pyrazinamide for prevention of tuberculosis in HIV-1 infections. Lancet 1998;351:786–92.

129 Gordin FM, Chaisson RE, Matts JP, et al. Rifampin and pyrazinamide vs. isoniazid for prevention of tuberculosis in HIV-infected persons: an international randomized trial. JAMA 2000;283:1445–50.

130 Jasmer RM, Saukkonen JJ, Blumberg HM, et al. Short course rifampin and pyrazinamide for latent tuberculosis infection: a multicenter clinical trial. Ann Intern Med 2002;137:640–7.

131 Update: fatal and severe liver injuries associated with rifampin and pyrazinamide for latent tuberculosis infection, and revisions in American Thoracic Society/CDC recommendations – United States, 2001. MMWR 2001;50:733–5.

132 From the Centers for Disease Control and Prevention. Update: fatal and severe liver injuries associated with rifampin and pyrazinamide treatment for latent tuberculosis infection. JAMA 2002;288:2967.

133 Papastavros T, Dolovich LR, Holbrook A, Whitehead L, Loeb M. Adverse events associated with pyrazinamide and levofloxacin in the treatment of latent multidrugresistant tuberculosis. CMAJ 2002;167:131–6.

134 Fraser A, Paul M, Attamna A, Leibovici L. Drugs for preventing tuberculosis in people at risk of multiple-drug-resistant pulmonary tuberculosis. Cochrane Database Syst Rev 2006 (2), CD005435, DOI 10.1002/14651858.

135 Fraser A, Paul M, Attamna A, Leibovici L. Treatment of latent tuberculosis in persons at risk for multidrug-resistant tuberculosis: systematic review. Int J Tuberc Lung Dis 2006;10(1):19–23.

CHAPTER 8

Diarrhea

Guy De Bruyn & Alain Bouckenooghe

Case presentation 1

A 52-year-old previously healthy woman is brought to the emergency room with symptoms of vomiting, severe abdominal cramps, and bloody diarrhea. About 3 days prior she developed abdominal pains and diarrhea, that was watery at the time of onset and for which she was given amoxicillin by her family healthcare provider. She got sicker with abdominal cramping and the stools became bloody over the 24 hours preceding admission. Earlier she had twice had spontaneous nose bleeding with loss of only small amounts of blood. No other family members are currently ill, but several co-workers who had eaten lunch with the patient at a local fast-food restaurant developed diarrhea around the same time. She has not traveled outside of her city of residence in the last 6 months.

On physical examination, she appears ill. She complains of severe abdominal pain. Her vital signs indicate she is afebrile, has a mild tachycardia with normal blood pressure. There is remarkable pallor of the conjunctiva. Her abdomen is mildly tender to palpation. Laboratory analysis is as follows: hemoglobin 84 g/L (8.4 mg/dL), hematocrit 24%, platelets 70 × 10^9/L, lactate dehydrogenase 855 U/L, liver function tests normal, urea 52.8 mmol/L (148 mg/dL), creatinine 548 μmol/L (6.2 mg/dL), reticulocyte count 5.2%, Coombs test negative, coagulation tests normal with exception of mildly elevated fibrin degradation products.

Evidence-Based Infectious Diseases, 2nd edition. Edited by Mark Loeb, Fiona Smaill and Marek Smieja. © 2009 Wiley-Blackwell Publishing, ISBN: 978-1-4051-7026-0

Diagnosis

Epidemiology

Diarrhea is a syndrome that is readily recognized. Definitions for diarrhea typically use duration as an organizing principle (see glossary at end of chapter), although pathophysiologic or anatomic definitions are also common. In general, the clinical concern is discerning infectious from noninfectious causes, as well as likely pathogens that may be encountered in infectious cases.

Globally, diarrheal diseases are a major cause of mortality and morbidity, accounting for an estimated 1.78 million deaths and 58.7 million disability-adjusted life-years (DALYs) lost [1]. Estimates of incidence of acute infectious diarrhea vary between 0.8 and 100 cases per 100 person-years (Table 8.1). Studies based in general practice settings tend to have lower incidence estimates, reflecting the large number of symptomatic persons who do not seek medical care as well as underascertainment of cases. For every person attending their primary care provider, a further five to six [2] or more symptomatic cases may not seek care [3]. Incidence rates also vary by age, with a bimodal distribution. Infants have the highest rates, with lowest rates in the late teens, rising slightly in early adulthood. Although recent data are scarce, prior reports indicate very high peak age-specific rates of disease in developing countries of 9.7 cases per person year [4]. Healthcare-seeking behavior is modified by age, symptom severity, and duration, and the presence of particular alarm symptoms such as fever or blood in the stool. One study found that in a multivariable logistic regression model, only age, fever, and abdominal cramps were independently associated with seeking medical consultation [3].

Table 8.1 Population-based estimates of diarrheal disease incidence

Location, period	Cohort	Incidence [cases/100 person years] (95% confidence interval)	Reference
Cleveland, 1948–57	Community	150	[158]
Tecumseh, 1965–71	Community	100	
Brazil (urban), 1978–80	Community	143	[159]
Egypt (rural), 1980–1	Community	100	[160]
England, 1993–6	Community	19.4 (18.1–20.8)	[2]
	General practice	3.3 (2.94–3.75)	
Netherlands, 1998–9	Community	28.3 (25.2–31.5)	[3]
	General practice	0.8	

Globally, poor water, sanitation, and hygiene are the greatest risk factors for diarrheal disease [5]. Aside from age, other personal characteristics such as underlying medical conditions (HIV infection, prior gastric surgery, intake of medications that lower gastric acidity) are associated with elevated risk of acquiring diarrhea [6,7], as are other factors including sexual practices [6].

In travelers to tropical or subtropical destinations, diarrhea is amongst the commonest of acute ailments encountered [8]. The attack rate of traveler's diarrhea varies by location, season of travel, consumption of high-risk food or beverages (e.g. tap water, ice cubes, ice cream, food from street vendors, salads, raw or uncooked shellfish), and other factors [8–14]. Rates in expatriates from developed nations may approach that for children under 5 years of age in these locations [12].

Vaccines have been developed against some of these pathogens, with variable degrees of efficacy. The most commonly used traveler's vaccines against specific enteric pathogens include various candidates against *Salmonella typhi* and *Vibrio cholerae*.

Clinical findings

Inquiry regarding certain physical symptoms may assist in defining patients in whom stool cultures are likely to yield pathogenic organisms. Clinicians should enquire regarding duration of symptoms; characteristics of stool (consistency, frequency, volume, and presence of blood or mucus); symptoms of hypovolemia, abdominal cramps, or fever; travel history; recent medications; and ingestion of raw or undercooked meat, unpasteurized dairy products, or raw seafood.

Physical examination should identify hypovolemia. However, the clinical diagnosis of hypovolemia in adults has best been validated in acute blood loss, and remains unproved in volume loss from diarrhea [15]. Therefore, physical findings such as postural vital signs, dry tongue, dry axillae, decreased skin turgor, or prolonged capillary refill time may need to be supplemented by measurement of serum electrolytes, urea, and creatinine to confirm the diagnosis.

The time to clinical presentation varies with causative agent, a point emphasized by data from the GeoSentinel Database. Presentation with acute diarrheal illness due to parasitic infections was more common in returning travelers than bacterial illness [8].

Laboratory findings

A metaanalysis of 25 studies of the diagnostic utility of fecal screening tests as a predictor of a stool culture positive for a known invasive enteropathogen reported the superior performance of fecal lactoferrin over fecal leukocytes or stool occult blood [16]. However, joint maximum sensitivity and specificity, as estimated from summary receiver operating characteristic (ROC) curves were only 86%, 63%, and 68%, respectively. Subsequent studies have indicated that lactoferrin has a sensitivity of 85–93% with a corresponding likelihood ratio positive (LR+) of 4.0–5.5 [17,18] and fecal leukocytes a sensitivity of 57% with LR+ 5.0 (95% CI 2.9–8.8) among outpatients [19]. These studies do not highlight the operational issues in using these tests in the clinical setting, including need for an experienced microscopist (in the case of fecal leukocytes), need for a fresh specimen (for fecal leukocytes), and integration into clinical care.

Initial work-up should therefore include a fecal lactoferrin measurement or, if microscopy can be performed on a fresh stool sample, presence of fecal leukocytes. If this is positive, a stool culture is indicated as the probability of finding an invasive pathogen is increased and this information is relevant towards further therapy of the patient and is also important from a public health standpoint.

Stool culture

Culture of fresh stool specimens remains the standard for determining an etiologic diagnosis. The rationale for continued use of stool culture includes directed antimicrobial therapy, and assistance with public health goals, such as disease surveillance, identification of outbreaks, further evaluation in cases of suspected inflammatory enteritis, and protection from secondary transmission from ill food service workers [20–22]. The yield of stool cultures in the evaluation of diarrhea in recent travelers is typically below 50% and in the case of community-acquired diarrhea in developed regions this is significantly less (1.5–6%), due to relative increased importance of viral pathogens. Because acute diarrheal disease is often self-limited, and because of the delay in receiving culture results, the contribution of culture results to therapeutic decision-making is often limited. This must be balanced with the need for identification of invasive pathogens and pathogens of public health importance, and also with the need to minimize empiric therapy which may be inappropriate. Most guidelines advise obtaining stool cultures selectively when the patient is moderately or severely ill, in cases with clinical signs of fever, mucus or blood visible in the stool, tenesmus, severe abdominal cramping, or treatment failure [23–25]. For public health reasons, stool cultures should also be tested for specific subpopulations: food handlers, daycare attendees, daycare employees, and any time an outbreak is suspected.

Treatment

Fluid management

Although the goal of fluid management is to reduce morbidity and mortality, most trials of these interventions have assessed other endpoints, such as stool output or need for intravenous rehydration. A direct comparison of intravenous versus oral rehydration has been reported in one small randomized controlled trial (RCT) among 20 adults with cholera and severe dehydration that compared enteral rehydration through a nasogastric tube versus intravenous rehydration [26]. Both groups received initial intravenous fluids. The RCT found no significant difference in the total duration of diarrhea (44 h with IV fluids vs 37 h with nasogastric fluids; difference +7 h, 95% CI −6 to +20 h), total volume of stool passed (8.2 L vs 11.0 L; difference 2.8 L, 95% CI 8 L to +3 L), or duration of *Vibrio* excretion (1.1 days vs 1.4 days; difference 0.3 days, 95% CI 0 to 1 day).

Many subsequent modifications to the formulation of oral rehydration solution (ORS) have been tested in prospective studies. These include amino acid ORS, bicarbonate free ORS, citrate-containing ORS, reduced osmolarity ORS, rice-based solutions [27] and zinc-based solutions [28]. Amino acid-containing ORS were found to reduce the total duration of diarrhea and the total volume of stool in two RCTs [29,30]. Replacing ORS bicarbonate with chloride was not found to be beneficial in one small RCT [31], nor was any significant effect of replacing ORS bicarbonate with citrate found in three RCTs [32–34]. Reduced osmolarity ORS was found to be associated with fewer unscheduled intravenous infusions in a systematic review of trials in children [35]. Fewer trials have examined the efficacy in adults, and among available trials, no consistent effect has been demonstrated. The risk of asymptomatic hyponatremia is higher among those receiving reduced osmolarity ORS in one study (OR 2.1, 95% CI 1.1–4.1) [36], but not in another [37]. The World Health Organization recently changed the formulation of standard oral rehydration solution to a reduced osmolarity formulation [38].

One systematic review (search date 1998, 22 RCTs conducted in Bangladesh, India, Indonesia, Pakistan, Egypt, Mexico, Chile, and Peru) in people with cholera and noncholera diarrhea found that rice-based ORS significantly reduced the 24-h stool volume compared to standard ORS (adults: 4 RCTs, WMD 51 mL/kg, 95% CI 66 mL/kg to 35 mL/kg; children: 5 RCTs, WMD 67 mL/kg, 95% CI 94 mL/kg to 41 mL/kg) [39]. The Cochrane review of this topic has been withdrawn from the Cochrane Library pending a substantive update.

One RCT found that both rice-based ORS and low sodium rice-based ORS reduced stool output compared with standard ORS (4 L for rice based ORS vs 5 L for standard ORS, $P < 0.02$; 3 L for low sodium rice-based ORS vs 5 L for standard ORS, $P < 0.05$) [40]. A second recent RCT demonstrated shortening of the duration of diarrhea with a starch-based ORS formulation, compared to glucose-based ORS [41]. The addition of zinc to ORS was found to be moderately efficacious in reducing severity of acute diarrhea without increasing vomiting or reducing ORS uptake in a trial in India [42].

Antimicrobial therapy

The use of antibiotics for treatment of domestically acquired diarrhea has been evaluated in at least eleven RCTs comparing one or more antibiotics with placebo or control [43–52]. These trials have evaluated fluoroquinolones ($n = 9$), trimethoprim/sulfamethoxazole (TMP/SMX) ($n = 4$), clioquinol ($n = 1$) (no longer widely used; drug is not available in the United States and available for otic and dermatologic use in several countries), and nifuroxazide ($n = 1$). Six RCTs found that antibiotics reduced illness duration or decreased number of liquid stools at 48 hours, while three RCTs found no benefit in reducing illness duration. One RCT found reduced duration of diarrhea for ciprofloxacin but not for TMP/SMX.

Antibiotics have been extensively investigated for the treatment of traveler's diarrhea. A systematic review [53] and three additional RCTs [54–56] describing the effects of treatment have been reported. The review (search date 1999) compared empirical use of antibiotics versus placebo and found 12 RCTs, among 1474 people with travelers' diarrhea, including students, package tourists, military personnel, and volunteers. Antibiotics evaluated in these trials included aztreonam, bicozamycin, ciprofloxacin, fleroxacin, norfloxacin, ofloxacin, TMP/SMX, and trimethoprim alone. The duration of therapy varied from a single dose to 5 days. The review found that antibiotics significantly increased the cure rate at 72 hours (defined as cessation of unformed stools, or less than one unformed stool per 24 hours without additional symptoms; OR 5.9, 95% CI 4.1–8.6). The additional RCT (598 people, 70% of whom had traveled recently) compared norfloxacin versus placebo. It found that norfloxacin significantly increased the number of people cured after 6 days (34/46 [74%] with norfloxacin vs 18/48 [38%] with placebo; RR 2.0, 95% CI 1.3–3.0).

The systematic review found that the rate of adverse effects varied with each antibiotic, ranging from 2% to 18%. Gastrointestinal, dermatologic, and respiratory symptoms were most frequently reported. The emergence of resistance of the infecting organism to the agent was also documented in a number of the trials. Antimicrobial resistance is clearly of concern for public health. One small RCT included in the review found a significant association between taking ciprofloxacin and isolation of resistant bacteria at 48 hours from these patients' stool samples (ciprofloxacin vs placebo; absolute risk increase [ARI] 50%, 95% CI 15–85%). Another RCT in the review (181 adults with acute diarrhea) reported three cases of continued excretion of *Shigella* in people taking TMP/SMX vs one person taking placebo [57]. Two of these isolates selected for resistance to the drug, although the participants were clinically well. One additional RCT found that people with salmonella infection treated with norfloxacin versus placebo had significantly prolonged excretion of *Salmonella* species (median time to clearance of *Salmonella* species from stool: 50 days with norfloxacin vs 23 days with placebo; CI not provided). In addition, six of nine *Campylobacter* isolates obtained after treatment showed some degree of resistance to norfloxacin.

The continued evolution of antimicrobial resistance among enteropathogens has meant that agents previously found to be effective in clinical trials, such as trimethoprim-sulfamethoxazole or ampicillin, no longer show in vitro activity [58,59]. Further active-control trials, not mentioned above, have evaluated a number of additional candidates, which could be considered. These include aztreonam [60], azithromycin [61–63], and rifaximin [64,65].

Antidiarrheals

A number of antidiarrheal compounds, drugs that generally act by prolonging intestinal transit time through an effect on bowel motility, have been evaluated in clinical trials. These agents include difenoxin, diphenoxylate-atropine [66], lidamidine [67,68], loperamide [68–71], and loperamide-oxide [70–74].

These trials of patients with acute diarrhea have generally been conducted among general practice networks. Trials evaluating loperamide or loperamide oxide have generally used "time to first relief" and "time to complete relief" as endpoints, the latter indicating the time between taking the loading dose and the start of the 24-h period in which no watery or loose stool were passed. The majority of these reports have indicated a benefit of antidiarrheals on symptoms. Some have reported the benefit being experienced in the early phase of the illness, with no impact on total duration of symptoms. The most common adverse effect of these medications is constipation. Two RCTs found that constipation was significantly more frequent in people taking loperamide versus placebo (25% vs 7%; ARI 18%, 95% CI 8–28%; number needed to harm [NNH] 5, 95% CI 3–12 [71]; 22% vs 10.3%; ARI 12%, 95% CI 5–29%; NNH 5, 95% CI 3–18 [70]). Another RCT (230 people) found that symptom scores for tiredness and sleepiness were significantly higher in people taking loperamide oxide 1 mg compared with placebo [73]. Other feared complications such as toxic megacolon have not been reported in clinical trials.

Antisecretory agents

A number of compounds have been developed that modify intestinal fluid secretion and thereby produce a clinical benefit. These include racecadotril, an inhibitor of enkephalinase which prolongs the antisecretory effect of endogenous enkephalins, and octreotide. At least seven trials of racecadotril compared with placebo or another active agent have been reported [75–81]. Placebo-controlled trials indicate that racecadotril shortens the duration of diarrhea. Active controlled trials show similar rates of resolution of symptoms of diarrhea to loperamide, however the rate of constipation is lower following racecadotril compared with loperamide (8.1% for racecadotril 100 mg three times daily vs 31.3% for loperamide 1.33 mg three times daily in one trial) [79]. Octreotide has been reported to shorten the duration of diarrhea due to *Vibrio cholerae* in one small study, although it did not affect the purging rate [82].

Other modalities

Probiotic agents, which are dietary supplements of living commensal microorganisms of low or no pathogenicity, have been proposed as potential therapy for a number of clinical indications [83]. A few small trials of therapy in adults with acute enteric infections have been reported, although the results appear conflicting.

Dietary modification, although frequently recommended for patients with acute diarrheal illnesses, has been evaluated in only small pilot studies, which have not demonstrated additional benefits to patients [84,85].

Supplementation of certain micronutrients has been evaluated as adjunctive therapy in acute diarrhea. The use of zinc supplementation has been extensively evaluated in children although not in adults.

Prognosis

Duration of symptoms

Acute diarrhea in adults is typically self-limited. Among travelers, symptoms typically last 3 to 5 days, may persist for over a week in 8 to 15%, and 2% develop chronic diarrhea [86], although some data suggests that chronic intestinal symptoms may occur more frequently [87,88].

Need for hospitalization

Based on hospital discharge data from the US, approximately 452 000 persons per year were hospitalized with acute diarrhea between 1979 and 1995. This represents <1% of all cases of diarrhea, and approximately 1.5% of all hospitalizations [89].

Other serious adverse outcomes

One particular concern in those patients with diarrhea due to *Eschericia coli* O157:H7 (EHEC) and other shiga-toxin-producing *E.coli* strains is the development of hemolytic uremic syndrome (HUS), a disorder characterized by hemolytic anemia, thrombocytopenia, and acute renal failure [90]. A recent metaanalysis assessed the risk of HUS after antibiotic treatment of EHEC in nine studies [91]. No association between antibiotic use and HUS were demonstrated (pooled OR 1.04, 95% CI 0.59–1.82). However, the authors reported significant heterogeneity of effect among the studies included in the metaanalysis. As a result, the topic remains controversial, and the value of antibiotics in this setting remains unresolved, hence the use of antibiotics is not advised [92].

Reactive arthritis and Reiter syndrome are further serious potential complications of enteric infection. The risk of these complications has been documented in the setting of outbreaks of enteric infection with *Salmonella typhimurium* or *S. enteritidis*, *Shigella flexneri*, *Yersinia pseudotuberculosis*, and sporadic cases of *Campylobacter* species or ETEC [93–95]. The prevalence of joint symptoms after infection has been reported to be as high as 37%, although most estimates are in the range of 1–15%. Reiter syndrome usually affects less than 3%. The prevalence of certain high-risk HLA types (such as HLA-B27) in the affected population has generally not been reported, although is clearly relevant to the development of joint symptoms.

Death

Worldwide, death from acute diarrhea remains a major cause of mortality, particularly in children under 5. Mortality trends from diarrhea for the US for the period 1979–87 showed a significant decline in deaths among young children, but rates for those 75 years or older remain around 15 deaths per 100 000 persons. Mortality from dysentery in hospitalized patients in Rwanda in the setting of a nationwide outbreak during the civil war was associated with age less than 5 years or greater than 50 years, severe dehydration on admission (assessed clinically), edema of the legs, and prescription of nalidixic acid (resistance to this agent emerged rapidly during the outbreak) [96,97].

Case presentation 2

A 73-year-old woman with diabetes, which was controlled by diet and oral medication, was admitted to the intensive care service of a hospital after she was admitted 10 days earlier with a clinical picture of community-acquired pneumonia. She had been admitted with high fever up to 40°C, had an elevated peripheral white blood cell count of 14.5×10^9/L without bands, and had dyspnea requiring oxygen support of 4 L/minute O_2 by face mask. She was started on a sliding scale of insulin to control moderate hyperglycemic values. Her condition did not require intubation,

and she was started on antibiotics (a third-generation cephalosporin with a respiratory fluoroquinolone), intravenous fluids and nonsteroidal medication for fever upon admission. A chest radiograph taken on admission showed a left lower lobe infiltrate.

She gradually improved: she had defervesced on day 5 and was coughing less. Her blood sugars normalized without additional insulin and she was markedly less dyspneic by day 7. Her WBC count had also normalized by the 5th day, and the chest radiograph showed a similar but perhaps more dense lung infiltrate in the same area of the left lower lobe. On day 8 she developed watery offensive diarrhea with severe abdominal cramping. She was anorexic and hypoglycemic. Her temperature increased to 38.5°C, her heart rate increased to 135 beats/minute, she became hypotensive, and on her peripheral blood smear she had 22.4×10^9 WBC/L with 15% bands. Given her worsening clinical picture, she was transferred to the intensive care unit.

Diagnosis

Epidemiology

Diarrhea occurring during hospitalization may be due to a number of infectious or noninfectious causes. The leading cause of infectious nosocomial diarrhea is cytotoxin-producing *Clostridium difficile*. Other infectious pathogens account for only a small proportion of nosocomial diarrhea, but may be important in outbreak settings. The patient population and locally prevalent pathogens are additional influences on the spectrum of pathogenic organisms encountered. Antibiotic-associated diarrhea may be caused not only by disruption of normal intestinal flora, but also by overgrowth of pathogenic organisms such as *C. difficile*. The effects of the antibiotic may be directly on the intestinal mucosa, gastrointestinal motility, or mediated through alteration of colonic metabolism induced through changes in the normal resident bacterial flora [98].

The rates of nosocomial diarrhea vary, in part due to the definition of diarrhea; rates of above 30% of admission have been reported [99]. Among a large cohort of antibiotic-treated hospitalized patients, the frequency of diarrhea was 12% [100]. *C. difficile* accounts for approximately 25% of cases of antibiotic-associated diarrhea [100,101]. Risk factors for *C. difficile* symptomatic infection include advanced age, length of hospitalization, and antibiotic use [102,103]. Proton pump inhibitors have been associated with increased risk for community-acquired *C. difficile*-associated diarrhea [104].

Clinical findings

Clinical findings often start shortly after use of an antibiotic although a delayed onset of up to 8 weeks is possible. Most patients have foul-smelling, watery, greenish diarrhea, the presence of mucus and blood in the stool, with signs of focal abdominal tenderness or tenesmus often present. However, milder presentations without diarrhea occur, and fulminant colitis is estimated to occur in 1–3% of cases [101]. Leukocytosis is common, and may even be markedly elevated [105].

Stool culture

A widely used policy in microbiology laboratories is to reject stool specimens obtained more than 3 days after admission (the "three-day rule"). The rationale for this is illustrated by the difference in stool culture yield for specimens taken <72 hours after admission compared with specimens taken 72 hours or more after admission: 3.3% vs 0.5% [106]. A recent prospective study to derive guidelines for stool culture of inpatients proposed a modification to the three-day rule, suggesting that cultures be obtained in the case of nosocomial diarrhea (>72 hours after admission) if at least one of the following criteria are met: age ≥65 years, HIV infection, neutropenia, or a nosocomial outbreak suspected. This would have resulted in only two missed positive cultures for enteropathogens (other than *C. difficile*) of 65 positive cultures from over 27 000 stool cultures obtained in three hospitals over a cumulative period of 14 years. The rule would have led to a reduction in workload for the microbiology laboratory of between 47% and 62% in these hospitals. The detection of nosocomial outbreaks may have been delayed in some instances, especially if cases were widely distributed across hospital wards.

Identification of *C. difficile* in a stool culture is not sufficient as strains that do not produce toxins are not pathogenic, and the presence of one or both of the toxins must be established. In addition, isolation of *C. difficile* may take 48–72 hours, which delays the diagnosis. Some strains of *C. difficile* have been associated with higher virulence leading to increased morbidity and mortality; in particular the strains BI, NAP1 or ribotype 027 – which are all synonymous – have been observed to lead to disease that is more severe, more prolonged, more refractory to therapy, and more likely to relapse [107–109].

Special examinations

The use of stool biomarkers has been examined as an aid to identification of patients with a higher likelihood of positive tests for *C. difficile*. The odds of a positive stool cytotoxin assay in persons with positive tests for stool leukocytes have been reported to be increased, whether detection is by lactoferrin assay (OR 3.7, 95% CI 1.8–7.8) or by light microscopy (OR 2.4, 95% CI 1.1–5.4) [110]. Both have imperfect sensitivity, although stool microscopy may be the less sensitive screening test [19,111].

The gold standard test is a cell culture-based cytotoxin assay, which takes 24 to 48 hours. The impetus for alternative diagnostic tests has been the diagnostic delay and requirement for a tissue culture facility. A variety of rapid assays have been developed to address these needs. Enzyme immunoassays (EIA) have been developed for toxin A and B, or the combination of both, with reduced sensitivity (72–94% compared with tissue culture), but results are available in a few hours [112]. If the initial test is negative and diarrhea persists, a second or even a third sample should be evaluated to compensate for limited sensitivity. The combined toxin A/B tests have superior sensitivity to EIAs that test for toxin A alone, possibly owing to the detection of toxin A−/B+ strains [113]. Realtime PCR on toxin B and immunochromatography assays on toxin A and B have some potential as rapid screening tests but are not better than the gold standard cytotoxicity test; use of PCR remains limited [114,115]. The use of latex agglutination assays that detect glutamate dehydrogenase has been discouraged by the Society for Healthcare Epidemiology in America because of the low sensitivity of the test, despite the ease of performance of the test, low cost, and high specificity [112]. Radiographic studies lack both sensitivity and specificity but toxic megacolon or thumbprinting can be suggestive of infection with *C. difficile*. Abdominal computed tomography scanning typically shows thickening of the mucosa, yet this is not a pathognomonic sign [116,117].

When a diagnosis needs to be made more rapidly, flexible sigmoidoscopy should be considered. This is particularly useful in situations where ileus has developed and stool studies cannot be obtained. In severe cases, pseudomembranous colitis may be visualized on examination. The typical appearance is of yellow adherent plaques about 10 mm in diameter scattered over the colonic mucosa and separated by hyperemic areas. Biopsies of the area show plentiful neutrophils in a classic "volcano" exudate of fibrin. About 10% of the cases of pseudomembranous colitis are in the proximal parts of the colon and can be visualized by a full colonoscopy.

Treatment

Usual interventions that are applicable to the management of diarrhea in other settings, such as correction of volume deficits and electrolyte imbalance, are important. Beyond this, the first consideration in therapy is to stop the offending antibiotic, whenever possible. This will often be sufficient to resolve the symptoms promptly. If the antibiotic needs to be continued or if symptoms are more severe, antibiotic therapy can be considered. Several effective therapies are available including vancomycin, teicoplanin, fusidic acid, metronidazole, and bacitracin [118–120]. Even though the efficacy of several antibiotics is similar [121,122], it did appear that oral vancomycin was superior in one small placebo-controlled trial [123]; the drug of choice is metronidazole 500 mg orally three times daily for 10–14 days, as it is recommended that vancomycin use be restricted where possible [112]. Where available, teicoplanin might be a good first choice [123]. Metronidazole failure could possibly be attributed to a slower and less consistent microbiologic response [124]. Sometimes longer therapy is required, particularly when the offending antibiotic is still given. When therapy is needed, patients usually improve within 72 hours of the first dose of metronidazole. Vancomycin given orally at a dose of 125 mg four times daily is effective [125] but, due to its higher cost and because of efforts to limit the spread of vancomycin-resistant organisms, metronidazole is preferred. Vancomycin can be considered for patients who have not responded to at least two courses of metronidazole, patients with allergies or intolerance to metronidazole, pregnant women, and children. If there is no adequate clinical response, the oral dose of vancomycin can be increased to 500 mg orally four times daily. For patients who are toxic or unable to take oral medication and in absence of a feeding tube, intravenous metronidazole at a dose of 500 to 750 mg every 6 hours can be used, although intravenous therapy is inferior and parenteral vancomycin is ineffective. Alternatives are under further study. Linezolid shows in vitro sensitivity but needs further clinical testing. Antimotility agents (e.g. loperamide, etc.) are contraindicated. Tolevamer, a polymer that binds the toxins, seems effective in mild to moderate cases and is under development [126]. Fusidic acid has been reported to be as effective as metronidazole [127].

Relapses can occur in up to 20% despite appropriate therapy. Reinfection can also occur. A second course of metronidazole is usually sufficient but prolonged courses of vancomycin can be considered in the face of multiple relapses with clinical signs, e.g., oral vancomycin courses followed by a slow taper over 6 weeks [128]. Use of probiotics with, e.g., *Saccharomyces boulardii* may be useful, although the evidence remains equivocal [129–132]. Historically, fecal enemas from healthy donors have been tried in an effort to restore normal healthy bowel flora in an effort to competitively displace enteric pathogens [133]. In a small study, serial therapy with vancomycin and rifaximin was given in persistent recurrent *C. difficile*-associated diarrhea episodes with success in terminating recurrent symptoms in 7 out of 8 cases [134].

Case presentation 3

A 27-year-old man is seen in the outpatient department for symptoms of diarrhea over the last 3 months. He reports stools every 2–3 hours that are watery or consist of poorly digested food he had consumed over the previous day. Occasionally the stool has an oily consistency. He has noted no fever, blood in the stool, tenesmus, or other abdominal complaints. He is known to be HIV-positive, although had declined close monitoring of his immune and virologic status, and has not been receiving antiretroviral therapy. He is taking no regular medications apart from multivitamins and a herbal supplement. He has not traveled recently, has not been sexually active for several months preceding the onset of symptoms, and has no pets.

continued

Case presentation 3 (continued)

On examination he is afebrile, with stable vital signs. His abdominal examination is unremarkable. His laboratory studies disclose: sodium 137 mmol/L, potassium 3.6 mmol/L, urea 3.6 mmol/L (10 mg/dL), creatinine 71 μmol/L (0.8 mg/dL), and CD4+ T-lymphocyte count 27 × 10^6/L (27 cells/μL).

Diagnosis

Epidemiology

Chronic diarrhea is a heterogeneous illness, encompassing symptoms caused by infection, inflammatory bowel disease, functional bowel syndromes, malabsorption, and other idiopathic syndromes. A consequence of this heterogeneity is a complex epidemiology, which remains relatively poorly defined. Methodologic flaws in the criteria for assembly of study cohorts, definition of diarrhea, and definition of "chronic" may all be important. The age- and sex-adjusted prevalence of this symptom have been estimated at 6.0 cases per 100 persons (95% CI 4.4–7.7) [135–139].

Persons infected with the human immunodeficiency virus (HIV) are commonly affected by diarrhea. The incidence of chronic diarrhea among participants in the Swiss HIV Cohort study was 8.5 per 100 person-years (95% CI 7.4–9.9) between July 1992 and June 1994, and 9.1 (95% CI 7.8–10.7) between July 1994 and March 1996 [140]. Among participants in the Adult/Adolescent Spectrum of HIV Disease study, conducted in the US, the incidence of diarrhea caused by bacterial pathogens known to be causes of enteric illness was 7.2 cases per 1000 person-years between 1992 and 2002 [141]. This is likely to represent a minimal estimate, given the study design. In this same study the most commonly identified bacterial cause of diarrhea was *C. difficile*, with the highest incidence rates in the most severely immunosuppressed symptomatic AIDS patients [127]. Prior studies have demonstrated that the risk of chronic diarrhea is related to degree of immunosuppression [141–143], transmission category [142], receipt of antiretroviral therapy [140,144], or prophylaxis against opportunistic infections [145,146].

Clinical findings

Limited data are available regarding the utility of physical findings for making an etiologic diagnosis in patients presenting with chronic diarrhea. Among HIV-infected patients, the history and physical examination have been reported not to be helpful in determining whether or not an enteropathogen will be identified [147], with the exception that abdominal tenderness was commoner in patients with CMV [148]. The American Gastroenterological Association have recommended that complete evaluation of persons seeking care for chronic diarrhea include evaluation of fluid balance, nutritional status, presence of flushing or rashes, mouth ulcers, thyroid masses, wheezing, arthritis, cardiac murmurs, hepatomegaly, abdominal masses, ascites, and edema. Attention should be paid during anorectal examination to the anal sphincter tone and the presence of perianal fistula or abscess [137].

Stool culture

The utility of stool studies for detection of enteric pathogens is well documented for the evaluation of chronic diarrhea in HIV infection. The yield of stool studies (including culture for enteric bacteria and mycobacteria, and microscopy for parasite ova) varies depending on the patient characteristics of the study population and the intensity of the diagnostic evaluation (Table 8.2).

Recommendations regarding the most appropriate diagnostic strategy for patients infected with HIV have not been formally tested in prospective studies examining a broad range of outcomes, including quality of life. Strategies range from an intensive work-up, including upper endoscopy and colonoscopy with mucosal biopsy, to a minimal evaluation involving only stool cultures [149]. The American Gastroenterological Association guidelines, published in 1996, propose a stepwise approach, which may be modified according to the clinical judgement of the physician [150]. The initial step identifies enteric bacteria and parasites through stool studies. Three samples should be submitted initially.

Laboratory tests

The use of fecal biomarkers as screening tools to detect gastrointestinal pathology have not been extensively evaluated in the setting of chronic diarrhea. The prototypic biomarker, occult blood, has not been extensively validated as a marker of intestinal

Table 8.2 Prevalence of enteric pathogens causing diarrhea in HIV-infected patients

Reference	N (%)[†]	Evaluation[‡]	Prevalence of pathogens		Pathogens[§]
			Patients with diarrhea (%)	Patients without diarrhea (%)	
Dworkin [162]	22 (55)	Stools	75	10	MAC *Cryptosporidia*
Laughon [163]	77 (64)	Stools	50	11	*Cryptosporidia* *Campylobacter* species
Smith [164]	30 (67)	Stools, EGD, colonoscopy	85	10	CMV *Entamoeba histolytica*
Antony [165]	66 (100)	Stools	55	–	MAC CMV
Rene [166]	132 (52)	Stools, EGD, colonoscopy	59	28	*Cryptosporidia* CMV
Cotte [167]	81 (73)	Stools	64	15	*Cryptosporidia* CMV
Kotler [168]	194 (73)	Stools	83	2	*Microsporidia* *Cryptosporidia*
Blanshard [148]	155 (100)	Stools, EGD, sigmoidoscopy	83	–	*Cryptosporidia* *Microsporidia*
Prasad [169]	59 (44)	Stools	73*	–	*Isospora Cryptosporidia*
Manatsathit [161]	45 (100)	Stools, EGD, colonoscopy	64		*Cryptosporidia* Tuberculosis

Adapted from references [150] and [161].
[†] Number of patients studied and proportion with diarrhea (%).
[‡] Endoscopic procedures listed only if performed in all patients.
[§] Two most common organisms are listed.
* Prevalence of pathogens not reported separately for patients with and without diarrhea.

inflammation in chronic diarrhea. When compared to another biomarker, the leukocyte-derived protein calprotectin, against a criterion standard of direct visualization at colonoscopy with biopsy among patients undergoing evaluation for chronic diarrhea of unknown cause or chronic colitis of unknown activity, fecal hemoglobin was of poor discriminatory value for the presence of intestinal inflammation (area under ROC curve (AUC) = 0.58, 95% CI 0.46–0.70) [151]. Fecal calprotectin levels were elevated and significantly associated with the presence of intestinal inflammation (AUC 0.89, 95% CI 0.81–0.97). Fecal lactoferrin, another leukocyte-derived protein, was reported to have sensitivity of 90%, specificity of 98%, positive predictive value (PPV) 82%, and negative predictive value (NPV) 99% for ulcerative colitis and Crohn's disease in patients being investigated for

chronic diarrhea with biomarkers and "an extensive evaluation" that included endoscopy [152].

Treatment

Antimicrobial therapy

Given the broad differential diagnosis, empiric antimicrobial therapy without initial evaluation is not recommended in this population. If no enteric pathogens are identified on stool studies, an empiric course of oral antibiotics may be considered. This may include a fluoroquinolone or a macrolide. Antiprotozoal therapy can also be considered such as empiric use of trimethoprim-sulfamethoxazole if *Cyclospora* or *Isospora* infections are suspected. Empiric use of metronidazole is indicated when the suspected pathogens include *Giardia lamblia* or *Entamoeba histolytica*, and

Table 8.3 Special pathogens and therapy

Cyclospora	TMP/SMX* 800 mg/160 mg twice daily × 7 d
Isospora	TMP/SMX 800 mg/160 mg twice daily × 10 d None (self-limited disease in immunocompetent host)
Cryptosporidium	In AIDS patients: Nitazoxanide plus antiretroviral therapy
Giardia	Metronidazole 250 mg three times daily × 5 d Tinidazole 2000 mg daily × 1 d Quinacrine 100 mg three times daily × 7 d Furazolidone 100 mg four times daily × 7–10 d Albendazole 400 mg daily × 7 d
Entamoeba	Metronidazole 250 mg four times daily × 7 d
MAC	Ethambutol and clarithromycin
HSV	Acyclovir
HIV	Antiretroviral combination therapy
CMV	Ganciclovir Valganciclovir

* Trimethoprim-sulfamethoxazole.

would also be of benefit in cases of *Clostridium difficile* colitis. Directed therapy may be available against identified pathogens (Table 8.3). Treatment of cryptosporidiosis in a normal host is typically not necessary, as this is a self-limiting disease; although a high clearance rate from stools has been reported with use of nitazoxanide and paromomycin. Use of nitazoxanide in HIV-positive subjects can be considered, even though effectiveness has not been proven [153].

Antidiarrheals

Nonspecific treatment with antidiarrheals, such as loperamide, loperamide oxide, diphenoxylate-atropine, codeine, or tincture of opium, may be considered for empirical therapy. The situations in which such use is tenable include: as a temporizing measure prior to a planned diagnostic evaluation; if diagnostic evaluation does not identify a specific etiology; if a diagnosis is made for which no effective therapy is known or for which specific treatment fails [138]. Antidiarrheals may also be considered in HIV-infected persons who have nonbloody diarrhea and a negative initial evaluation on stool testing, although these recommendations have not been evaluated in prospective studies [150].

The somatostatin analog octreotide has been evaluated as a potential therapy for HIV-associated diarrhea, but has not been found to be superior to placebo [154].

Other therapy

The evidence for the efficacy of probiotic agents in chronic diarrhea is limited. Dietary modifications, such as a diet based on medium chain triglycerides, have been evaluated as adjunctive therapy in HIV-infected patients with chronic diarrhea, and may be of value [155]. Use of moderate amounts of lactose-containing products does not appear to worsen symptoms of diarrhea [156]. Zinc does not reduce the proportion of patients with chronic diarrhea after 2 weeks of supplementation, although the evidence from one study is limited by high rates of loss to follow-up, perhaps reflecting, in part, a lack of efficacy or poor tolerability of the supplement [157].

Prognosis

Duration of symptoms

Remission rates of chronic diarrhea have been estimated to be 282 per 1000 person-years [135]. Given a similar incidence rate, the overall prevalence of chronic diarrhea was stable in the survey.

Survival

Chronic diarrhea among HIV-infected persons in the Swiss HIV Cohort study was found to be an independent predictor of death (risk ratio 1.5, 95% CI 1.2–1.8) [140].

Glossary

(per definitions used in Infectious Diseases Society of America guidelines)

Acute diarrhea: Diarrheal episode lasting less than 14 days.

Chronic diarrhea: Diarrheal episode lasting more than 30 days.

Diarrhea: Alteration of normal bowel movement, associated with increase in stool volume or water content or frequency. Also decreased stool consistency (unformed or liquid stools).

Infectious diarrhea: Diarrheal episode due to infection with an enteropathogenic organism.

Persistent diarrhea: Diarrheal episode lasting more than 14 days.

References

1 Lopez AD, Mathers CD, Ezzati M, Jamison DT, Murray CJ. Global and regional burden of disease and risk factors, 2001: systematic analysis of population health data. Lancet 2006;367(9524):1747–57.

2 Wheeler JG, Sethi D, Cowden JM, et al. Study of infectious intestinal disease in England: rates in the community, presenting to general practice, and reported to national surveillance. The Infectious Intestinal Disease Study Executive. BMJ 1999;318(7190):1046–50.

3 De Wit MA, Kortbeek LM, Koopmans MP, et al. A comparison of gastroenteritis in a general practice-based study and a community-based study. Epidemiol Infect 2001;127(3):389–97.

4 Guerrant RL, Hughes JM, Lima NL, Crane J. Diarrhea in developed and developing countries: magnitude, special settings, and etiologies. Rev Infect Dis 1990;12 Suppl 1:S41–50.

5 Murray CJ, Lopez AD. Global mortality, disability, and the contribution of risk factors: Global Burden of Disease Study. Lancet 1997;349(9063):1436–42.

6 Baer JT, Vugia DJ, Reingold AL, Aragon T, Angulo FJ, Bradford WZ. HIV infection as a risk factor for shigellosis. Emerg Infect Dis 1999;5(6):820–3.

7 Cobelens FG, Leentvaar-Kuijpers A, Kleijnen J, Coutinho RA. Incidence and risk factors of diarrhoea in Dutch travellers: consequences for priorities in pre-travel health advice. Trop Med Int Health 1998;3(11):896–903.

8 Freedman DO, Weld LH, Kozarsky PE, et al. Spectrum of disease and relation to place of exposure among ill returned travelers. N Engl J Med 2006;354(2):119–30.

9 Kollaritsch H. Traveller's diarrhea among Austrian tourists in warm climate countries: I. Epidemiology. Eur J Epidemiol 1989;5(1):74–81.

10 von Sonnenburg F, Tornieporth N, Waiyaki P, et al. Risk and aetiology of diarrhoea at various tourist destinations. Lancet 2000;356(9224):133–4.

11 Mattila L, Siitonen A, Kyronseppa H, et al. Seasonal variation in etiology of travelers' diarrhea. Finnish-Moroccan Study Group. J Infect Dis 1992;165(2):385–8.

12 Herwaldt BL, de Arroyave KR, Roberts JM, Juranek DD. A multiyear prospective study of the risk factors for and incidence of diarrheal illness in a cohort of Peace Corps volunteers in Guatemala. Ann Intern Med 2000;132(12):982–8.

13 Steffen R, Collard F, Tornieporth N, et al. Epidemiology, etiology, and impact of traveler's diarrhea in Jamaica. JAMA 1999;281(9):811–7.

14 Riddle MS, Sanders JW, Putnam SD, Tribble DR. Incidence, etiology, and impact of diarrhea among long-term travelers (US military and similar populations): a systematic review. Am J Trop Med Hyg 2006;74(5):891–900.

15 McGee S, Abernethy WB, 3rd, Simel DL. The rational clinical examination. Is this patient hypovolemic? JAMA 1999;281(11):1022–9.

16 Huicho L, Campos M, Rivera J, Guerrant RL. Fecal screening tests in the approach to acute infectious diarrhea: a scientific overview. Pediatr Infect Dis J 1996;15(6):486–94.

17 Choi SW, Park CH, Silva TM, Zaenker EI, Guerrant RL. To culture or not to culture: fecal lactoferrin screening for inflammatory bacterial diarrhea. J Clin Microbiol 1996;34(4):928–32.

18 Silletti RP, Lee G, Ailey E. Role of stool screening tests in diagnosis of inflammatory bacterial enteritis and in selection of specimens likely to yield invasive enteric pathogens. J Clin Microbiol 1996;34(5):1161–5.

19 Savola KL, Baron EJ, Tompkins LS, Passaro DJ. Fecal leukocyte stain has diagnostic value for outpatients but not inpatients. J Clin Microbiol 2001;39(1):266–9.

20 Slutsker L, Ries AA, Greene KD, Wells JG, Hutwagner L, Griffin PM. *Escherichia coli* O157:H7 diarrhea in the United States: clinical and epidemiologic features. Ann Intern Med 1997;126(7):505–13.

21 Koplan JP, Fineberg HV, Ferraro MJ, Rosenberg ML. Value of stool cultures. Lancet 1980;2(8191):413–6.

22 Feldman RA, Banatvala N. The frequency of culturing stools from adults with diarrhoea in Great Britain. Epidemiol Infect 1994;113(1):41–4.

23 Guerrant RL, Van Gilder T, Steiner TS, et al. Practice guidelines for the management of infectious diarrhea. Clin Infect Dis 2001;32(3):331–51.

24 Manatsathit S, Dupont HL, Farthing M, et al. Guideline for the management of acute diarrhea in adults. J Gastroenterol Hepatol 2002;17 Suppl:S54–71.

25 DuPont HL. Guidelines on acute infectious diarrhea in adults. The Practice Parameters Committee of the American College of Gastroenterology. Am J Gastroenterol 1997;92(11):1962–75.

26 Pierce NF, Sack RB, Mitra RC, et al. Replacement of water and electrolyte losses in cholera by an oral glucose-electrolyte solution. Ann Intern Med 1969;70(6):1173–81.

27 De Bruyn G. Diarrhoea. Clin Evid 2002;(7):627–35.

28 Robberstad B, Strand T, Black RE, Sommerfelt H. Cost-effectiveness of zinc as adjunct therapy for acute childhood diarrhoea in developing countries. Bulletin of the World Health Organization 2004;82(7):523–31.

29 Nalin DR, Cash RA, Rahman M, Yunus M. Effect of glycine and glucose on sodium and water adsorption in patients with cholera. Gut 1970;11(9):768–72.

30 Patra FC, Sack DA, Islam A, Alam AN, Mazumder RN. Oral rehydration formula containing alanine and glucose for treatment of diarrhoea: a controlled trial. BMJ 1989;298(6684):1353–6.

31 Sarker SA, Mahalanabis D. The presence of bicarbonate in oral rehydration solution does not influence fluid absorption in cholera. Scand J Gastroenterol 1995;30(3):242–5.

32 Ahmed SM, Islam MR, Butler T. Effective treatment of diarrhoeal dehydration with an oral rehydration solution containing citrate. Scand J Infect Dis 1986;18(1):65–70.

33 Mazumder RN, Nath SK, Ashraf H, Patra FC, Alam AN. Oral rehydration solution containing trisodium citrate for treating severe diarrhoea: controlled clinical trial. BMJ 1991;302(6768):88–9.

34 Hoffman SL, Moechtar MA, Simanjuntak CH, et al. Rehydration and maintenance therapy of cholera patients in Jakarta: citrate-based versus bicarbonate-based oral rehydration salt solution. J Infect Dis 1985;152(6):1159–65.

35 Hahn S, Kim Y, Garner P. Reduced osmolarity oral rehydration solution for treating dehydration due to diarrhoea in children: systematic review. BMJ 2001;323(7304):81–5.

36 Alam NH, Majumder RN, Fuchs GJ. Efficacy and safety of oral rehydration solution with reduced osmolarity in adults with cholera: a randomised double-blind clinical trial. CHOICE study group. Lancet 1999;354(9175):296–9.

37 Pulungsih SP, Punjabi NH, Rafli K, et al. Standard WHO-ORS versus reduced-osmolarity ORS in the management of cholera patients. J Health Popul Nutr 2006;24(1):107–12.

38 Hirschhorn N, Nalin DR, Cash RA, Greenough WB, 3rd. Formulation of oral rehydration solution. Lancet 2002;360(9329):340–1.

39 Fontaine O, Gore SM, Pierce NF. Rice-based oral rehydration solution for treating diarrhoea. Cochrane Database Syst Rev. 2000(2):CD001264. Withdrawn.

40 Bhattacharya MK, Bhattacharya SK, Dutta D, et al. Efficacy of oral hyposmolar glucose-based and rice-based oral rehydration salt solutions in the treatment of cholera in adults. Scand J Gastroenterol 1998;33(2):159–63.

41 Ramakrishna BS, Subramanian V, Mohan V, et al. A Randomized controlled trial of glucose versus amylase resistant starch hypo-osmolar oral rehydration solution for adult acute dehydrating diarrhea. PLoS ONE 2008;3(2): e1587.

42 Bahl R, Bhandari N, Saksena M, et al. Efficacy of zinc-fortified oral rehydration solution in 6- to 35-month-old children with acute diarrhea. J Pediatrics 2002;141(5):677–82.

43 de la Cabada FJ, DuPont HL, Gyr K, Mathewson JJ. Antimicrobial therapy of bacterial diarrhea in adult residents of Mexico – lack of an effect. Digestion 1992;53(3–4):134–41.

44 Ellis-Pegler RB, Hyman LK, Ingram RJ, McCarthy M. A placebo controlled evaluation of lomefloxacin in the treatment of bacterial diarrhoea in the community. J Antimicrob Chemother 1995;36(1):259–63.

45 Pichler HE, Diridl G, Stickler K, Wolf D. Clinical efficacy of ciprofloxacin compared with placebo in bacterial diarrhea. Am J Med 1987;82(4A):329–32.

46 Goodman LJ, Trenholme GM, Kaplan RL, et al. Empiric antimicrobial therapy of domestically acquired acute diarrhea in urban adults. Arch Intern Med 1990;150(3):541–6.

47 Noguerado A, Garcia-Polo I, Isasia T, et al. Early single dose therapy with ofloxacin for empirical treatment of acute gastroenteritis: a randomised, placebo-controlled double-blind clinical trial. J Antimicrob Chemother 1995;36(4):665–72.

48 Dryden MS, Gabb RJ, Wright SK. Empirical treatment of severe acute community-acquired gastroenteritis with ciprofloxacin. Clin Infect Dis 1996;22(6):1019–25.

49 Butler T, Lolekha S, Rasidi C, et al. Treatment of acute bacterial diarrhea: a multicenter international trial comparing placebo with fleroxacin given as a single dose or once daily for 3 days. Am J Med 1993;94(3A):187S–94S.

50 Lolekha S, Patanachareon S, Thanangkul B, Vibulbandhitkit S. Norfloxacin versus co-trimoxazole in the treatment of acute bacterial diarrhoea: a placebo controlled study. Scand J Infect Dis Suppl 1988;56:35–45.

51 Troselj-Vukic B, Poljak I, Milotic I, Slavic I, Nikolic N, Morovic M. Efficacy of pefloxacin in the treatment of patients with acute infectious diarrhoea. Clin Drug Investig 2003;23(9):591–6.

52 Bouree P, Chaput JC, Krainik F, Michel H, Trepo C. [Double-blind controlled study of the efficacy of nifuroxazide versus placebo in the treatment of acute diarrhea in adults]. Gastroenterol Clin Biol 1989;13(5):469–72.

53 De Bruyn G, Hahn S, Borwick A. Antibiotic treatment for travellers' diarrhoea. Cochrane Database Syst Rev 2000 (3), CD002242, DOI: 10.1002/14651858.

54 Wistrom J, Jertborn M, Ekwall E, et al. Empiric treatment of acute diarrheal disease with norfloxacin. A randomized, placebo-controlled study. Swedish Study Group. Ann Intern Med 1992;117(3):202–8.

55 Steffen R, Sack DA, Riopel L, et al. Therapy of travelers' diarrhea with rifaximin on various continents. Am J Gastroenterol 2003;98(5):1073–8.

56 Taylor DN, Bourgeois AL, Ericsson CD, et al. A randomized, double-blind, multicenter study of rifaximin compared with placebo and with ciprofloxacin in the treatment of travelers' diarrhea. Am J Trop Med Hyg 2006;74(6):1060–6.

57 Ericsson CD, Johnson PC, Dupont HL, Morgan DR, Bitsura JA, de la Cabada FJ. Ciprofloxacin or trimethoprim-sulfamethoxazole as initial therapy for travelers' diarrhea. A placebo-controlled, randomized trial. Ann Intern Med 1987;106(2):216–20.

58 Isenbarger DW, Hoge CW, Srijan A, et al. Comparative antibiotic resistance of diarrheal pathogens from Vietnam and Thailand, 1996–1999. Emerg Infect Dis 2002;8(2):175–80.

59 Gomi H, Jiang ZD, Adachi JA, et al. In vitro antimicrobial susceptibility testing of bacterial enteropathogens causing traveler's diarrhea in four geographic regions. Antimicrob Agents Chemother 2001;45(1):212–6.

60 DuPont HL, Ericsson CD, Mathewson JJ, de la Cabada FJ, Conrad DA. Oral aztreonam, a poorly absorbed yet effective

therapy for bacterial diarrhea in US travelers to Mexico. JAMA 19928;267(14):1932–5.

61 Kuschner RA, Trofa AF, Thomas RJ, et al. Use of azithromycin for the treatment of *Campylobacter* enteritis in travelers to Thailand, an area where ciprofloxacin resistance is prevalent. Clin Infect Dis 1995;21(3):536–41.

62 Tribble DR, Sanders JW, Pang LW, et al. Traveler's diarrhea in Thailand: randomized, double-blind trial comparing single-dose and 3-day azithromycin-based regimens with a 3-day levofloxacin regimen. Clin Infect Dis 2007;44(3):338–46.

63 Adachi JA, Ericsson CD, Jiang ZD, et al. Azithromycin found to be comparable to levofloxacin for the treatment of US travelers with acute diarrhea acquired in Mexico. Clin Infect Dis 2003;37(9):1165–71.

64 DuPont HL, Jiang ZD, Ericsson CD, et al. Rifaximin versus ciprofloxacin for the treatment of traveler's diarrhea: a randomized, double-blind clinical trial. Clin Infect Dis 2001;33(11):1807–15.

65 Dupont HL, Jiang ZD, Belkind-Gerson J, et al. Treatment of travelers' diarrhea: randomized trial comparing rifaximin, rifaximin plus loperamide, and loperamide alone. Clin Gastroenterol Hepatol 2007;5(4):451–6.

66 Lustman F, Walters E.G., Shroff NE, Akbar FA. Diphenoxylate hydrochloride (Lomotil) in the treatment of acute diarrhoea. Br J Clin Pract 1987;41(3):648–51.

67 Heredia Diaz JG, Alcantara I, Solis A. [Evaluation of the safety and effectiveness of WHR-1142A in the treatment of non-specific acute diarrhea]. Rev Gastroenterol Mex 1979;44(4):167–73.

68 Heredia Diaz JG, Kajeyama Escobar ML. [Double-blind evaluation of the effectiveness of lidamidine hydrochloride (WHR-1142A) vs loperamide vs. placebo in the treatment of acute diarrhea]. Salud Publica Mex 1981;23(5):483–91.

69 Van Loon FP, Bennish ML, Speelman P, Butler C. Double blind trial of loperamide for treating acute watery diarrhoea in expatriates in Bangladesh. Gut 1989;30(4):492–5.

70 Van den Eynden B, Spaepen W. New approaches to the treatment of patients with acute, nonspecific diarrhea: a comparison of the effects of loperamide and loperamide oxide. Curr Ther Res 1995;56:1132–41.

71 Hughes IW. First-line treatment in acute non-dysenteric diarrhoea: clinical comparison of loperamide oxide, loperamide and placebo. UK Janssen Research Group of General Practitioners. Br J Clin Pract 1995;49(4):181–5.

72 Cardon E, Van Elsen J, Frascio M, et al. Gut-selective opiates: the effect of loperamide oxide in acute diarrhoea in adults. The Diarrhoea Trialists Group. Eur J Clin Res 1995;7:135–44.

73 Dettmer A. Loperamide oxide in the treatment of acute diarrhea in adults. Clin Ther 1994;16(6):972–80.

74 Dreverman JW, Van der Poel AJ. Loperamide oxide in acute diarrhoea: a double-blind, placebo-controlled trial. The Dutch Diarrhoea Trialists Group. Aliment Pharmacol Ther 1995;9(4):441–6.

75 Alam NH, Ashraf H, Khan WA, Karim MM, Fuchs GJ. Efficacy and tolerability of racecadotril in the treatment of cholera in adults: a double blind, randomised, controlled clinical trial. Gut 2003;52(10):1419–23.

76 Baumer P, Danquechin Dorval E, Bertrand J, Vetel JM, Schwartz JC, Lecomte JM. Effects of acetorphan, an enkephalinase inhibitor, on experimental and acute diarrhoea. Gut 1992;33(6):753–8.

77 Hamza H, Ben Khalifa H, Baumer P, Berard H, Lecomte JM. Racecadotril versus placebo in the treatment of acute diarrhoea in adults. Aliment Pharmacol Ther 1999;13 Suppl 6:15–9.

78 Prado D. A multinational comparison of racecadotril and loperamide in the treatment of acute watery diarrhoea in adults. Scand J Gastroenterol 2002;37(6):656–61.

79 Roge J, Baumer P, Berard H, Schwartz JC, Lecomte JM. The enkephalinase inhibitor, acetorphan, in acute diarrhoea. A double-blind, controlled clinical trial versus loperamide. Scand J Gastroenterol 1993;28(4):352–4.

80 Vetel JM, Berard H, Fretault N, Lecomte JM. Comparison of racecadotril and loperamide in adults with acute diarrhoea. Aliment Pharmacol Ther 1999;13 Suppl 6:21–6.

81 Wang HH, Shieh MJ, Liao KF. A blind, randomized comparison of racecadotril and loperamide for stopping acute diarrhea in adults. World J Gastroenterol 2005;11(10):1540–3.

82 Abbas Z, Moid I, Khan AH, et al. Efficacy of octreotide in diarrhoea due to *Vibrio cholerae*: a randomized, controlled trial. Ann Trop Med Parasitol 1996;90(5):507–13.

83 Alvarez-Olmos MI, Oberhelman RA. Probiotic agents and infectious diseases: a modern perspective on a traditional therapy. Clin Infect Dis 2001;32(11):1567–76.

84 Lamers HJ, Jamin RH, Zaat JO, Van Eijk JT. Dietary advice for acute diarrhoea in general practice: a pilot study. Br J Gen Pract 1998;48(437):1819–23.

85 Huang DB, Awasthi M, Le BM, et al. The role of diet in the treatment of travelers' diarrhea: a pilot study. Clin Infect Dis 2004;39(4):468–71.

86 Ericsson CD, DuPont HL. Travelers' diarrhea: approaches to prevention and treatment. Clin Infect Dis 1993;16(5):616–24.

87 Okhuysen PC, Jiang ZD, Carlin L, Forbes C, DuPont HL. Post-diarrhea chronic intestinal symptoms and irritable bowel syndrome in North American travelers to Mexico. Am J Gastroenterol 2004;99(9):1774–8.

88 Connor BA. Sequelae of traveler's diarrhea: focus on postinfectious irritable bowel syndrome. Clin Infect Dis 2005;41 Suppl 8:S577–86.

89 Mounts AW, Holman RC, Clarke MJ, Bresee JS, Glass RI. Trends in hospitalizations associated with gastroenteritis among adults in the United States, 1979–1995. Epidemiol Infect 1999;123(1):1–8.

90 Gerber A, Karch H, Allerberger F, Verweyen HM, Zimmerhackl LB. Clinical course and the role of shiga toxin-producing *Escherichia coli* infection in the hemolytic-uremic syndrome in pediatric patients, 1997–2000, in Germany and Austria: a prospective study. J Infect Dis 2002;186(4):493–500.

91 Safdar N, Said A, Gangnon RE, Maki DG. Risk of hemolytic uremic syndrome after antibiotic treatment of *Escherichia coli* O157:H7 enteritis: a meta-analysis. JAMA 2002;288(8):996–1001.

92 Zimmerhackl LB. E. coli, antibiotics, and the hemolytic-uremic syndrome. N Engl J Med 2000;342(26):1990–1.

93 Locht H, Krogfelt KA. Comparison of rheumatological and gastrointestinal symptoms after infection with *Campylobacter jejuni/coli* and enterotoxigenic *Escherichia coli*. Ann Rheum Dis 2002;61(5):448–52.

94 Fendler C, Laitko S, Sorensen H, et al. Frequency of triggering bacteria in patients with reactive arthritis and undifferentiated oligoarthritis and the relative importance of the tests used for diagnosis. Ann Rheum Dis 2001;60(4):337–43.

95 Dworkin MS, Shoemaker PC, Goldoft MJ, Kobayashi JM. Reactive arthritis and Reiter's syndrome following an outbreak of gastroenteritis caused by *Salmonella enteritidis*. Clin Infect Dis 2001;33(7):1010–4.

96 Lew JF, Glass RI, Gangarosa RE, Cohen IP, Bern C, Moe CL. Diarrheal deaths in the United States, 1979 through 1987. A special problem for the elderly. JAMA 1991;265(24):3280–4.

97 Legros D, Paquet C, Dorlencourt F, Saoult E. Risk factors for death in hospitalized dysentery patients in Rwanda. Trop Med Int Health 1999;4(6):428–32.

98 Hogenauer C, Hammer HF, Krejs GJ, Reisinger EC. Mechanisms and management of antibiotic-associated diarrhea. Clin Infect Dis 1998;27(4):702–10.

99 McFarland LV. Epidemiology of infectious and iatrogenic nosocomial diarrhea in a cohort of general medicine patients. Am J Infect Control 1995;23(5):295–305.

100 Wistrom J, Norrby SR, Myhre EB, et al. Frequency of antibiotic-associated diarrhoea in 2462 antibiotic-treated hospitalized patients: a prospective study. J Antimicrob Chemother 2001;47(1):43–50.

101 Mylonakis E, Ryan ET, Calderwood SB. *Clostridium difficile*-associated diarrhea: A review. Arch Intern Med 2001;161(4):525–33.

102 Bartlett JG, Gerding DN. Clinical recognition and diagnosis of *Clostridium difficile* infection. Clin Infect Dis 2008;46 Suppl 1:S12–8.

103 Thomas C, Stevenson M, Riley TV. Antibiotics and hospital-acquired *Clostridium difficile*-associated diarrhoea: a systematic review. J Antimicrob Chemother 2003;51(6):1339–50.

104 Dial S, Alrasadi K, Manoukian C, Huang A, Menzies D. Risk of *Clostridium difficile* diarrhea among hospital inpatients prescribed proton pump inhibitors: cohort and case-control studies. CMAJ 2004;171(1):33–8.

105 Wanahita A, Goldsmith EA, Musher DM. Conditions associated with leukocytosis in a tertiary care hospital, with particular attention to the role of infection caused by *Clostridium difficile*. Clin Infect Dis 2002;34(12):1585–92.

106 Bauer TM, Lalvani A, Fehrenbach J, et al. Derivation and validation of guidelines for stool cultures for enteropathogenic bacteria other than *Clostridium difficile* in hospitalized adults. JAMA 2001;285(3):313–9.

107 Loo VG, Poirier L, Miller MA, et al. A predominantly clonal multi-institutional outbreak of *Clostridium difficile*-associated diarrhea with high morbidity and mortality. N Engl J Med 2005;353(23):2442–9.

108 Bartlett JG. Narrative review: the new epidemic of *Clostridium difficile*-associated enteric disease. Ann Intern Med 2006;145(10):758–64.

109 Pepin J, Valiquette L, Alary ME, et al. *Clostridium difficile*-associated diarrhea in a region of Quebec from 1991 to 2003: a changing pattern of disease severity. CMAJ 2004;171(5):466–72.

110 Manabe YC, Vinetz JM, Moore RD, Merz C, Charache P, Bartlett JG. *Clostridium difficile* colitis: an efficient clinical approach to diagnosis. Ann Intern Med 1995;123(11):835–40.

111 Schleupner MA, Garner DC, Sosnowski KM, et al. Concurrence of *Clostridium difficile* toxin A enzyme-linked immunosorbent assay, fecal lactoferrin assay, and clinical criteria with *C. difficile* cytotoxin titer in two patient cohorts. J Clin Microbiol 1995;33(7):1755–9.

112 Gerding DN, Johnson S, Peterson LR, Mulligan ME, Silva J, Jr. *Clostridium difficile*-associated diarrhea and colitis. Infect Control Hosp Epidemiol 1995;16(8):459–77.

113 Lyerly DM, Barroso LA, Wilkins TD, Depitre C, Corthier G. Characterization of a toxin A-negative, toxin B-positive strain of *Clostridium difficile*. Infect Immun 1992;60(11):4633–9.

114 van den Berg RJ, Vaessen N, Endtz HP, Schulin T, van der Vorm ER, Kuijper EJ. Evaluation of real-time PCR and conventional diagnostic methods for the detection of *Clostridium difficile*-associated diarrhoea in a prospective multicentre study. J Med Microbiol 2007;56(Pt 1):36–42.

115 van den Berg RJ, Bruijnesteijn van Coppenraet LS, Gerritsen HJ, Endtz HP, van der Vorm ER, Kuijper EJ. Prospective multicenter evaluation of a new immunoassay and real-time PCR for rapid diagnosis of Clostridium difficile-associated diarrhea in hospitalized patients. J Clin Microbiol 2005;43(10):5338–40.

116 Boland GW, Lee MJ, Cats AM, Gaa JA, Saini S, Mueller PR. Antibiotic-induced diarrhea: specificity of abdominal CT for the diagnosis of *Clostridium difficile* disease. Radiology 1994;191(1):103–6.

117 Kawamoto S, Horton KM, Fishman EK. Pseudo membranous colitis: spectrum of imaging findings with clinical and pathologic correlation. Radiographics 1999;19(4):887–97.

118 Wenisch C, Parschalk B, Hasenhundl M, Hirschl AM, Graninger W. Comparison of vancomycin, teicoplanin, metronidazole, and fusidic acid for the treatment of *Clostridium difficile*-associated diarrhea. Clin Infect Dis 1996;22(5):813–8.

119 The Swedish CDAD Study Group. Treatment of *Clostridium difficile* associated diarrhea and colitis with an oral preparation of teicoplanin; a dose finding study. The Swedish CDAD Study Group. Scand J Infect Dis 1994;26(3):309–16.

120 Dudley MN, McLaughlin JC, Carrington G, Frick J, Nightingale CH, Quintiliani R. Oral bacitracin vs vancomycin therapy for *Clostridium difficile*-induced diarrhea. A randomized double-blind trial. Arch Intern Med 1986;146(6):1101–4.

121 Teasley DG, Gerding DN, Olson MM, et al. Prospective randomised trial of metronidazole versus vancomycin for *Clostridium*-difficile-associated diarrhoea and colitis. Lancet 1983 5;2(8358):1043–6.

122 de Lalla F, Nicolin R, Rinaldi E, et al. Prospective study of oral teicoplanin versus oral vancomycin for therapy of pseudomembranous colitis and *Clostridium difficile*-associated diarrhea. Antimicrob Agents Chemother 1992;36(10):2192–6.

123 Nelson RL. Antibiotic treatment for *Clostridium difficile*-associated diarrhea in adults. Cochrane Database Syst Rev 2007 (3), CD004610, DOI: 10.1002/14651858.

124 Al-Nassir WN, Sethi AK, Nerandzic MM, Bobulsky GS, Jump RL, Donskey CJ. Comparison of clinical and microbiological response to treatment of *Clostridium difficile*-associated disease with metronidazole and vancomycin. Clin Infect Dis 2008;47(1):56–62.

125 Fekety R, Silva J, Kauffman C, Buggy B, Deery HG. Treatment of antibiotic-associated *Clostridium difficile* colitis with oral vancomycin: comparison of two dosage regimens. Am J Med 1989;86(1):15–9.

126 Louie TJ, Peppe J, Watt CK, et al. Tolevamer, a novel non-antibiotic polymer, compared with vancomycin in the treatment of mild to moderately severe *Clostridium difficile*-associated diarrhea. Clin Infect Dis 2006;43(4):411–20.

127 Wullt M, Odenholt I. A double-blind randomized controlled trial of fusidic acid and metronidazole for treatment of an initial episode of *Clostridium difficile*-associated diarrhoea. J Antimicrob Chemother 2004;54(1):211–16.

128 Fekety R, McFarland LV, Surawicz CM, Greenberg RN, Elmer GW, Mulligan ME. Recurrent *Clostridium difficile* diarrhea: characteristics of and risk factors for patients enrolled in a prospective, randomized, double-blinded trial. Clin Infect Dis 1997;24(3):324–33.

129 Lewis SJ, Potts LF, Barry RE. The lack of therapeutic effect of *Saccharomyces boulardii* in the prevention of antibiotic-related diarrhoea in elderly patients. J Infect 1998;36(2):171–4.

130 Surawicz CM, McFarland LV, Greenberg RN, et al. The search for a better treatment for recurrent *Clostridium difficile* disease: use of high-dose vancomycin combined with *Saccharomyces boulardii*. Clin Infect Dis 2000;31(4):1012–7.

131 Dendukuri N, Costa V, McGregor M, Brophy JM. Probiotic therapy for the prevention and treatment of *Clostridium difficile*-associated diarrhea: a systematic review. CMAJ 2005;173(2):167–70.

132 McFarland LV. Meta-analysis of probiotics for the prevention of antibiotic associated diarrhea and the treatment of *Clostridium difficile* disease. Am J Gastroenterol 2006101(4):812–22.

133 Gustafsson A, Berstad A, Lund-Tonnesen S, Midtvedt T, Norin E. The effect of faecal enema on five microflora-associated characteristics in patients with antibiotic-associated diarrhoea. Scand J Gastroenterol 1999;34(6):580–6.

134 Johnson S, Schriever C, Galang M, Kelly CP, Gerding DN. Interruption of recurrent *Clostridium difficile*-associated diarrhea episodes by serial therapy with vancomycin and rifaximin. Clin Infect Dis 2007;44(6):846–8.

135 Talley NJ, Weaver AL, Zinsmeister AR, Melton LJ, 3rd. Onset and disappearance of gastrointestinal symptoms and functional gastrointestinal disorders. Am J Epidemiol 1992;136(2):165–77.

136 American Gastroenterological Association medical position statement: guidelines for the management of malnutrition and cachexia, chronic diarrhea, and hepatobiliary disease in patients with human immunodeficiency virus infection. Gastroenterology 1996;111(6):1722–3.

137 American Gastroenterological Association medical position statement: guidelines for the evaluation and management of chronic diarrhea. Gastroenterology 1999;116(6):1461–3.

138 Fine KD, Schiller LR. AGA technical review on the evaluation and management of chronic diarrhea. Gastroenterology 1999;116(6):1464–86.

139 Huttly SR, Hoque BA, Aziz KM, et al. Persistent diarrhoea in a rural area of Bangladesh: a community-based longitudinal study. Int J Epidemiol 1989;18(4):964–9.

140 Weber R, Ledergerber B, Zbinden R, et al. Enteric infections and diarrhea in human immunodeficiency virus-infected persons: prospective community-based cohort study. Swiss HIV Cohort Study. Arch Intern Med 1999;159(13):1473–80.

141 Sanchez TH, Brooks JT, Sullivan PS, et al. Bacterial diarrhea in persons with HIV infection, United States, 1992–2002. Clin Infect Dis 2005;41(11):1621–7.

142 Rabeneck L, Crane MM, Risser JM, Lacke CE, Wray NP. Effect of HIV transmission category and CD4 count on the occurrence of diarrhea in HIV-infected patients. Am J Gastroenterol 1993;88(10):1720–3.

143 Kaslow RA, Phair JP, Friedman HB, et al. Infection with the human immunodeficiency virus: clinical manifestations and their relationship to immune deficiency. A report from the Multicenter AIDS Cohort Study. Ann Intern Med 1987;107(4):474–80.

144 Eisenberg JN, Wade TJ, Charles S, et al. Risk factors in HIV-associated diarrhoeal disease: the role of drinking water, medication and immune status. Epidemiol Infect 2002;128(1):73–81.

145 Becker ML, Cohen CR, Cheang M, Washington RG, Blanchard JF, Moses S. Diarrheal disease among HIV-infected adults in Karnataka, India: evaluation of risk factors and etiology. Am J Trop Med Hyg 2007;76(4):718–22.

146 Johnson JL, Okwera A, Horter L, Whalen CC, Mugerwa RD. Rifampicin-containing regimens for the treatment of latent tuberculosis infection also prevented diarrheal illnesses in HIV-infected Ugandan adults. Aids 2004;18(4):706–8.

147 Carcamo C, Hooton T, Wener MH, et al. Etiologies and manifestations of persistent diarrhea in adults with HIV-1 infection: a case-control study in Lima, Peru. J Infect Dis 2005;191(1):11–9.

148 Blanshard C, Francis N, Gazzard BG. Investigation of chronic diarrhoea in acquired immunodeficiency syndrome. A prospective study of 155 patients. Gut 1996;39(96):824–32.

149 Datta D, Gazzard B, Stebbing J. The diagnostic yield of stool analysis in 525 HIV-1-infected individuals. Aids 2003;17(11):1711–3.

150 Wilcox CM, Rabeneck L, Friedman S. AGA technical review: malnutrition and cachexia, chronic diarrhea, and hepatobiliary disease in patients with human immunodeficiency virus infection. Gastroenterology 1996;111(6):1724–52.

151 Limburg PJ, Ahlquist DA, Sandborn WJ, et al. Fecal calprotectin levels predict colorectal inflammation among patients with chronic diarrhea referred for colonoscopy. Am J Gastroenterol 2000;95(10):2831–7.

152 Fine KD, Ogunji F, George J, Niehaus MD, Guerrant RL. Utility of a rapid fecal latex agglutination test detecting the neutrophil protein, lactoferrin, for diagnosing inflammatory causes of chronic diarrhea. Am J Gastroenterol 1998;93(8):1300–5.

153 Abubakar I, Aliyu SH, Arumugam C, Usman NK, Hunter PR. Treatment of cryptosporidiosis in immunocompromised individuals: systematic review and meta-analysis. Br J Clin Pharmacol 2007;63(4):387–93.

154 Simon DM, Cello JP, Valenzuela J, et al. Multicenter trial of octreotide in patients with refractory acquired immunodeficiency syndrome-associated diarrhea. Gastroenterology 1995;108(6):1753–60.

155 Wanke CA, Pleskow D, Degirolami PC, Lambl BB, Merkel K, Akrabawi S. A medium chain triglyceride-based diet in patients with HIV and chronic diarrhea reduces diarrhea and malabsorption: a prospective, controlled trial. Nutrition 1996;12(11–12):766–71.

156 Tinmouth J, Kandel G, Tomlinson G, Walmsley S, Steinhart AH, Glazier R. The effect of dairy product ingestion on human immunodeficiency virus-related diarrhea in a sample of predominantly gay men: a randomized, controlled, double-blind, crossover trial. Arch Intern Med 2006;166(11):1178–83.

157 Carcamo C, Hooton T, Weiss NS, et al. Randomized controlled trial of zinc supplementation for persistent diarrhea in adults with HIV-1 infection. J Acquir Immune Defic Syndr 2006;43(2):197–201.

158 Garthright WE, Archer DL, Kvenberg JE. Estimates of incidence and costs of intestinal infectious diseases in the United States. Public Health Rep 1988;103(2):107–15.

159 Guerrant RL, Kirchhoff LV, Shields DS, et al. Prospective study of diarrheal illnesses in northeastern Brazil: patterns of disease, nutritional impact, etiologies, and risk factors. J Infect Di. 1983;148(6):986–97.

160 el Alamy MA, Thacker SB, Arafat RR, Wright CE, Zaki AM. The incidence of diarrheal disease in a defined population of rural Egypt. Am J Trop Med Hyg 1986;35(5):1006–12.

161 Manatsathit S, Tansupasawasdikul S, Wanachiwanawin D, et al. Causes of chronic diarrhea in patients with AIDS in Thailand: a prospective clinical and microbiological study. J Gastroenterol 1996;31(4):533–7.

162 Dworkin B, Wormser GP, Rosenthal WS, et al. Gastrointestinal manifestations of the acquired immunodeficiency syndrome: a review of 22 cases. Am J Gastroenterol 1985;80(10):774–8.

163 Laughon BE, Druckman DA, Vernon A, et al. Prevalence of enteric pathogens in homosexual men with and without acquired immunodeficiency syndrome. Gastroenterology 1988;94(4):984–93.

164 Smith PD, Lane HC, Gill VJ, et al. Intestinal infections in patients with the acquired immunodeficiency syndrome (AIDS). Etiology and response to therapy. Ann Intern Med 1988;108(3):328–33.

165 Antony MA, Brandt LJ, Klein RS, Bernstein LH. Infectious diarrhea in patients with AIDS. Dig Dis Sci 1988;33(9):1141–6.

166 Rene E, Marche C, Regnier B, et al. Intestinal infections in patients with acquired immunodeficiency syndrome. A prospective study in 132 patients. Dig Dis Sci 1989;34(5):773–80.

167 Cotte L, Rabodonirina M, Piens MA, Perreard M, Mojon M, Trepo C. Prevalence of intestinal protozoans in French patients infected with HIV. J Acquir Immune Defic Syndr 1993;6(9):1024–9.

168 Kotler DP, Orenstein JM. Prevalence of intestinal microsporidiosis in HIV-infected individuals referred for gastroenterological evaluation. Am J Gastroenterol 1994;89(11):1998–2002.

169 Prasad KN, Nag VL, Dhole TN, Ayyagari A. Identification of enteric pathogens in HIV-positive patients with diarrhoea in northern India. J Health Popul Nutr 2000;18(1):23–6.

CHAPTER 9

Urinary tract infections

Thomas Fekete

Case presentation 1

A 35-year-old woman is seen in the outpatient clinic for a 2-day history of worsening urinary burning and frequency. She is a healthy woman with no medical problems. She has two children at home and is currently using oral contraceptives. She recalls a urinary tract infection (UTI) from about 6 years earlier that responded to a 3-day course of antibiotics, and she has had no sequelae of UTI since. She has no symptoms of vaginal itching or discharge. On examination she looks mildly uncomfortable but otherwise in no distress. She is afebrile and has normal vital signs. There is no costovertebral angle tenderness. There is slight discomfort with deep palpation over the pubis, but the bladder is not enlarged. The patient refuses a pelvic examination since she has just seen her gynecologist 2 weeks earlier for a routine check-up and was told everything was normal.

UTIs are a common medical problem, with costs estimated at more than US$1.6 billion in 1995 in the United States [1]. While many people with serious underlying illnesses develop UTIs in healthcare facilities as a consequence of bladder dysfunction and catheterization, women are especially vulnerable to getting UTIs even in the absence of underlying illness. About 40% of adult women report having had a previous UTI [2]. In young, sexually active women the rate of UTIs has been reported to be as high as 0.5 episodes per woman year [3]. Moreover, in a random

Evidence-Based Infectious Diseases, 2nd edition. Edited by Mark Loeb, Fiona Smaill and Marek Smieja. © 2009 Wiley-Blackwell Publishing, ISBN: 978-1-4051-7026-0

telephone dialing survey, nearly 11% of women reported at least one UTI in the past 12 months [1]. For the more specific diagnosis of pyelonephritis, the estimated annual population based rate was 15–17 per 10 000 for women and 4–6 per 10 000 for men [4]. The incidence of all these urinary infections has been stable for the past 15 years.

Case presentation 1 (continued)

Urine dipstick testing is done in the office. It is strongly positive for leukocyte esterase and nitrites but negative for blood, protein, and glucose. Is there sufficient evidence to make a clinical diagnosis of UTI in this patient?

Diagnosis

In the case presentation, this woman has a short history of dysuria and frequency with no prior known urinary pathology. A systematic review assessing the accuracy of history-taking and physical examination for diagnosing acute uncomplicated UTI in women reveals that dysuria and frequency without vaginal discharge or irritation raises the probability of UTI from about 48% to more than 90% [5]. While a positive urine dipstick can raise this probability even higher, a negative result will still leave a high post-test probability of UTI. The clinical elements in our patient (dysuria, frequency) along with history of hematuria, back pain, and costovertebral angle tenderness all tend to increase the likelihood that the woman has a UTI, as do the lack of vaginal complaints (discharge, irritation). Since the pretest

Table 9.1 Likelihood ratios (LR) for some important UTI clinical features

Clinical features	Positive LR	Negative LR
Dysuria	1.5	0.5
Frequency	1.8	–
Hematuria	2.0	–
Vaginal discharge	0.3	–
Vaginal irritation	0.2	–
Back pain	1.6	0.8
Vaginal discharge on examination	0.7	–
Costovertebral angle tenderness	1.7	–

probability of UTI in an otherwise healthy woman coming to the clinic with a suspicion of UTI is so high (48%), it would be a fair question to ask how low a probability would argue against the initiation of therapy. The study made a formal evaluation of clinical features of UTI by a systematic review of the literature (464 articles) and focused on nine that met rigorous inclusion criteria. These individual studies were chosen because they allowed an assessment of individual features such as dysuria or vaginal irritation so that each one could be given a likelihood ratio for the presence of a UTI. This likelihood ratio could be applied to a prior probability of UTI (as determined by the patient or the physician) so that a reasonable clinical diagnosis could be made. The likelihood ratios for some of the most important clinical features (where the 95% CI did not include 1.0) are in Table 9.1.

The two most common tests used on the commercial dipstick to assess possible UTI are the nitrite (nitrate reductase) and the leukocyte esterase tests [6]. The nitrite test measures the presence of the enzyme nitrate reductase – a bacterial enzyme present in many though not all gram-negative bacteria. False positives are rare, but the rate of false negatives ranges from 10% to 30% and is especially high in infections caused by nitrite-negative organisms, when the urine has a low pH or a large amount of urobilinogen or ascorbic acid. Leukocyte esterase measures the presence of white blood cells in the urine. While other conditions can cause pyuria, the clinical setting is usually sufficiently clear to rule out these infections. False-negative results can be found with low

concentrations of urinary leukocytes, the presence of ascorbic acid, phenazopyridine, or large amounts of protein. One of the problems of these rapid tests for UTI is that they are affected by spectrum bias [7]. What this means is that the sensitivity of the test is influenced by the underlying characteristics of the population being studied. In this example, the sensitivity of a positive dipstick test was 0.92 (95% CI 0.82–0.98) whereas, if the prior probability was low, the sensitivity would be reduced to 0.56 (0.03–0.79). When the presence of a positive urine culture is used as the reference standard of a UTI, the performance characteristics of various components of the urinalysis can be disappointing [8]. The clinical benefit of treatment for symptomatic women with a negative dipstick test in the absence of cultures has been evaluated in a double-blind randomized controlled trial. Suitable women with negative nitrite and leukocyte esterase dipstick tests were randomized to a 3-day course of trimethoprim vs placebo [9]. The speed and degree of improved dysuria strongly favored the trimethoprim-treated patients suggesting an infectious entity despite negative screening tests (and no urine culture). This result would not be expected given a systematic review of dipstick testing that indicates negative dipstick results have the capacity to rule out even low levels (about 10^2) of bacteriuria [10]. Perhaps using cultures as the marker for likelihood of improvement in this setting misses some people destined to respond clinically to antibiotics.

In terms of noninvasive diagnostic tests that can be done in the ambulatory setting, there are two options: microscopic analysis of the urinary sediment and urine culture. Urine microscopy (determining in a semiquantitative manner the concentration of leukocytes in the urine) is done as a routine part of the urinalysis in many hospital laboratories, but the urine dipstick is almost as reliable in confirming UTI as the microscopic analysis [11] and is quicker and less expensive than microscopy. Both tests are imperfect but, in an Emergency Room study, each test had roughly the same number of false negatives and false positives when compared with the results of urine culture [12]. In pregnancy, the urine culture is the test of choice, since even a negative urinalysis does not ablate the need for culture. Less is known about the usefulness of dipstick testing in hospitalized patients, who experience higher rates of pyuria and UTI than ambulatory patients. Zaman and colleagues found high specificity using >10 WBC/µL and >5 WBC/µL (94% and 90%), but lower sensitivity with these values (57% and 84% respectively) [13]. The positive predictive values were 91% and 77% and the negative predictive values were 68% and 93%, respectively. Quantitative determination of pyuria in uncentrifuged urine (as contrasted with the usual semiquantitative assessment of WBC in centrifuged urine) can be a useful tool for research [11] to assure a consistent definition of UTI, but it is time-consuming and rarely done. Gram stain of uncentrifuged urine is a test seldom done in most clinical laboratories, but when positive, it has positive likelihood ratios of 7.0 and 8.1 for confirming the presence of infection by gram-positive cocci and gram-negative rods, respectively [14].

A management strategy that does not include any kind of urine testing might be appealing as a way of reducing costs and perhaps avoiding clinic visits. Unfortunately, this could result in considerable overtreatment. In a cohort of 231 Canadian women presenting with dysuria, about 80% thought that they had a UTI [15]. Physician diagnosis of a UTI occurred in 92% of cases; however, UTIs were documented in only 53%. As a result, unnecessary antibiotics were frequently prescribed. Combining clinical features and urine testing for pyuria and nitrates could have reduced the number of unnecessary treatment courses considerably. Unfortunately, it would have delayed the treatment of infection in a number of women with true cystitis (positive urine culture but negative dipstick test). The lesson from this set of observations is that, in the case of a very common problem like UTI, there can be diagnostic uncertainty comparable to that of other problems seen in the ambulatory setting. The careful clinician might interpret this as a choice between overtreatment and overdiagnosis. Luckily the consequences of either approach are modest both economically (since the drugs and the diagnostic tests are fairly inexpensive) and in toxicity (since the medications are well tolerated and a short delay in the treatment of UTI almost never leads to serious sequelae). The McIsaac paper algorithm led to a reduction in unnecessary antibiotic use from 40% of all drugs used to 27%, and a reduction in total urine cultures obtained from 87% to 40%; however, it also led to a reduction in the sensitivity for UTI from 92% to 81%. These guidelines would result in one delay of therapy in every 13 women with UTI.

Treatment guidelines for telephone-based prescription strategies might have the same problem of overtreatment. In a large study of women in the Group Health Cooperative in Washington state, who stated on the telephone that they had dysuria and met certain clinical criteria, the use of nurse prescribers of antibiotics resulted in very few clinic visits for UTI [16]. Sparing office visits might be cost-effective even at the expense of excess antibiotic prescriptions.

By strict definition, a UTI should have >10^3 colony forming units of microbe per mL of urine [17], but urine cultures demand time for processing and growth (at least 18 hours) and further time for identification of the microbe and determination of antimicrobial susceptibility. A treatment delay while these results are awaited can increase the morbidity of UTI, and the culture itself increases the cost of diagnosis. However, there are no RCTs that have randomized patients with presenting UTI symptoms to urine culture versus no culture.

Obtaining urine cultures in patients who require hospitalization, who are allergic to first-line antibiotics, or who fail therapy is done in anticipation of possible changes in treatment based on resistance or drug intolerance. Severely ill patients may also benefit from a urine culture insofar as it might guide appropriate changes in treatment if there is a failure to respond to initial therapy. Withholding treatment until a culture report is available is reasonable only for those patients with a low suspicion of infection or significant drug allergy. The only benefit of obtaining a culture when there is a plan to initiate treatment is to help interpret treatment failure. In most studies to date of healthy ambulatory women, this is rare (<5%) but changing resistance patterns could affect this strategy [18].

Other diagnostic testing

UTI can be defined as simple or complicated based on the respective absence or presence of documented or suspected structural or physiologic abnormalities of the urinary tract. There is no information in Case 1 to suggest abnormal urinary anatomy and physiology and thus no need for radiological localization of the infection [19].

Case presentation 1 (continued)

After checking to make sure the patient had no drug allergies, the physician prescribed a 3-day course of trimethoprim-sulfamethoxazole (TMP-SMX) (160/800 mg orally twice a day). A phone call to the patient 2 days after the completion of therapy showed that her symptoms were totally resolved and that she had experienced only mild nausea on antimicrobial therapy.

Therapy for the ambulatory patient

The results of urine cultures in ambulatory patients with UTIs show a great preponderance for *Escherichia coli*. Although *E. coli* is a common commensal of the gastrointestinal tract, the strains that cause UTIs are a subset of gastrointestinal-adapted strains that are also able to adhere to the periurethral area and to the cells lining the urinary tract. Similarly other gram-negative bacteria (such as *Klebsiella* spp., *Proteus* spp.) with uropathogenic attributes can also cause UTIs in otherwise healthy people.

There are two important gram-positive uropathogens of ambulatory women. The first is *Staphylococcus saprophyticus*, a coagulase-negative staphylococcus present in young women especially during the summer months. The gene sequence of *S. saprophyticus* has revealed differences from *S. aureus* and *S. epidermidis* that favor survival of *S. saprophyticus* in the uroepithelial environment [20]. These include enhanced adherence to bladder cells, adaptive ion transport pathways (to adapt to varied urinary ion concentrations) and the elaboration of urease. The second gram-positive pathogen, *Enterococcus*, is the third most common genus after *Escherichia* and *Klebsiella* and tends to cause infection in people who have received antibiotics previously.

The threshold concentration of organisms in the urine distinguishing contamination from infection has been the source of some disagreement in the past. While quantitative cultures usually show a large number of organisms present ($>10^5$/mL), about 25–30% of UTIs will have fewer organisms ($>10^3$/mL) [21].

There are many choices of antimicrobials for the treatment of UTIs and a number of potential treatment durations. The patient in Case 1 had resolution

of symptoms of her first UTI after a 3-day course of therapy. An older approach, single-dose treatment, has a higher failure rate and early recurrence as compared to short-course (usually 3-day) treatments [22,23]. A systematic review of the relative efficacy of single-dose versus 3-day or longer therapy shows better outcomes with the 3-day or longer therapy. The question of whether prolonged treatment (a week of more) is superior to 3-day therapy has been addressed in a systematic review [24]. Unsurprisingly, in the management of uncomplicated cystitis in women, 3-day courses have fewer side effects but slightly inferior bacteriologic efficacy as compared to prolonged courses. The symptomatic clinical response is indistinguishable in the individual studies as well as in the combined analysis ($n = 5000$) so there is no compelling reason to use more expensive and potentially toxic durations of antibiotic treatment for uncomplicated cystitis.

Studies of single-dose therapy using β-lactams, TMP, TMP-SMX, and fluoroquinolones have essentially been halted, not only because the clinical outcomes are worse, but also because the total costs (including time off from work, repeated visits to healthcare providers, etc.) are magnified by relatively small differences in the recurrence rate [25,26]. The only drug still given in a single dose is fosfomycin which has a long half-life (5.7 hours) and high urinary levels (a single 3 g dose is given as a sachet dissolved in water) [27]. The use of single-dose fosfomycin or longer courses of nitrofurantoin (5–7 days) gives a more reduced cure rate than TMP-SMX or fluoroquinolones [25,28–30]. Therefore these agents find their greatest use in salvage regimens or when patients have significant drug allergies or intolerance. Furthermore, fosfomycin (about US$38 in 2007) and nitrofurantoin (about US$27 in 2007) are more expensive than generic trimethoprim-sulfamethoxazole or ciprofloxacin [31].

Numerous studies have demonstrated the inferiority of β-lactams for UTI [25,32]. That is not to say that some patients do not respond well to inexpensive β-lactams such as amoxicillin but that the overall rates of response and relapse are disappointing as compared with other drugs even in the absence of β-lactam resistance in uropathogens. Thus expanding the β-lactam spectrum by using amoxicillin/clavulanate does not provide robust initial improvement or prevention of recurrence. A randomized trial of 3-day regimens of amoxicillin/clavulanate or ciprofloxacin showed a clinical cure rate of 58% for the β-lactam and 77% for ciprofloxacin ($P < 0.001$) [33]. Surprisingly, the durability of response seemed equal regardless of the initial susceptibility of the organism to amoxicillin/clavulanate. The authors speculate that a large share of failure is attributable to a failure to eradicate the organism from the genitals (45% vs 10% persistent colonization respectively). However, β-lactams are recommended for the treatment of UTI during pregnancy given their favorable safety profile and the concerns about toxicity for the alternative first-line agents.

It is important to interpret the results of clinical trials of antimicrobial agents for UTIs in the context of the local antimicrobial resistance patterns. Changing patterns of resistance of uropathogens occur constantly [34]. Therefore, changes in strains and resistance patterns of bacteria causing UTI, as well as differences in dosages of antimicrobials used, make the interpretation of older studies challenging. An example is a large, well-designed study comparing the outcome of treatment with either ciprofloxacin, ofloxacin, or TMP-SMX in women with UTI [18]. Although a large number of women were in this study (866 were recruited and 688 were available for analysis), there were no significant differences among the three study drugs in terms of outcome or adverse reactions. The study was powered to show significance assuming a success rate of 93% for ciprofloxacin, 80% for TMP-SMX, and 90% for ofloxacin. The actual clinical success rates were 93% for ciprofloxacin, 95% for TMP-SMX, and 96% for ofloxacin. Of note, the patient outcomes were as good as or better than expected (bacteriologic responses of 92–97% and clinical responses of 93–96%). Resistance to any of the drugs used was quite low; therefore the results may not apply in situations where resistance to one or more of the drugs is higher. In that situation, the outcome might be less good with the drug to which resistance has now emerged. Finally, the overall "better-than-expected" outcome might reflect especially mild disease in the patients enrolled in this study – thus true differences in outcome (or even adverse events) might be underestimated as compared with a sicker population with less capacity for spontaneous or aided recovery. A Cochrane review about fluoroquinolones

for uncomplicated cystitis in women indicates that, although as a class fluoroquinolones have shown good clinical outcomes in the published literature, there might be clinically important differences in efficacy and tolerability within the class or compared with other agents [35].

As drug resistance patterns change, it is important to identify predictors of resistance to avoid ineffective empiric therapy. A study from the San Francisco bay area showed that recurrent UTI and prior fluoroquinolone use were strong predictors for fluoroquinolone resistance (OR of 8.1 and 30.4, respectively) [36]. This study also indicated that 92% of the ciprofloxacin-resistant strains were also TMP/SMX resistant. A large study looking at nearly 2000 ciprofloxacin-resistant strains of *E. coli* obtained in 2004–5 from outpatient urine cultures from 40 North American medical centers showed that isolated fluoroquinolone resistance was present in only 10% [37]. Cross-resistance to ampicillin and TMP/SMX was common; resistance to cefdinir and nitrofurantoin was much less common. Resistance is even more of a problem in long-term care facilities where prior fluoroquinolone use and urinary catheterization were strongly associated with fluoroquinolone resistance with odds ratios of 22 and 19, respectively [38]. The use of fluoroquinolones seems to have a short-term effect on the acquisition of fluoroquinolone-resistant UTI pathogens, but an Italian study showed that the odds ratio of having a ciprofloxacin-resistant *E. coli* was 20 in the first month after a course of fluoroquinolones, 7.2 for the next 2 months and 3.3 for the next 3 months [39].

A potential limitation of guidelines is that they may not keep up with changes in microbial resistance. Failure to follow guidelines has been documented, but the consequences are unclear. In a large primary care setting, of the 30% of patients with UTIs who would have met criteria for guideline directed therapy only 25% were treated in a manner compatible with the 1999 IDSA guideline [40]. A national, ongoing survey of prescribing practices shows that fluoroquinolone use is steadily increasing, in fact fluoroquinolones have now surpassed TMP/SMX as the preferred treatment for uncomplicated UTIs in ambulatory women [41]. While there are some regional differences, the overall trend appears to be an increase in the use of fluoroquinolones to treat older women. There is debate about whether fluoroquinolones are appropriate first-line agents (especially with the reduced acquisition cost of generic ciprofloxacin) particularly given the potential problem of unnecessary use leading to increased resistance. A more nuanced approach of using TMP/SMX as first-line therapy for uncomplicated cystitis and having roles for nitrofurantoin and fosfomycin as fluoroquinolone sparing agents has been proposed but not formally tested in clinical trials [42].

Prognosis

While withholding therapy from an otherwise healthy ambulatory woman with dysuria and a positive urine culture would be difficult for most clinicians, there are some data on the expected outcome. A randomized trial in Belgium studied the benefit of a 3-day course of nitrofurantoin (100 mg orally every 6 hours) with a similar schedule of placebo [43]. Although 166 women were screened, only 78 had pyuria and agreed to participate. Thirty-five women in each group were evaluable at the conclusion of therapy and 77% of the nitrofurantoin recipients were better as compared with 54% of the placebo recipients. Excluding women with negative urine cultures showed that 17/23 (74%) of the nitrofurantoin recipients versus 9/22 (41%) of the placebo recipients were better at the 7-day evaluation. While this confirms a considerable benefit of antimicrobials for UTI (NNT for various favorable outcomes ranged from 1.7 to 4.4), clinical and microbial success was fairly common without any active treatment. In one metaanalysis of six double-blind clinical trials (over 3000 patients), the following four factors were associated with better outcomes [44]:
- not using a diaphragm
- treatment for ≥3 days
- symptoms for <2 days
- African-American race.

Patients infected with bacteria categorized as *Klebsiella* or "other" had a worse prognosis.

Response to treatment is usually fast although it may take days for all symptoms to resolve. There is even some clinical success in women with organisms that are reported to be resistant to the drug chosen for treatment. This might result from spontaneous cure or from achieving high enough a concentration of antimicrobial in the urine to result in cure

despite apparent resistance. In an Israeli study [45], all patients received a 5-day course of TMP-SMX and, in the patients with strains that were susceptible, the success rate was 82% as compared with 42% in whom the organism was resistant. In a large British study showing a relatively low incidence of trimethoprim resistance (14%), half the patients with in vitro resistance to trimethoprim receiving a 3-day course of trimethoprim were symptomatically resolved in 1 week [46]. The time to resolution of symptoms was longer (when it occurred), but given the rate of resistance and the fairly good clinical response even in patients with resistant strains, the authors calculate that they would need to treat 23 patients to find one who returned for retreatment. Thus they make the case for continued empiric therapy with TMP/SMX without the need for a pretreatment urine culture. In areas where resistance is more frequent to usual first-line agents, the approach is to use a second-line agent such as fosfomycin or an alternative (but perhaps more expensive) first-line agent such as a fluoroquinolone. The same would be true for women who are allergic or cannot tolerate the usual medical interventions. Differences in resistance patterns can be associated with geographic location, patient age, and gender. A large multicenter study of antibiotic resistance in outpatients with UTI looking at nearly 2000 uropathogens collected in the US and Canada between 2003 and 2004 illustrates some of these differences [47]. The 175 patients under the age of 15 had almost no fluoroquinolone-resistant bacteria although they were more likely to have bacteria with ampicillin, nitrofurantoin, or TMP/SMX resistance than was found in adults. Younger adults (15–50) had less fluoroquinolone resistance than older adults (>50). Regional and gender differences likely reflect variations in circulating strains of potential uropathogens in the gastrointestinal tract as well as the selective pressure of antimicrobial use.

Pathogenesis

The sequence of events that follow the entry of uropathogens into the bladder is now better understood. The host innate immune process, using Toll-like receptors, begins a variety of nonspecific consequences including more rapid shedding of bladder mucosa to avoid infection [48]. The proper physiologic functioning of Toll-like receptors seems to coordinate the inflammatory response. In an animal model, mice with defective Toll-like receptors could not marshal a neutrophil response to a kidney infection and did not develop the pathologic features of pyelonephritis [49]. A similar phenomenon can be shown in the bladders of animals with defective Toll-like receptors after local challenge with bacteria. However the uropathogen can hide within the cells of the bladder and create a large number of copies within a biofilm coat. This accounts for the difficulty for some people to clear the infection despite a paucity of initial symptoms. On the other side of the ledger, we know that bacteria in the process of causing infection upregulate a variety of virulence genes such as adhesins (e.g., type 1 fimbriae) and iron acquisition systems while downregulating motility and chemotaxis-related genes as a way to maintain colonization/infection once in the uroepithelium [50].

Case presentation 2

A 63-year-old woman is seen in the office for a 2-day history of dysuria. She had recently retired from her secretarial job because of complications of her diabetes (early cataracts and mild, painful neuropathy) that had made it difficult for her to travel to work. She had recently completed a course of cefadroxil for cellulitis of the left foot with clinical improvement. Her current voiding symptoms were moderately severe. She thought she might have had a fever and some mild sweats but at the time of the clinic visit she was afebrile. The remainder of the examination was unremarkable except for mild left costovertebral angle tenderness and diminished sensation in both feet. A pelvic examination was normal. A urine specimen was obtained: the dipstick test was positive for leukocyte esterase and glucose and negative for all other tests including nitrite.

Like the previous patient, this woman also has a short history of irritative voiding symptoms, but there are some important distinctions. In addition to being older, this patient has longstanding diabetes with complications. As a result, bladder dysfunction due to diabetic neuropathy is a possibility. This patient's previous course of antibiotics (cephalosporins) may have changed the specific potential uropathogens, and may specifically have selected a more antibiotic-resistant flora [51]. The presence of significant diabetic peripheral neuropathy might portend autonomic neuropathy and incomplete bladder emptying. Significant residual bladder urine increases the risk of upper tract infection and treatment failure as well as the intrinsic risk for cystitis [52,53]. There are two potential strategies with respect to obtaining urine cultures for this patient:

- obtain a culture before initiating antibiotics (early culture)
- obtain a culture only if there is a clinical failure of therapy (late culture).

Early culture is reasonable when urine can be obtained in the office and if culture reports are promptly and reliably available. On the other hand, a late culture strategy makes sense if cultures are difficult to obtain and if adherence with medication and follow-up is likely to be excellent. These strategies have not been formally compared in clinical trials.

Case presentation 2 (continued)

Because of the patient's recent antibiotic course, a urine culture was requested. While culture results were awaited, the patient began a course of antibiotics with TMP-SMX (160/800 mg orally twice a day) with the intention of giving a 14-day course of treatment. The laboratory report on the culture showed that she had an *E. coli* that was resistant to ampicillin and tetracycline but susceptible to all the other agents tested. The patient responded clinically within 2 days of starting treatment. At the conclusion of her 14-day course of therapy, she was asymptomatic and, at the time of follow-up clinic visit, had no symptoms or physical findings of UTI.

Follow-up

Follow-up for the woman with a symptomatic UTI is simple. If all symptoms have resolved, the treatment is considered successful and no further visit or diagnostic testing is needed. Both of the cases presented had good responses and would not need follow-up. It would be sufficient to have telephone contact to assure that the treatment was successful. The success rate with TMP-SMX in the IDSA study [54] was 93%, and the majority of treatment failures were symptomatic. In a large primary care database (104 099 infections) in the UK, the failure rate (i.e., need for a second course of therapy) was 14% at 28 days of follow-up after the diagnosis of UTI was first made [51]. This study included women treated in 1992–99. Of all the drugs used, TMP-SMX was the least likely to fail with a hazard ratio (HR) for failure of 1.39 for amoxicillin and 1.23 for nitrofurantoin, although ciprofloxacin (HR for failure of 1.12; 95% CI 0.90–1.40) and cefadroxil (HR 1.17; 95% CI 0.93–1.48) were of comparable efficacy but were used much less often than TMP-SMX. There are certainly limitations of this nonrandomized study design, but the large number of women studied gives some indication of the likelihood of a successful outcome, even though treatment was assigned by physician preference and not controlled. Since this study did not look at the result of follow-up cultures, but only at the need for another course of antimicrobials, it is difficult to know whether to look for early failure with scheduled culture before the recurrence of symptoms. Since failure requiring retreatment is expected in about one in seven patients, and these failures can occur within a few days of the conclusion of the original therapy to a month later, the usefulness of routine follow-up cultures is questionable.

Asymptomatic bacteriuria

Asymptomatic bacteriuria refers to the presence of significant numbers of bacteria in the urine in the absence of symptoms such as urinary burning, frequency, or urgency. In young, healthy women, the prevalence of asymptomatic bacteriuria is 5–6% [55]. In this study, it was shown that, in the vast majority of cases of asymptomatic bacteriuria, the bacteriuria resolves spontaneously. However, the likelihood of developing cystitis within a week of the detection of asymptomatic bacteriuria is eight times higher than the risk within a week of having a sterile urine culture. Thus, in this setting, asymptomatic bacteriuria is an uncommon and unalarming entity that has a small chance of progressing to symptomatic disease. Underlying conditions known to be associated with higher rates of asymptomatic bacteriuria are

pregnancy, post-bladder catheter removal, advanced age (>65 years), and diabetes mellitus. There is evidence favoring treatment of asymptomatic bacteriuria during pregnancy [56,57] and following bladder catheter removal [58]. A Cochrane review of bacteriuria in pregnancy showed substantial benefits of treatment for asymptomatic bacteriuria during pregnancy. The elimination of bacteriuria was much greater with antibiotics than with placebo or no treatment (OR 0.07; 95% CI 0.05–0.10), the reduction of pyelonephritis was impressive (OR 0.24; 95% CI 0.19–0.32), and the pregnancy outcome (fewer preterm or low birthweight babies) was enhanced (OR 0.60; 95% CI 0.45–0.80). A randomized controlled clinical trial demonstrated that bacteriuria resolved spontaneously within 14 days of bladder catheterization in 36% and after a single dose of antibiotics in 81% [58]. More importantly, of the women who received no treatment, seven of 42 developed symptomatic UTIs. In general, untreated women under the age of 65 did better at clearing their bacteriuria (74%) than older women (4%). Without controlled trials, this could be interpreted as a suggestion to promptly treat bacteriuria after catheter removal in older people but to wait for symptoms to emerge in younger ones. Post-procedure bacteriuria can occur after cystoscopy. Patients with known bacteriuria are often treated before invasive procedures (including surgery and cystoscopy). There is evidence that prophylaxis with a single dose of pre-procedure ciprofloxacin can appreciably reduce the risk of post-cystoscopy bacteriuria in women with negative urine cultures undergoing diagnostic cystoscopy [59]. In other settings such as diabetes and old age, attempted treatment of bacteriuria is unhelpful in preventing subsequent infections and exposes patients to the potential toxicity of antimicrobials and the cost of repeated clinic visits and urine tests [60,61]. A recent prospective, randomized trial of treatment of asymptomatic bacteriuria in diabetic women showed no net benefit for a 14-day course of antibiotics directed at the organism isolated [62]. There was no reduction in symptomatic UTI in a 3-year follow-up, but there was a considerable excess in the use of antibiotics (5-fold increase) and in treatment-related adverse effects (3-fold increase). A minor side note: a 3-day course of antibiotics for the eradication of asymptomatic bacteriuria was ineffective in all six cases in which it was tried, so that regimen was dropped from the study.

Case presentation 2 (continued)

Three months later, the patient noted the onset of dysuria and urinary frequency over a period of 2 days. At the time of the office visit, she was uncomfortable but had no fever or constitutional symptoms. Her urinalysis again showed a positive leukocyte esterase on the dipstick and a large number of white blood cells on microscopic analysis. She was given another course of TMP-SMX after a urine culture was sent. This time, the culture showed >100 000 colony-forming units of *Klebsiella pneumoniae*. This organism was resistant to ampicillin but susceptible to all other antibiotics tested.

In this situation, the patient had a new infection after cure of the previous UTI. Recurrence of UTI is a common problem with rates reported as high as 44% at one year [63]. Recurrent symptoms following apparent cure of a UTI can represent a relapse of the previous infection or a reinfection. In this case, the patient clearly had a reinfection since the organism isolated was a different species from that of the prior infection. To document a relapse, it is essential to demonstrate not only the same species of bacteria in both infections but also the same strain. This can be done using molecular typing.

Case presentation 2 (continued)

Although she felt completely well at the conclusion of her second course of antibiotics, the patient is frustrated and asks, "Why does this keep happening to me? Can't something be done to prevent another one of these infections?"

Prevention

Although the reservoir for organisms causing UTIs is the lower gastrointestinal tract, it is unclear exactly how uropathogens become part of our flora. A large multi-state study done among attendees of college health services showed that variants of an *E. coli* clone were circulating as uropathogens in at least three US states [64]. Women with UTIs were not acquainted with each other. Men from the same campuses were also colonized by these strains although there was no reported excess of UTIs among them. These clones had in common a resistance to TMP/SMX, but it is likely that more common strains are in national circulation causing epidemics of UTIs. In a follow-on study in the same general population, the clonal group found in all three geographic regions was still present but had decreased by 38% within 2 years of the original collection [65]. On a smaller scale, it has been shown that members of a household (including the family dog) can also be part of a gastrointestinal tract uropathogen-sharing network even if most of them have no UTI [66]. Individual susceptibility to pyelonephritis seems to be partially familial. In addition to variations in cellular adhesins that make genital and bladder colonization more common (e.g., secretor status and blood type O), it appears that expression of CXCR1 is lower in pyelonephritis patients and their relatives than in controls or people with cystitis but no upper tract involvement [67].

The timing and frequency of recurrent UTI is unpredictable. Most of the known risk factors for UTI are difficult to control. Efforts to reduce the adhesion of uropathogenic bacteria to the genitourinary epithelium by the ingestion of cranberry juice have been mildly effective while the use of a lactobacillus GG beverage was not helpful in preventing UTI [68]. Women who were at risk of recurrent UTIs were randomized to receive a cranberry/lingonberry juice daily or lactobacillus GG for 5 days/week. The study was not blinded, although the investigators were not informed which treatment the women were getting. In a 6-month period, the women using the cranberry beverage had a 20% absolute reduction in the rate of UTIs (95% CI 3–36). There was a very slight increase in the absolute rate of UTIs in the group taking the lactobacillus beverage. Cranberry juice prophylaxis was studied as a preventive measure for hospitalized, elderly patients although the 50% reduction in symptomatic UTIs was not statistically significant [69]. Cranberry juice prophylaxis for ambulatory women was studied in a Cochrane systematic review and found to be somewhat helpful for those who can tolerate it [70]. Change in vaginal pH, in particular the use of spermicide (often accompanying diaphragms), has been associated with an increased risk of UTI in several studies [3,71]. Sexual activity can predispose to UTIs [3] and this may be especially problematic with newer sex partners. In postmenopausal women, not taking estrogen replacement therapy is a risk factor for recurrent UTI [52]. Topical or systemic estrogens will reduce the rate of recurrent UTI in these women [72]. Clearly, the use of systemic estrogens should be informed by their risk/benefit for medical problems other than UTI.

The controversy over seeking an anatomic explanation for recurrent UTI is not fully resolved, but in adults it is rare to identify correctable lesions [73]. In this study, 104 adult women referred to Urology for UTI consultation were evaluated with excretory urography and 74 of them also had cystoscopy. These women had a heterogeneous history of UTI, but most had had two or more UTIs in the past year. The radiographic work-up showed only 12 abnormalities of which perhaps five were related to (but not likely to be causal of) UTI. The cystoscopies showed that 18% of the women had abnormalities (most of which were mucosal inflammation) and that only 4% had a potentially treatable problem (urethral diverticula). For our patient, bladder function could be abnormal if she also has an autonomic neuropathy from diabetes. Obstructions to urine flow, poor emptying of the bladder and ureters, reflux of urine from the bladder to the ureter, and anatomic variations of the urethra can be found as causes of recurrent infection. However, standard techniques (radiographic imaging, cystoscopy, etc.) have a low yield in identifying such lesions [73]. Relatively common problems such as incomplete bladder emptying because of neural injury or disease are often difficult or impossible to correct.

Evidence exists to support antimicrobial prevention of recurrent infections. Women with frequent, uncomplicated recurrences (usually two or more infections in a 6-month period) may benefit from one of three antibiotic use strategies:

- continuous low-dose prophylaxis [74,75]
- postcoital prophylaxis [76]
- pre-emptive short course treatment (without medical consultation) at first sign of infection [77].

Each of these strategies reduces the frequency and morbidity of UTI, but there are no controlled trials comparing them. Postcoital prophylaxis with trimethoprim-sulfamethoxazole (TMP-SMX) was studied in a randomized, placebo-controlled trial and shown to reduce UTIs by 12-fold (from 3.6 per patient year to 0.3 per patient year) [76]. However, the very small number of women studied (16 in the TMP-SMX group and 11 in the placebo group) limits precision. Self-directed therapy appeals to many women, and there is evidence that women who have experienced UTI can self-diagnose and treat with impressive accuracy and good outcomes [78]. In this study, 172 women were given the opportunity to initiate levofloxacin therapy at the first indication of a UTI. There was no control group since all women were eligible to initiate therapy after obtaining a urine specimen for analysis and culture. Roughly 50% of the women studied had one or more UTIs after enrolling in the study (on average, two per woman for those who had UTI), and the urinalysis and/or urine culture was positive in 95% of these episodes. Clinical and microbiologic cures were attained in 92% and 96% of cases, respectively. Old trials of daily prophylaxis with TMP/SMX or fluoroquinolones showed benefits over placebo, but a newer placebo-controlled study of 317 women showed potential benefit of fosfomycin for women with at least three UTIs in the prior 12 months [79]. A single sachet of 3 g of fosfomycin was dissolved in water and taken orally every 10 days for 6 months and the infection rate of 0.14 infections per patient year was much lower than the 2.97 infections per patient year of placebo recipients ($P < 0.001$).

Whether prophylaxis is offered or not, there tends to be a slow trend towards cessation of recurrent infections in women without anatomic or physiologic reasons to have recurrent UTI. For women on continuing prophylaxis or postcoital prophylaxis, it might make sense to stop this treatment every year or so to see if the propensity to recurrent infections has faded. The patient in Case 2 will need to be aware of her urinary infection pattern and attend to her possible bladder dysfunction. This may entail consultation with a urologist who can assess her urodynamics and help determine the best way to maintain good voiding patterns.

The use of special silver-coated catheters in people who need short-term bladder catheterization has been studied and been shown to reduce the risk of UTI. A randomized crossover study in hospitalized patients showed that the relative risk of infection per

100 catheters used was 0.68 (95% CI 0.54–0.86) [80]. A report prepared for the US Agency for Healthcare Research and Quality indicated that silver-coated catheters could prevent bacteriuria and complications of UTI such as bacteremia, although these benefits might be somewhat vitiated with a long duration of catheterization [81]. This paper describes a number of randomized controlled trials of various silver-coated catheters versus standard silicon urinary catheters. The range of benefits is broad from a 4-fold reduction (at most) to no meaningful reduction. This large variation is related in part to differences in the patient populations and in the duration of catheterization. A systematic review of antimicrobial urinary catheters emphasized the lack of conclusive evidence that can be derived from 12 trials comparing nitrofurazone- or silver-coated catheters with standard ones [82]. The largest and newest studies showed the smallest effect on bacteriuria, and none of them showed an effect on clinically important outcomes such as hospital stay, antibiotic administration, or other morbidity. On the other hand, a careful bladder management plan in the perioperative setting was shown to have a substantial reduction in bacteriuria among orthopedic patients [83]. Even 2 years after the formal intervention period the 60% reduction in bacteriuria persisted, which suggests that an easy-to-implement protocol can have lasting benefits.

The problem of UTI in people with spinal cord injury has also led to the study of preventive measures. The US Agency for Health Care Policy initiated a metaanalysis of the role of prophylactic antibiotics in adults and adolescents with neurogenic bladder secondary to spinal cord injury [84]. They showed a reduction in the number of episodes of asymptomatic bacteriuria but not in the number of symptomatic UTIs. This calls into question the practice of aggressive prophylaxis, especially in an environment of rising rates of *Clostridium difficile* colitis. Patients with spinal cord injuries are also a target population for a new concept in infection prevention: bacterial interference. *E. coli* strain 83972 isolated from a child with persistent, symptom-free bacteriuria has been shown to reduce both bacteriuria and UTI in a placebo-controlled trial where it was instilled into the bladder and established colonization [85]. Other trials are under way, and this may be an attractive option in other patient groups with a risk for recurrent UTI [86].

Urinary tract infections in men

Case presentation 3

A 40-year-old man presented to his physician with a 3-day history of dysuria. The pain was moderately severe but only present during voiding. He had no urethral discharge and he had no pelvic pain. He had not been sexually active for over 1 month prior to his dysuria. On examination, his temperature was 37.4°C and the general physical examination was normal. The rectal examination showed a mildly enlarged but nontender prostate. Urine analysis showed pyuria and bacteriuria. Urine culture was obtained and he was given ciprofloxacin 750 mg every 12 hours pending culture results. The culture eventually showed 10^5 colony forming units per mL of *Escherichia coli* susceptible to ciprofloxacin.

Clinical presentation

The presentation in this case is comparable to UTIs that are seen in women. However, in men it is important to consider involvement of the prostate gland as well as the bladder, ureters, and kidneys. The literature on UTI in men is limited and groups together urinary infections, such as cystitis and pyelonephritis, with prostatitis. It is easy to "rule in" prostatitis with a variety of clinical features (prostate tenderness, post-prostate examination urethral discharge) because acute prostatitis is often defined as a UTI in a man with additional features supporting prostate inflammation [87]. However, in men with features of UTI, it can be impossible to rule out some degree of prostatitis at the time of initial diagnosis since there may be only subtle or subclinical features of prostate involvement, which would only be revealed by prostate biopsy or culture of prostatic secretions. Thus the absence of prostate tenderness or post-prostate examination urethral discharge does not exclude the possibility of prostatitis in a man with dysuria and positive urine cultures [87]. Because of this overlap, acute prostatitis and UTI can be considered to form a continuum in men. Some older literature refers to this as "recurrent UTI in men" or chronic prostatitis because of the incomplete response to the short courses of antibiotics used at the time [88].

Prostatitis

Prostatitis is a common condition and has protean manifestations. Several classification schemes have been devised to account for the variable characteristics that can be present. An NIH consensus classification has been developed to standardize prostatitis variants and permit more meaningful research [89]. This system creates four categories:

- acute bacterial prostatitis
- chronic bacterial prostatitis
- chronic prostatitis/pelvic pain syndrome (with inflammatory and noninflammatory subtypes)
- asymptomatic inflammatory prostatitis.

Although having reproducible definitions for the advancement of clinical research is reasonable, this division is difficult to translate into everyday clinical practice. Acute and chronic bacterial prostatitis share similarities with UTI since all three are infections. However, it is much less clear what the relationship is between infection and the other two forms of prostate disease. The exact distinction between acute and chronic bacterial prostatitis in this working definition is imprecise and does not specify the number of days of symptoms needed to invoke a diagnosis of prostatitis. This difficulty is also reflected in clinical trials of bacterial prostatitis. Of interest, it is widely believed that the chronic bacterial and nonbacterial forms of prostatitis account for about 90% of cases of prostatitis. A large population-based study in Canada showed that nearly 10% of men (aged 20–74) had symptoms consistent with prostatitis other than acute bacterial prostatitis and there was a fairly smooth age distribution throughout the group [90]. A similar survey in Minnesota also showed that 9% of men (aged 40–70) had symptoms typical of prostatitis other than acute bacterial prostatitis [91]. However, among men with prior prostatitis (including acute bacterial prostatitis), there was a significant increase in the age-related risk of prostatitis (20% at age 40, 38% at age 60, and 50% at age 50), suggesting that the various chronic prostatitis syndromes can have a remitting/relapsing form that tends not to resolve completely irrespective of the intervention.

Diagnosis

The diagnosis of UTI in men is made in a similar fashion to that in women. Urine collection is less likely to be compromised by contamination from skin flora. Pyuria and bacteriuria are both highly predictive of significant positive cultures. The lower limit of a positive quantitative culture is 10^3 colony-forming units per mL [92]. The sensitivity and specificity of this cut-off were both 97%, and it was unimportant as to whether a clean-catch mid-stream specimen or an uncleansed first void specimen was used.

Other investigations

The evaluation of the cause of UTI in men differs from that in women since it is believed that there should be some diagnosable anatomic or physiologic factor to account for the UTI in men [93]. Recent studies in this area mostly come from referral centers and thus may suffer from referral bias. For example, a Scandinavian study of 83 men with UTI showed that 19 men had some upper tract finding and 35 men had lower tract problems [94]. There was a correctable defect in only one man with an upper tract lesion, but 41% of the men had a lower tract abnormality. Only 18% of the men were found to have previously unrecognized, correctable abnormalities with the multiple modalities used to study the lower tract: cystourethroscopy, uroflowmetry, digital rectal examination, and measurement of postvoid residual by abdominal ultrasound. There is no mention of how many of these men actually underwent a corrective procedure. A study designed to compare intravenous urography (IVU) with ultrasound and plain film showed that half of the men studied had some abnormality (most of which were not correctable) [95]. The most common problem found was bladder outflow obstruction that was actually diagnosed by urodynamics (which was not part of the formal study protocol but was available for many but not all of the patients). There was no mention of how many men received treatment for any abnormality found. A community-based study from Australia showed that of gay men with UTI (one-third of whom were HIV positive), clinical management was satisfactory and, of the men who underwent further investigation, only 14% had detectable abnormalities [96]. Again there was no report on how many of these men underwent a corrective procedure. One thing lacking in all these studies is a sense of the rate of baseline abnormalities in similar populations of men without UTIs. Given the high rate of prostate symptoms recorded in community-based surveys [90,91], UTIs might simply coexist with some of the voiding problems and other prostate complaints seen in so many men. An additional issue that might be contributory is the referral bias of the studies performed by urologists [94,95]. If the primary care providers suspected some anatomic or physiologic problem in these men, they might have referred them for evaluation more quickly than for men with UTIs who evinced no symptoms.

Treatment strategies for men

The organisms that cause urinary tract infections in men (including acute and chronic prostatitis) are essentially the same as those found in women although the relative rates will vary [14]]. The same virulence factors (P fimbriae, adhesins, hemolysins) that make bacteria good uropathogens in women (particularly as a cause of pyelonephritis) also make them uropathogenic in men [97–99]. Thus, E. coli, Klebsiella spp., Enterococcus spp., Proteus spp., and various other gram-negative bacteria comprise the vast majority of uropathogens in men.

There are few studies comparing treatment strategies for male urinary tract infection or prostatitis in randomized controlled trials. There are no systematic reviews. Because of the possibility of concurrent prostatitis in men with UTI, the drugs selected for initial therapy are often those that penetrate into the prostate gland. These include TMP and the fluoroquinolones. Whilst other classes of drugs may be effective in the treatment of UTI in men, these drugs are active against most uropathogens. TMP is often given in a fixed combination with SMX. Clinical trials of TMP-SMX for UTI in males have, however, been disappointing. In an effort to compare a short course (10 days) to a long course (12 weeks) for recurrent UTI, the investigators of a multicenter US Veterans Administration study tried to recruit appropriate patients to randomize [100]. Of the 306 patients screened, only 38 were randomized and only 30 were available for analysis at the end of the study period. Of the men screened, 17% were excluded because of comorbidity, 28% for paramorbidity, 6% for comedication, 24% for lack of compliance, and 9% for miscellaneous reasons. This left 46 men to study. Four of them did not have meaningful outcome on localization tests (which would likely not be considered very important today, but were required for study entry). Of the 42 remaining men, four could not be randomized.

Eight more were dropped from the study for a variety of protocol violations, leaving a total of 30. Notably, fewer than half of the men studied were symptomatic from their UTI, and two did not even have pyuria. Of interest, the long course of therapy was superior – 60% success for 12 weeks and only 20% for 10 days (RR 3; 95% CI 1.01–8.95). Recurrent infections were from the same organism in the majority of cases. Another study of 42 men with recurrent UTI showed that a longer course of treatment (6 weeks vs 2 weeks) had a lower failure rate at a 6-week post-treatment follow-up visit (68% vs 32%; RR 2·2; 95% CI 1.05–4.49) [101].

In contrast to TMP-SMX, the clinical response to fluoroquinolones in men with UTI is much better. Fluoroquinolones have good prostate penetration in animal models, and agents studied appear comparable in the treatment of male UTI/prostatitis. When norfloxacin was compared with TMP-SMX in 109 men in a randomized controlled trial, the bacterial eradication rate of 93% with norfloxacin compared with 67% with TMP-SMX ($P < 0.05$) [102].

Ofloxacin, a drug that has largely been replaced by its L-isomer, levofloxacin, was studied in an unblinded comparison to indanyl carbenicillin (an oral form of the drug that has an FDA indication for UTI/prostatitis) and to TMP-SMX [103]. The population included men and women in equal numbers; however, treatment arms were not stratified by gender, an important limitation. Treatment failure with carbenicillin was 25% compared with no treatment failures with ofloxacin (0%) ($P = 0.048$). The comparison with TMP-SMX was done in a larger group (173 patients) and the outcomes were similar in both treatment arms, although the trend for clinical cure favored ofloxacin. Only 117 patients were evaluable for clinical cure: 93% of ofloxacin-treated patients were cured as compared with 85% of TMP-SMX-treated patients for an RR of 0.92 (95% CI 0.81–1.04).

In another study, ciprofloxacin was compared with TMP-SMX in men with UTI [104]. There was no significant difference in outcomes at late follow-up (4–6 weeks), but the early bacterial eradication rate (days 5–9 following antibiotics) favored ciprofloxacin (82% vs 52%, $P = 0.035$). The drug doses used in the study were low (ciprofloxacin 250 mg orally every 12 hours, and TMP-SMX 160/800 mg orally every 12 hours) and the duration was brief (mean of 7 days).

An open-label study of ciprofloxacin for chronic bacterial prostatitis showed a good outcome with a 4-week course [105]. The bacteriologic cure rate was 92% at 3 months after the end of therapy and 70% at 2 years post therapy. A randomized trial comparing 2 vs 4 weeks of ciprofloxacin for men with febrile UTIs showed no significant difference in either early response or at 1-year follow-up [106].

How does this evidence apply to the example of the patient in Case 3 above? The treatment with ciprofloxacin is rational and should be of at least 2 weeks' duration. Assuming that he makes a good recovery and has no further symptoms, he does not need investigative studies, but incomplete resolution or relapse should occasion a work-up. An ultrasound and plain abdominal radiograph can look for structural lesions such as kidney stones or hydronephrosis. A urologic evaluation could find problems with bladder emptying or structural disease of the lower urinary tract (including the prostate gland). While his prognosis is good, he may require a longer course of antibiotics for subsequent UTI. Treatment benefit is less optimistic for men with chronic prostatitis/chronic pelvic pain syndrome. A multicenter 6-week trial of levofloxacin vs placebo in 80 men showed some improvement in both groups but no benefit of the antibiotic over the placebo [107]. A double-blind, randomized trial of nearly 200 men compared ciprofloxacin plus tamsulosin, ciprofloxacin plus placebo, tamsulosin plus placebo, and two placebos [108]. The four groups were indistinguishable in terms of clinical response or measurement of disease using the NIH scoring system.

Severe and complex urinary tract infections

Case presentation 4

A 59-year-old diabetic woman with no other prior medical problems was seen in the Emergency Department with a 36-hour history of fever, chills, and flank pain. She attempted to go to work that day, but after 2 hours at the office, her co-workers became alarmed when she nearly fainted on the way to the copier. In the ED, she was slightly confused and sweaty. Her oral temperature was 38.9°C, pulse 110, and respiratory rate 24. Her blood pressure was 92/60 mmHg. She had right flank tenderness on palpation. Urine obtained by bladder catheterization was cloudy and had numerous WBC and bacteria on microscopic examination. She had a WBC of 22 000 with 80% PMNs, 14% bands, and 6% lymphocytes. Her fingerstick blood glucose was 21 mmol/L and her creatinine was 100 μmol/L.

This patient has a severe urinary tract infection requiring hospital admission [5]. In addition to fever and flank tenderness, she has signs of possible sepsis with hypotension, rapid heart and respiratory rates, and mental clouding. Furthermore, her diabetes is out of control and she is dehydrated. Based on her clinical presentation, she has upper urinary tract disease (kidney, renal pelvis, or ureter), otherwise known as pyelonephritis.

Because this woman is diabetic, she could be presenting with a complicated UTI. This is defined as either a disruption of the normal anatomy or physiology (as in this patient) of the urinary tract. Obstructions to urine flow such as stones, tumors, or strictures can lead to more clinically severe infections. Alterations to barriers that normally maintain the unidirectional flow of urine such as vesicoureteral reflux and external bladder catheters can also predispose to severe infections. The presence of stones or catheters can also contribute a surface for the growth of microbes as well as some protection from host defenses such as complement and phagocytosis. Physiologic problems such as incomplete bladder emptying with residual urine or poor ureteral muscular function can contribute to UTI complexity. Risk factors for pyelonephritis are similar to those of cystitis: sexual activity, family history, diabetes, and incontinence [109].

Diagnosis of severe urinary tract infections

The diagnosis of severe UTI starts with urine collection for urinalysis and culture. Quantitation of pyuria or bacteriuria cannot distinguish mild from severe UTI. A review of quantitative pyuria in 1983 showed a sensitivity of 97% and a specificity of 98% for the finding of concomitant bacteriuria [110]. Pyuria and UTI in the setting of an indwelling bladder catheter is still a topic of interest, but a recent study has shown that the high specificity of pyuria for bacteriuria (90%) is offset by a low sensitivity (37%) [111]. In a British hospital study, urine dipstick testing on hospitalized patients was highly sensitive (98.3%) for bacteriuria; negative results on leukocyte esterase, nitrite, blood, and protein had a 98.3% NPV [112].

Blood cultures are commonly performed in patients with severe UTI. The rate of blood culture positivity varies, but is rarely in excess of 20–25%, even in the most severe hospitalized cases [113]. In almost all cases, positive blood cultures have the same organism that is found in the urine and thus may add little to the determination of the specific etiology of the UTI [114]. Whether positive blood cultures are systematically associated with worse outcomes, such as prolonged hospitalization, has not been determined [115]. There is some evidence from a retrospective chart review that young women with severe UTI and positive blood cultures do have higher rates of genitourinary abnormality, persistent fever, and abnormal heart rate than women without bacteremia [116]. A study of pregnant women with severe UTI showed that those who were bacteremic had a longer hospital stay than those who were not [117]. The management implications for patients with positive blood cultures is hard to assess since they often have other markers of severity that call for more intensive treatment [118]. Positive blood cultures rarely surprise the clinician or independently change the therapeutic approach [119].

Site of care

The initial management of severe UTI includes a decision about hospitalization, which is based generally on the need for intravenous fluids, pressors, close nursing care, and adherence to a medical regimen. The patient in Case 4 might be stabilized in the Emergency Department, but would likely require hospital admission for assessment and treatment of her hemodynamic instability.

For patients with uncomplicated severe UTI, the choice of hospital admission greatly increases the cost of treatment. It is difficult to ascertain whether it improves outcome, however. This topic has not been studied in a controlled fashion except to show that for patients who can be managed in the ambulatory environment with oral therapy, there is no advantage

to parenteral medications [120,121]. A retrospective survey of women evaluated in an Emergency Department showed that patients who were admitted (28 out of a total of 111) were older, had higher degrees of fever, were more likely to be diabetic or to have some genitourinary abnormality, or to be vomiting than women who were managed as outpatients [122]. The presence of vomiting was highly associated with admission (OR 12). It is notable that 12% of the patients initially discharged from the Emergency Department returned. A large population-based study of pyelonephritis in the Seattle area showed that the majority were managed in the ambulatory environment [4]. However the outpatient site of care was much more commonly chosen for women between 15–54 as compared to children, older women, or men of any age.

Treatment

After obtaining cultures and other laboratory tests, antibiotics are given empirically until susceptibility results are available.

The bacterial species that cause serious UTI are similar to those that cause cystitis. There is a preponderance of *E. coli* and other gram-negative rods. There are different phylogenetic characteristics and excess virulence factors in uropathogens causing pyelonephritis as compared to those causing cystitis or just found in normal fecal flora [123]. These bacteria usually have the same adherence properties as the ones that cause lower tract infection but may have additional virulence attributes that permit ascent of the ureter and in some cases deeper invasion such as bacteremia. The implication is that only a subset of cystitis strains are destined to cause pyelonephritis and this subset is not commonly present in the normal fecal flora. For the very ill patient in whom even a short delay in treatment could be significant, broad therapy is appropriate until culture results permit a narrowing. In many cases, fluoroquinolones will still be effective for treatment of UTIs, but prior exposure to fluoroquinolones is the most significant risk factor for the presence of a drug-resistant flora. This is true for resistance in gram-positive [124] as well as gram-negative [125] bacteria and irrespective of the indication for the previous course of fluoroquinolones. Many clinicians start with combination therapy to address the changing resistance patterns in patients with severe pyelonephritis – usually the combination include two of the following three classes: broad-spectrum β-lactam, fluoroquinolone and aminoglycoside.

So long as there is no contraindication such as vomiting or hypotension, oral antibiotics are effective. In one study, route of administration of ciprofloxacin was randomized to intravenous or oral therapy with about 70 patients per arm [120]. Over one-third of the patients were bacteremic. There was no discernable difference in any of the outcome measures between oral and intravenous therapy, although the study was not powered to show modest superiority of either regimen. Because of the excellent bioavailability of oral ciprofloxacin, this outcome was not surprising. The presence of enterococci required a change in regimen in both groups, although the patients were doing well clinically at the time of the change. Among specific fluoroquinolones, there is no clear evidence as to which is most effective. This is largely because the comparative clinical trials have been powered for equivalence. For example, gatifloxacin was shown to be as effective as ciprofloxacin in a randomized trial evaluating 372 adults with complicated UTI and/or pyelonephritis [126]. In a smaller study, levofloxacin and lomefloxacin (the latter is no longer available in the USA) were comparable to ciprofloxacin [127]. Both of these studies used oral therapy.

There is evidence to suggest that for severe UTI, fluoroquinolones are superior to TMP-SMX. A randomized controlled trial comparing a 7-day course of ciprofloxacin with a 14-day course of TMP-SMX showed a better microbiologic and clinical outcome for ciprofloxacin at early (4–11 days) and late (22–48 days) follow-up [128]. The magnitude of the difference was roughly that for every 9–10 patients treated with ciprofloxacin there would be one less failure than if they were treated with TMP-SMX (NNT about 9–10). This was likely due to a fairly high rate of TMP-SMX resistance in the bacterial strains collected in this multicenter (25 centers) US study. While >90% of bacteria were E. coli as would be expected, 16% of the patients in the TMP-SMX arm had E. coli that were TMP-SMX-resistant. About half of these patients failed therapy (clinically and microbiologically) at the time of early follow-up. Although TMP-SMX is a very inexpensive drug, the pharmaco-economic analysis showed that the cost of treatment failures (such as repeat courses of therapy and repeat laboratory tests) made the TMP-SMX arm more expensive than the ciprofloxacin arm.

A similar study today might show a different outcome depending on the relative frequency of isolation of bacteria resistant to these classes of antibiotics.

Aminoglycosides are another therapeutic option for severe UTIs. Almost all uropathogens from ambulatory patients are still susceptible to aminoglycosides (with the exception of Enterococcus spp.). However, careful monitoring is required because of the possibility for nephrotoxicity and ototoxicity. Modern once-a-day dosing schedules for aminoglycosides can reduce the risk of nephrotoxicity of a 7-day treatment course without sacrificing efficacy [129].

Other classes of drugs have been studied in equivalence trials for the treatment of severe UTI. In one study, piperacillin/tazobactam and imipenem were equivalent for severe UTI with a microbiologic success rate of about 50% for each [130]. In another study, patients were randomized to a single dose of intravenous ceftriaxone followed by oral cefixime versus daily intravenous ceftriaxone. Both groups of patients received a 10-day course of therapy and their outcomes were nearly identical. This cohort of patients was well enough to tolerate oral therapy after the first day and had a good outcome overall (about 75% bacteriologic and 90% clinical cure for each arm). Our patient in Case 4 might well be able to be discharged home after one or just a few doses of parenteral antibiotics.

Durability of response is a concern with severe UTI. In a comparison of hospitalized patients with severe UTI who received a short course of intravenous cefuroxime (for 2–3 days), patients who had follow-up with norfloxacin (a fluoroquinolone) did better microbiologically than those who had ceftibuten (a cephalosporin) [131]. The relative probability of bacterial eradication at 7–14-day follow up after the conclusion of therapy was 0.84 (95% CI 0.74–0.97) with ceftibuten being less effective. This seems to parallel the experience of β-lactams and fluoroquinolones for simple cystitis. This study did not explain why the responses were shorter lived for the cephalosporin, but it would be logical to assume that failure to eradicate the organism in other gastrointestinal and genital sites might have led to recurrence despite the 10-day course of therapy and the initial use of a parenteral cephalosporin. In some patients, duration alone may account for differences in outcomes. Patients with spinal cord injuries are prone to developing UTIs but there may be difficulty in correlating clinical response with microbial response since the bacteriuria associated with relapse can be variably symptomatic. Nevertheless, a randomized trial comparing 3 vs 14 days of ciprofloxacin therapy for adults with symptomatic UTI in the presence of spinal cord injury showed a much higher rate of relapse in those who got the shorter course (RR 2.5 for early relapse and 2.1 for late relapse) [132].

As is the case with less severe UTIs, the prospect of more resistance can influence choices of initial therapy and may limit alternatives in the face of drug allergy. There is clearly an increase in resistance to TMP-SMX in the USA. Between 1992 and 1996 there was a doubling in the prevalence of TMP-SMX resistance in the Seattle area [133]. In the international arena, there is considerable variability of resistance – even within the USA, the range of resistance varies by region of the country [34]. In a review of resistance rates in the 1990s outside the USA, percentage of *E. coli* isolates resistant to TMP-SMX varied from 12% in Holland to 60% in Bangladesh, and resistance to fluoroquinolones varied from 0% to 13% in Spain and 18% in Bangladesh [134]. Bacteria with resistance patterns typical of hospital-acquired strains now threaten women with community-acquired UTIs. In addition to fluoroquinolone resistance, some community-acquired strains show extended-spectrum β-lactamase (ESBL) resistance to cephalosporins. In a Spanish study, there was a 3-fold increase between 2000 and 2003 in the isolation of ESBL-producing *E. coli* among ambulatory women with UTIs [135]. The strains were from several different clones but shared a CTX-M ESBL gene, suggesting that carrying this gene does not interfere with colonization of the healthy gastrointestinal and genital tracts. The only antibiotic exposure risk factor in this case–control study was exposure to a second-generation cephalosporin, cefuroxime (OR = 21), not third-generation cephalosporins or fluoroquinolones. In this study and others, the presence of ESBL genes was strongly associated with other resistance markers including those for fluoroquinolones and trimethoprim.

How quickly should a severe UTI respond to therapy?

This leads to a reasonable question of how quickly a woman with severe UTI should respond to therapy. Considering fever duration as an easily measured indicator of response, the answer is that there is a wide range of rates of improvement. A large retrospective survey of patients admitted with fever and UTI showed that the mean duration of fever (T > 37.5°C at some point during a 12-hour interval) was 39 hours with a median of 34 hours [136]. At 48 hours, about a quarter of the patients were still febrile. Elements associated with longer fever were increased serum creatinine, younger age, higher initial white blood cell counts, and the presence of *E. coli* as the causative agent. The interpretation of this data is difficult since the choice of hospital admission and initial antibiotics were completely uncontrolled. At the least it demonstrates that it is possible to see persistent temperature elevations in people who do well on therapy and have no underlying problems that predispose them to severe UTI. In fact the presence of persistent fever in a patient making a good clinical response is a poor reason to initiate a more detailed work-up for potentially complicated UTI, since fever was weakly correlated with abnormal results of imaging studies of the urinary tract that were done at the physician's request in some patients in this study.

References

1 Foxman B, Barlow R, D'Arcy H, Gillespie B, Sobel JD. Urinary tract infection: self-reported incidence and associated costs. Ann Epidemiol 2000;10:509–15.

2 Kunin CM. An overview of urinary infections. In: Kunin CM (ed.) Urinary Tract Infections: Detection, Prevention and Management, 5th edn, Baltimore: Williams & Wilkins, 1997.

3 Hooton TM, Scholes D, Hughes JP, et al. A prospective study of risk factors for symptomatic urinary tract infection in young women. N Engl J Med 1996;335:468.

4 Czaja CA, Scholes D, Hooton TM, Stamm WE. Population-based epidemiologic analysis of acute pyelonephritis. Clin Infect Dis. 2007;45;273–80.

5 Bent S, Nallamothu BK, Simel DL, Fihn SD, Saint S. Does this woman have an acute uncomplicated urinary tract infection? JAMA 2002;287:2701–10.

6 Pezzlo M. Detection of urinary tract infections by rapid methods. Clin Microbiol Rev 1988;1:268–80.

7 Lachs MS, Nachamkin I, Edelstein PH, Goldman J, Feinstein AR, Schwartz JS. Spectrum bias in the evaluation of diagnostic tests: lessons from the rapid dipstick test for urinary tract infection. Ann Intern Med 1993;117:135–40.

8 Van Nostrand JD, Junkins AD, Bartholdi RK. Poor predictive ability of urinalysis and microscopic examination to detect urinary tract infection. Am J Clin Pathol 2000;113:709–13.

9 Richards D, Toop L, Chambers S, Fletcher L. Response to antibiotics of women with symptoms of urinary tract infection but negative dipstick urine test results: double blind randomized controlled trial. BMJ 2005;331;143–7.

10 St. John A, Boyd JC, Lowes AJ, Price CP. The use of urinary dipstick tests to exclude urinary tract infection: a systematic review of the literature. Am J Clin Path 2006;126;428–36.

11 Komaroff AL. Urinalysis and urine culture in women with dysuria. Ann Intern Med 1986;104:212–18.

12 Lammers RL, Gibson S, Kovacs D, Sears W, Strachan G. Comparison of test characteristics of urine dipstick and urinalysis at various test cutoff points. Ann Emerg Med 2001;38:505–12.

13 Zaman Z, Borremans A, Verhaegen J, Verbist L, Blanckaert N. Disappointing dipstick screening for urinary tract infection in hospital inpatients. J Clin Pathol 1998;51: 471–2.

14 Cornia PB, Takahashi TA, Lipsky BA. The microbiology of bacteriuria in men: a 5-year study at a Veteran's Affairs hospital. Diag Microbiol Infect Dis 2006;56;25–30.

15 McIsaac WJ, Low DE, Biringer A, Pimlott N, Evans M, Glazier R. The impact of empirical management of acute cystitis on unnecessary antibiotic use. Arch Intern Med 2002;162:600–5.

16 Saint S, Scholes D, Fihn SD, et al. The effectiveness of a clinical practice guideline for the management of presumed uncomplicated urinary tract infection in women. Am J Med 1999;106:636–41.

17 Rubin RH, Shapiro ED, Andriole VT, Davis RJ, Stamm WE. Evaluation of new anti-infective drugs for the treatment of urinary tract infection. Clin Infect Dis 1992;15 (Suppl.): S216–27.

18 McCarty JM, Richard G, Huck W, et al. A randomized trial of short course ciprofloxacin, ofloxacin or trimethoprim-sulfamethoxazole for the treatment of acute urinary tract infection in women. Am J Med 1999;106:292–9.

19 Sandler CM, Amis ES, Bigongiari LR, et al. Imaging in acute pyelonephritis. American College of Radiology. ACR Appropriateness Criteria. Radiology 2000;215(Suppl.1): 677–81.

20 Kuroda M, Yamashita A, Hirakawa H, Kumano M, Morikawa K, Higashide M, Maruyama A, Inose Y, Matoba K, Toh H, Kuhara S, Hattora M, Ohta T. Whole genome sequence of Staphylococcus saprophyticus reveals the pathogenesis of urinary tract infections. Proc Nat Acad Sci 2005;37;13272–7.

21 Stamm WE. Quantitative urine cultures revisited (editorial). Eur J Clin Microbiol Infect Dis 1984;3:279–81.

22 Norrby SR. Short-term treatment of uncomplicated lower urinary tract infections in women. Rev Infect Dis 1990;12:458–67.

23 Leibovici L, Wysenbeek AJ. Single-dose antibiotic treatment for symptomatic urinary tract infections in women: a meta-analysis of randomized trials. Q J Med 1991;78:43–57.

24 Katchman EA, Milo G, Paul M, Christiaens T, Baerheim A, Leibovici L. Three-day vs longer duration of antibiotic treatment for cystitis in women: systematic review and meta-analysis. Am J Med 2005;118:1196–1207.

25 Hooton TM, Winter C, Tiu F, Stamm WE. Randomized comparative trial and cost analysis of 3-day antimicrobial regimens for treatment of acute cystitis in women. JAMA 1995;273:41–5.

26 Fekete T. Review of three-day trimethoprimsulfamethoxazole was best for acute cystitis. ACP J Club, 1995;123:15.

27 Patel SS, Balfour JA, Bryson HM. Fosfomycin tromethamine. A review of its antibacterial activity, pharmacokinetic properties and therapeutic efficacy as a single-dose oral treatment for acute uncomplicated lower urinary tract infections. Drugs 1997;53:637–56.

28 Huang ES, Stafford RS. National patterns in the treatment of urinary tract infections in women by ambulatory care physicians. Arch Intern Med 2002;162:41–7.

29 Iravani A, Klimberg I, Briefer C, Munera C, Kowalsky SF, Echols RM. A trial comparing low-dose, short-course ciprofloxacin and standard 7 day therapy with cotrimoxazole or nitrofurantoin in the treatment of uncomplicated urinary tract infection. J Antimicrob Chemother 1999; 43(Suppl. A):67–75.

30 Gupta K, Hooton TM, Roberts PL, Stamm WE. Short-course nitrofurantoin for the treatment of acute uncomplicated cystitis in women. Arch Intern Med 2007;167;2207–12.

31 Fosfomycin for urinary tract infections. Med Lett Drugs Ther 1997;39:66–8.

32 Stamm WE, McKevitt M, Counts GW. Acute renal infection in women: treatment with trimethoprim sulfamethoxazole or ampicillin for two or six weeks. Ann Intern Med 1987; 106:341–5.

33 Hooton TM, Scholes D, Gupta K, Stapleton AE, Roberts PL, Stamm WE. Amoxicillin-clavulanate vs ciprofloxacin for the treatment of uncomplicated cystitis in women. JAMA 2005;293:949–55.

34 Gupta K, Sahm DF, Mayfield D, Stamm WE. Antimicrobial resistance among uropathogens that cause community acquired urinary tract infections in women: a nationwide analysis. Clin Infect Dis 2001;33:89–94.

35 Rafalsky V, Andreeva I, Rjabkova E. Quinolones for uncomplicated acute cystitis in women. Cochrane Database Syst Rev, 2006 (3), CD003597, DOI: 10/1002/14651858.

36 Killgore KM, Maarch KL, Guglielmo BJ. Risk factors for community-acquired ciprofloxacin-resistant Escherichia coli urinary tract infection. Ann Pharmacotherapy 2004;38;1148–52.

37 Karlowsky JA, Hoban DJ, DeCorby MR, Laing NM, Zhanel GG. Fluoroquinolone-resistant urinary isolates of Escherichia coli from outpatients are frequently multidrug resistant: results from the North American urinary tract infection collaborative alliance-quinolone resistance study. Antimicrob Agents Chemother 2006;50;2251–4.

38 Cohen AE, Lautenbach E, Morales KH, Linkin DR. Fluoroquinolone-resistant Escherichia coli in the long-term care setting. Am J Med 2006;119;958–63.

39 Gagliotti C, Nobilio L, Moro ML. Emergence of ciprofloxacin resistance in Escherichia coli isolates from outpatient urine samples. Clin Microbiol Infect 2007;13;328–31.

40 Grover ML, Bracamonte JD, Kanodia AK, Bryan MJ, Donahue SP, Warner A-M, Edwards FD, Weaver AL. Assessing adherence to evidence-based guidelines for the

diagnosis and management of uncomplicated urinary tract infection. Mayo Clin Proc 2007;82;181–185.

41 Kallen AJ, Welch HG, Sirovich BE. Current antibiotic therapy for isolated urinary tract infections in women. Arch Int Med 2006;166;635–39.

42 Hooton TM, Besser R, Foxman B, Fritsche TR, Nicolle LE. Acute uncomplicated cystitis in an era of increasing antibiotic resistance: a proposed approach to empirical therapy. Clin Infect Dis 2004;39;75–80.

43 Christiaens TC, De Meyere M, Verschraegen G, Peersman W, Heytens S, De Maseneer JM. Randomized controlled trial of nitrofurantoin versus placebo in the treatment of uncomplicated urinary tract infection in adult women. Br J Gen Pract 2002;52:708–10.

44 Echols RM, Tosiello RL, Haverstock DC, Tice AD. Demographic, clinical and treatment parameters influencing the outcome of acute cystitis. Clin Infect Dis 1999;29:113–19.

45 Raz R, Chazan B, Kennes Y, et al.; Israeli Urinary Tract Infection Group. Empiric use of trimethoprim-sulfamethoxazole (TMP-SMX) in the treatment of women with uncomplicated urinary tract infections in a geographical area with a high prevalence of TMP-SMX resistant uropathogens. Clin Infect Dis 2002;34:1165–9.

46 McNulty CAM, Richards J, Livermore DM, Little P, Charlett A, Freeman E, Harvey I, Thomas M. Clinical relevance of laboratory-reported antibiotic resistance in acute uncomplicated urinary tract infection in primary care. J Antimicrob Chemother 2006;58;1000–8.

47 Zhanel GG, Hisanaga TL, Laing NM, et al. Antibiotic resistance in outpatient urinary isolates: Final results from North American Urinary Tract Infection Collaborative Alliance (NAUTICA). Int J Antimicrob Agents 2005;26(5):380–8.

48 Anderson GG, Palermo JJ, Schilling JD, Roth R, Heuser J, Hultgren SJ. Intracellular bacterial biofilm-like pods in urinary tract infections. Science 2003;301;105–107.

49 Anders H-J, Patole PS. Toll-like receptors recognize uropathogenic Escherichia coli and trigger inflammation in the urinary tract. Nephrol Dial Transplant 2005;20;1529–32.

50 Snyder JA, Haugen BJ, Buckles EL, et al. Transcriptosome of uropathogenic Escherichia coli during urinary tract infection. Infect Immun 2004;72;6373–6381.

51 Lawrenson RA, Logie JW. Antibiotic failure in the treatment of urinary tract infections in young women. J Antimicrob Chemother 2001;48:895–901.

52 Stamm WE, Raz R. Factors contributing to susceptibility of postmenopausal women to recurrent urinary tract infections. Clin Infect Dis 1999;28:723–5.

53 Beylot M, Marion D, Noel G. Ultrasonographic determination of residual urine in diabetic subjects: relationship to neuropathy and urinary tract infection. Diabetes Care 1982;5:501–5.

54 Warren JW, Abrutyn E, Hebel JR, et al. Guidelines for antimicrobial treatment of uncomplicated acute bacterial cystitis and acute pyelonephritis in women. Clin Infect Dis 1999;29:745–58.

55 Hooton TM, Scholes D, Stapleton AE, et al. A prospective study of asymptomatic bacteriuria in sexually active young women. N Engl J Med 2000;343;992–7.

56 Smaill F, Vazquez JC. Antibiotics for asymptomatic bacteriuria in pregnancy. Cochrane Database Syst Rev 2007 (2), CD000490, DOI: 10.1002/14651858.

57 Gratacos E, Torres P-J, Vila J, Alonso PL, Cararach V. Screening and treatment of asymptomatic bacteriuria in pregnancy prevent pyelonephritis. J Infect Dis 1994; 169:1390–2.

58 Harding GKM, Nicolle LE, Ronald AR, et al. How long should catheter acquired urinary tract infection in women be treated? Ann Intern Med 1991;114:713–19.

59 Kartal ED, Yenilmez A, Kiremitca A, Meric H, Kale M, Usluer G. Effectiveness of ciprofloxacin prophylaxis in preventing bacteriuria caused by urodynamics study: a blind, randomized study of 192 patients. Urology 2006;67;1149–53.

60 Forland M, Thomas VL. The treatment of urinary tract infections in women with diabetes mellitus. Diab Care 1985;8:499–506.

61 Abrutyn E, Berlin J, Mossey J, Pitsakis P, Levison M, Kaye D. Does treatment of asymptomatic bacteriuria in older ambulatory women reduce subsequent symptoms of urinary tract infections? J Am Geriatr Soc 1996;44:293–5.

62 Harding GKM, Zhanel GG, Nicolle LE, Cheang M. Antimicrobial treatment in diabetic women with asymptomatic bacteriuria. N Engl J Med 2002;347:1576–83.

63 Ikaheimo R, Siitonen A, Heiskanen T, et al. Recurrence of urinary tract infection in a primary care setting: analysis of a 1-year follow up of 179 women. Clin Infect Dis 1996;22:91–9.

64 Manges AR, Johnson JR, Foxman B, O'Bryan TT, Fullerton KE, Riley LW. Widespread distribution of urinary tract infections caused by a multidrug-resistant Escherichia coli clonal group. New Engl J Med 2001;345;1007–13.

65 Manges AR, Natarajan P, Solberg OD, Dietrich PS, Riley LW. The changing prevalence of drug-resistant Escherichia coli clonal groups in a community: evidence for community outbreaks of urinary tract infections. Epidemiol Infect 2006;134;425–31.

66 Johnson JR, Clabots C. Sharing of virulent Escherichia coli clones among household members of a woman with acute cystitis. Clin Infect Dis 2006;43;e101–8.

67 Lundstet A-C, Leijonhufvud I, Ragnarsdottir B, Karpman D, Andersson B, Svanborg C. Inherited susceptibility to acute pyelonephritis: a family study of urinary tract infection. J Infect Dis 2007;195;1227–34.

68 Kontiokari T, Sundqvist K, Nuutinen M, et al. Randomized trial of cranberry–lingonberry juice and Lactobacillus GG drink for the prevention of urinary tract infection in women. BMJ 2001;30:1571.

69 McMurdo ME, Bissett LY, Price RJG, Phillips G. Does ingestion of cranberry juice reduce symptomatic urinary tract infections in older people in hospital? A double-blind, placebo-controlled trial. Age Ageing 2005;34;256–61.

70 Jepson RG, Craig J. Cranberries for preventing urinary tract infections. Cochrane Database Syst Rev 2008 (1), CD001321, DOI: 10.1002/14651858.

71 Fihn SD, Boyko EJ, Normand EH, et al. Association between use of spermicide coated condoms and Escherichia coli urinary tract infections in young women. Am J Epidemiol 1996;144:512.

72 Raz R, Stamm WE. A controlled trial of intravaginal estriol in postmenopausal women with recurrent urinary tract infection. N Engl J Med 1993;329:753–6.

73 Fowler JE, Pulaski ET. Excretory urography, cystography, and cystoscopy in the evaluation of women with urinary tract infection. N Engl J Med 1981;304:462–5.

74 Nicolle LE. Prophylaxis: recurrent urinary tract infection in women. Infection 1992;20(Suppl. 3):S203–10.

75 Nicolle LE, Harding GKM, Thomson M, Kennedy J, Urias B, Ronald AR. Efficacy of five years of continuous low-dose trimethoprim-sulfamethoxazole prophylaxis for urinary tract infection. J Infect Dis 1988;157:1239–42.

76 Stapleton A, Latham RH, Johnson C, Stamm WE. Postcoital antimicrobial prophylaxis for recurrent urinary tract infection. A randomized, double-blind, placebo controlled trial. JAMA 1990;264:703–6.

77 Chew LD, Fihn SD. Recurrent cystitis in nonpregnant women. West J Med 1999;170:274–7.

78 Gupta K, Hooton TM, Roberts PL, Stamm WE. Patient-initiated treatment of uncomplicated recurrent urinary tract infections in young women. Ann Intern Med 2001;135:9–16.

79 Rudenko N, Dorofeyev A. Prevention of recurrent lower urinary tract infections by long-term administration of fosfomycin trometrol. Double blind, randomized, parallel group placebo controlled study. Arzneimittel-Forschung 2005;55:420–7.

80 Karchmer TB, Gianetta ET, Muto CA, Strain BA, Farr BM. A randomized crossover study of silver coated urinary catheters in hospitalized patients. Arch Int Med 2000;160:3294–8.

81 Saint S. Prevention of nosocomial urinary tract infections. Agency for Healthcare Research and Quality, Contract No. 290–97–0013 (http://www.ahcpr.gov/clinic/ptsafety/pdf/chap15.pdf).

82 Johnson JR, Kuskowski MA, Wilt TJ. Systematic review: antimicrobial urinary catheters to prevent catheter-associated urinary tract infection in hospitalized patients. Ann Intern Med 2006;144;116–26.

83 Stephan F, Sax H, Wachsmuth M, Hoffmeyer P, Clergue F, Pittet D. Reduction of urinary tract infection and antibiotic use after surgery: a controlled, prospective, before-after intervention study. Clin Infect Dis 2006;42;1544–51.

84 Vickrey BG, Shekelle P, Morton S, Clark K, Pathak M, Kamberg C. Prevention and management of urinary tract infections in paralyzed persons. Evidence Report/Technology Assessment No. 6 (prepared by the Southern California Evidence-Based Practice Center/RAND under Contract No. 290–97–0001). AHCPR Publication No. 99–E008. Rockville, MD: Agency for Health Care Policy and Research, February 1999.

85 Darouiche R, Thornby JI, Cerra-Stewart C, Donovan WH, Hull RA. Bacterial interference for prevention of urinary tract infection: a prospective, randomized placebo-controlled, double-blind pilot trial. Clin Infect Dis 2005;41;1535–6.

86 Sunden F, Hakansson L, Ljunggren E, Wullt B. Bacterial interference – is deliberate colonization with Escherichia coli 83972 an alternative treatment for patients with recurrent urinary tract infection? Int J Antimicrob Agents 2006;28S;S26–S29.

87 Lipsky BA. Prostatitis and urinary tract infection in men: What's new?; what's true? Am J Med 1999;106:327–34.

88 Lipsky BA. Urinary tract infections in men: Epidemiology, pathophysiology, diagnosis and treatment. Ann Intern Med 1989;110:138–50.

89 Krieger JN, Nyberg L, Nickel JC. NIH consensus definition and classification of prostatitis. JAMA 1999;282:236–7.

90 Nickel JC, Downey J, Hunter D, Clark J. Prevalence of prostatitis-like symptoms in a population-based study using the National Institutes of Health chronic prostatitis symptom index. J Urol 2001;165:842–5.

91 Roberts RO, Lieber MM, Rhodes T, Girman CJ, Bostwick DG. Jacobsen SJ. Prevalence of a physician-assigned diagnosis of prostatitis: the Olmsted County Study of Urinary Symptoms and Health Status Among Men. Urology 1998;51:578–84.

92 Lipsky BA, Ireton RC, Fihn SD, Hackett R, Berger RE. Diagnosis of bacteriuria in men: specimen collection and culture interpretation. J Infect Dis 1987;155:847–54.

93 Sobel JD, Kaye D. Urinary tract infections. In: Mandell GL, Bennett JE, Dolin R, eds. Principles and Practice of Infectious Diseases, 5th edn. Philadelphia: Churchill Livingstone, 2000.

94 Ulleryd P, Zackrisson B, Aus G, Bergdahl S, Hugosson J, Sandberg T. Selective urological evaluation in men with febrile urinary tract infection. BJU Int 2001;88:15–20.

95 Andrews SJ, Brooks PT, Hanbury DC, et al. Ultrasonography and abdominal radiography versus intravenous urography in investigation of urinary tract infection in men: prospective incident cohort study. BMJ 2002;324:454–6.

96 Russell DB, Roth NJ. Urinary tract infections in men in a primary care population. Aust Fam Phys 2001;30:177–9.

97 Ulleryd P, Lincoln K, Scheutz F, Sandberg T. Virulence characteristics of Escherichia coli in relation to host response in men with symptomatic urinary tract infection. Clin Infect Dis 1994;18:579–84.

98 Mitsumori K, Terai A, Yamamoto S, Ishitoya S, Yoshida O. Virulence characteristics of Escherichia coli in acute bacterial prostatitis. J Infect Dis 1999;180:1378–81.

99 Andreu A, Stapleton AE, Fennell C, et al. Urovirulence determinants in Escherichia coli strains causing prostatitis. J Infect Dis 1997;176:464–9.

100 Smith JW, Jones SR, Reed WP, Tice AD, Deupress RH, Kaijser B. Recurrent urinary tract infections in men. Ann Intern Med 1979;91:544–8.

101 Gleckman R, Crowley M, Natsios GA. Therapy of recurrent invasive urinary-tract infections of men. N Engl J Med 1979;301:878–80.

102 Sabbaj J, Hoagland VL, Cook T. Norfloxacin versus cotrimoxazole in the treatment of recurring urinary tract infections in men. Scand J Infect Dis 1986;48:S48–S53.

103 Cox CE. Ofloxacin in the management of complicated urinary tract infections, including prostatitis. Am J Med 1989;87: 61S–68S.

104 Allais JM, Preheim LC, Cuevas TA, Roccaforte JS, Mellencamp MA, Bittner MJ. Randomized, double-blind comparison of ciprofloxacin and trimethoprimsulfametho

xazole for complicated urinary tract infections. Antimicrob Agents Chemother 1988;32:1327–30.

105 Weidner W. Ludwig M. Brahler E. Schiefer HG. Outcome of antibiotic therapy with ciprofloxacin in chronic bacterial prostatitis. Drugs 1999;58(Suppl. 2):103–6.

106 Ulleryd P, Sandberg T. Ciprofloxacin for 2 or 4 weeks in the treatment of febrile urinary tract infection in men: a randomized trial with a 1 year follow-up. Scand J Infect Dis 2003;35;34–9.

107 Nickel JC, Downey J, Clark J, et al. Levofloxacin for chronic prostatitis/chronic pelvic pain syndrome in men: a randomized placebo-controlled multicenter trial. Urology 2003;62;614–17.

108 Alexander RB, Propert KJ, Schaeffer AJ, et al. Ciprofloxacin or tamsulosin in men with chronic prostatitis/chronic pelvic pain syndrome: a randomized, double-blind trial. Ann Intern Med 2004;141;581–9.

109 Scholes D, Hooton TM, Roberts PL, Gupta K, Stapleton AE, Stamm WE. Risk factors associated with acute pyelonephritis in healthy women. Annals Int Med 2005;142;20–7.

110 Stamm WE. Measurement of pyuria and its relation to bacteriuria. Am J Med 1983;75 (Suppl. 1B):53–8.

111 Tambyah PA, Maki DG. The relationship between pyuria and infection in patients with indwelling urinary catheters. Arch Intern Med 2000;160:673–7.

112 Patel HD, Livsey SA, Swann RA, Bukhari SS. Can urine dipstick testing for urinary tract infection at point of care reduce laboratory workload? J Clin Pathol 2005;58;951–4.

113 McMurry BR, Wrenn KD, Wright SW. Usefulness of blood cultures in pyelonephritis. Am J Emerg Med 1997;15:137–40.

114 Thanassi M. Utility of urine and blood cultures in pyelonephritis. Acad Emerg Med 1997;4:797–800.

115 Grover SA, Komaroff AL, Weisberg M, et al. The characteristics and hospital course of patients admitted for presumed acute pyelonephritis. J Gen Intern Med 1987;2:5–10.

116 Smith WR, McClish DK, Poses RM, et al. Bacteremia in young urban women admitted with pyelonephritis. Am J Med Sci 1997;313:50–7.

117 Wing DA, Park AS, Debuque L, Millar LK. Limited clinical utility of blood and urine cultures in the treatment of acute pyelonephritis during pregnancy. Am J Obst Gynecol 2000;182:1437–40.

118 Hsu C-Y, Fang H-C, Chou K-J, Chen C-L, Lee P-T, Chung H-M. The clinical impact of bacteremia in complicated acute pyelonephritis. Am J Med Sci 2006;332;175–80.

119 Chen Y, Nitzan O, Saliba W, Chazan B, Colodner R, Raz R. Are blood cultures necessary in the management of women with complicated pyelonephritis? J Infect 2006;53;235–40.

120 Mombelli G, Pezzoli R, Pinoja-Lutz G, Monotti R, Marone C, Franciolli M. Oral v intravenous ciprofloxacin in the initial management of severe pyelonephritis or complicated urinary tract infections: a prospective randomized clinical trial. Arch Intern Med 1999;159:53–58.

121 Sanchez M, Collvinent B, Miro O, et al. Short-term effectiveness of ceftriaxone single dose in the initial treatment of acute uncomplicated pyelonephritis in women. A randomized controlled trial. Emerg Med J 2002;19:19–22.

122 Pinson AG, Philbrick JT, Lindbeck GH, Schorling JB. ED management of acute pyelonephritis in women: a cohort study. Am J Emerg Med 1994;12:271–8.

123 Johnson JR, Owens K, Gajewski A, Kuskowski MA. Bacterial characteristics in relation to clinical source of Escherichia coli isolates from women with acute cystitis or pyelonephritis and uninfected women. J Clin Microbiol 2005;43;6064–72.

124 Goldstein EJ, Garabedian-Ruffalo SM. Widespread use of fluoroquinolones versus emerging resistance in pneumococci. Clin Infect Dis 2002;35:1501–11.

125 Lautenbach E, Fishman NO, Bilker WB, et al. Risk factors for fluoroquinolone resistance in nosocomial Escherichia coli and Klebsiella pneumoniae infections. Arch Intern Med 2002;162:2469–77.

126 Cox CE, Marbury TC, Pittman WG, et al. A randomized, double-blind multicenter comparison of gatifloxacin versus ciprofloxacin in the treatment of complicated urinary tract infection and pyelonephritis. Clin Ther 2002;24:223–36.

127 Richard GA, Klimberg IN, Fowler CL, Callery-D'Amico S, Kim SS. Levofloxacin versus ciprofloxacin versus lomefloxacin in acute pyelonephritis. Urology 1998;52:51–5.

128 Talan DA, Stamm WE, Hooton TM, et al. Comparison of ciprofloxacin (7 days) with trimethoprim sulfamethoxazole (14 days) for acute uncomplicated pyelonephritis in women: a randomized trial. JAMA 2000;283:1583–90.

129 Drusano GL, Ambrose PG, Bhavnani SM, Bertino JS, Nafziger AN, Louie A. Back to the future: using aminoglycosides again and how to dose them optimally. Clin Infect Dis 2007;45;753–60.

130 Naber KG, Savov O, Salmen HC. Piperacillin 2g/tazobactam 0.5g is as effective as imipenem 0.5g/cilastatin 0.5g for the treatment of acute uncomplicated pyelonephritis and complicated urinary tract infections. Int J Antimicrob Agents 2002;19:95–103.

131 Cronberg S, Banke S, Bergman B, et al. Fewer bacterial relapses after oral treatment with norfloxacin than with ceftibuten in acute pyelonephritis initially treated with intravenous cefuroxime. Scand J Infect Dis 2001;33:339–43.

132 Dow G, Rao P, Harding G, et al. A prospective, randomized trial of 3 or 14 days of ciprofloxacin treatment for acute urinary tract infection in patients with spinal cord injury. Clin Infect Dis 2004;39;658–66.

133 Gupta K, Scholes D, Stamm WE. Increasing prevalence of antimicrobial resistance among uropathogens causing acute uncomplicated cystitis in women. JAMA 1999;281:736–8.

134 Gupta K, Hooton TM, Stamm WE. Increasing antimicrobial resistance and the management of uncomplicated community-acquired urinary tract infections. Ann Intern Med 2001;135:41–50.

135 Calbo E, Romani V, Xercavins M, et al. Risk factors for community-onset urinary tract infections due to Escherichia coli harbouring extended-spectrum beta-lactamases. J Antimicrob Chemother 2006;57;780–3.

136 Behr MA, Drummond R, Libman M, Delaney S, Dylewski JS. Fever duration in hospitalized acute pyelonephritis patients. Am J Med 1996;101:277–80.

CHAPTER 10
Sexually transmitted infections

Kaede Ota, Darrell H. S. Tan, Sharmistha Mishra & David N. Fisman

Case presentation

A 17-year-old girl presents to the city sexual health clinic with vaginal discharge. She has a new boyfriend and is "on the pill"; she and her partner do not use condoms as their relationship "is monogamous." On examination, she has mild lower abdominal tenderness to palpation, cervicitis, and cervical discharge. There is cervical motion tenderness and left adnexal tenderness on bimanual examination. Her 17-year-old boyfriend has accompanied her to the clinic and is assessed separately; he reports a small amount of urethral discharge and mild dysuria. Examination reveals copious urethral discharge with meatal edema. A Gram stain of discharge reveals gram-negative intracellular diplococci. You review the literature to determine the following.

- How accurate is the clinical diagnosis of sexually transmitted infections (STI)?
- Do laboratory test results change the range of diagnostic possibilities in an individual with a possible STI?
- How helpful are historical and clinical findings in the diagnosis of pelvic inflammatory disease?
- Do condoms reduce the likelihood of transmission of STI?

STI are caused by a large and heterogeneous group of pathogens. Many of these pathogens can be transmitted by nonsexual as well as sexual routes; for example, enteric pathogens can be transmitted through food and water as well as via sexual intercourse. This chapter will focus on those infectious agents that are

principally or exclusively transmitted via sexual contact, although the general principles described below can be applied to the larger group of STI. This chapter will not focus on human immunodeficiency virus (HIV) infection, which is discussed in Chapter 11.

STI are distinguished from other infectious diseases by several clinical and epidemiologic features. Perhaps most notable is the extremely high incidence of these infections; not withstanding likely underdiagnosis, *Chlamydia trachomatis* infection is the most common reportable infectious disease in the USA and Canada [1,2]. Herpes simplex virus type 2 (HSV-2) infection and human papillomavirus (HPV) infections are also extremely common: approximately 22% of adults in the USA have serologic evidence of HSV-2 infection [3]. Transient HPV infection is acquired through sexual activity by 33–55% of young adults in the USA and Europe [4–6]. Worldwide, it is estimated that over 330 million cases of syphilis, gonorrhea, trichomoniasis, and genital chlamydia infection occur annually [7]. The high incidence and prevalence of infection results in a high burden of disease, as well as large economic costs [8–11].

The burden of disease associated with these infections is further augmented by the synergistic relationship between non-HIV STI and HIV infection, owing to physical disruption of host mucosa, recruitment of immunologically active cells to the genital tract, and increases in HIV viral burden in genital secretions. A metaanalysis of observational studies generated a summary estimate of the relative risk of HIV acquisition in the context of another sexually transmitted infection to be 3.7 (95% CI 2.7–5.0%) (Fig. 10.1) [12].

However, STI other than HIV infection may also result in chronic medical illness or long-term complications. Genital chlamydia infection is associated with tubal infertility [13], ectopic pregnancies [14,15], and

Evidence-Based Infectious Diseases, 2nd edition. Edited by Mark Loeb, Fiona Smaill and Marek Smieja. © 2009 Wiley-Blackwell Publishing, ISBN: 978-1-4051-7026-0

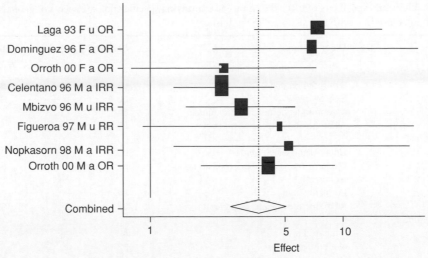

Figure 10.1 The impact of other sexually transmitted infections (STI) on risk of acquiring human immunodeficiency virus (HIV) infection. Forest plot showing the effect of other STI on HIV risk in individuals initially uninfected with HIV. Studies are listed on the vertical axis, with labels connoting author, year of publication, gender of initially uninfected partner, adjustment (a) or lack of adjustment (u) of effect estimate for other variables, and effect measure (OR, odds ratio; IRR, incidence rate ratio; RR, relative risk). Estimate of effect is plotted on the horizontal axis. The size of black boxes is proportional to study statistical precision, and horizontal lines represent 95% confidence intervals. The diamond represents the summary estimate of effect of sexually transmitted infection on HIV acquisition, and 95% confidence interval. Modified from reference [12]: Rottingen J, Cameron D, Garnett G. A systematic review of the epidemiologic interactions between classic sexually transmitted diseases and HIV. Sex Transm Dis 2001;28(10):579–97 with permission of Lippincott Williams & Wilkins.

chronic pelvic pain [16,17]. HPVs are strongly associated with cervical and anal cancers [18,19]. Infection of pregnant individuals with sexually transmitted pathogens may increase the risk of premature delivery, and may cause severe illness in the newborn [20–25]. This chapter will review the evidence for the clinical and microbiologic diagnosis of these infections, including evidence related to syndromic management (i.e., the use of more broadly targeted therapy in response to a clinical constellation of symptoms or signs). Evidence related to the interaction between contraceptive choice and STI is also reviewed. The second part of the chapter focuses on empiric and targeted management of STI, including some issues related to management in pregnancy. Finally, evidence of effectiveness for population-based STI prevention strategies is discussed.

Diagnosis of STI

Clinical and syndromic diagnosis

Sexually transmitted pathogens cause several common syndromes. Infection with *Neisseria gonorrhoea*

or *Chlamydia trachomatis* frequently results in urethritis, cervicitis, or the constellation of symptoms and signs that suggest the presence of pelvic inflammatory disease. HSV, *Treponema pallidum*, and *Haemophilus ducreyi* are common agents of ulcerative genital disease, while vaginal discharge is commonly caused by infection with *Trichomonas vaginalis* or *Candida* species or by bacterial vaginosis.

The ability of clinicians to accurately diagnose infections caused by specific pathogens without the use of diagnostic tests appears poor. For example, a study involving a cohort of 446 men presenting to a New Orleans clinic found the clinical diagnosis of the causative agents of genital ulcer disease to be highly sensitive (94–98%), but nonspecific (31–35%) when compared with culture, microscopy, and serologic diagnosis (Table 10.1) [26]. Studies comparing clinical diagnosis of genital ulcer disease with the use of multiplex PCR have found similar limitations in clinician diagnostic accuracy [27–29].

The accuracy of bedside diagnosis of vaginitis based on clinical features and simple bedside tests

Table 10.1 Sensitivity and specificity of ulcer appearance in identifying specific etiologic agents of genital ulcer disease (modified from reference [26] with permission of the publisher)

Pathogen	Ulcer feature	Sensitivity (%)	Specificity (%)
Herpes simplex virus			
	3 or more lesions	63	64
	Shallow ulcer	60	88
	Moderate tenderness on examination	60	50
	All of the above features present	35	94
Hemophilus ducreyi			
	Undermined lesion border	85	68
	Moderate or severe tenderness on examination	57	52
	Purulent ulcer	64	75
	All of the above features present	34	94
Treponema pallidum			
	Indurated ulcer	47	95
	Nonpurulent ulcer	82	53
	Ulcer painless or minimally painful	67	58
	All of the above features present	31	98

(e.g., pH testing, whiff test, microscopic evaluation of "wet preps") also appears limited when compared with more comprehensive laboratory-based evaluations [30]. In a study performed in 153 women presenting to a clinic in Israel with vaginal discharge, only the finding of vaginal pH <4.5 was associated with infection by a particular pathogen (yeast); the positive predictive value of low vaginal pH for vaginal candidiasis was 68%.

Nonetheless, the limited availability of laboratory diagnostics in areas where STI are prevalent, combined with concern that patients will not return for treatment, has resulted in the development of the "syndromic" approach to diagnosis and treatment. In this approach, the presence of a given clinical history or constellation of physical examination findings results in the provision of broad-spectrum therapy targeting multiple treatable organisms [31,32].

Relatively simple diagnostic algorithms exist for such syndromes as genital ulceration, lower abdominal discomfort, and genital discharge. The term "sensitivity" as applied to these algorithms indicates the proportion of individuals with infections diagnosed by laboratory methods who receive appropriate therapy as a result of algorithm use.

A review published in 2000 evaluated studies of syndromic diagnosis and management of STI; this review included no controlled trials comparing diagnostic approaches [33]. Rather, attempts were made to validate algorithms using more comprehensive laboratory testing as a gold standard. Algorithms used alone have been associated with high sensitivity for urethral discharge (91–97%), genital ulcer diseases from syphilis or chancroid (68–100%), and vaginal discharge syndromes. However, diagnostic sensitivity is achieved at a cost of low specificity (as low as 7% in diagnosis of urethral discharge) and low positive predictive values. Thus the decision to use algorithms in settings where diagnostic tests are unavailable needs to be based on the prevalence and health impact of a given infection in the local population, and balanced against the potential consequences and costs of unnecessary antibiotic treatment.

Basic laboratory testing for urethritis and cervicitis

Nonspecific laboratory tests for the presence of gonorrheal and chlamydial cervicitis and urethritis include assessment of cervical, urethral, and vaginal white blood cell counts, urine leukocyte esterase testing, and the use of Gram stains. Most of these modalities have proven disappointing. For example, a study evaluating the use of cervical or vaginal white blood cell counts for the identification of gonorrheal

Table 10.2 Use of urine leukocyte esterase for the diagnosis of gonorrhea or chlamydia in men

Population or specimen source	Prevalence	Study gold standard	Sensitivity (%)	Specificity (%)	Reference
55 male STD clinic patients, Mwanza Region, Tanzania	Gonorrhea: 40% Chlamydia: 7%	Gonorrhea detected by culture, chlamydia by EIA	96	38	[370]
1095 ambulatory emergency room patients, Atlanta, Georgia	Gonorrhea: 2.5% Chlamydia: 3.9%	Gonorrhea and chlamydia detected by culture	41	90	[371]
479 male college students, Songkla Province, Thailand	Gonorrhea: 0.2% Chlamydia: 4.0%	Gonorrhea and chlamydia detected by PCR	26	11	[40]

or chlamydial cervicitis found no white blood cell cut-off to be both sensitive and specific. The area under the receiver operating curves created using a range of white blood cell cut-offs was less than or equal to 0.6 for the presence of either type of infection, suggesting that such tests provide little additional information (i.e., a random guess would have a value of 0.5) [34]. Although specificity can be enhanced by the use of white blood cell cut-offs in concert with clinical findings of cervical erythema and mucopus, sensitivity of such testing remains poor, especially for chlamydia (sensitivity 41–52% for greater than or equal to 10 polymorphonuclear cells per high powered field) [35,36].

In men, urine leukocyte esterase testing has had variable sensitivity and specificity in the diagnosis of urethritis (Table 10.2), while the evaluation of urethral Gram stain findings for leukocytes has low sensitivity (~67%) for the presence of chlamydia [37].

In experienced hands, the use of urethral Gram stain for the identification of gram-negative diplococci appears to be an extremely sensitive and specific tool for the identification of gonorrhea in men. An extremely high degree of correlation between Gram stain results and nucleic acid amplification-based testing was reported in more than 7000 specimens submitted to a sexually transmitted disease program in Houston (kappa = 0.99) [38]. The ability to perform Gram stain evaluations on clinical specimens may markedly enhance the diagnostic usefulness of clinical algorithms, as described above. For example, in a study evaluating the diagnostic performance of an algorithm for urethritis, the addition of the Gram stain on urethral discharge markedly improved the specificity of algorithm diagnosis of gonorrhea (from 15% to 99%) [39].

The so-called "two glass test" (passage of about 50 mL of urine into the first glass, with the remainder passed into the second) has traditionally been used to distinguish infection in the anterior urethra from more proximal infection (anterior urethritis is thought to be present when only the first glass specimen has a cloudy appearance). The sensitivity and specificity of this test for the diagnosis of either gonococcal or chlamydial infection were 57% and 83% respectively in a cohort of Thai men [40].

Identification of individual pathogens

Recent years have seen an explosion in the use of molecular diagnostic tests, particularly nucleic acid amplification tests (NAAT), in the clinical diagnosis of STI. Commonly used NAAT include polymerase chain reaction (PCR), strand displacement amplification (SDA), and transmission-mediated amplification (TMA). NAAT not only improve test sensitivity in the diagnosis of STI caused by fastidious pathogens, but also permit the use of specimen collection techniques that overcome traditional barriers for STI testing. For example, newer tests may yield satisfactory results when specimens are obtained via self-sampling, which may increase test acceptability [41,42]. NAAT-based urine testing also has satisfactory sensitivity and specificity for the diagnosis of gonorrhea and chlamydial infection, such that the discomfort associated with urethral swabs (in men) and speculum examination (in women) need no longer act as barriers to STI testing [43].

However, because newer tests may be more sensitive than the traditional "gold standards" (culture or microscopic visualization of an individual pathogen), calculation of sensitivity and specificity relative to a gold standard has become problematic. Furthermore, the use of additional tests to resolve discrepancies between negative culture tests and positive nonculture tests may introduce a form of verification bias, resulting in overestimation of sensitivity and specificity [44]. Such difficulties need to be taken into account in the interpretation of the data provided below. Emerging statistical methodologies, including latent class analysis and the use of composite reference standards, may improve future efforts to estimate test characteristics when gold standard tests are absent [45].

Neisseria gonorhoeae

Culture has long been considered the gold standard test for diagnosis of *N. gonorrhoeae* infections. The sensitivity of *N. gonorrhoeae* culture is relatively low in genital specimens when compared to nucleic acid amplification testing (Table 10.3) [46–49]. The poor sensitivity is due in part to loss of viability associated with delays in transport. A decline in sensitivity of culture testing from 89% to 78% was seen when onsite and off-site cultures were compared [48]. Specimen source also contributes to the sensitivity of culture, which is as low

as 55% when specimens are obtained from the pharynx and 49% for rectal specimens [50,51].

More sensitive, nonculture methods for the diagnosis of gonococcal infection include nucleic acid hybridization ("probe") tests and NAAT. These tests have been the subject of a recent systematic review [52]. NAAT identified in this review were highly sensitive and specific in the diagnosis of gonococcal infections of the cervix (sensitivity 91–100%, specificity 97–100%), male urethra (sensitivity 98–100%, specificity 98–100%), and in male urine specimens (94–100%, specificity 98–100%). Studies of NAAT not included in this review have reported similar test characteristics [46,47,53–56]. Female urine specimens have demonstrated variable sensitivity for the detection of *N. gonorrhoeae* (65–91% sensitivity, specificity 99%) [43,53,55].

Although not approved for use on samples from nongenital sources, such as pharynx and rectum, certain NAAT have shown superior sensitivity compared to culture in the detection of *N. gonorrhoeae* in pharyngeal and rectal sites. A recent study demonstrated a sensitivity of 88% in the pharynx and 89–92% in the rectum. Specificity was consistently >97% [57].

Nucleic acid hybridization or "probe" tests were also highly sensitive and specific in the diagnosis of gonococcal infections of the cervix (sensitivity 91–100%, specificity 97–100%), male urethra (sensitivity 98–100%, specificity 98–100%), and in urine testing (94–100%, specificity 98–100%) [58,59].

Table 10.3 Estimated sensitivity of culture for *Neisseria gonorrhoea* relative to newer nucleic-acid-based tests

Population	Culture source	% Gonorrhea prevalence	% Sensitivity of culture (95% CI)	Reference
Female commercial sex-trade workers in Benin, South Africa, and Thailand	Endocervical	5	70 (57–81)	[46]
Male STD clinic attendees, Baltimore, Maryland	Urethral	22	77 (66–86)	[47]
Female STD clinic attendees, Baltimore, Maryland	Endocervical	18	65 (46–80)	[47]
Female hospital emergency department attendees, Omaha, Nebraska	Endocervical	7	89 (71–98)	[48]
Females using Duke University health system, North Carolina	Endocervical	4	93 (76–99)	[49]

Chlamydia trachomatis

Sensitivity of culture for the recovery of *C. trachomatis* is more limited than in *N. gonorrhoeae*, as the former must be grown in cell culture. Recovery is influenced by the expertise of the testing laboratory, composition of the collection swab, and timely transport to the microbiology laboratory. The limited sensitivity of culture has resulted in substantial efforts being devoted to the development of nonculture methods for the diagnosis of *C. trachomatis* infection. Such methods include antigen detection methods such as direct fluorescent antigen testing (DFA), enzyme immunoassay (EIA), and NAAT.

DFA and EIA perform with demonstrably lower sensitivity compared to culture and NAAT (though DFA still finds clinical application in the diagnosis of acute inclusion conjunctivitis related to vertical *C. trachomatis* infection in the newborn) [60,61]. NAAT have shown high sensitivity and specificity in the diagnosis of *C. trachomatis* infections of the cervix (sensitivity 90–94%, specificity 98–99%), in the male urethra (sensitivity 89–98%, specificity 96–99%), and in male urine testing (90–96%, specificity 94–98%). Sensitivity in female urine specimens has ranged from 81% to 95% [43,53,62,63].

Available evidence suggests that the sensitivity and specificity of certain NAAT for both *C. trachomatis* and *N. gonorrhoeae* detection using self-collected vaginal specimens are similar to that seen with clinician-collected cervical specimens [64]. Self-collection may have the advantage of greater acceptability or convenience in some circumstances [65–68]. The use of self-collected specimens may open the way to approaches such as mail-in sampling for population-based screening. In a study performed in general practices in Denmark, testing of pooled self-collected mail-in specimens had a sensitivity and specificity comparable to that seen with testing of pooled physician-collected cervical and urethral swabs (sensitivity 96–100%, specificity of 93–100% with self-collected specimens; sensitivity 91%, specificity 100% with clinician-collected specimens) [69].

Pelvic inflammatory disease

Clinical assessment remains the mainstay of diagnosis of pelvic inflammatory disease (PID), a spectrum of pathologic conditions including endometritis, salpingitis, tubo-ovarian abscess, and pelvic peritonitis. "Gold standard" tests (e.g., endometrial biopsy, laparoscopy) are invasive and not readily available in many clinical settings. The triad of lower abdominal discomfort, cervical motion tenderness, and adnexal tenderness has been suggested to represent minimal diagnostic criteria for PID [70].

A systematic review evaluated the sensitivity and specificity of historical, clinical, and laboratory findings for PID, when compared with laparoscopic diagnosis [71]. This review found no evidence that historical information (e.g., history of irregular menses or history of intrauterine device use) can reliably identify the presence of PID in cohorts of women with abdominal pain and other signs of genital tract infection. The presence of individual clinical signs, such as purulent vaginal discharge or a palpable adnexal mass on examination in an individual with a complaint of abdominal tenderness, was both insensitive and nonspecific [71]. In a study performed in Sweden in the 1960s, the presence of at least four clinical signs (such as pelvic tenderness, pelvic mass, fever, and abnormal vaginal discharge) was found to be specific (91%) for laparoscopically diagnosed PID but had a sensitivity of only 39% [72].

The detection of gonorrhea or chlamydia may be helpful in the diagnosis of PID in individuals with compatible signs and symptoms. In a study performed in a cohort of women with abdominal pain and tenderness on bimanual examination, the isolation of one of these organisms from the lower genital tract had a sensitivity and specificity of 77% for the presence of PID [73].

Two recent studies have used the presence of plasma cell endometritis, rather than laparoscopic evidence of PID, as the gold standard for the diagnosis of PID [74,75]. One study found the US Centers for Disease Control and Prevention (CDC) "minimal diagnostic criteria" to be only 33% sensitive for the presence of plasma cell endometritis, but 88% specific [74], while a second study found the CDC criteria to be more sensitive (83%) but less specific (22%) [75].

When available, ultrasonography may aid in the diagnosis of PID. The finding of fluid-filled fallopian tubes on ultrasound appears to be specific for the presence of PID, although the sensitivity of this finding has varied between studies (Table 10.4).

Table 10.4 Sensitivity and specificity of ultrasonographic detection of fluid-filled fallopian tubes in the diagnosis of pelvic inflammatory diseases

Population	Type of sonography	Study gold standard	% Sensitivity (95% CI)	% Specificity (95% CI)	Reference
51 nonpregnant outpatients in Helsinki, Finland	Transvaginal	Plasma cell endometritis on biopsy	85 (55–98)	100 (91–100)	[372]
30 consecutive individuals hospitalized for suspected PID in Helsinki, Finland	Transvaginal	Presence of PID at laparoscopy	81 (58–95)	78 (40–97)	[373]
55 women with suspected PID in Providence, Rhode Island	Transvaginal	Presence of PID at laparoscopy or histological endometritis on biopsy or culture of *N. gonorrhoeae* or *C. trachomatis* from upper genital tract specimen	32 (13–57)	97 (85–100)	[374]

Trichomonas vaginalis

Trichomomas vaginalis is a unicellular flagellated organism that causes vaginitis in women and urethritis in men. The importance of diagnosis and treatment relates to the association between infection with this organism and adverse outcomes in pregnancy, as well as enhanced HIV transmission [20,76]. A meta-analysis of test characteristics associated with simple bedside tests, such as the use of "wet mounts," and the use of Papanicolaou smear testing, found the sensitivity of these methods to be low (wet mount sensitivity 68%, 95% CI 62–74%; Papanicolaou smear sensitivity 58%, 95% CI 43–73%) [77].

Superior sensitivity is seen with other testing modalities, including culture and PCR-based testing. A systematic review and metaanalysis found that culture using special media has a sensitivity of 90% (95% CI 77–93%), while PCR has a sensitivity of 95% (95% CI 91–99%) and specificity of 98% (95% CI 96–100%) relative to culture. Other nonculture tests, including DFA testing (sensitivity 85%, specificity 99%) and ELISA (sensitivity 80–82%, specificity 73–98%) also have good test performance, and are less expensive than culture methods [78,79]. A novel ELISA-based "dipstick" can be used for diagnosis at the point of care [79].

The impact of delays in transport and inoculation onto special media on recovery of *T. vaginalis* by culture is controversial [80–82]. The relative expense of culture methods, but its superior test sensitivity relative to wet mount, has led to the suggestion that a two-step process might be more efficient, with inexpensive and highly specific "wet mount" testing used initially, and more expensive and sensitive tests reserved for specimens that test negative by wet mount [83]. It should be noted that such an approach would provide few advantages in settings where the prevalence of *T. vaginalis* infection is low. Another evolving facet of testing for trichomoniasis relates to the development of multiplex nucleic acid amplification tests which can be used to identify *T. vaginalis* as well as gonorrhea and *Chlamydia* with reasonable sensitivity and specificity [84].

Chancroid

Chancroid is an ulcerative genital disease caused by *Haemophilus ducreyi*. This organism has a distinct microscopic appearance, and direct Gram staining of purulent material from the ulcer base may reveal chains of short, gram-negative bacilli. Such a finding had a sensitivity of 60% compared with culture in a cohort of individuals with genital ulcer disease attending a sexually transmitted diseases clinic in Nairobi, Kenya [85]. Of 37 individuals who did not have *H. ducreyi* isolated by culture, 18 had Gram stain findings suggestive of *H. ducreyi*, suggesting either lack of sensitivity of culture or lack of specificity of Gram stain. When compared with the use of concurrent PCR assays for *H. ducreyi*-specific sequences, culture for *H. ducreyi* had a sensitivity ranging from 63% to 87% [86–88].

Initial studies evaluating the use of PCR for the identification of *H. ducreyi* in clinical settings estimated sensitivity to be as low as 62% relative to culture [89]. However, subsequent technical improvements in specimen preparation have increased the sensitivity of PCR [90], and more current estimates of the sensitivity of PCR for detection of *H. ducreyi* range from 79–98%, with specificity of 92–100% relative to culture [87,88,91].

The use of PCR for the identification of *H. ducreyi* has provided important insights into the epidemiology of chancroid; for example, it has been observed that *H. ducreyi* may be present in ulcers coinfected with herpes viruses or *T. pallidum* [27–29,88]. Further, the phenomenon of asymptomatic carriage of *H. ducreyi* has been observed in 2% of commercial sex workers in the Gambia without signs or symptoms of chancroid [92].

Other diagnostic modalities, including an indirect immunofluorescent assay, and an enzyme immunoassay, may also have value in the diagnosis of chancroid [86].

Herpes simplex viruses

Herpes simplex viruses (HSV) are the most common agents of ulcerative genital disease in the developed world, and are increasingly recognized in the developing world as well [93]. Although genital herpes has traditionally been associated with HSV-2, recent studies from several industrialized world settings have shown that the incidence of genital HSV-1 infection has increased [94–96]. For instance, 78% of newly diagnosed genital herpes in a sample of US college students was attributable to HSV-1 [96]. However, HSV-2 accounts for the majority of recurrent genital herpes lesions because genital HSV-1 infection reactivates less frequently than HSV-2 [97,98].

The gold standard test for diagnosis of genital herpes has traditionally been culture of virus from genital lesions. If viral culture is not available, infection may be diagnosed by evaluating ulcer scrapings for the presence of multinucleated giant cells ("Tzank smear"). The sensitivity of Tzank smear relative to culture is 52–80% in anogenital lesions, with higher sensitivity in men than in women; the corresponding specificity is reported as 93% [99]. When used for orolabial herpes, the Tzanck smear has a reported sensitivity of 54% and a specificity of 100% relative to culture [100].

Enzyme immunoassays provide a rapid and sensitive alternative to culture for identification of HSV. The sensitivity of these tests has been estimated to be 80–96%, while their specificity has been reported as 93–100% [101–104]. Direct immunofluorescent assays may also be useful for the diagnosis of HSV in the genital tract, and provide a more timely diagnosis than culture. Reported sensitivity is 74–80%, and specificity is 85–98% relative to culture [105,106].

As has been noted, the quantification of the sensitivity and specificity of newer assays (e.g., nucleic acid amplification-based assays) is difficult, since these assays are more sensitive than culture, the traditional gold standard. For example, in studies using PCR as the gold standard, viral culture has a sensitivity of 72–88% [87,101,107,108], while EIA has a sensitivity of 65% [101]. A linear relationship exists between HSV detection by culture and the log copy number of HSV DNA detected by PCR, which may account for these differences [109]. In addition, the sensitivity of HSV culture relative to PCR may decline further if specimens are transported in warm weather conditions [109].

Older serologic assays for anti-herpes simplex antibody were unable to reliably distinguish between infection with HSV-1 and HSV-2 [110]. More recent serologic assays, such as glycoprotein G-based Western blot, can differentiate the response to infection with these two viruses, and are more than 90% sensitive if performed 21 days or more after primary infection [111]. Based on individuals prospectively followed in the setting of randomized controlled trials, it can be estimated that approximately 40% of those who acquire HSV-2 infection (as evidenced by seroconversion) actually develop genital herpes [112].

Newer FDA-approved, ELISA-based assays for type-specific antibodies against HSV-1 and HSV-2 such as HerpeSelect™ 1 and 2 (Focus Technology, Inc., Herndon, Virginia) have reported sensitivities and specificities of 96–100% and 97–100% respectively [113,114] when compared with Western blot assays, and are less expensive to perform. The role of antibody testing in the diagnosis of genital herpes remains poorly defined, but such tests might be used in diagnosing recurrent or atypical symptoms with negative culture results [115], in counseling couples [116], and in pregnancy-related screening [117,118].

Syphilis

Primary and secondary syphilis may be diagnosed by visualization of spirochetes from ulcers, condylomata lata, and mucous patches using dark-field microscopy. Such diagnostic methods require both technical competence and experience; in the hands of an experienced microscopist, the sensitivity of dark-field microscopy has been estimated to range from 74% to 81% when compared with various reference standards [87,119–121]. The finding of motile spirochetes by dark-field microscopy in a sample from a genital lesion might be expected to be pathognomonic for syphilis, but other nonpathogenic genital tract spirochetes may lead to false-positive test results [122]. Antibody-based assays and PCR may also be used to detect the presence of *T. pallidum* in lesions of primary or secondary syphilis, and may offer improved sensitivity in detection of treponemes (Table 10.5).

Serologic testing is the mainstay of syphilis diagnosis in adults with nonprimary disease; the characteristics of these tests have been reviewed in detail elsewhere [122,123]. Such tests can be classified as nontreponemal tests, which identify antibodies not directed against treponemes, and treponemal tests, which identify antibodies directed at treponemal components. Nontreponemal tests may be positive in the presence of a primary chancre, but are less than 90% sensitive in primary syphilis. Sensitivity is higher in secondary and early latent syphilis. By contrast, the fluorescent treponemal antibody absorbed assay (FTA Abs), a treponemal test, is usually positive within a week of the development of a primary chancre (Fig. 10.2).

A small proportion of individuals with syphilis have a negative nontreponemal test for syphilis due to "prozone" phenomena, which occur when extremely high titers of antibody disrupt the assay. This results in a false-negative test result, which becomes positive upon dilution [124]. Nontreponemal tests revert to negative over time in approximately 30% of untreated individuals [125]; treponemal tests may uncommonly revert to negative, a phenomenon that appears to be more common in individuals with HIV-associated immune dysfunction [126].

The specificity of nontreponemal tests is problematic, and reports of falsely positive nontreponemal tests in the presence of other infectious diseases, rheumatologic diseases, and pregnancy are common [127]. The relative risk of a false-positive nontreponemal test in individuals with underlying HIV infection was 8.4 (95% CI 4.2–13.6) in a Spanish cohort [128]. Nonetheless, nontreponemal tests remain useful as screening tests because of their low cost, and because a reduction in titer following treatment is a useful indicator of microbiologic cure [129]. Treponemal tests are more specific than nontreponemal tests, although false-positive test results are reported [127]. Treponeme-specific tests, such as syphilis ELISA and TPHA, can be used for automated, high-throughput testing [130,131], but this does not obviate the need for both confirmatory testing, and the ongoing use of nontreponemal tests, which can identify reinfection and which can be used to evaluate response to treatment [132]. Interpretation of results with reactive treponemal tests and negative nontreponemal test require a detailed clinical and epidemiologic history as well as physical examination to appropriately integrate the serologic result into the clinical picture. The notable disadvantage of serologic testing in nonprimary syphilis is the lack of a true gold standard test; this is particularly important in asympomatic patients and especially the patient with HIV coinfection. The characteristics of commonly used laboratory tests for the serologic diagnosis of syphilis are presented in further detail in Table 10.6.

In an effort to combat high rates of congenital syphilis in the developing world, rapid point-of-care syphilis tests have come into focus as a method of increasing access to onsite diagnosis (and targeted treatment). Sensitivity of these tests (compared to TPHA or TPPA) appears higher when used with whole blood (84–96%) than with serum (where sensitivity has been as low as 57%) [133]; specificity has been >95%. Sensitivity may also be worse in the field than in laboratory conditions [134]. Although empiric data on cost-effectiveness are not available, model-based estimates suggest that using these tests to target antimicrobial therapy may prevent congenital syphilis at a cost of $0.22 per case averted, a ratio that would be considered highly cost-effective in the developing-world context [135].

The diagnosis of neurosyphilis is challenging. While VDRL testing of cerebrospinal fluid (CSF VDRL)

Table 10.5 Diagnostic characteristics of commonly used tests for the detection of *Treponema pallidum* in early syphilis

Population or specimen source	Prevalence (%)	Comparator or study gold standard	Sensitivity (%)	Specificity (%)	Reference
Darkfield microscopy					
128 individuals with anogenital lesions attending an STD clinic in Edmonton, Alberta	52	Positive darkfield evaluation or positive serologic test for syphilis	79	100	[121]
350 specimens taken from individuals with lesions suggestive of syphilis (>1 specimen per individual)	34	"Subsequent diagnosis of syphilis"	74	97	[120]
302 individuals with genital ulcer disease in Pune, India	14	Multiplex PCR	39	82	[28]
188 individuals with genital lesions attending STD clinics in Brooklyn, New York, and Seattle, Washington	34	Direct fluorescent monoclonal antibody testing	85	96	[119]
295 men presenting to New Orleans sexually transmitted diseases clinic with genital ulcer	25	Multiplex PCR	81	100	[87]
241 individuals assessed at county clinics in San Francisco and Los Angeles with lesions suggestive of primary syphilis	22	Direct fluorescent antibody testing	85	97	[375]
Direct fluorescent antibody test					
241 Individuals assessed at county clinics in San Francisco and Los Angeles with lesions suggestive of primary syphilis	18	Darkfield microscopy	86	93	[375]
156 individuals with genital ulcer disease from Malawi	17	PCR with dot-blot hybridization	85	97	[376]
128 individuals with anogenital lesions attending an STD clinic in Edmonton, Alberta	52	Positive darkfield evaluation or positive serologic test for syphilis	79	100	[121]
350 specimens taken from individuals with lesions suggestive of syphilis (>1 specimen per individual)	34	"Subsequent diagnosis of syphilis"	86	100	[120]
188 individuals with genital lesions attending STD clinics in Brooklyn, New York, and Seattle, Washington	34	Darkfield microscopy	91	93	[119]
PCR					
295 men presenting to New Orleans sexually transmitted diseases clinic with genital ulcer	22	Darkfield microscopy	100	99	[87]
301 individuals tested for early syphilis in sexual health clinics in Melbourne, Australia	17	Concurrent serological testing for syphilis	80	98	[377]

Continued

Population or specimen source	Prevalence (%)	Comparator or study gold standard	Sensitivity (%)	Specificity (%)	Reference
98 individuals (86 male) with clinical signs and symptoms resulting in testing for syphilis at UK genitourinary medicine clinics	29	Diagnosis by clinicians, with consideration of all laboratory results (including serology)	95	99	[378]
112 individuals attending a public sexual health clinic in Amsterdam with suspected syphilis. Compared 3 different PCR-based assays	12	Darkfield microscopy and serology	94–100	99–100	[379]

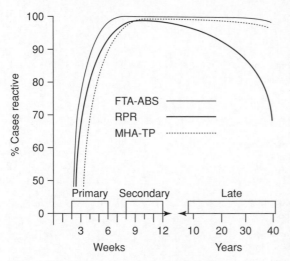

Figure 10.2 Timing of serologic test positivity in syphilis. Comparison of timing of test positivity for a nontreponemal test (rapid plasma regain or RPR), and two treponemal tests (fluorescent treponemal antibody absorbed (FTA-ABS) and microhemagglutination assay for *T. pallidum* (MHA-TP)). Both the RPR and FTA-ABS are positive in most individuals with a primary chancre, but FTA-ABS is more sensitive in primary syphilis. The two treponemal tests remain positive over time, while RPR will revert to negative in approximately one-third of untreated individuals. Reproduced from reference [122]: Larsen SA, Steiner BM, Rudolph AH. Laboratory diagnosis and interpretation of tests for syphilis. Clin Microbiol Rev 1995;8(1):1–21 with permission from the American Society for Microbiology.

is often advocated, the sensitivity of this test is poor. A retrospective study was performed in 38 individuals with positive cerebrospinal fluid FTA-Abs (a test thought to be sensitive but nonspecific for the diagnosis of neurosyphilis). Fifteen of 38 had likely neurosyphilis on the basis of a compatible clinical history and other CSF abnormalities (e.g., leukocytosis or elevated protein), but only four of these 15 individuals had a positive CSF VDRL (sensitivity 27%) [136].

The use of the "TPHA index" has been suggested as a more sensitive means of diagnosing neurosyphilis. This index is based on an antibody test (MHA-TP) that is more sensitive than CSF VDRL. False-positive test results are reduced by adjusting for CSF protein concentration, which in turn helps to control for blood contamination of the CSF sample [137]. However, a study in individuals coinfected with HIV and syphilis found high index values in only five of 40 individuals with possible neurosyphilis, and three of five individuals with positive CSF VDRL tests, suggesting that the TPHA index may also be relatively insensitive for active central nervous system infection [138].

Existing evidence does not support the routine use of PCR for the diagnosis of neurosyphilis in adults, and published studies have yielded inconsistent results [139,140]. In a study conducted in infants born to mothers with untreated syphilis in Dallas, Texas, CSF PCR had a sensitivity of 65% when compared with a gold standard of rabbit infectivity testing; in this study PCR of blood or serum was more sensitive than CSF

Table 10.6 Ranges of sensitivity and specificity reported for serological tests for syphilis by stage

Test	Sensitivity (%)				Specificity (%)	Reference
	Primary	Secondary	Latent	Late		
Nontreponemal tests						
VDRL	74–87	100	88–100	34–94	96–99	[125,380,381]
RPR	77–100	100	95–100	73	93–99	[125,381]
TRUST	77–86	100	95–100	–	98–99	[125]
USR	72–88	100	88–100	–	99	[125]
Treponemal tests						
FTA-ABS	70–100	100	99–100	96	84–100	[125,380–382]
MHA-TP	69–90	99–100	97–100	94	98–100	[125,380–382]
Nonstandard tests						
ELISA	82–100	91–100	86–100	100	89–100	[130,383–387]
Western blot	78–100	98–100	83–100	100	97–100	[388–390]

VDRL, Venereal Disease Research Laboratory; RPR, Rapid Plasma Reagin; TRUST, toluidine red unheated serum test; USR, unheated serum reagin; FTA-Abs, fluorescent treponemal antibody absorbed; MHA-TP, microhemagglutination assay for T. pallidum; ELISA, enzyme-linked immunosorbent assay.

Modified with permission from reference [125]: Larsen SA, Pope V, Johnson RE, Kennedy EJ, eds. A Manual of Tests for Syphilis, 9th ed. 13–18. Copyright © 1998 by American Public Health Association.

PCR for the presence of central nervous system disease (94%) [141].

Diagnosis of genital warts and human papillomavirus infection

The diagnosis of genital warts is usually made clinically, but rigorous studies of the sensitivity and specificity of clinical diagnosis are lacking. Although the intuition of experienced clinicians was more sensitive and specific than the use of a standardized diagnostic instrument in a small study of extragenital warts, the gold standard used in this study was the clinical judgment of one of the study investigators [142].

Acetic acid (3–5%) has been used as an adjunct to the clinical diagnosis of genital warts, and whitening with acid application is said to signify the presence of underlying HPV infection. The application of acetic acid has also been advocated for the identification of subclinical warty lesions. However, whitening appears to be nonspecific for the presence of HPV infection: in a cohort of Swedish army conscripts, HPV DNA was detected by PCR in only 17 of 39 biopsy specimens taken from aceto-white areas, and there was no difference in the detection of HPV DNA in urethral brushings from men with and without aceto-white lesions [143]. In another study HPV DNA was

detected in only 55 of 91 acetowhite lesions detected by penoscopy, with other aceto-white biopsy specimens having histology suggestive of eczema [144].

Furthermore, aceto-white lesions appear to be insensitive for the presence of HPV infection: in a cohort of Swedish women undergoing colposcopy, the finding of an aceto-white vulvar lesion had a sensitivity of 44% for the detection of HPV DNA by PCR [143]. Finally, many clinically typical genital warts do not turn white with the application of acetic acid. In a study of 202 men in Chandigarh, India, all hyperplastic warts turned white with the application of acetic acid, but only one of 12 typical verruca vulgaris-type lesions, and 15 of 59 flat warts, did so [145]. Thus, the poor sensitivity and specificity of acetic acid testing for small or subclinical genital warts, combined with the lack of evidence to suggest that treatment of such lesions changes long-term outcome, makes it difficult to advocate the routine use of acetic acid testing for external genital warts.

Similarly, no evidence exists currently to support the use of HPV DNA testing in the clinical diagnosis of external genital warts. However, such testing may contribute substantially to cervical cancer screening programs. The presence of "high-risk" HPV DNA in genital tract specimens of women with atypical squamous cells of undetermined significance (ASCUS) on Papanicolaou smear is highly sensitive for the presence of underlying cervical neoplasia [146–148]. Mathematical models based on available screening data suggest that the incorporation of HPV DNA testing into screening practices would likely be cost-effective relative to current practices [149–151]. A more complete review of the relationship between human papillomavirus and cervical neoplasia is available elsewhere [152].

Prevention of STI

Condoms and other contraceptives

Evidence exists to support the effectiveness of latex male condoms in preventing transmission of several different STI. A prospective study of the impact of condom use on acquisition of either HIV or other STI in a community in Uganda found consistent condom use to be associated with a reduced risk of acquiring HIV infection (RR 0.4, 95% CI 0.2–0.9), syphilis (OR 0.7, 95% CI 0.5–0.9), and gonorrhea or chlamydia (OR 0.5, 95% CI 0.3–1.0). These effects were seen despite the fact that condom users had riskier sexual practices than nonusers [153]. No reduction in risk was associated with inconsistent condom use. Another prospective cohort study in a cohort of Kenyan sex trade workers found consistent condom use to be associated with a decreased risk of chlamydia (HR 0.6, 95% CI 0.4–0.9); gonorrhea (HR 0.6, 95% CI 0.4–0.8), genital ulcer disease (HR 0.5, 95% CI 0.3–0.9), and PID (HR 0.6, 95% CI 0.4–0.9), after adjustment for such covariates as place of work and number of sexual encounters per week [154]. A prospective study in American sailors suggested that consistent condom use reduced the risk of gonorrhea acquisition during shore leave from 10% to 0%, although this difference was not statistically significant, perhaps as a result of the small number of sailors who actually reported using condoms [155].

The relationship between condom use and acquisition of genital herpes was studied in the context of a trial of a herpes vaccine in couples discordant for genital infection with HSV-2. Condom use by males during sexual intercourse in 25% of episodes or more was associated with a dramatic reduction in the hazard of acquisition of genital herpes by female partners (adjusted HR 0.09, 95% CI 0.01–0.7) [156]. No effect was seen on female-to-male transmission in this study, but the study likely lacked statistical power to find such an effect. A more recent cohort study found "frequent" condom use to decrease the risk of HSV-2 acquisition in both males and females (HR 0.74, 95% CI 0.59–0.95) [157].

A systematic review and metaanalysis evaluated the relationship between condom use and acquisition of HPV infection, or HPV-associated disease (e.g., genital warts or cervical intraepithelial neoplasia). The authors found no convincing evidence for a protective effect associated with condoms [158]. However, a more recent cohort study in newly sexually active university students identified a strong protection against HPV acquisition associated with consistent condom use (adjusted HR 0.3, 95% CI 0.1–0.5); condom use also reduced the incidence of cervical intraepithelial neoplasia [159]. Similar findings were reported in a recent study of HPV transmission in infection-discordant couples [160].

Other contraceptive practices, including the use of spermicides, oral contraceptive pills, and intrauterine contraceptive devices (IUD), may affect the risk of STI. Despite the fact that it is bactericidal in vitro, there is no consistent evidence to suggest that the spermicide nonoxynol-9 reduces the risk of genital gonorrheal or chlamydia infection [162–166]. Further, nonoxynol-9 may increase the risk of ulcerative genital disease, which may enhance HIV transmission [163,166].

A strong association between IUD and PID was noted in a multicenter case–control study conducted in the late 1970s [167], but subsequent analyses found the risk of PID to be most strongly associated with one particular type of IUD, the "Dalkon shield" (OR 15.6; 95% CI 8.1–30.0). The association of other types of IUD with PID is more controversial [168–173].

Hormonal contraception, particularly oral contraceptive pills, may enhance the risk of acquisition of cervicitis, particularly due to *C. trachomatis* [154], but a number of studies have found that symptomatic PID associated with *C. trachomatis* is less likely in women who use oral contraceptive pills [174,175]. This paradox may relate to the impact of oral contraceptive pills on recognition of PID: in a case–control study, individuals with asymptomatic PID were found to be 4.3 times as likely to use oral contraceptives as women with symptomatic disease (95% CI 1.6–11.7) [176].

Management of sexually transmitted infections

Case presentation (continued)

The male adolescent described above is treated syndromically for urethritis with 1 g of oral azithromycin, and 400 mg of oral cefixime. Because of the presence of abdominal discomfort, adnexal tenderness, and cervical motion tenderness, his female partner is treated for PID. Despite some misgivings related to the question of compliance, the treating physician opts to manage her as an outpatient, with a 2-week course of oral metronidazole and levofloxacin. Subsequent laboratory testing shows both to be infected with *Chlamydia trachomatis* as well as gonorrhea. The female patient subsequently fails to return for scheduled follow-up; when contacted by local public health personnel 2 weeks after presentation, she says that she took "all her medication," although she is still experiencing vaginal discharge and low abdominal discomfort. You wonder.

- How effective is syndromic management of STI?
- How effective is directed treatment of STI?
- Does treatment of sexual partners reduce the risk of relapse or reinfection?
- Are population-based interventions (including vaccination, screening, the use of mass antibiotic treatment) effective as control strategy for STI?
- Can behavioral interventions modify the future risk of sexually transmitted infection?

As discussed above, the syndromic diagnosis of STI is substantially less accurate than laboratory-based diagnosis. Nonetheless, evidence exists to support management based on syndromic diagnoses, as this approach results in receipt of treatment by most infected individuals, and eliminates concerns related to nontreatment as a result of loss to follow-up.

For example, despite the lack of accuracy of the clinical diagnosis of cervicitis, a study performed in female sex trade workers in Benin found that such a diagnosis was sufficient to warrant treatment for gonorrheal and chlamydial infections. The clinical diagnosis of cervicitis in this study was 48% sensitive and 75% specific for the presence of gonorrhea or chlamydia. This compared unfavorably to the 75% sensitivity and 100% specificity associated with laboratory diag-

nosis. However, the "effective sensitivity" of laboratory diagnosis, defined as the proportion of infected individuals detected by laboratory testing who actually returned to clinic within 30 days, was only 29%, worse than that seen with clinical diagnosis alone [177].

A single non-randomized, controlled clinical trial has compared outcomes following the use of a diagnostic algorithm (with speculum examination) to a diagnostic approach incorporating basic microbiologic testing in the evaluation of vaginal discharge. In this study, performed in a cohort of women in southern Thailand, the presence of gross cervical mucopus was a less sensitive indicator of cervical infection with gonorrhea and chlamydia than was the finding of microscopic mucopus on Gram stain (sensitivity 34% vs 64%). However, no significant differences were seen between groups in the proportion of women with gonococcal or chlamydial infection at follow-up, or in the proportion of women with persisting vaginal discharge 1–2 weeks after initial evaluation [178]. It should be noted that this study may have lacked statistical power to detect clinically significant differences in outcome.

Intensified syndromic management of STI has also been evaluated as a strategy for preventing HIV infection in two East African trials. In a randomized controlled trial of pairwise matched communities in Mwanza district, Tanzania, a strategy including syndromic STI treatment resulted in a slight, but nonstatistically significant, decrease in prevalence of syphilis (adjusted RR 0.92, 95% CI 0.78–1.07) and gonorrhea/chlamydia (adjusted RR 0.65; 95% CI 0.26–1.62), and successfully reduced HIV incidence (RR 0.58, 95% CI 0.42–0.79) [179]. In a cluster-randomized controlled trial in the Masaka district of Uganda, a similar syndromic STI management strategy decreased the incidence of syphilis (IRR 0.52, 95% CI 0.27–0.98) and prevalence of gonorrhea (PR 0.25, 95% CI 0.10–0.64), but had no impact on HIV incidence (IRR 1.00, 95% CI 0.63–1.58) [180]. The apparently contradictory results of these and other studies regarding HIV incidence have been attributed to epidemiologic differences in the stage of the HIV epidemic, as well as differences in prevalence of HSV-2 infection (see below) [180].

Treatment of *Neisseria gonorrhoeae* infections

A variety of drug regimens for the treatment of uncomplicated gonococcal urethritis and cervicitis have been assessed since the late 1960s via randomized controlled trials [181–183]. However, the relevance of early trials to current practice is limited, owing to the emergence of widespread antibiotic resistance in *N. gonorrhoeae*. Resistance to penicillins, tetracyclines, and macrolides have become commonplace throughout the world [184,185]. Although tetracycline and penicillin resistance have actually diminished in some areas in recent years, this probably reflects decreased selective pressure because of the nonuse of these agents by treating clinicians [184].

Prior to the emergence of widespread β-lactam resistance, the use of a single 3 g oral dose of ampicillin or amoxicillin, combined with 1 g of probenecid, was highly effective for the treatment of uncomplicated gonorrheal infections [182]. However, a randomized controlled trial performed in an area of Ethiopia with high rates of penicillin resistance demonstrated that in vitro resistance to penicillin was associated with clinical treatment failure; 19% of individuals treated with oral ampicillin and probenecid experienced clinical failure, while no failures were noted with a single 2 g intramuscular dose of spectinomycin [186].

A subsequent randomized trial in Thailand showed single-dose therapy with third-generation cephalosporins to be equivalent in efficacy to single-dose spectinomycin therapy [187]. Treatment with either a single 400 mg dose of cefixime orally, or 250 mg of ceftriaxone intramuscularly, reliably cured more than 95% of individuals with uncomplicated gonococcal urethritis or cervicitis in a randomized controlled trial performed in Nairobi, Kenya [188]. Single-dose cefixime and ceftriaxone have also been found to be highly effective and equivalent in a randomized controlled trial performed in the US [189].

Fluoroquinolones may be useful agents as single-dose therapy for uncomplicated gonococcal infections in some geographic areas. A US trial completed in the 1980s found single-dose ofloxacin (400 mg) to be equivalent to therapy with amoxicillin plus probenecid [190]. Comparison of a single 500 mg dose of ciprofloxacin with intramuscular ceftriaxone for urethritis treatment in an area of Zambia with a high prevalence of antibiotic-resistant *Neisseria gonorrhoeae* found the two treatment regimens to be equivalent [191]. However, resistance to fluoroquinolones has recently become widespread in many parts of the world [192,193]. The US CDC issued an advisory in 2007 indicating that fluorquinolone use should be avoided altogether for treatment of gonorrhea [194], leaving cefixime and ceftriaxone as the sole recommended agents for empiric treatment of *N. gonorrhoeae* infections in the US. There is strong evidence linking in vitro resistance to fluoroquinolones to clinical treatment failure. A randomized controlled trial compared the efficacy of ceftriaxone to that of ciprofloxacin in *N. gonorrhoeae*-infected sex-trade workers in the Philippines. The relative risk of clinical failure when individuals with a highly fluoroquinolone-resistant organism (defined by ciprofloxacine MIC greater than or equal to 0.4 μg/mL) were treated with ciprofloxacin was 13.1 (95% CI 1.8–93.0) [195].

A single 2 g dose of azithromycin may be an effective treatment for uncomplicated gonococcal infection. In a randomized trial both azithromycin and a single 250 mg intramuscular dose of ceftriaxone eradicated gonorrhea in more than 97% of participants; concomitant chlamydial infection was eradicated by azithromycin, but not by ceftriaxone [196]. The effectiveness of azithromycin outside the context of a clinical trial may be limited by the fact that over a third of trial participants experience gastrointestinal discomfort with high-dose azithromycin, and by the emergence of azithromycin resistance in gonococcal isolates [197]. Although resistance to spectinomycin and third-generation cephalosporins remains uncommon, resistance to these agents has been reported and may increase in coming years [198]. Because of the extremely dynamic nature of antimicrobial resistance in *N. gonorrhoeae*, clinicians should remain abreast of changes in antimicrobial resistance patterns; in North America, an excellent resource in this regard is the Gonorrhea Isolate Surveillance Project (GISP) (http://www.cdc.gov/std/GISP/default.htm).

Treatment of *Chlamydia trachomatis* infections and nongonococcal urethritis or cervicitis

The past three decades have seen an evolution in the understanding of so-called nongonococcal urethritis, postgonococcal urethritis, and mucopurulent cervicitis, with increasing recognition that these syndromes are most commonly caused by *C. trachomatis*. As such, early data on the treatment of chlamydial infections are derived from studies that did not explicitly identify this pathogen, or which grouped chlamydial infections with those caused by other nongonococcal organisms.

The efficacy of tetracyclines in the treatment of chlamydial infections has been demonstrated in several randomized controlled trials. An early trial compared spectinomycin to tetracycline for the treatment of gonorrhea, and found postgonococcal urethritis to occur less frequently with tetracycline [178]. Tetracyclines were subsequently found to be superior to sulfa drugs combined with spectinomycin in a randomized trial in men with nongonococcal urethritis [199]. Doxycycline was also significantly more efficacious than placebo in preventing postgonococcal urethritis (RR 0.6, 95% CI 0.4–0.8) [200].

Minocycline (100 mg twice daily), doxycycline (100 mg twice daily), and tetracycline (250 mg four times a day) had equal efficacy in the treatment of nongonococcal urethritis and mucopurulent cervicitis in randomized trials [201,202]. A 2 g total daily dose of tetracycline may be more efficacious than a single gram total dose [203].

Macrolide agents serve as a valuable alternative to the tetracyclines for the treatment of chlamydial infections. A week of therapy with 1 g per day of either erythromycin or tetracycline had equal efficacy in a randomized trial of treatment for men with chlamydial urethritis and their infected sex partners [204], and newer macrolides such as clarithromycin (250 mg twice daily for 7 days) and roxithromycin (300 mg once a day for 10 days) also appear to be equivalent to doxycycline in the treatment of uncomplicated genital chlamydia infections and nongonococcal urethritis and cervicitis [205,206].

The development of azithromycin has had a dramatic impact on the treatment of chlamydial infections in the clinic setting, with a single 1 g dose of azithromycin proved equivalent to a 7-day course of doxycycline in the eradication of chlamydial infection, and in the resolution of cervicitis and urethritis. A systematic review and metaanalysis of 12 randomized controlled trials comparing azithromycin and doxycycline for the treatment of urethritis or cervicitis found no difference between these regimens in microbiologic cure, or in the incidence of adverse drug events [207].

Fluoroquinolones have had variable efficacy in the treatment of chlamydial infections. Two randomized trials comparing ciprofloxacin (750–1000 mg twice daily) to doxycycline found that elimination of chlamydia occurred in only 46–62% of those treated with ciprofloxacin, in contrast to 75–100% of those treated with doxycycline [208,209]. In contrast, one week of ofloxacin at a dose of 300–400 mg twice daily appears to be equivalent in efficacy to doxycycline dosed at 100 mg twice daily, with both drugs reported to eradicate chlamydial infections in 97–100% of individuals with urethritis or cervicitis [208,209]. Newer quinolones, such as sparfloxacin, grepafloxacin, and trovafloxacin, have been proven efficacious for the treatment of uncomplicated chlamydial infections of the genital tract, but their use has been limited by severe adverse drug effects, including cardiac arrhythmias and hepatotoxicity [210–212].

Untreated lower genital tract chlamydial infection appears to be associated with adverse pregnancy outcomes including prematurity, low birthweight, stillbirth, postpartum endometritis, and pneumonitis and conjunctivitis in the newborn [213–221]. A retrospective cohort study found lower perinatal mortality associated with erythromycin treatment versus no treatment in pregnancies with a positive chlamydial culture [222]. A second retrospective cohort study found that women with successfully treated chlamydial cervicitis had lower frequencies of premature rupture of membranes and small-for-gestational-age infants compared with unsuccessfully treated women [22]. A randomized placebo-controlled trial evaluating chlamydia screening and erythromycin treatment in pregnancy found no differences between study arms, but this absence of effect may have occurred as a result of high rates of ancillary antibiotic use in the placebo arm [223].

Subsequently, randomized controlled trials have compared amoxicillin (500 mg three times a day for 7 days) to nonestolate preparations of erythromycin for the treatment of uncomplicated chlamydial infection in pregnant women. A metaanalysis of trials comparing amoxicillin and erythromycin found the two drugs to be similar in efficacy, although amoxicillin is associated with a lower incidence of adverse effects, especially nausea [224]. With increasing comfort related to the use of azithromycin in pregnancy, randomized trials have been performed comparing this agent to amoxicillin; the two agents appear to have equivalent efficacy [225,226].

Treatment of pelvic inflammatory disease

The agents of urethritis and cervicitis are strongly associated with the development of PID, a syndrome characterized clinically by the presence of lower abdominal pain, cervical motion tenderness, and uterine adnexal tenderness. However, while either *N. gonorrhoea* or *C. trachomatis* or both organisms are identifiable in cervical culture specimens of 70% of individuals with clinically diagnosed PID, this infection is typically polymicrobial, and therapeutic regimens include agents that are effective against these organisms, as well as gram-negative bacilli and anaerobes. A systematic review of 34 clinical trials and case series found most available drug regimens to be associated with cure in 80–100%, although the pooled probability of cure was less than 80% when doxycycline and metronidazole were used without other agents [227].

A key clinical branch point in the management of PID involves the question of whether individuals need to be admitted to hospital for therapy. A single randomized controlled trial (the "PEACH" trial) evaluated the question of inpatient versus outpatient therapy for women with moderate PID diagnosed clinically: 831 women received inpatient treatment with intravenous cefoxitin and doxycycline, or outpatient treatment with a single intramuscular injection of cefoxitin and oral doxycycline. No significant differences were seen in short-term cure rates, or in the development of longer-term sequelae, including infertility, pelvic pain, and ectopic pregnancy in the 808 women available for long-term follow-up. The average follow-up time in these women was 35 months [228].

Treatment of syphilis

Benzathine penicillin and aqueous penicillin G are the mainstays of therapy for syphilis, and are believed to be highly effective despite a lack of randomized controlled trials. Evidence supporting the use of tetracyclines as an alternative to penicillin for syphilis treatment is similarly based on descriptions of case series [229,230]. Recent randomized controlled trials of therapy for syphilis have compared alternative treatments to penicillin-based regimens.

Intramuscular ceftriaxone is commonly used as an alternative to benzathine penicillin for syphilis not affecting the central nervous system; however, there is little in the clinical trials literature to support this practice. A small randomized controlled trial compared a 15-day course of intramuscular penicillin to 1 g of intramuscular ceftriaxone given every other day

for 7 days (i.e., four doses in total) in 28 patients with early syphilis. This study found an adequate serologic and clinical response in all participants [231]. A small randomized controlled trial comparing a single 2.4 million unit dose of benzathine penicillin to a single 3 g intramuscular dose of ceftriaxone and to 2 g of ceftriaxone given intramuscularly for 5 days found either clinical cure or sustained clinical response in 16 of 17 participants available for follow-up. Although the single failure of treatment occurred with single-dose ceftriaxone, this study was too small to permit comparisons between treatment regimens [232].

A promising alternative to benzathine penicillin in the treatment of early syphilis was azithromycin, which when compared with benzathine penicillin in an open-label pilot study [233] had provided promising results. A total of 74 patients were randomized to receive standard dose benzathine penicillin, a single 2 g dose of azithromycin, or two 2 g doses of azithromycin 1 week apart. Of the 46 individuals available for evaluation a year after therapy, only three had experienced serologic evidence of relapse or failure of response (defined as a <2-fold reduction in RPR titers from pretreatment levels). In a similar study conducted in Tanzania, patients with primary or high-titre (RPR > 1:8) latent syphilis were randomized to benzathine penicillin 2.4 million units intramuscularly as a single dose or to a single oral dose of 2 g of azithromycin. At 9 months of follow-up, cure rates were equivalent.

However, the value of azithromycin for treatment of syphilis is threatened by the emergence of antimicrobial resistance in the US, Ireland, and Canada [234–236]. Treatment failure with azithromycin was first documented in San Francisco in 2002, when three patients with primary syphilis did not respond to azithromycin treatment, and five patients who were contacts of patients with early syphilis experienced clinical symptoms or seroconversion. Molecular evidence indicated that the A2058G mutation (previously linked to erythromycin resistance) conferred azithromycin resistance in *T. pallidum* [234]. Although surveillance for azithromycin resistance is in its infancy, in San Francisco, the proportion of specimens that harbor the resistance mutation has increased from 41% of 32 isolates in 2003, to 77.3% of 22 isolates in 2006 [234].

Case reports and series suggesting that HIV-infected individuals are more prone to relapse after treatment of syphilis with standard drug regimens [237,238] prompted investigators to initiate two randomized controlled trials comparing usual therapy with penicillin to alternate therapies. The first of these trials [239] compared a standard regimen of 2.4 million units of benzathine penicillin G intramuscularly with standard therapy plus a 10-day course of amoxicillin and probenicid in 541 individuals with primary, secondary, or early latent syphilis: 101 participants were HIV-infected, with one-third of these having very low CD4 cell counts. No differences were seen between groups in clinical outcomes, regardless of HIV status or treatment regimens. A second trial compared 10 days of intramuscular ceftriaxone (2 g per day) to aqueous penicillin G (24 million units per day) in 36 individuals with neurosyphilis and HIV coinfection [240]. No difference was seen in the proportion of individuals with improvement in CSF VDRL titers, white blood cell counts, or protein concentrations at 14–26 weeks after therapy, although ceftriaxone was associated with a greater decline in serum RPR titers.

Preventive therapy is usually recommended for sex contacts of individuals found to have infectious syphilis. A randomized, open-label trial compared azithromycin to benzathine penicillin for the prevention of syphilis in individuals with an infectious sex partner. None of the 96 participants was documented to have developed syphilis during follow-up, although fully one-third of participants were lost to follow-up before completing 3 months of post-treatment surveillance [241]. Syphilis incidence also appears to be reduced in cohorts treated for gonorrhea with tetracyclines or erythromycin, suggesting that these agents are also effective against incubating syphilis [242].

Intravenous penicillin G or intramuscular procaine penicillin have been recommended for the treatment of infants with clinical illness related to congenital syphilis [243]. However, a randomized controlled trial comparing a single dose of benzathine penicillin to a 10-day course of intramuscular procaine penicillin in 169 infants with asymptomatic congenital syphilis found no differences in efficacy between the two drug regimens. All 152 infants available for follow-up at 2–3 months had a 4-fold decrease in RPR titers, while 149 became RPR nonreactive [244]. A small clinical trial performed in South Africa randomized asymptomatic infants of mothers with untreated syphilis and high serum regain titers to single-dose benzathine penicillin or no therapy. While this study raises ethical concerns, it clearly demonstrated that nontreatment of such infants places them at high risk for the development of congenital syphilis. Congenital syphilis developed in four of eight infants randomized to no treatment, and none of the 11 infants who received penicillin ($P = 0.04$) [245].

Treatment of genital herpes

Genital herpes may have a broad spectrum of clinical manifestations. First episodes of genital herpes may be primary (no previous infection with HSV-1 or HSV-2), or nonprimary, with primary episodes often being more severe [246–248]. Among individuals with primary genital herpes infection, intravenous acyclovir at a dose of 5 mg/kg every 8 hours was shown to be superior to placebo in time to healing of genital ulcers and in speed of elimination of viral shedding [249]. Subsequently, oral acylovir at a dose of 200 mg five times per day was shown to be superior to placebo in individuals with first episodes of genital herpes, both primary and nonprimary [250,251]. Further increasing the dose of antiviral drug does not result in improved outcomes; a randomized trial comparing a total of 4 g of acyclovir per day with 1 g per day found no differences between treatment groups [252].

Treatment of recurrent genital herpes episodes with oral acyclovir at doses of 200 mg five times a day or 800 mg twice a day has been shown to be superior to placebo in the elimination of symptoms and viral shedding [253–255]. The related drugs famciclovir (125 mg orally twice a day) and valacyclovir (500 mg orally twice a day), are superior to placebo [256,257], and equivalent to acyclovir in efficacy [258,259]. Because many individuals with recurrent genital herpes recognize prodromal symptoms such as itching or tingling prior to experiencing an outbreak, patient-initiated therapy on the basis of such symptoms is often advocated, and appears effective in reducing outbreak duration and in aborting outbreaks [256,257,259]. More recently, evidence has emerged that traditional 5-day courses of therapy with antiviral drugs can be shortened. A 3-day course of valacyclovir appears equivalent in efficacy to a 5-day course [260], while a 2-day course of oral acyclovir (800 mg three times per day) is superior to placebo in the reduction of duration of lesions and viral shedding [261].

Individuals who experience frequent recurrences may prefer to use suppressive chronic therapy with antiviral drugs. The use of acyclovir at a dose of 400 mg twice a day is superior to placebo [262–264], and to lower doses of acyclovir [265], in the reduction of outbreak frequency. Treatment with daily acyclovir for as long as 6 years appears to be safe and well tolerated by patients, and the emergence of viral resistance does not appear to be a problem in immunocompetent hosts [266–268]. Famciclovir (125 or 250 mg orally twice daily) and valacyclovir (250 mg twice daily, 500 mg once daily, or 1 g once daily) are also superior to placebo for the prevention of recurrences [267,269–271]. A recent metaanalysis of 14 placebo-controlled randomized controlled trials of suppressive therapy with acyclovir, famciclovir, or valacyclovir for the prevention of genital herpes outbreaks showed a pooled relative risk of developing at least one outbreak during therapy of 0.53 (95% CI 51–55) [272]. Subgroup analyses showed a clear dose–response relationship for famciclovir between total daily doses of 250 and 750 mg. Two short-term randomized controlled clinical trials comparing famciclovir 250 mg orally twice

daily to valacyclovir 500 mg orally once daily demonstrated a similar time to first clinical recurrence (HR 1.17, 95% CI 0.78–1.76) but a shorter time to first virologically confirmed recurrence (HR 2.15, 95% CI 1.00–4.60) and high rate of HSV shedding (RR 2.33, 95% CI 1.18–4.89) with famciclovir [273].

Suppressive antiviral therapy appears to markedly reduce the frequency of asymptomatic viral shedding between recurrences as well [274]. To determine whether suppressive antiviral therapy could therefore decrease transmission of genital herpes, the Valacyclovir HSV Transmission Study randomized the HSV-2 seropositive partner in 1484 heterosexual, monogamous, HSV-2 serodiscordant couples to valacyclovir 500 mg orally daily versus matching placebo. This trial showed a significant reduction in both symptomatic (HR 0.25, 95% CI 0.08–0.75) and serologically confirmed (HR 0.52, 95% CI 0.27–0.99) HSV-2 infections among susceptible partners (Fig. 10.3) [275]. There was no difference between transmitters and nontransmitters in frequency of symptomatic reactivations in either the valacyclovir or the placebo arm of this trial, underlining the importance of asymptomatic

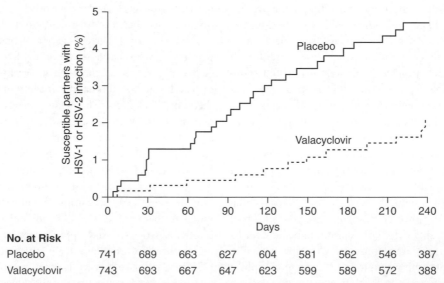

No. at Risk									
Placebo	741	689	663	627	604	581	562	546	387
Valacyclovir	743	693	667	647	623	599	589	572	388

Figure 10.3 Kaplan-Meier curve depicting time to transmission of HSV-1 or HSV-2 from an infected individual to an uninfected sex partner, based on the use of suppressive valacyclovir (500 mg orally 4 times daily) or placebo in the infected individual. Valacyclovir suppression reduces the risk of HSV transmission by approximately 50% (HR 0.45, 95% CI 0.24–0.84). Similar effects were seen in prevention of symptomatic HSV-2 infection in the initially uninfected partner. Reproduced from reference [275]: Corey L, Wald A, Patel R, et al. Once-daily valacyclovir to reduce the risk of transmission of genital herpes. N Engl J Med 2004;350:11–20 © 2004 Massachusetts Medical Society. All rights reserved.

viral shedding in determining risk of HSV-2 transmission [276]. Suppressive antiviral therapy in individuals with frequent recurrences does appear to significantly improve health-related quality of life, and also reduces anxiety and depression scores on standardized instruments [277,278].

The epidemiology of maternal–fetal HSV transmission is complex. Available epidemiologic evidence from a large cohort of women in Washington State suggests that the highest risk of maternal–fetal HSV transmission occurs with maternal acquisition of genital HSV infection in the third trimester of pregnancy (adjusted OR 59.3, 95% CI 6.7–525) [25,279]. No randomized controlled trials exist to support the recommendation that women undergo cesarean section if herpetic lesions are present at the time of delivery [280]. However, among women in the Washington cohort with detectable HSV at delivery, a trend towards reduced transmission was seen in those who underwent cesarean delivery (adjusted OR 0.14, 95% CI 0.02–1.26). This is consistent with population-level data from California between 1995 and 2003, which identified a stable incidence of neonatal herpes over that time period in conjunction with an increase in the rate of genital herpes complicating labor and a concomitant increase in cesarean section due to herpes [281]. Randomized controlled trials have found that suppressive antiviral drugs in pregnancy reduce the risk of cesarean section, by reducing the likelihood that active herpetic lesions are present at delivery [282–284] (pooled RR of cesarean section 0.49, 95% CI 0.33–0.74). However, the question of whether antiviral drugs in pregnancy can actually reduce peripartum HSV transmission remains unresolved.

Treatment of chancroid

A variety of drug regimens have proven efficacious in the treatment of chancroid in randomized controlled trials. However, the development of drug resistance in *H. ducreyi* has made some treatment options obsolete in certain geographic areas. Traditional agents of choice for the treatment of chancroid included tetracyclines and sulfonamides, but resistance to these agents is now extremely common, and macrolides, fluoroquinolones, and third-generation cephalosporins are now preferred for the treatment of chancroid [285–290]. The results of randomized controlled trials evaluating the efficacy of these agents are presented in Table 10.7.

Of note, single-dose therapies with ciprofloxacin (500 g) or azithromycin (1 g) have been proven equivalent to multiple-dose antibiotic regimens, while ceftriaxone (250 mg intramuscularly) appears equivalent to single-dose azithromycin [88,291–293].

Other antibiotic classes, including penicillins and aminoglycosides, may be useful in the treatment of chancroid. Although resistance to ampicillin by *H. ducreyi* is well described, resistance is mediated by β-lactamase production, and chancroid can be effectively treated with the addition of a β-lactamase inhibitor [294]. A single 2 g dose of spectinomycin is a useful alternative. A trial comparing spectinomycin to trimethoprim-sulfamethoxazole in Thailand found spectinomycin to be more likely to result in cure (RR of cure with spectinomycin 2.0, 95% CI 1.7–2.0) [295]. However, a randomized trial comparing erythromycin (500 mg orally three times a day for 5 days) to a single 2 g dose of spectinomycin found higher rates of cure with erythromycin (RR of cure with spectinomycin 0.9, 95% CI 0.8–1.0) [296].

Chancroid may be complicated by the development of fluctuant inguinal buboes. A small randomized trial compared aspiration to incision and drainage for the management of buboes during an outbreak of chancroid in New Orleans. Both forms of management appeared to be efficacious and acceptable, although six of 15 individuals who underwent aspiration experienced reaccumulation of purulent material, and required reaspiration ($P = 0.05$) [297].

Treatment of genital warts

A number of treatment modalities are available for the management of genital warts. These include topical agents, cryotherapy, surgical modalities (including scissors excision, laser ablation, and electrocautery), and interferon. While it is often suggested that genital warts involute spontaneously over time, it has been pointed out that there is little evidence to support this contention [298,299]. Important clinical outcomes in the study of genital wart treatment include reductions in wart area and rates of relapse, as well as rates of wart clearance.

Podophyllotoxin and imiquimod are both patient-applied topical therapies that have been proven efficacious in the treatment of genital warts in randomized, placebo-controlled trials (Table 10.8). A randomized trial comparing thrice-weekly application of 5% imiquimod cream with more frequent applications

Table 10.7 Randomized controlled trials evaluating macrolides, fluoroquinolones, and third-generation cephalosporins for the treatment of chancroid

Study population	Treatment arms	Primary outcome measure	Results	Comments	Reference
245 men and women attending an urban STD clinic in Nairobi, Kenya with genital ulcer disease compatible with chancroid	Single 500 mg dose of ciprofloxacin vs erythromycin 500 mg tid for 7 days	Ulcer healing or improvement among individuals proven to have chancroid by culture or PCR	No difference between treatment arms in healing or improvement (RR of cure with ciprofloxacin 1.0, 95% CI 0.8–1.2)	Double-blind, placebo-controlled	[88]
46 Indian men with clinical diagnosis of chancroid presenting to an outpatient specialty clinic	Ciprofloxacin 500 mg bid for 3 days vs erythromycin 500 mg qid for 7 days vs trimethoprim-sulfamethoxazole 160/800 mg bid for 7 days	Complete healing of ulcer 21 days after initial presentation	Cure in 29 of 31 individuals randomized to either erythromycin or ciprofloxacin. Relative risk of failure with trimethoprim-sulfamethoxazole 1.7, 95% CI 1.1–2.8	Open label trial. *H ducreyi* isolates resistant to trimethoprim-sulfamethoxazole. Individuals who failed initial therapy cured with ciprofloxacin or erythromycin	[289]
98 HIV-seronegative men presenting to a Nairobi clinic with culture-positive chancroid and negative syphilis evaluation	Single 400 mg oral dose of fleroxacin or trimethoprim-sulfamethoxazole 160/800 mg bid for 3 days	Clinical cure, defined as complete re-epithelialization at 1–2 weeks	Trend towards improved outcome with fleroxacin (RR of cure with fleroxacin 1.4, 95% CI 0.9–2.3)	Study performed as trimethoprim-sulfamethoxazole resistance being recognized in East Africa	[290]
204 men presenting to a Nairobi clinic with purulent genital ulcers	Azithromycin 1 gram orally vs erythromycin 500 mg qid for 7 days	Complete cure, defined as re-epithelialization of the ulcer base, ≤21 days after initial treatment	No differences between treatment regimens in outcome (cure in 73/82 with azithromycin and 41/45 with erythromycin	HIV seropositivity associated with increased risk of failed therapy (OR 4.5, 95% CI 1.4–14.7)	[291]
139 men presenting to a Nairobi clinic with culture-positive chancroid and negative syphilis evaluation	500 mg ciprofloxacin as a single dose vs 500 mg ciprofloxacin or trimethoprim-sulfamethoxazole 160/800 mg bid for 3 days	Complete cure, defined as re-epithelialization of the ulcer base, ≤21 days after initial treatment, and resolution of buboes	No differences between treatment regimens (cure seen in 28/46 with trimethoprim-sulfamethoxazole, 28/46 with single-dose ciprofloxacin, and 27/43 with 3-day ciprofloxacin regimen	Double-blind, placebo-controlled	[292]
197 men and women presenting to clinics in 4 US cities with genital ulcer but without evidence for syphilis	Single 1 g oral dose of azithromycin vs 250 mg ceftriaxone given intramuscularly	Complete healing of ulcer ≥18 days after treatment in individuals with culture-proven chancroid	High rates of cure in both groups (32/32 with azithromycin, 29/33 with ceftriaxone), but azithromycin more efficacious (RR of cure 1.1, 95% CI 1.0–1.3)	High rates of healing among individuals with ulcers of uncertain etiology in both arms	[293]
48 men presenting to a Nairobi clinic with negative syphilis evaluation	Cefotaxime (1 g intramuscularly) with 1 g of probenecid orally, single treatment vs once-daily treatment for 3 days	Complete healing of ulcer at 28 days of follow-up	Total dose of 3 g cefotaxime superior to 1 g (RR of healing 1.4, 95% CI 1.0–2.0 with 3 g dose)	Double-blind, placebo-controlled	[391]

Table 10.8 Randomized placebo-controlled trials of selected therapeutic modalities for the treatment of genital warts

Study population	Intervention	Results	Reference
Podophyllotoxin			
60 men with a clinical diagnosis of genital warts attending government-affiliated clinics in Punjab region of Pakistan	Subjects randomized to treatment with podophyllotoxin 0.5% cream, interferon-alpha cream, or placebo up to 9 times per week for up to 4 weeks	Podophllotoxin cured more individuals at 4 weeks than placebo (RR of cure 3.0, 95% CI 1.2–7.7), but less efficacious than interferon-alpha (RR of cure 0.7, 95% CI 0.5–1.0)	[308]
60 men with a clinical diagnosis of genital warts attending government-affiliated clinics in Punjab region of Pakistan	Subjects randomized to treatment with podophyllotoxin 0.5% cream, interferon-alpha cream, or placebo up to 9 times per week for up to 4 weeks	Podophllotoxin cured more individuals at 4 weeks than placebo (RR of cure 3.7, 95% CI 1.2–11.2), but less efficacious than interferon-alpha (RR of cure 0.6, 95% CI 0.4–0.9)	[309]
57 men and women at several US centers, with prior complete resolution of genital warts	Participants randomized to receive 0.5% podophyllotoxin or placebo once daily, 3 days per week, for 8 weeks	Reduction in recurrence with podophyllotoxin 8 weeks after enrollment (RR of recurrence 0.4, 95% CI 0.1–1.0)	[392]
57 Swedish men with previously untreated genital warts	Subjects randomly assigned to receive up to 2 courses of 0.25% or 0.5% podophyllotoxin, or placebo, twice daily for 3 days	No resolution seen in placebo arm. Warts cleared after 2 cycles of treatment in 13/18 patients receiving 0.25% and 13/16 patients receiving 0.5% podophyllotoxin	[393]
109 men with at several US centers, with a clinical diagnosis of genital warts	Subjects randomly assigned to 0.5% podophyllotoxin or placebo for 3 consecutive days, followed by 4 days without treatment. Applications repeated for 2–4 weeks	25/56 podophyllotoxin treated men wart-free at some point during study; no individual was wart-free In placebo arm. Reduction in total wart area also seen with podophyllotoxin	[394]
72 women with a clinical diagnosis of exophytic vulvar condyloma	Subjects randomly assigned to 0.5% podopyllotoxin in either alcohol or cream formulation or placebo, 2 applications per day, 3 consecutive days per week, for up to 4 weeks	Trend towards greater efficacy with podophyllotoxin at 10 weeks (RR for clearance 2.1, 95% CI 0.9–4.7)	[395]
38 men with genital warts in Seattle, Washington	Subjects randomly assigned to 0.5% podophyllotoxin or placebo applied 3 consecutive days per week for up to 4 weeks	11/19 podophyllotoxin treated men wart-free at some point during study; no individual was wart-free in placebo arm. Reduction in total wart area also seen with podophyllotoxin	[396]
Imiquimod			
311 men and women with anogenital warts at multiple US centers	Subjects randomized to 5% or 1% imiquimod cream or placebo, 3 applications per week for up to 16 weeks	Higher rates of clearance of warts seen with 5% imiquimod (RR of clearance 4.5, 95% CI 2.5–8.1) and 1% imiquimod than with placebo. 5% imiquimod more efficacious than 1% imiquimod (RR of clearance 2.4, 95% CI 1.6–3.7)	[397]

Continued

Study population	Intervention	Results	Reference
279 men and women with 2 or more biopsy-proven external genital warts at multiple centers in the US	Subjects randomized to daily application of 5% or 1% imiquimod cream or placebo, for up to 16 weeks	Higher rates of clearance of warts seen with 5% imiquimod (RR of clearance 16.3, 95% CI 5.3–51.1) and 1% imiquimod than with placebo. 5% imiquimod more efficacious than 1% imiquimod (RR of clearance 3.6, 95% CI 2.1–6.2)	[398]
60 women with genital warts in Punjab region of Pakistan	Subjects randomly assigned to 2% imiquimod or placebo, up to 10 applications per week for 6 weeks	Higher rates of clearance seen with 2% imiquimod than placebo after 6 weeks (RR of clearance 25, 95% CI 3.6–172.6)	[399]
60 men with genital warts attending public health centers and municipal dispensaries in Punjab region of Pakistan	Subjects randomized to 2% imiquimod cream or placebo, 3 applications weekly for 4 weeks	Higher rates of clearance seen with 2% imiquimod (RR of clearance 7.0, 95% CI 2.3–21.0)	[400]
Intralesional interferon 296 men and women with a clinical diagnosis of genital warts attending multiple centers in the US	Subjects randomized to 3 weekly intralesional injections of interferon alpha-2b or placebo, into up to 3 warts per subject, for 3 weeks	Higher rates of clearance of treated warts with interferon than with placebo at 16 weeks (RR for clearance of treated lesions 2.5, 95% CI 1.5–4.1). Higher percentage of interferon-treated subjects had a 50% or greater reduction in total wart area ($P < 0.001$)	[401]
158 men and women with a clinical diagnosis of at least 2 genital warts, covering at least 10 mm^2 in area, treated at 4 US centers	Warts injected with interferon alpha or placebo twice weekly for up to eight weeks, or until disappearance of warts	Interferon alpha more efficacious than placebo three months after last injection (RR of clearance with interferon 2.9, 95% CI 1.8–4.8)	[402]
76 men and women from multiple US centers, with genital warts present despite the use of conventional therapy	A single wart from each patient was injected 3 times per week for 4 weeks with one of 3 interferon preparations or placebo	Significant difference between interferon preparations and placebo in resolution of injected warts over 16-week follow-up period ($P = 0.02$). No difference in efficacy between interferon preparations. Interferon did not affect noninjected warts	[403]
114 men and women with genital warts treated at six centers in the US	Single wart injected intralesionally with high dose interferon alpha, low dose interferon alpha, or placebo, 3 times weekly for 3 weeks	Both high dose interferon alpha more efficacious than low dose interferon alpha (RR of clearance 2.8, 95% CI 1.3–6.3), and placebo (RR of clearance 3.8, 95% CI 1.5–10.2) at 12 weeks. Low dose interferon alpha no better than placebo (RR of clearance 1.4, 95% CI 0.4–4.3)	[404]
41 women and 1 man aged 16 to 65 treated at a clinic in North Carolina	6 to 9 injections of interferon alpha-2b or placebo over a period of up to 29 days	Trend towards greater efficacy with interferon than placebo after 1 month (RR of clearance 3.0, 95% CI 0.9–10.0)	[405]

found no benefit with more frequent applications, and identified an increase in the incidence of adverse events [300].

Cryotherapy is commonly used for the treatment of genital warts, but has not been evaluated in placebo-controlled trials. This modality was superior to podophyllin in a randomized trial (RR of clearance 3.2; 95% CI 1.7–6.1), although this trial had high rates of loss to follow-up [301]. More prolonged application of liquid nitrogen (~10 s) increased the probability of wart clearance, but was associated with an increased risk of pain during treatment in a randomized trial (RR of clearance 1.7, 95% CI 1.2–2.4; RR of pain 2.3, 95% CI 1.4–3.9) [302].

Two randomized trials have compared the efficacy of cryotherapy to trichloroacetic acid (TCAA), with no significant difference seen in rates of clearance (pooled RR for wart clearance with cryotherapy 1.0, 95% CI 0.7–1.4) [303,304]. However, cryotherapy may also be less likely to cause genital ulceration than TCAA (OR of ulceration with cryotherapy 0, 95% CI 0–0.3) [304].

No placebo-controlled trials of surgical modalities for genital wart treatment have been performed to date. Randomized trials comparing laser surgery with conventional scissors excision, and electrocautery with cryotherapy, have failed to find any difference between modalities in terms of efficacy [305,306]. However, scissors excision of perianal warts was superior to podophyllin application both in initial wart clearance and in subsequent recurrence rates (RR of recurrence after scissors excision 0.3, 95% CI 0.2–0.7) [307].

Topical, intralesional and systemic interferon preparations have been evaluated for the treatment of genital warts. Both topical and intralesional interferon are more efficacious than placebo in the eradication of genital warts (Table 10.8). Topical interferon-alpha was more efficacious than podophyllotoxin in two randomized trials (pooled RR of clearance with interferon-alpha 1.6, 95% CI 1.2–2.1) [308,309]. A randomized trial comparing podophyllin plus intralesional interferon-alpha to podophyllin alone found a higher rate of wart clearance with interferon, but a high rate of relapse was seen in both treatment groups, and intralesional interferon was associated with adverse effects including fever, myalgia, gastrointestinal distress, and headache [310]. Although systemic interferons have been more efficacious than placebo in the clearance of genital warts, the addition of systemic interferon to such standard therapies as cryotherapy or podophyllin has been no more efficacious than standard therapies alone [311–316]. Further, the expense and potential toxicity of systemic interferon limits its practical value in most clinical situations.

Treatment of genital warts in immunocompromised individuals, including those with HIV infection, may be particularly challenging. A randomized trial comparing imiquimod 5% to placebo in individuals with HIV infection and CD4+ T-lymphocyte counts <100 cells/mL found no difference between the two arms in rates of wart clearance [317]. Cidofovir 1% gel may be a useful therapeutic option in HIV-infected individuals; a small randomized trial found higher rates of clearance with cidofovir (9/19 individuals) than with placebo (0/9 individuals, $P = 0.006$). A second randomized trial found the combination of cidofovir 1% gel and scissors excision to be more efficacious than either scissors excision or cidofovir gel alone in a population of individuals with HIV infection [318].

Patient factors other than immunocompromise may influence clearance of genital warts. An observational study carried out on individuals with genital warts in Leeds, UK, found increasing wart numbers associated with decreased clearance in response to therapy (hazard ratio for every 2-fold increase in wart numbers 0.70, 95% CI 0.45–0.86). Smoking was evaluated as a possible predictor of persistence in this study, and was not found to be predictive of wart persistence [319].

Treatment of trichomoniasis

Metronidazole appears to be a highly effective agent for the treatment of vaginal trichomoniasis. Double-blind randomized controlled trials have found no significant difference in efficacy between a single 2 g dose of metronidazole and 5- to 7-day courses of the drug dosed at 750–800 mg per day. Both regimens appear to result in parasitologic cure in over 85% of individuals [320,321]. Single-dose metronidazole for the treatment of trichomoniasis appears less efficacious if the drug is given as a single 1 g dose, although a single 1.5 g dose may be equivalent to a 2 g dose [297,298]. A single 2 g dose of tinidazole is equivalent in efficacy to 2 g of metronidazole for the treatment of vaginal trichomoniasis [322,323]. Tinidazole appears to be efficacious in individuals with prior failure of therapy associated with metronidazole-resistant trichomonads, and eradicated infection in 22 of 24 women who had previously failed therapy with metronidazole for trichomonal vaginitis [324].

Topical therapies for trichomoniasis have been disappointing to date. A multicenter, open-label randomized trial comparing single-dose oral metronidazole to intravaginal clotrimazole or sulfanilamide-allantoin-aminacrine hydrochloride suppositories found metronidazole to be curative in 34/45 of subjects, while suppositories were associated with microbiologic failure in over 80% of participants [325]. Intravaginal 0.75% metronidazole gel was significantly less efficacious than oral metronidazole in a small randomized trial (RR of cure with gel 0.4, 95% CI 0.3–0.8) [326]. Topical nonoxynol-9 was ineffective in the treatment of vaginal trichomoniasis [327].

The association between asymptomatic carriage of *T. vaginalis* and preterm delivery led investigators to hypothesize that screening for and treating subclinical infections in pregnancy could reduce the risk of preterm delivery. However, in a randomized placebo-controlled trial, the incidence of preterm delivery was significantly higher in women treated with metronidazole than among those treated with placebo (RR 3.0, 95% CI 1.5–5.9). Screening for trichomoniasis in asymptomatic pregnant women cannot be recommended at this time [20].

Treatment of partners for prevention of reinfection

The importance of treating sex partners for the prevention of repeated infection has been demonstrated for several curable sexually transmitted infections, including trichomonal vaginitis, genital chlamydia, and gonorrheal infection in women. In a study in which partners of women with trichomoniasis were randomized to receive either tinidazole or placebo, reinfection was strongly associated with the receipt of placebo (RR 4.7, 95% CI 1.3–25.3) [328]. Additionally, analysis of data from a randomized controlled trial of a behavioral intervention in women with a baseline sexually transmitted infection found reinfection with gonorrhea or chlamydia to be strongly associated with sex with a partner who was not adequately treated (OR 5.6, 95% CI 3.0–10.5) [329].

Patient delivery of medications to sex partners might help ensure partner treatment. Non-randomized studies have found lower rates of reinfection with chlamydia in women who delivered medications to their partners [330,331], and these findings have now been replicated in randomized controlled trials. A trial conducted in Seattle found that expedited delivery of therapy to sex partners reduced the risk of persistent or recurrent *Chlamydia* infection or gonorrhea in women and heterosexual men (RR for reinfection 0.75, 95% CI 0.57–0.97) [332]. A study restricted to men with urethritis found an even stronger protection against persistent infection with patient-delivered partner therapy (adjusted OR 0.38, 95% CI 0.19–0.74) [333]. A third trial restricted to women with *Chlamydia* cervicitis failed to find significant protection, but this may have been due to inadequate statistical power (OR of reinfection 0.80, 95% CI 0.62–1.05) [330].

Strategies for control of STI in the community

Vaccination

The past 5 years have witnessed a remarkable change in the extent to which vaccination is regarded as a mainstay of STI prevention strategies. While vaccination as a strategy for the prevention of bacterial STI has been unsuccessful to date, conjugate virus-like particle (VLP) vaccines against both oncogenic and wart-associated strains of human papillomaviruses (HPV 16 and 18, and HPV 6 and 11, respectively) are now in clinical use in many countries. In published randomized, placebo-controlled trials, these vaccines have been highly immunogenic (Fig. 10.4) [334–336], extremely effective at preventing acquisition of vaccine HPV strains by sexually active women [337–339], and have consistently been shown to reduce the risk of HPV-associated cervical dysplasia by >90% [338,340,341]. These vaccines are likely to reduce the risk of both future cervical cancer, and (not insignificantly) invasive follow-up testing for women with abnormal Papanicolau smears. Furthermore, in randomized trials, these vaccines prevent vulvar, vaginal, and perianal HPV-related lesions and neoplasia [342,343]. Unfortunately, effectiveness is limited to women without preexisting HPV infection [344], necessitating vaccination before or shortly after initiation of coitarche.

Although VLP HPV vaccines are associated with a risk of anaphylaxis higher than other conjugate vaccines, severe adverse events are rare (true anaphylaxis

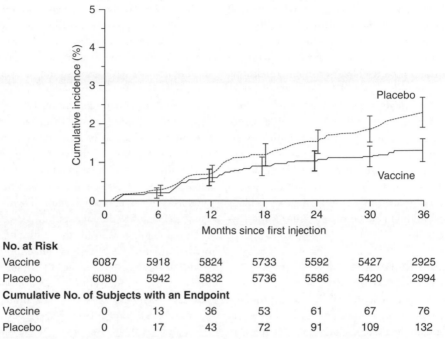

No. at Risk							
Vaccine	6087	5918	5824	5733	5592	5427	2925
Placebo	6080	5942	5832	5736	5586	5420	2994
Cumulative No. of Subjects with an Endpoint							
Vaccine	0	13	36	53	61	67	76
Placebo	0	17	43	72	91	109	132

Figure 10.4 Effectiveness of a 4-valent virus-like particle human papillomavirus (HPV) vaccine against development of HPV-associated cervical intraepithelial neoplasia. In the intention-to-treat analysis depicted here, women were analyzed according to randomization, regardless of whether or not they had prevalent vaccine-strain HPV infection at the time of vaccination or whether they received vaccination. The overall risk reduction for cervical lesions associated with any HPV type was 20% (95% CI 8–31%) in the intention-to-treat analysis. Vaccination was also associated with a 34% (95% CI 15–49%) reduction in anogenital HPV lesions of any viral type in intention-to-treat analyses. Reproduced from reference [340]: Quadrivalent vaccine against human papillomavirus to prevent high-grade cervical lesions. N Engl J Med 2007;356:1915–27, © 2007 Massachusetts Medical Society. All rights reserved.

occurs in approximate 2.6 per 100 000 vaccinations, 95% CI 1.0–5.3) [344]. Given the long latency of cervical cancer following HPV infection, data proving reductions in cervical cancer incidence as a result of vaccination, and trials of vaccine effectiveness in males, are still pending. However, a mathematical model synthesizing the best available data suggests that HPV vaccination is likely to be highly cost-effective relative to currently available health interventions; furthermore, cost-effectiveness would be enhanced by considering noncervical cancers prevented by these vaccines, and by modifying existing cervical screening regimens to account for the additional protection they provide[345].

A novel glycoprotein-conjugate vaccine may be efficacious for the prevention of genital herpes in women without prior serologic evidence of either HSV-1 or HSV-2 (RR 0.26, 95% CI 0.09–0.93), but has not been

shown to be effective in men [346]. Effective vaccines are also available for hepatitis A and B virus infections, which may be sexually transmitted [347–351]. A single small randomized, placebo-controlled trial failed to identify protection associated with postexposure vaccination for sex partners of individuals with acute hepatitis B infection [352].

Population-based screening programs

Screening and use of curative or suppressive antibacterial and antiviral agents may provide an effective means of disrupting disease transmission, particularly if infections are asymptomatic or unrecognized in the absence of therapy. In nonpregnant populations, limited evidence exists to guide policy related to population-based screening for most pathogens. An exception is *C. trachomatis*, which is likely to be markedly underdiagnosed if testing is limited to those with symptoms [353,354]. A randomized controlled trial of screening for genital chlamydia infection in women enrolled in a Washington State health maintenance organization found a significant reduction in the incidence of PID after 1 year of follow-up among screened women (RR 0.44, 95% CI 0.20–0.90) [355]. Screening for chlamydia has been suggested to be a cost-saving health intervention in high-prevalence populations [356], but a recent systematic review found numerous limitations in health economic evaluations of chlamydia screening [357]. Mathematical models that account for transmissibility do suggest that inclusion of males in screening programs is likely to provide additional gains in women's health at reasonable cost [358].

Mass antibiotic treatment in high-risk populations and outbreaks

Mass antibiotic treatment for STI has been proposed for outbreak control, prevention of HIV acquisition in high-risk populations, and for prevention of sequelae in pregnant women at increased risk of STI. Good evidence exists to support the use of such treatment in the latter population; in two randomized, placebo-controlled trials conducted in Kenya, the empiric administration of third-generation cephalosporins to women at 28–32 weeks of gestation found a reduced risk of stillbirth (pooled RR 0.54, 95% CI 0.36–0.81) and postpartum endometritis (pooled RR 0.50, 95% CI 0.31–0.81) [359,360]; and in a subgroup analysis restricted to pregnant women participating in the "Rakai study" (described below), empiric STI therapy was associated with a significant reduction in neonatal death (RR 0.83, 95% CI 0.71–0.97), as well as low birthweight, ophthalmia neonatorum, and maternal carriage of *T. vaginalis*, gonococcus, and *C. trachomatis* [361].

However, the primary endpoint in the Rakai study was prevention of HIV infection through treatment of non-HIV STI. This cluster-randomized controlled trial, in the Rakai district of Uganda, applied community-wide antibiotic treatment in an effort to slow HIV transmission. No impact was seen on HIV infection, but this trial did document significant reductions in syphilis (RR 0.8, 95% CI 0.7–0.9%) and trichomoniasis (RR 0.6, 95% CI 0.4–0.9%) in communities that received mass antibiotic therapy. Similar results were found in a randomized controlled trial of monthly azithromycin prophylaxis among HIV-seronegative

female sex workers in Nairobi, Kenya: significant reductions in syphilis, gonorrhea and trichomoniaisis occurred without reduction in HIV risk [362]. The modest effect of these interventions and the potential impact of such a strategy on local antimicrobial susceptibility patterns argue against the use of such a strategy for primary control of STI other than HIV [179]. Indeed, other efforts to apply mass antibiotic therapy for reduction of STI risk have shown limited short-term effects, with rebound to baseline levels following discontinuation of mass therapy for gonorrhea [363], or in the case of mass antibiotic therapy for syphilis control, rebound in rates to levels higher than those seen prior to the intervention [364].

One possible reason for the failure of mass antibiotic treatment to reduce HIV infection in the Rakai study was suggested to be the high background prevalence of genital HSV-2 infection (which would not have been controlled by the antimicrobial agents administered) [365]. However, recent randomized trials that evaluated suppressive acyclovir therapy for HSV-2 seropositive African women [366,367], and men who have sex with men in the US and Peru [366], found no protective effect against HIV acquisition associated with anti-herpes therapy (pooled HR 1.14, 95% CI 0.86–1.51) [366,367].

Counseling and behavioral interventions

Several randomized controlled trials have evaluated behavioral interventions targeting groups perceived to be at increased risk of acquiring STI [368]. A recent systematic review identified marked between-study heterogeneity with respect to populations, interventions, and estimated effectiveness. However, behavioral and counseling interventions that are more extensive (e.g., multiple sessions, incorporate multiple modalities) do appear to have a moderate effect in reducing STI risk in adults and adolescents, with no increase in sexual risk-taking noted as a result of counseling [368]. For example, in one multicenter trial (Project RESPECT) conducted in publicly funded clinics in five US cities, evaluated changes in behavior and incidence of infection in individuals receiving a brief didactic message, brief counseling, or extended counseling. Both brief and extended counseling reduced the risk of laboratory-confirmed sexually transmitted infection at 6 months (RR for brief intervention 0.7, 95% CI 0.6–0.9, RR for enhanced intervention 0.7; 95% CI

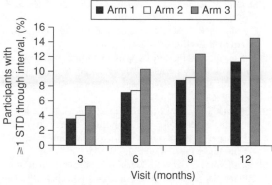

Figure 10.5 Effectiveness of clinic-based counseling interventions in the prevention of sexually transmitted infections. Clinic attendees enrolled in a multicenter trial were randomized to receive four interactive counseling sessions (Arm 1), two interactive counseling sessions (Arm 2), or didactic message on sexually transmitted infection risk-reduction (Arm 3). Reductions in sexually transmitted infection risk were seen with both counseling interventions, and persisted 12 months after initial counseling ($P = 0.008$). Reproduced from reference [369]: Kamb ML, et al. Efficacy of risk reduction counseling to prevent human immunodeficiency virus and sexually transmitted diseases: a randomized controlled trial. Project RESPECT Study Group. JAMA 1998;280(13):1165. Copyright © 1998, American Medical Association. All rights reserved.

0.5–0.9); a transient increase in condom use was also seen (Fig. 10.5). However, these effects diminished over time [369].

References

1 1998/1999 Canadian Sexually Transmitted Diseases (STD) Surveillance Report. Can Commun Dis Rep 26S6. 2000.

2 Centers for Disease Control and Prevention. Sexually Transmitted Disease Surveillance, 2000, 2001. Atlanta, GA, US Department of Health and Human Services.

3 Fleming D, McQuillan G, Nahmias A, Aral S, Lee F, St Louis M. Herpes simplex virus type 2 in the United States, 1976 to 1994. N Engl J Med 1997;337:1105–11.

4 Wikstrom A, Popescu C, Forslund O. Asymptomatic penile HPV infection: a prospective study. Int J STD AIDS 2000;11:80–4.

5 Winer RL, Lee SK, Hughes JP, Adam DE, Kiviat NB, Koutsky LA. Genital human papillomavirus infection: incidence and risk factors in a cohort of female university students. Am J Epidemiol 2003;157:218–26.

6 Woodman CB, Collins S, Winter H, Bailey A, Ellis J, Prior P, et al. Natural history of cervical human papillomavirus infection in young women: a longitudinal cohort study. Lancet 2001;357:1831–6.

7 Gerbase A, Rowley J, Heymann D, Berkley S, Piot P. Global prevalence and incidence estimates of selected curable STDs. Sex Transm Infect 1998;74(Suppl 1):S12–S16.

8 Szucs T, Berger K, Fisman D, Harbarth S. The estimated economic burden of genital herpes in the United States: an analysis using two costing approaches. BMC Infect Dis 2001;1:5.

9 Washington A, Johnson R, Sanders L. Chlamydia trachomatis infections in the United States: what are they costing us? JAMA 1987;257:2070–2.

10 Washington A, Katz P. Cost of and payment source for pelvic inflammatory disease: trends and projections, 1983 through 2000. JAMA 1991;266:2565–9.

11 Siegel J. The economic burden of sexually transmitted diseases in the United States. In Holmes K, Sparling P, Mardh P, Lemon S, Stamm W, Piot P et al, eds. Sexually Transmitted Diseases, pp 1367–79. New York: McGraw Hill, 1999.

12 Rottingen J, Cameron D, Garnett G. A systematic review of the epidemiologic interactions between classic sexually transmitted diseases and HIV. Sex Transm Dis 2001;28:579–97.

13 World Health Organization Task Force on the Prevention and Management of Infertility. Tubal infertility: serologic relationship to past chlamydial and gonococcal infection. Sex Transm Dis 1995;22:71–7.

14 Coste J, Laumon B, Bremond A, Collet P, Job-Spira N. Sexually transmitted diseases as major causes of ectopic pregnancy: results from a large case-control study in France. Fertil Steril 1994;62:289–95.

15 Ankum W, Mol B, Van der Veer F, Bossuyt P. Risk factors for ectopic pregnancy: a meta-analysis. Fertil Steril 1996;65:1093–9.

16 Stacey CM, Munday PE, Taylor-Robinson D, et al. A longitudinal study of pelvic inflammatory disease. Br J Obstet Gynaecol 1992;99:994–9.

17 Safrin S, Schachter J, Dahrouge D, Sweet RL. Long-term sequelae of acute pelvic inflammatory disease. A retrospective cohort study. Am J Obstet Gynecol 1992;166:1300–5.

18 Mitchell H, Drake M, Medley G. Prospective evaluation of risk of cervical cancer after cytological evidence of human papilloma virus infection. Lancet 1986;1:573–5.

19 Palefsky JM, Holly EA, Ralston ML, Arthur SP, Hogeboom CJ, Darragh TM. Anal cytological abnormalities and anal HPV infection in men with Centers for Disease Control group IV HIV disease. Genitourin Med 1997;73:174–80.

20 Klebanoff MA, Carey JC, Hauth JC, et al. Failure of metronidazole to prevent preterm delivery among pregnant women with asymptomatic Trichomonas vaginalis infection. N Engl J Med 2001;345:487–93.

21 Sliverman N, Sullivan M, Hochman M, Womack M, Jugnkind D. A randomized, prospective trial comparing amoxicillin and erythromycin for the treatment of

Chlamydia trachomatis in pregnancy. Am J Obstet Gynecol 1994;170:829–32.

22 Cohen I, Veille JC, Calkins BM. Improved pregnancy outcome following successful treatment of chlamydial infection. JAMA 1990;263:3160–3.

23 Temmerman M, Gichangi P, Fonck K, et al. Effect of a syphilis control programme on pregnancy outcome in Nairobi, Kenya. Sex Transm Infect 2000;76:117–21.

24 Rotchford K, Lombard C, Zuma K, Wilkinson D. Impact on perinatal mortality of missed opportunities to treat maternal syphilis in rural South Africa: baseline results from a clinic randomized controlled trial. Trop Med Int Health 2000;5:800–4.

25 Brown ZA, Wald A, Morrow RA, Selke S, Zeh J, Corey L. Effect of serologic status and cesarean delivery on transmission rates of herpes simplex virus from mother to infant. JAMA 2003;289:203–9.

26 DiCarlo R, Martin D. The clinical diagnosis of genital ulcer disease in men. Clin Infect Dis 1997;25:292–8.

27 Behets F, Andriamiadana J, Randrianasolo D, et al. Chancroid, primary syphilis, genital herpes and lymphogranuloma venereum in Antananarivo, Madagascar. J Infect Dis 1999;180:1382–5.

28 Risbud A, Chan-Tack K, Gadkari D, et al. The etiology of genital ulcer disease by multiplex polymerase chain reaction and relationship to HIV infection among patients attending sexually transmitted disease clinics in Pune, India. Sex Transm Dis 1998;26:55–62.

29 Behets F, Braitwaith A, Hylton-Kong T, et al. Genital ulcers: etiology, clinical diagnosis, and associated human immunodeficiency virus infection in Kingston, Jamaica. Clin Infect Dis 1999;28:1086–90.

30 Bornstein J, Lakovsky Y, Lavi I, Bar-Am A, Abramovici H. The classic approach to diagnosis of vulvovaginitis: a critical approach. Infect Dis Obstet Gynecol 2001;9:105–11.

31 World Health Organization. Report of a WHO Study Group: management of patients with sexually transmitted diseases. 810. 1991. Geneva, WHO. WHO Technical Reports Series.

32 Dallabetta G, Gerbase A, Holmes K. Problems, solutions, and challenges in syndromic management of sexually transmitted diseases. Sex Transm Infect 1998;74(Suppl 1): S1–S11.

33 Pettifor A, Walsh J, Wilkins V, Raghunathan P. How effective is syndromic management of STDs? A review of current studies. Sex Transm Dis 2000;27:371–85.

34 Moore SG, Miller WC, Hoffman IF, et al. Clinical utility of measuring white blood cells on vaginal wet mount and endocervical gram stain for the prediction of chlamydial and gonococcal infections. Sex Transm Dis 2000;27:530–8.

35 Myziuk L, Romanowski B, Brown M. Endocervical Gram stain smears and their usefulness in the diagnosis of *Chlamydia trachomatis*. Sex Transm Infect 2001;77:103–6.

36 Sellors J, Howard M, Pickard L, Jang D, Mahony J, Chernesky M. Chlamydial cervicitis: testing the practice guidelines for presumptive diagnosis. CMAJ 1998;158: 41–6.

37 Stamm W, Koutsky L, Benedetti J, Jourden J, Holmes K. *Chlamydia trachomatis* urethral infections in men. Prevalence, risk factors, and clinical manifestations. Ann Intern Med 1984;100:47–51.

38 Juchau SV, Nackman R, Ruppart D. Comparison of Gram stain with DNA probe for detection of *Neisseria gonorrhoeae* in urethras of symptomatic males. J Clin Microbiol 1995;33:3068–9.

39 Moherdaui F, Vuylsteke B, Siqueira LF, et al. Validation of national algorithms for the diagnosis of sexually transmitted diseases in Brazil: results from a multicentre study. Sex Transm Infect 1998;74 Suppl 1:S38–S43.

40 Chandeying V, Skov S, Tabrizi SN, Kemapunmanus M, Garland S. Can a two-glass urine test or leucocyte esterase test of first-void urine improve syndromic management of male urethritis in southern Thailand? Int J STD AIDS 2000;11:235–40.

41 Wiesenfeld H, Lowry D, Heine R, et al. Self-collection of vaginal swabs for the detection of chlamydia, gonorrhea, and trichomoniasis. Sex Transm Dis 2001;28:321–5.

42 Sellors J, Lorincz A, Mahony J, et al. Comparison of self-collected vaginal, vulvar and urine samples with physician-collected cervical samples for human papillomavirus testing to detect high-grade squamous intraepithelial lesions. CMAJ 2000;163:513–18.

43 Gaydos CA, Quinn TC, Willis D, et al. Performance of the APTIMA Combo 2 assay for detection of *Chlamydia trachomatis* and *Neisseria gonorrhoeae* in female urine and endocervical swab specimens. J Clin Microbiol 2003; 41:304–9.

44 Hadgu A. Bias in the evaluation of DNA-amplification tests for detecting *Chlamydia trachomatis*. Stat Med 1997; 16:1391–9.

45 Baughman AL, Bisgard KM, Cortese MM, Thompson WW, Sanden GN, Strebel PM. Utility of composite reference standards and latent class analysis in evaluating the clinical accuracy of diagnostic tests for pertussis. Clin Vaccine Immunol 2008;15:106–14.

46 Van Dyck E, Ieven M, Pattyn S, Van Damme L, Laga M. Detection of *Chlamydia trachomatis* and *Neisseria gonorrhoeae* by enzyme immunoassay, culture, and three nucleic acid amplification tests. J Clin Microbiol 2001;39:1751–6.

47 Crotchfelt KA, Welsh LE, DeBonville D, Rosenstraus M, Quinn TC. Detection of *Neisseria gonorrhoeae* and *Chlamydia trachomatis* in genitourinary specimens from men and women by a coamplification PCR assay. J Clin Microbiol 1997;35:1536–40.

48 Iwen PC, Walker RA, Warren KL, Kelly DM, Linder J, Hinrichs SH. Effect of off-site transportation on detection of *Neisseria gonorrhoeae* in endocervical specimens. Arch Pathol Lab Med 1996;120:1019–22.

49 Livengood CH, III, Wrenn JW. Evaluation of COBAS AMPLICOR (Roche): accuracy in detection of *Chlamydia trachomatis* and *Neisseria gonorrhoeae* by coamplification of endocervical specimens. J Clin Microbiol 2001;39:2928–32.

50 Page-Shafer K, Graves A, Kent C, Balls JE, Zapitz VM, Klausner JD. Increased sensitivity of DNA amplification

testing for the detection of pharyngeal gonorrhea in men who have sex with men. Clin Infect Dis 2002;34:173–6.

51 Stary A, Ching SF, Teodorowicz L, Lee H. Comparison of ligase chain reaction and culture for detection of *Neisseria gonorrhoeae* in genital and extragenital specimens. J Clin Microbiol 1997;35:239–42.

52 Koumans E, Johnson R, Knapp J, St Louis M. Laboratory testing for *Neisseria gonorrhoeae* by recently introduced nonculture tests: a performance review with clinical and public health considerations. Clin Infect Dis 1998; 27:1171–80.

53 Van Der Pol B, Ferrero DV, Buck-Barrington L, et al. Multicenter evaluation of the BDProbeTec ET System for detection of *Chlamydia trachomatis* and *Neisseria gonorrhoeae* in urine specimens, female endocervical swabs, and male urethral swabs. J Clin Microbiol 2001;39:1008–16.

54 Mahony J, Luinstra KE, Tyndall M, Sellors J, Krepel J, Chernesky M. Multiplex PCR for detection of *Chlamydia trachomatis* and *Neisseria gonorrhoeae* in genitourinary specimens. J Clin Microbiol 1995;33:3049–53.

55 Martin DH, Cammarata C, Van Der Pol B, et al. Multicenter evaluation of AMPLICOR and automated COBAS AMPLICOR CT/NG tests for *Neisseria gonorrhoeae*. J Clin Microbiol 2000;38:3544–9.

56 Xu K, Glanton V, Johnson S, et al. Detection of *Neisseria gonorrhoeae* infection by ligase chain reaction testing of urine among adolescent women with and without Chlamydia trachomatis infection. Sex Transm Dis 1998; 25:533–8.

57 Schachter J, Moncada J, Liska S, Shayevich C, Klausner JD. Nucleic acid amplification tests in the diagnosis of chlamydial and gonococcal infections of the oropharynx and rectum in men who have sex with men. Sex Transm Dis 2008;35:637–42.

58 Lewis JS, Fakile O, Foss E, et al. Direct DNA probe assay for *Neisseria gonorrhoeae* in pharyngeal and rectal specimens. J Clin Microbiol 1993;31:2783–5.

59 Young H, Anderson J, Moyes A, McMillan A. Non-cultural detection of rectal and pharyngeal gonorrhoea by the Gen-Probe PACE 2 assay. Genitourin Med 1997;73:59–62.

60 Elnifro EM, Storey CC, Morris DJ, Tullo AB. Polymerase chain reaction for detection of *Chlamydia trachomatis* in conjunctival swabs. Br J Ophthalmol 1997;81:497–500.

61 Roblin PM, Hammerschlag MR, Cummings C, Williams TH, Worku M. Comparison of two rapid microscopic methods and culture for detection of *Chlamydia trachomatis* in ocular and nasopharyngeal specimens from infants. J Clin Microbiol 1989;27:968–70.

62 Chernesky MA, Martin DH, Hook EW, et al. Ability of new APTIMA CT and APTIMA GC assays to detect *Chlamydia trachomatis* and *Neisseria gonorrhoeae* in male urine and urethral swabs. J Clin. Microbiol 2005;43:127–31.

63 Van der Pol B, Quinn TC, Gaydos CA, Crotchfelt K, Schachter J, Moncada J, et al. Multicenter evaluation of the AMPLICOR and automated COBAS AMPLICOR CT/NG tests for detection of *Chlamydia trachomatis*. J.Clin. Microbiol 2000;38:1105–12.

64 Schachter J, Chernesky MA, Willis DE, et al. Vaginal swabs are the specimens of choice when screening for *Chlamydia trachomatis* and *Neisseria gonorrhoeae*: results from a multicenter evaluation of the APTIMA assays for both infections. Sex Transm Dis 2005;32:725–8.

65 Gaydos C, Crotchfelt K, Shah N, et al. Evaluation of dry and wet transported intravaginal swabs in detection of *Chlamydia trachomatis* and *Neisseria gonorrhoeae* infections in female soldiers by PCR. J Clin Microbiol 2002;40:758–61.

66 Domeika M, Bassiri M, Butrimiene I, Venalis A, Ranceva J, Vasjanova V. Evaluation of vaginal introital sampling as an alternative approach for the detection of genital *Chlamydia trachomatis* infection in women. Acta Obstet Gynecol Scand 1999;78:131–6.

67 Knox J, Tabrizi SN, Miller P, et al. Evaluation of self-collected samples in contrast to practitioner-collected samples for detection of *Chlamydia trachomatis*, *Neisseria gonorrhoeae*, and *Trichomonas vaginalis* by polymerase chain reaction among women living in remote areas. Sex Transm Dis 2002;29:647–54.

68 Quigley M, Munguti K, Grosskurth H, et al. Sexual behaviour patterns and other risk factors for HIV infection in rural Tanzania: a case-control study. AIDS 1997;11:237–48.

69 Ostergaard L, Moller J, Andersen B, Olesen F. Diagnosis of urogenital *Chlamydia trachomatis* infection in women based on mailed samples obtained at home: multipractice comparative study. BMJ 1996;313:1186–9.

70 Centers for Disease Control and Prevention 1998 Guidelines for treatment of Sexually Transmitted Diseases. MMWR Morb Mortal Wkly Rep 1998;47(RR-1):1–118.

71 Kahn J, Walker C, Washington A, Landers D, Sweet R. Diagnosing pelvic inflammatory disease: a comprehensive analysis and considerations for developing a new model. JAMA 1991;266:2594–604.

72 Jacobson L, Westrom L. Objectivized diagnosis of acute pelvic inflammatory disease: diagnostic and prognostic value of laparoscopy. Am J Obstet Gynecol 1969;105:1088–98.

73 Wasserheit J, Bell T, Kiviat N. Microbial causes of proven pelvic inflammatory disease and efficacy of clindamycin and tobramycin. Ann Intern Med 1986;104:187–93.

74 Korn AP, Hessol N, Padian N, et al. Commonly used diagnostic criteria for pelvic inflammatory disease have poor sensitivity for plasma cell endometritis. Sex Transm Dis 1995;22:335–41.

75 Peipert JF, Ness RB, Blume J, et al. Clinical predictors of endometritis in women with symptoms and signs of pelvic inflammatory disease. Am J Obstet Gynecol 2001;184:856–63.

76 Sorvillo F, Smith L, Kerndt P, Ash L. *Trichomonas vaginalis*, HIV, and African-Americans. Emerg Infect Dis 2001;7: 927–32.

77 Wiese W, Patel SR, Patel SC, Ohl CA, Estrada CA. A meta-analysis of the Papanicolaou smear and wet mount for the diagnosis of vaginal trichomoniasis. Am J Med 2000;108:301–8.

78 Patel SR, Wiese W, Patel SC, Ohl C, Byrd JC, Estrada CA. Systematic review of diagnostic tests for vaginal trichomoniasis. Infect Dis Obstet Gynecol 2000;8:248–57.

79 Kurth A, Whittington WL, Golden MR, Thomas KK, Holmes KK, Schwebke JR. Performance of a new, rapid assay for detection of *Trichomonas vaginalis*. J Clin Microbiol 2004;42:2940–3.

80 Kingston MA, Bansal D, Carlin EM. "Shelf life" of *Trichomonas vaginalis*. Int J STD AIDS 2003;14:28–9.

81 Beverly A, Venglarik M, Cotton B, Schwebke JR. Viability of *Trichomonas vaginalis* in transport medium. J Clin Microbiol 1999;37:3749–50.

82 Schwebke JR, Venglarik M, Morgan S. Delayed versus immediate bedside inoculation of culture media for diagnosis of vaginal trichomoniasis. J Clin Microbiol 1999;37:2369–70.

83 Schwebke JR. Cost-effective screening for trichomoniasis. Emerg Infect Dis 2002;8:749–50.

84 Huppert JS, Mortensen JE, Reed JL, Kahn JA, Rich KD, Miller WC et al. Rapid antigen testing compares favorably with transcription-mediated amplification assay for the detection of *Trichomonas vaginalis* in young women. Clin Infect Dis 2007;45:194–8.

85 Nsanze H, Fast M, D'Costa L, Tukei P, Curran J, Ronald A. Genital ulcers in Kenya: a clinical and laboratory study. Br J Vener Dis 1981;59:378–81.

86 Ahmed HJ, Borrelli S, Jonasson J, et al. Monoclonal antibodies against *Haemophilus ducreyi* lipooligosaccharide and their diagnostic usefulness. Eur J Clin Microbiol Infect Dis 1995;14:892–8.

87 Orle K, Gates C, Martin D, Body B, Weiss J. Simultaneous PCR detection of *Haemophilus ducreyi*, *Treponema pallidum*, and herpes simplex virus types 1 and 2 from genital ulcers. J Clin Microbiol 1996;34:49–55.

88 Malonza I, Tyndall M, Ndinya-Achola J, et al. A randomized, double-blind, placebo-controlled trial of single-dose ciprofloxacin versus erythromycin for the treatment of chancroid in Nairobi, Kenya. J Infect Dis 1999;180:1886–93.

89 Johnson SR, Martin DH, Cammarata C, Morse SA. Development of a polymerase chain reaction assay for the detection of *Haemophilus ducreyi*. Sex Transm Dis 1994;21:13–23.

90 Johnson SR, Martin DH, Cammarata C, Morse SA. Alterations in sample preparation increase sensitivity of PCR assay for diagnosis of chancroid. J Clin Microbiol 1995;33:1036–8.

91 Parsons LM, Waring AL, Otido J, Shayegani M. Laboratory diagnosis of chancroid using species-specific primers from *Haemophilus ducreyi* groEL and the polymerase chain reaction. Diagn Microbiol Infect Dis 1995;23:89–98.

92 Hawkes S, West B, Wilson S, Whittle H, Mabey D. Asymptomatic carriage of *Haemophilus ducreyi* confirmed by the polymerase chain reaction. Genitourin Med 1995;71:224–7.

93 Corey L, Handsfield HH. Genital herpes and public health: addressing a global problem. JAMA 2000;283:791–4.

94 Lowhagen GB, Tunback P, Bergstrom T. Proportion of herpes simplex virus (HSV) type 1 and type 2 among genital and extragenital HSV isolates. Acta Derm Venereol 2002;82:118–20.

95 Janier M, Scieux C, Meouchi R, et al. Virological, serological and epidemiological study of 255 consecutive cases of genital herpes in a sexually transmitted disease clinic of Paris (France): a prospective study. Int J STD AIDS 2006;17:44–9.

96 Roberts C, Pfister J, Spear S. Increasing proportion of herpes simplex virus type 1 as a cause of genital herpes infection in college students. Sex Transm Dis 2003;30:797–800.

97 Lafferty WE, Coombs RW, Benedetti J, Critchlow C, Corey L. Recurrences after oral and genital herpes simplex virus infection. Influence of site of infection and viral type. N Engl J Med 1987;316:1444–9.

98 Wald A, Zeh J, Selke S, Ashley RL, Corey L. Virologic characteristics of subclinical and symptomatic genital herpes infections. N Engl J Med 1995;333:770–5.

99 Folkers E, Oranje AP, Duivenvoorden JN, van der Veen JP, Rijlaarsdam JU, Emsbroek JA. Tzanck smear in diagnosing genital herpes. Genitourin Med 1988;64:249–54.

100 Bagg J, Mannings A, Munro J, Walker DM. Rapid diagnosis of oral herpes simplex or zoster virus infections by immunofluorescence: comparison with Tzanck cell preparations and viral culture. Br Dent J 1989;167:235–8.

101 Slomka MJ, Emery L, Munday PE, Moulsdale M, Brown DW. A comparison of PCR with virus isolation and direct antigen detection for diagnosis and typing of genital herpes. J Med Virol 1998;55:177–83.

102 Kudesia G, Van Hegan A, Wake S, Van Hegan RJ, Kinghorn GR. Comparison of cell culture with an amplified enzyme immunoassay for diagnosing genital herpes simplex infection. J Clin Pathol 1991;44:778–80.

103 Nerurkar LS, Namba M, Brashears G, Jacob AJ, Lee YJ, Sever JL. Rapid detection of herpes simplex virus in clinical specimens by use of a capture biotin-streptavidin enzyme-linked immunosorbent assay. J Clin Microbiol 1984;20:109–14.

104 Skar AG, Middeldorp J, Gundersen T, Rollag H, Degre M. Rapid diagnosis of genital herpes simplex infection by an indirect ELISA method. NIPH Ann 1988;11:59–65.

105 Chan EL, Brandt K, Horsman GB. Comparison of Chemicon SimulFluor direct fluorescent antibody staining with cell culture and shell vial direct immunoperoxidase staining for detection of herpes simplex virus and with cytospin direct immunofluorescence staining for detection of varicella-zoster virus. Clin Diagn Lab Immunol 2001;8:909–12.

106 Lafferty WE, Krofft S, Remington M, et al. Diagnosis of herpes simplex virus by direct immunofluorescence and viral isolation from samples of external genital lesions in a high-prevalence population. J Clin Microbiol 1987;25:323–6.

107 Scoular A, Gillespie G, Carman WF. Polymerase chain reaction for diagnosis of genital herpes in a genitourinary medicine clinic. Sex Transm Infect 2002;78:21–5.

108 Marshall DS, Linfert DR, Draghi A, McCarter YS, Tsongalis GJ. Identification of herpes simplex virus genital infection: comparison of a multiplex PCR assay and traditional viral isolation techniques. Mod Pathol 2001;14:152–6.

109 Wald A, Huang ML, Carrell D, Selke S, Corey L. Polymerase chain reaction for detection of herpes simplex virus (HSV) DNA on mucosal surfaces: comparison with HSV isolation in cell culture. J Infect Dis 2003;188:1345–51.

110 Ashley R, Cent A, Maggs V, Nahmias A, Corey L. Inability of enzyme immunoassays to discriminate between infections with herpes simplex virus types 1 and 2. Ann Intern Med 1991;115:520–6.

111 Ashley RL, Militoni J, Lee F, Nahmias A, Corey L. Comparison of Western blot (immunoblot) and glycoprotein G-specific immunodot enzyme assay for detecting antibodies to herpes simplex virus types 1 and 2 in human sera. J Clin Microbiol 1988;26:662–7.

112 Langenberg AG, Corey L, Ashley RL, Leong WP, Straus SE. A prospective study of new infections with herpes simplex virus type 1 and type 2. Chiron HSV Vaccine Study Group. N Engl J Med 1999;341:1432–8.

113 Wald A, Ashley-Morrow R. Serological testing for herpes simplex virus (HSV)-1 and HSV-2 infection. Clin Infect Dis 2002;35:S173–S182.

114 Scoular A. Using the evidence base on genital herpes: optimising the use of diagnostic tests and information provision. Sex Transm Infect 2002;78:160–5.

115 Workowski KA, Berman SM. Sexually transmitted diseases treatment guidelines, 2006. MMWR Recomm Rep 2006;55:1–94.

116 Fisman DN, Hook EW, III, Goldie SJ. Estimating the costs and benefits of screening monogamous, heterosexual couples for unrecognised infection with herpes simplex virus type 2. Sex Transm Infect 2003;79:45–52.

117 Lipsitch M, Davis G, Corey L. Potential benefits of a serodiagnostic test for herpes simplex virus type 1 (HSV-1) to prevent neonatal HSV-1 infection. Sex Transm Dis 2002;29:399–405.

118 Barnabas RV, Carabin H, Garnett GP. The potential role of suppressive therapy for sex partners in the prevention of neonatal herpes: a health economic analysis. Sex Transm Infect 2002;78:425–9.

119 Cummings MC, Lukehart SA, Marra C, et al. Comparison of methods for the detection of Treponema pallidum in lesions of early syphilis. Sex Transm Dis 1996;23:366–9.

120 Daniels K, Ferneyhough H. Specific direct fluorescent antibody detection of Treponema pallidum. Health Lab Sci 1977;14:164–71.

121 Romanowski B, Forsey E, Prasad E, Lukehart S, Tam M, Hook EW. Detection of Treponema pallidum by a fluorescent monoclonal antibody test. Sex Transm Dis 1987;22:156–9.

122 Larsen SA, Steiner BM, Rudolph AH. Laboratory diagnosis and interpretation of tests for syphilis. Clin Microbiol Rev 1995;8:1–21.

123 Hart G. Syphilis tests in diagnostic and therapeutic decision making. Ann Intern Med 1986;104:368–76.

124 Spangler A, Jackson J, Fiumara N, Warthin T. Syphilis with a negative blood test reaction. JAMA 1964;189:87–90.

125 Larsen S, Johnson R. Diagnostic tests. In Larsen S, Pope V, Johnson R, Kennedy E, eds. A Manual of Tests for Syphilis, pp 1–52. Washington, DC: American Public Health Association, 1998.

126 Haas JS, Bolan G, Larsen SA, Clement MJ, Bacchetti P, Moss AR. Sensitivity of treponemal tests for detecting prior treated syphilis during human immunodeficiency virus infection. J Infect Dis 1990;162:862–6.

127 Hook EW, III, Marra CM. Acquired syphilis in adults. N Engl J Med 1992;326:1060–9.

128 Joyanes P, Borborio M, Arquez J, Perea E. The association of false-positive rapid plasma reagin results and HIV infection. Sex Transm Dis 1998;25:569–71.

129 Romanowski B, Sutherland R, Fick GH, Mooney D, Love EJ. Serologic response to treatment of infectious syphilis. Ann Intern Med 1991;114:1005–9.

130 Castro R, Prieto E, Santo I, Azevedo J, Exposto F. Evaluation of an enzyme immunoassay technique for detection of antibodies against Treponema pallidum. J Clin Microbiol 2003;41:250–3.

131 Schmidt BL, Edjlalipour M, Luger A. Comparative evaluation of nine different enzyme-linked immunosorbent assays for determination of antibodies against Treponema pallidum in patients with primary syphilis. J Clin Microbiol 2000;38:1279–82.

132 Egglestone SI, Turner AJ. Serological diagnosis of syphilis. PHLS Syphilis Serology Working Group. Commun Dis Public Health 2000;3:158–62.

133 Mabey D, Peeling RW, Ballard R, et al. Prospective, multicentre clinic-based evaluation of four rapid diagnostic tests for syphilis. Sex Transm Infect 2006;82 Suppl 5: v13–v16.

134 Campos PE, Buffardi AL, Chiappe M, et al. Utility of the Determine Syphilis TP rapid test in commercial sex venues in Peru. Sex Transm Infect 2006;82 Suppl 5:v22–v25.

135 Blandford JM, Gift TL, Vasaikar S, Mwesigwa-Kayongo D, Dlali P, Bronzan RN. Cost-effectiveness of on-site antenatal screening to prevent congenital syphilis in rural eastern Cape Province, Republic of South Africa. Sex Transm Dis 2007;34:S61–S66.

136 Davis LE, Schmitt JW. Clinical significance of cerebrospinal fluid tests for neurosyphilis. Ann Neurol 1989;25:50–5.

137 Luger A, Schmidt BL, Steyrer K, Schonwald E. Diagnosis of neurosyphilis by examination of the cerebrospinal fluid. Br J Vener Dis 1981;57:232–7.

138 Tomberlin MG, Holtom PD, Owens JL, Larsen RA. Evaluation of neurosyphilis in human immunodeficiency virus-infected individuals. Clin Infect Dis 1994;18:288–94.

139 Marra CM, Gary DW, Kuypers J, Jacobson MA. Diagnosis of neurosyphilis in patients infected with human immunodeficiency virus type 1. J Infect Dis 1996;174:219–21.

140 Noordhoek GT, Wolters EC, de Jonge ME, van Embden JD. Detection by polymerase chain reaction of Treponema pallidum DNA in cerebrospinal fluid from neurosyphilis patients before and after antibiotic treatment. J Clin Microbiol 1991;29:1976–84.

141 Michelow IC, Wendel GD, Jr., Norgard MV, et al. Central nervous system infection in congenital syphilis. N Engl J Med 2002;346:1792–8.

142 Young R, Jolley D, Marks R. Comparison of the use of standardized diagnostic criteria and intuitive clinical diagnosis in the diagnosis of common viral warts (verrucae vulgaris). Arch Dermatol 1998;134:1586–9.

143 Jonsson M, Karlsson R, Evander M, Gustavsson A, Rylander E, Wadell G. Acetowhitening of the cervix and vulva as a predictor of subclinical human papillomavirus infection: sensitivity and specificity in a population-based study. Obstet Gynecol 1997;90:744–7.

144 Wikstrom A, Hedblad M, Johansson B, et al. The acetic acid test in evaluation of subclinical genital papillomavirus infection: a comparative study on penoscopy, histopathology, virology, and scanning electron microscopy findings. Genitourin Med 1992;68:90–9.

145 Kumar B, Gupta S. The acetowhite test in genital human papillomavirus infection in men: what does it add? J Eur Acad Dermatol Venereol 2001;15:27–9.

146 Manos MM, Kinney WK, Hurley LB, et al. Identifying women with cervical neoplasia: using human papillomavirus DNA testing for equivocal Papanicolaou results. JAMA 1999;281:1605–10.

147 Kuhn L, Denny L, Pollack A, Lorincz A, Richart RM, Wright TC. Human papillomavirus DNA testing for cervical cancer screening in low-resource settings. J Natl Cancer Inst 2000;92:818–25.

148 Results of a randomized trial on the management of cytology interpretations of atypical squamous cells of undetermined significance. Am J Obstet Gynecol 2003;188:1383–92.

149 Kim J, Wright T, Goldie S. Cost-effectiveness of alternative triage strategies for atypical squamous cells of undetermined significance. JAMA 2002;287:2382–90.

150 Goldie SJ, Weinstein MC, Kuntz KM, Freedberg KA. The costs, clinical benefits, and cost-effectiveness of screening for cervical cancer in HIV-infected women. Ann Intern Med 1999;130:97–107.

151 Goldie SJ, Kuhn L, Denny L, Pollack A, Wright TC. Policy analysis of cervical cancer screening strategies in low-resource settings: clinical benefits and cost-effectiveness. JAMA 2001;285:3107–15.

152 Burd EM. Human papillomavirus and cervical cancer. Clin Microbiol Rev 2003;16:1–17.

153 Ahmed S, Lutaloa T, Wawer M, et al. HIV incidence and sexually transmitted disease prevalence associated with condom use: a population study in Rakai, Uganda. AIDS 2002;15:2171–9.

154 Baeten J, Nyange P, Richardson B, et al. Hormonal contraception and risk of sexually transmitted disease acquisition: results from a prospective study. Am J Obstet Gynecol 2002;185:380–5.

155 Hooper R. Cohort study of venereal disease. I: The risk of gonorrhea transmission from infected women to men. Am J Epidemiol 1978;108:136–44.

156 Wald A, Langenberg A, Link K, et al. Effect of condoms on reducing the transmission of herpes simplex virus type 2 from men to women. JAMA 2001;285:3100–6.

157 Wald A, Langenberg AG, Krantz E, et al. The relationship between condom use and herpes simplex virus acquisition. Ann Intern Med 2005;143:707–13.

158 Manhart LE, Koutsky LA. Do condoms prevent genital HPV infection, external genital warts, or cervical neoplasia? A meta-analysis. Sex Transm Dis 2002;29:725–35.

159 Winer RL, Hughes JP, Feng Q, et al. Condom use and the risk of genital human papillomavirus infection in young women. N Engl J Med 2006;354:2645–54.

160 Hernandez BY, Wilkens LR, Zhu X, et al. Transmission of human papillomavirus in heterosexual couples. Emerg Infect Dis 2008;14:888–94.

161 Niruthisard S, Roddy R, Chutivongse S. Use of nonoxynol-9 and reduction in rate of gonococcal and chlamydial cervical infections. Lancet 1992;339:1371–5.

162 Louv W, Austin H, Alexander W, Stagno S, Cheeks J. A clinical trail of nonoxynol-9 for preventing gonococcal and chlamydial infections. J Infect Dis 1988;158:518–23.

163 Kreiss J, Ngugi E, Holmes K, et al. Efficacy of nonoxynol 9 contraceptive sponge use in preventing heterosexual acquisition of HIV in Nairobi prostitutes. JAMA 1992;268:477–82.

164 Richardson B, Lavreys L, Martin H, et al. Evaluation of a low-dose nonoxynol-9 gel for the prevention of sexually transmitted diseases. Sex Transm Dis 2001;28:394–400.

165 Roddy R, Zekeng L, Ryan K, Tamoufe U, Tweedy K. Effect of nonoxynol-9 on urogenital gonorrhea and chlamydia infection: a randomized controlled trial. JAMA 2002;287:1117–22.

166 Roddy R, Zekeng L, Ryan K, Tamoufe U, Weir S, Wong E. A controlled trial of nonoxynol 9 film to reduce male-to-female transmission of sexually transmitted diseases. N Engl J Med 1998;339:504–10.

167 Burkman RT. Association between intrauterine device and pelvic inflammatory disease. Obstet Gynecol 1981;57:269–76.

168 Grimes DA. Intrauterine device and upper-genital-tract infection. Lancet 2000;356:1013–19.

169 Lee NC, Rubin GL, Ory HW, Burkman RT. Type of intrauterine device and the risk of pelvic inflammatory disease. Obstet Gynecol 1983;62:1–6.

170 Farley T, Rosenberg M, Rowe P, Chen J, Meirik O. Intrauterine devices and pelvic inflammatory disease: an international perspective. Lancet 1992;339:785–8.

171 Kronmal RA, Whitney CW, Mumford SD. The intrauterine device and pelvic inflammatory disease: the Women's Health Study reanalyzed. J Clin Epidemiol 1991;44:109–22.

172 Gareen IF, Greenland S, Morgenstern H. Intrauterine devices and pelvic inflammatory disease: meta-analyses of published studies, 1974–1990. Epidemiology 2000;11:589–97.

173 Hubacher D, Lara-Ricalde R, Taylor DJ, Guerra-Infante F, Guzman-Rodriguez R. Use of copper intrauterine devices

and the risk of tubal infertility among nulligravid women. N Engl J Med 2001;345:561–7.

174 Kimani J, Maclean IW, Bwayo JJ, et al. Risk factors for *Chlamydia trachomatis* pelvic inflammatory disease among sex workers in Nairobi, Kenya. J Infect Dis 1996;173:1437–44.

175 Wolner-Hanssen P, Eschenbach DA, Paavonen J, et al. Decreased risk of symptomatic chlamydial pelvic inflammatory disease associated with oral contraceptive use. JAMA 1990;263:54–9.

176 Ness RB, Keder LM, Soper DE, et al. Oral contraception and the recognition of endometritis. Am J Obstet Gynecol 1997;176:580–5.

177 Mukenge-Tshibaka L, Alary M, Lowndes C, et al. Syndromic versus laboratory-based diagnosis of cervical infections among female sex workers in Benin: implications of nonattendance for return visits. Sex Transm Dis 2002;29:324–30.

178 Chandeying V, Skov S, Kemapunmanus M, Law M, Geater A, Rowe P. Evaluation of two clinical protocols for the management of women with vaginal discharge in southern Thailand. Sex Transm Infect 1998;74:194–201.

179 Wawer MJ, Sewankambo NK, Serwadda D, et al. Control of sexually transmitted diseases for AIDS prevention in Uganda: a randomised community trial. Rakai Project Study Group. Lancet 1999;353:525–35.

180 Korenromp EL, White RG, Orroth KK, et al. Determinants of the impact of sexually transmitted infection treatment on prevention of HIV infection: a synthesis of evidence from the Mwanza, Rakai, and Masaka intervention trials. J Infect Dis 2005;191 Suppl 1:S168–S178.

181 Waugh MA, Cooke EM, Nehaul BB, Brayson J. Comparison of minocycline and ampicillin in gonococcal urethritis. Br J Vener Dis 1979;55:411–14.

182 Brathwaite AR. Double-blind trial of amoxicillin and ampicillin plus probenecid in the treatment of gonorrhoea in men. Br J Vener Dis 1979;55:340–2.

183 Berry E. Treatment of gonorrheal urethritis evaluated in 230 men. JAMA 1967;202:657–9.

184 Nissinen A, Jarvinen H, Liimatainen O, Jahkola M, Huovinen P. Antimicrobial resistance in *Neisseria gonorrhoeae* in Finland, 1976 to 1995. The Finnish Study Group For Antimicrobial Resistance. Sex Transm Dis 1997;24:576–81.

185 Rahman M, Sultan Z, Monira S, et al. Antimicrobial susceptibility of *Neisseria gonorrhoeae* isolated in Bangladesh (1997 to 1999): rapid shift to fluoroquinolone resistance. J Clin Microbiol 2002;40:2037–40.

186 Habte-Gabr E, Geyid A, Serdo D, Biddle J, Perine PL. Single-dose treatment of uncomplicated acute gonococcal urethritis in Ethiopian men: comparison of rosoxacin, spectinomycin, penicillin, and ampicillin. Sex Transm Dis 1987;14:153–5.

187 Panikabutra K, Ariyarit C, Chitwarakorn A, Saensanoh C, Wongba C. Randomised comparative study of ceftriaxone and spectinomycin in gonorrhoea. Genitourin Med 1985;61:106–8.

188 Plourde PJ, Tyndall M, Agoki E, et al. Single-dose cefixime versus single-dose ceftriaxone in the treatment of antimicrobial-resistant *Neisseria gonorrhoeae* infection. J Infect Dis 1992;166:919–22.

189 Handsfield HH, McCormack WM, Hook EW, III, et al. A comparison of single-dose cefixime with ceftriaxone as treatment for uncomplicated gonorrhea. The Gonorrhea Treatment Study Group. N Engl J Med 1991;325:1337–41.

190 Black JR, Long JM, Zwickl BE, et al. Multicenter randomized study of single-dose ofloxacin versus amoxicillin-probenecid for treatment of uncomplicated gonococcal infection. Antimicrob Agents Chemother 1989;33:167–70.

191 Bryan JP, Hira SK, Brady W, et al. Oral ciprofloxacin versus ceftriaxone for the treatment of urethritis from resistant *Neisseria gonorrhoeae* in Zambia. Antimicrob Agents Chemother 1990;34:819–22.

192 Kilmarx P, Knapp J, Xia M, et al. Intercity spread of gonococci with decreased susceptibility to fluoroquinolones: a unique focus in the United States. J Infect Dis 1998;177:677–82.

193 Trees D, Sandul A, Neal S, Higa H, Knapp J. Molecular epidemiology of *Neisseria gonorrhoeae* exhibiting decreased susceptibility and resistance to ciprofloxacin in Hawaii, 1991–1999. Sex Transm Dis 2001;309–14.

194 Update to CDC's sexually transmitted diseases treatment guidelines, 2006: fluoroquinolones no longer recommended for treatment of gonococcal infections. MMWR Morb Mortal Wkly Rep 2007;56:332–6.

195 Aplasca de los Reyes M, Pato-Mesola V, Klausner J, et al. A randomized trial of ciprofloxacin versus cefixime for treatment of gonorrhea after rapid emergence of gonococcal ciprofloxacin resistance in the Phillipines. Clin Infect Dis 2001;32:1313–8.

196 Handsfield HH, Dalu ZA, Martin DH, Douglas JM, Jr., McCarty JM, Schlossberg D. Multicenter trial of single-dose azithromycin vs. ceftriaxone in the treatment of uncomplicated gonorrhea. Azithromycin Gonorrhea Study Group. Sex Transm Dis 1994;21:107–11.

197 Zarantonelli L, Borthagaray G, Lee EH, Veal W, Shafer WM. Decreased susceptibility to azithromycin and erythromycin mediated by a novel mtr(R) promoter mutation in *Neisseria gonorrhoeae*. J Antimicrob Chemother 2001;47:651–4.

198 Guoming L, Qun C, Shengchun W. Resistance of *Neisseria gonorrhoeae* epidemic strains to antibiotics: report of resistant isolates and surveillance in Zhanjiang, China: 1998 to 1999. Sex Transm Dis 2000;27:115–18.

199 Karney W, Pedersen A, Nelson M, Adams H, Pfeifer R, Holmes K. Spectinomycin versus tetracycline for the treatment of gonorrhea. N Engl J Med 1977;296:889–94.

200 McLean K, Evans B, Lim J, Azadin B. Postgonococcal urethritis: a double-bline study of doxycycline vs placebo. Genitourin Med 1990;66:20–3.

201 Turnbull B, Stringer H, Meech R. Tetracycline and minocycline in the management of non-gonococcal urethritis: a comparison. N Z Med J 1982;95:460–2.

202 Romanowski B, Talbot H, Stadnyk M, Kowalchuck P, Bowie W. Minocycline compared with doxycycline in the treatment of non-gonococcal urethritis and mucopurulent cervicitis. Ann Intern Med 1993;119:16–22.

203 Bowie W, Yu J, Fawcett A, Jones H. Tetracycline in non-gonococcal urethritis. Comparison of 2 g and 1 g daily for seven days. Br J Vener Dis 1980;56:332–6.

204 Scheibel J, Kristensen J, Hentzer B, et al. Treatment of chlamydial urethritis in men and Chlamydia trachomatis-positive female partners: comparison of erythromycin and tetracycline in treatment courses of one week. Sex Transm Dis 1982;9:128–31.

205 Lidbrink P, Bygdeman S, Emtestam L, Gajecki M, Lapins J, Weden U. Roxithromycin compared to doxycycline in the treatment of genital chlamydial infection and non-specific urethritis. Int J STD AIDS 1993;4:110–3.

206 Stein GE, Mummaw NL, Havlichek DH. A preliminary study of clarithromycin versus doxycycline in the treatment of nongonococcal urethritis and mucopurulent cervicitis. Pharmacotherapy 1995;15:727–31.

207 Lau C,.Qureshi A. Azithromycin versus doxycycline for genital chalmydial infections: a meta-analysis of randomized clinical trials. Sex Transm Dis 2002;29:497–502.

208 Fong I, Linton W, Simbul M, et al. Treatment of non-gonococcal urethritis with ciprofloxacin. Am J Med 1987;82:311–16.

209 Hooton T, Rogers M, Medina T, et al. Ciprofloxacin compared with doxycycline for nongonococcal urethritis. Ineffectiveness against Chlamydia trachomatis due to relapsing infection. JAMA 1990;264:1418–21.

210 Phillips I, Dimian C, Barlow D, Moi H, Stolz E, Weidner W et al. A comparative study of two different regimens of sparfloxacin versus doxycycline in the treatment of nongonococcal urethritis in men. J Antimicrob Chemother 1996;37 Suppl A:123–34.

211 McCormack WM, Dalu ZA, Martin DH, et al. Double-blind comparison of trovafloxacin and doxycycline in the treatment of uncomplicated chlamydial urethritis and cervicitis. Trovafloxacin Chlamydial Urethritis/Cervicitis Study Group. Sex Transm Dis 1999;26:531–6.

212 McCormack WM, Martin DH, Hook EW, III, Jones RB. Daily oral grepafloxacin vs. twice daily oral doxycycline in the treatment of Chlamydia trachomatis endocervical infection. Infect Dis Obstet Gynecol 1998;6:109–15.

213 Martin DH, Koutsky L, Eschenbach DA, et al. Prematurity and perinatal mortality in pregnancies complicated by maternal Chlamydia trachomatis infections. JAMA 1982;247:1585–8.

214 Rastogi S, Kapur S, Salhan S, Mittal A. Chlamydia trachomatis infection in pregnancy: risk factor for an adverse outcome. Br J Biomed Sci 1999;56:94–8.

215 Rastogi S, Salhan S, Mittal A. Detection of Chlamydia trachomatis antigen in spontaneous abortions. Is this organism a primary or secondary indicator of risk? Br J Biomed Sci 2000;57:126–9.

216 Claman P, Toye B, Peeling RW, Jessamine P, Belcher J. Serologic evidence of Chlamydia trachomatis infection and risk of preterm birth. CMAJ 1995;153:259–62.

217 Witkin SS,.Ledger WJ. Antibodies to Chlamydia trachomatis in sera of women with recurrent spontaneous abortions. Am J Obstet Gynecol 1992;167:135–9.

218 Berman SM, Harrison HR, Boyce WT, Haffner WJ, Lewis M, Arthur JB. Low birth weight, prematurity, and postpartum endometritis. Association with prenatal cervical Mycoplasma hominis and Chlamydia trachomatis infections. JAMA 1987;257:1189–94.

219 Hammerschlag MR, Anderka M, Semine DZ, McComb D, McCormack WM. Prospective study of maternal and infantile infection with Chlamydia trachomatis. Pediatrics 1979;64:142–8.

220 Schachter J, Lum L, Gooding CA, Ostler B. Pneumonitis following inclusion blennorrhea. J Pediatr 1975;87:779–80.

221 Wager GP, Martin DH, Koutsky L, et al. Puerperal infectious morbidity: relationship to route of delivery and to antepartum Chlamydia trachomatis infection. Am J Obstet Gynecol 1980;138:1028–33.

222 Ryan GM, Jr., Abdella TN, McNeeley SG, Baselski VS, Drummond DE. Chlamydia trachomatis infection in pregnancy and effect of treatment on outcome. Am J Obstet Gynecol 1990;162:34–9.

223 Martin DH, Eschenbach DA, Cotch M, Nugent R, Rao A, Klebanoff MA, et al. Double-blind placebo-controlled treatment trial of Chlamydia trachomatis endocervical infections in pregnant women. Infect Dis Obstet Gynecol 1997;5:10–17.

224 Turrentine M, Newton E. Amoxicillin or erythromycin for the treatment of antenatal chlamydial infection: a meta-analysis. Obstet Gynecol 1995;86:1025.

225 Kacmar J, Cheh E, Montagno A, Peipert JF. A randomized trial of azithromycin versus amoxicillin for the treatment of Chlamydia trachomatis in pregnancy. Infect Dis Obstet Gynecol 2001;9:197–202.

226 Jacobson GF, Autry AM, Kirby RS, Liverman EM, Motley RU. A randomized controlled trial comparing amoxicillin and azithromycin for the treatment of Chlamydia trachomatis in pregnancy. Am J Obstet Gynecol 2001;184:1352–4.

227 Walker C, Kahn J, Washington A, Peterson H, Sweet R. Pelvic inflammatory disease: meta-analysis of antimicrobial regimen efficacy. J Infect Dis 2002;168:969–78.

228 Ness R, Soper D, Peipert J, et al. Effectiveness of inpatient and outpatient treatment strategies for women with pelvic inflammatory disease: results from the Pelvic Inflammatory Disease Evaluation and Clinical Health (PEACH) Randomized Trial. Am J Obstet Gynecol 2002;186:929–37.

229 Fiumara NJ. Treatment of secondary syphilis: an evaluation of 204 patients. Sex Transm Dis 1977;4:96–9.

230 Fiumara NJ. Treatment of seropositive primary syphilis: an evaluation of 196 patients. Sex Transm Dis 1977;4:92–5.

231 Schofer H, Vogt HJ, Milbradt R. Ceftriaxone for the treatment of primary and secondary syphilis. Chemotherapy 1989;35:140–5.

232 Moorthy TT, Lee CT, Lim KB, Tan T. Ceftriaxone for treatment of primary syphilis in men: a preliminary study. Sex Transm Dis 1987;14:116–18.

233 Hook E, Martin D, Stephens J, Smith B, Smith K. A randomized, comparative pilot study of azithromycin versus benzathine penicillin G for treatment of early syphilis. Sex Transm Dis 2002;29:486–90.

234 Mitchell SJ, Engelman J, Kent CK, Lukehart SA, Godornes C, Klausner JD. Azithromycin-resistant syphilis infection: San Francisco, California, 2000–2004. Clin Infect Dis 2006;42:337–45.

235 Lukehart SA, Godornes C, Molini BJ, et al. Macrolide resistance in Treponema pallidum in the United States and Ireland. N Engl J Med 2004;351:154–8.

236 Morshed MG, Jones HD. Treponema pallidum macrolide resistance in BC. CMAJ 2006;174:349.

237 Gordon S, Eaton M, George R, et al. The response of sypmptomatic neurosyphilis to high-dose intravenous penicillin G in patients with human immunodeficiency virus infection. N Engl J Med 1994;331:1469–73.

238 Berry C, Hooton T, Collier A, Lukehart S. Neurologic relapse after benzathine penicillin therapy for secondary syphilis in a patient with HIV infection. N Engl J Med 1987;316:1587–9.

239 Rolfs R, Joesoef M, Hendershot E, et al. A randomized trial of enhanced therapy for early syphilis in patients with and without human immunodeficiency virus infection. N Engl J Med 1997;337:307–14.

240 Marra C, Boutin P, McArthur J, et al. A pilot study evaluating ceftriaxone and penicillin G as treatment agents for neurosyphilis in human immunodeficiency virus-infected individuals. Clin Infect Dis 2000;30:540–4.

241 Hook E, Stephens J, Ennis D. Azithromycin compared to penicillin G benzathine for treatment of incubating syphilis. Ann Intern Med 1999;131:434–7.

242 Peterman T, Zaidi A, Lieb S, Wroten J. Incubating syphilis in patients treated for gonorrhea: a comparison of treatment regimens. J Infect Dis 1994;170:689–92.

243 Centers for Disease Control and Prevention. Sexually transmitted diseases treatment guidelines 2002. MMWR Morb Mortal Wkly Rep 2002;51 (No. RR-6):26–8.

244 Paryani SG, Vaughn AJ, Crosby M, Lawrence S. Treatment of asymptomatic congenital syphilis: benzathine versus procaine penicillin G therapy. J Pediatr 1994;125:471–5.

245 Radcliffe M, Meyer M, Roditi D, Malan A. Single-dose benzathine penicillin in infants at risk of congenital syphilis – results of a randomised study. S Afr Med J 1997;87:62–5.

246 Benedetti JK, Zeh J, Selke S, Corey L. Frequency and reactivation of nongenital lesions among patients with genital herpes simplex virus. Am J Med 1995;98:237–42.

247 Reeves WC, Corey L, Adams HG, Vontver LA, Holmes KK. Risk of recurrence after first episodes of genital herpes. Relation to HSV type and antibody response. N Engl J Med 1981;305:315–9.

248 Vontver LA, Reeves WC, Rattray M, et al. Clinical course and diagnosis of genital herpes simplex virus infection and evaluation of topical surfactant therapy. Am J Obstet Gynecol 1979;133:548–54.

249 Corey L, Fife K, Benedetti J, et al. Intravenous acyclovir for the treatment of primary genital herpes. Ann Intern Med 1983;98:914–21.

250 Bryson Y, Dillon M, Lovett M, et al. Treatment of first episodes of genital herpes simplex virus infection with oral acyclovir. A randomized double-blind controlled trial. N Engl J Med 1983;308:916–21.

251 Mertz G, Critchlow C, Benedetti J, et al. Double-blind placebo-controlled trial of oral acyclovir in first-episode genital herpes simplex virus infection. JAMA 1984;252:1147–51.

252 Wald A, Benedetti J, Davis G, Remington M, Winter C, Corey L. A randomized, double-blind, comparative trial comparing high- and standard-dose oral acyclovir for first-episode genital herpes infections. Antimicrob Agents Chemother 1994;38:174–6.

253 Ruhnek-Forsbeck M, Sandstrom E, Andersson B, et al. Treatment of recurrent genital herpes simplex virus infections with oral acyclovir. J Antimicrob Chemother 1985;16:621–8.

254 Reichman R, Badger G, Mertz G, et al. Treatment of recurrent genital herpes simplex infections with oral acyclovir. A controlled trial. JAMA 1984;251:2103–7.

255 Stone K, Whittington W. Treatment of genital herpes. Rev Infect Dis 1990;12 (suppl 6):610–19.

256 Spruance S, Tyring S, Degregorio B, Miller C, Beutner K. A large-scale, placebo-controlled, dose-ragning trial of peroral valacyclovir for episodic treatment of recurrent genital herpes. Arch Intern Med 1996;156:1729–35.

257 Sacks S, Aoki F, Diaz-Mitoma F, Sellors J, Shafran S. Patient-initiated, twice-daily oral famciclovir for early recurrent genital herpes: a randomized, double-blind multicenter trial. JAMA 1996;276:44–9.

258 Chosidow O, Drouault Y, Leconte-Veyriac F, et al. Famciclovir vs. aciclovir in immunocompetent patients with recurrent genital herpes infections: a parallel groups, randomized, double-blind clinical trial. Br J Dermatol 2001;144:818–24.

259 Bodsworth N, Crooks R, Borelli S, et al. Valacyclovir versus acyclovir in patient initiated treatment of recurrent genital herpes: a randomised, double blind clinical trial. Genitourin Med 1997;73:110–16.

260 Leone P, Trottier S, Miller J. Valacyclovir for episodic treatment of genital herpes: a shorter 3-day treatment course compared with 5-day treatment. Clin Infect Dis 2002;34:958–62.

261 Wald A, Carrell D, Remington M, Kexel E, Zeh J, Corey L. Two-day regimen of acyclovir for treatment of recurrent genital herpes simplex virus type 2 infection. Clin Infect Dis 2002;34:944–8.

262 Mertz G, Jones C, Mills J, et al. Long-term acyclovir suppression of frequently recurring genital herpes simplex virus infection. A multicenter double-blind trial. JAMA 1988;260:201–6.

263 Kaplowitz L, Baker D, Gelb L, et al. Prolonged continuous acyclovir treatment of normal adults with frequently recurring genital herpes simplex virus infection. JAMA 1991;265:747–51.

264 Mattison H, Reichman R, Benedetti J, et al. Double-blind, placebo-controlled trial comparing long-term suppressive with short-term oral acyclovir therapy for management of recurrent genital herpes. Am J Med 1988;85:20–5.

265 Mindel A, Faherty A, Carney O, Patou G, Freris M, Williams P. Dosage and safety of long-term suppressive acyclovir therapy for recurrent genital herpes. Lancet 1988;1:926–8.

266 Goldberg L, Kaufman R, Kurtz T, et al. Long-term suppression of recurrent genital herpes with acyclovir: a 5-year benchmark study. Arch Dermatol 1993;1993: 582–7.

267 Mertz G, Loveless M, Levin M, et al. Oral famciclovir for suppression of recurrent genital herpes simplex virus infection in women. A multicenter, double-blind, placebo-controlled trial. Arch Intern Med 1997;157:343–9.

268 Fife KH, Crumpacker CS, Mertz GJ, Hill EL, Boone GS. Recurrence and resistance patterns of herpes simplex virus following cessation of > or = 6 years of chronic suppression with acyclovir. Acyclovir Study Group. J Infect Dis 1994;169:1338–41.

269 Patel R, Bobsworth N, Woolley P, et al. Valacyclovir for the suppression of recurrent genital HSV infection: a placebo controlled study of once daily therapy. Genitourin Med 1997;73:105–9.

270 Reitano M, Tyring S, Lang W, et al. Valacyclovir for the suppression of recurrent genital herpes simplex virus infection: a large-scale dose range-finding study. J Infect Dis 1998;178:603–10.

271 Diaz-Mitoma F, Sibbald R, Shafran S, Boon R, Saltzman R. Oral famciclovir for the suppression of recurrent genital herpes: a randomized controlled trial. JAMA 1998;280:887–92.

272 Lebrun-Vignes B, Bouzamondo A, Dupuy A, Guillaume JC, Lechat P, Chosidow O. A meta-analysis to assess the efficacy of oral antiviral treatment to prevent genital herpes outbreaks. J Am Acad Dermatol 2007;57:238–46.

273 Wald A, Selke S, Warren T, et al. Comparative efficacy of famciclovir and valacyclovir for suppression of recurrent genital herpes and viral shedding. Sex Transm Dis 2006;33:529–33.

274 Wald A, Zeh J, Barnum G, Davis L, Corey L. Suppression of subclinical shedding of herpes simplex virus type 2 with acyclovir. Ann Intern Med 1996;124:8–15.

275 Corey L, Wald A, Patel R, et al. Once-daily valacyclovir to reduce the risk of transmission of genital herpes. N Engl J Med 2004;350:11–20.

276 Kim HN, Wald A, Harris J, Almekinder J, Heitman C, Corey L. Does frequency of genital herpes recurrences predict risk of transmission? Further analysis of the valacyclovir transmission study. Sex Transm Dis 2008;35:124–8.

277 Patel R, Tyring S, Strand A, Price M, Grant D. Impact of suppressive antiviral therapy on the health related quality of life of patients with recurrent genital herpes infection. Sex Transm Infect 1999;75:398–402.

278 Carney O, Ross E, Ikkos G, Mindel A. The effect of suppressive oral acyclovir on the psychological morbidity associated with recurrent genital herpes. Genitourin Med 1993;69:457–9.

279 Brown Z, Selke S, Zeh J, et al. The acquisition of herpes simplex virus during pregnancy. N Engl J Med 1997;337:515.

280 Prober CG, Corey L, Brown ZA, et al. The management of pregnancies complicated by genital infections with herpes simplex virus. Clin Infect Dis 1992;15:1031–8.

281 Morris SR, Bauer HM, Samuel MC, Gallagher D, Bolan G. Neonatal herpes morbidity and mortality in California, 1995–2003. Sex Transm Dis 2008;35:14–1.

282 Watts DH, Brown ZA, Money D, Selke S, Huang ML, Sacks SL et al. A double-blind, randomized, placebo-controlled trial of acyclovir in late pregnancy for the reduction of herpes simplex virus shedding and cesarean delivery. Am J Obstet Gynecol 2003;188:836–43.

283 Brocklehurst P, Kinghorn G, Carney O, et al. A randomised placebo controlled trial of suppressive acyclovir in late pregnancy in women with recurrent genital herpes infection. Br J Obstet Gynaecol 1998;105:275–80.

284 Stray-Pedersen B. Acyclovir in late pregnancy to prevent neonatal herpes simplex. Lancet 1990;336:756.

285 Hammond G, Slutchuk M, Lian C, Wilt J, Ronald A. The treatment of chancroid: comparison of one week of sulfisoxazole with single dose doxycycline. J Antimicrob Chemother 1979;5:261–5.

286 Meheus A, Ursi J, Van Dyck E, Ballard R. Treatment of chancroid with single-dose doxycycline compared with a two-day course of co-trimoxazole. Ann Soc Belg Med Trop 1981;61:119–24.

287 Rutanarugsa A, Vorachit M, Polnikorn N, Jayanetra P. Drug resistance of Haemophilus ducreyi. Southeast Asian J Trop Med Public Health 1990;21:185–93.

288 Fast M, Nsanze H, D'Costa LJ, et al. Antimicrobial therapy of chancroid: an evaluation of five treatment regimens correlated with in vitro sensitivity. Sex Transm Dis 1983;10:1–6.

289 D'Souza P, Pandhi RK, Khanna N, Rattan A, Misra RS. A comparative study of therapeutic response of patients with clinical chancroid to ciprofloxacin, erythromycin, and cotrimoxazole. Sex Transm Dis 1998;25:293–5.

290 Plourde PJ, D'Costa LJ, Agoki E, et al. A randomized, double-blind study of the efficacy of fleroxacin versus trimethoprim-sulfamethoxazole in men with culture-proven chancroid. J Infect Dis 1992;165:949–52.

291 Tyndall M, Agoki E, Plummer FA, Malisa W, Ndinya-Achola J, Ronald A. Single dose azithromycin for the treatment of chancroid: a randomized comparison of erythromycin. Sex Transm Dis 1994;21:213–34.

292 Naamara W, Plummer F, Greenblatt R, D'Costa L, Ndinya-Achola J, Ronald A. Treatment of chancroid with ciprofloxacin. A prospective, randomized clinical trial. Am J Med 1987;82:317–20.

293 Martin D, Sargent S, Wendel G, McCormack WM, Johnson RB. Comparison of azithromycin and ceftriaxone for the treatment of chancroid. Clin Infect Dis 1995;21:409–14.

294 Fast M, Nsanze H, D'Costa L, et al. Treatment of chancroid by clavulanic acid with amoxycillin in patients with beta-lactamase-positive Haemophilus ducreyi infection. Lancet 1982;2:509–11.

295 Traisupa A, Ariyarit C, Metheeprapha C, Buatiang A, Sungthong P. Treatment of chancroid with spectinomycin or co-trimoxazole. Clin Ther 1990;12:200–5.

296 Ballard R, da L'Exposto F, Dangor Y, Fehler H, Miller S, Koornhof H. A comparative study of spectinomycin and erythromycin in the treatment of chancroid. J Antimicrob Chemother 1990;26:429–34.

297 Ernst AA, Marvez-Valls E, Martin DH. Incision and drainage versus aspiration of fluctuant buboes in the emergency department during an epidemic of chancroid. Sex Transm Dis 1995;21:217–20.

298 Handsfield HH. Clinical presentation and natural course of anogenital warts. Am J Med 1997;102:16–20.

299 Oriel D. Genital human papillomavirus infection. In Holmes K, Mardh PA, Sparling P, et al, eds. Sexually Transmitted Diseases, pp 433–42. New York: McGraw-Hill, 1990.

300 Fife K, Ferenczy A, Douglas JM, Jr., Brown D, Smith M, Owens M. Treatment of external genital warts in men using 5% imiquimod cream applied three times a week, once daily, twice daily, or three times daily. Sex Transm Dis 2001;28:226–31.

301 Stone K, Becker T, Hadgu A, Kraus S. Treatment of external genital warts: a randomised clinical trial comparing podophyllin, cryotherapy, and electrodessication. Genitourin Med 1990;66:16–19.

302 Connolly M, Bazmi K, O'Connell M, Lyons JF, Bourke JF. Cryotherapy of viral warts: a sustained 10-s freeze is more effective than the traditional method. Br J Dermatol 2001;145:554–7.

303 Godley M, Bradbeer C, Gellan M, Thin R. Cryotherapy compared with trichloroacetic acid in treating genital warts. Genitourin Med 1987;63:390–2.

304 Abdullah A, Walzman M, Wade A. Treatment of external genital warts comparing cryotherapy (liquid nitrogen) and trichloroacetic acid. Sex Transm Dis 1993;20:344–5.

305 Duus B, Philipsen T, Christensen J, Lundvall F, Sondergaard J. Refractory condylomata acuminata: a controlled clinical trial of carbon dioxide laser versus conventional surgical treatment. Genitourin Med 1985;61:59–61.

306 Simmons P, Langlet F, Thin R. Cryotherapy versus electrocautery in the treatment of genital warts. Br J Vener Dis 1981;57:273–4.

307 Jensen S. Comparison of podophyllin application with simple surgical excision in clearance and recurrence of perianal condyloma acuminata. Lancet 1985;2:1146–8.

308 Syed TA, Khayyami M, Kriz D, et al. Management of genital warts in women with human leukocyte interferon-alpha vs. podophyllotoxin in cream: a placebo-controlled, double-blind, comparative study. J Mol Med 1995;73:255–8.

309 Syed TA, Cheema KM, Khayyami M, et al. Human leukocyte interferon-alpha versus podophyllotoxin in cream for the treatment of genital warts in males. A placebo-controlled, double-blind, comparative study. Dermatology 1995;191:129–32.

310 Douglas JM, Jr., Eron LJ, Judson FN, et al. A randomized trial of combination therapy with intralesional interferon alpha 2b and podophyllin versus podophyllin alone for the therapy of anogenital warts. J Infect Dis 1990;162:52–9.

311 Olmos L, Vilata J, Rodriguez PA, Lloret A, Ojeda A, Calderon MD. Double-blind, randomized clinical trial on the effect of interferon-beta in the treatment of condylomata acuminata. Int J STD AIDS 1994;5:182–5.

312 Gentile G, Formelli G, Busacchi P, Pelusi G. Systemic interferon therapy for female florid genital condylomata. Clin Exp Obstet Gynecol 1994;21:198–202.

313 Reichman RC, Oakes D, Bonnez W, et al. Treatment of condyloma acuminatum with three different interferon-alpha preparations administered parenterally: a double-blind, placebo-controlled trial. J Infect Dis 1990;162:1270–6.

314 Armstrong DK, Maw RD, Dinsmore WW, et al. Combined therapy trial with interferon alpha-2a and ablative therapy in the treatment of anogenital warts. Genitourin Med 1996;72:103–7.

315 Armstrong DK, Maw RD, Dinsmore WW, et al. A randomised, double-blind, parallel group study to compare subcutaneous interferon alpha-2a plus podophyllin with placebo plus podophyllin in the treatment of primary condylomata acuminata. Genitourin Med 1994;70:389–93.

316 Bonnez W, Oakes D, Bailey-Farchione A, et al. A randomized, double-blind, placebo-controlled trial of systemically administered interferon-alpha, -beta, or -gamma in combination with cryotherapy for the treatment of condyloma acuminatum. J Infect Dis 1995;171:1081–9.

317 Gilson RJ, Shupack JL, Friedman-Kien AE, et al. A randomized, controlled, safety study using imiquimod for the topical treatment of anogenital warts in HIV-infected patients. Imiquimod Study Group. AIDS 1999;13:2397–404.

318 Orlando G, Fasolo MM, Beretta R, Merli S, Cargnel A. Combined surgery and cidofovir is an effective treatment for genital warts in HIV-infected patients. AIDS 2002;16:447–50.

319 Wilson JD, Brown CB, Walker PP. Factors involved in clearance of genital warts. Int J STD AIDS 2001;12:789–92.

320 Thin RN, Symonds MA, Booker R, Cook S, Langlet F. Double-blind comparison of a single dose and a five-day course of metronidazole in the treatment of trichomoniasis. Br J Vener Dis 1979;55:354–6.

321 Hager WD, Brown ST, Kraus SJ, Kleris GS, Perkins GJ, Henderson M. Metronidazole for vaginal trichomoniasis.

Seven-day vs single-dose regimens. JAMA 1980; 244:1219–20.

322 Austin TW, Smith EA, Darwish R, Ralph ED, Pattison FL. Metronidazole in a single dose for the treatment of trichomoniasis. Failure of a 1-g single dose. Br J Vener Dis 1982;58:121–3.

323 Spence MR, Harwell TS, Davies MC, Smith JL. The minimum single oral metronidazole dose for treating trichomoniasis: a randomized, blinded study. Obstet Gynecol 1997;89:699–703.

324 Sobel JD, Nyirjesy P, Brown W. Tinidazole therapy for metronidazole-resistant vaginal trichomoniasis. Clin Infect Dis 2001;33:1341–6.

325 duBouchet L, Spence MR, Rein MF, Danzig MR, McCormack WM. Multicenter comparison of clotrimazole vaginal tablets, oral metronidazole, and vaginal suppositories containing sulfanilamide, aminacrine hydrochloride, and allantoin in the treatment of symptomatic trichomoniasis. Sex Transm Dis 1997;24:156–60.

326 duBouchet L, McGregor JA, Ismail M, McCormack WM. A pilot study of metronidazole vaginal gel versus oral metronidazole for the treatment of *Trichomonas vaginalis* vaginitis. Sex Transm Dis 1998;25:176–9.

327 Antonelli NM, Diehl SJ, Wright JW. A randomized trial of intravaginal nonoxynol 9 versus oral metronidazole in the treatment of vaginal trichomoniasis. Am J Obstet Gynecol 2000;182:1008–10.

328 Lyng J, Christensen J. A double-blind study of the value of treatment with a single dose tinidazole of partners to females with trichomoniasis. Acta Obstet Gynecol Scand 1981;60:199–201.

329 Shain RN, Perdue ST, Piper JM, et al. Behaviors changed by intervention are associated with reduced STD recurrence: the importance of context in measurement. Sex Transm Dis 2002;29:520–9.

330 Kissinger P, Brown R, Reed K, et al. Effectiveness of patient delivered partner medication for preventing recurrent *Chlamydia trachomatis*. Sex Transm Infect 1998;74:331–3.

331 Ramstedt K, Forssman L, Johannisson G. Contact tracing in the control of genital *Chlamydia trachomatis* infection. Int J STD AIDS 1991;2:116–8.

332 Golden MR, Whittington WL, Handsfield HH, et al. Effect of expedited treatment of sex partners on recurrent or persistent gonorrhea or chlamydial infection. N Engl J Med 2005;352:676–85.

333 Kissinger P, Mohammed H, Richardson-Alston G, et al. Patient-delivered partner treatment for male urethritis: a randomized, controlled trial. Clin Infect Dis 2005;41:623–9.

334 Koutsky LA, Ault KA, Wheeler CM, et al. A controlled trial of a human papillomavirus type 16 vaccine. N Engl J Med 2002;347:1645–51.

335 Joura EA, Kjaer SK, Wheeler CM, et al. HPV antibody levels and clinical efficacy following administration of a prophylactic quadrivalent HPV vaccine. Vaccine 2008;26:6844–51.

336 Villa LL, Ault KA, Giuliano AR, et al. Immunologic responses following administration of a vaccine targeting human papillomavirus Types 6, 11, 16, and 18. Vaccine 2006;24:5571–83.

337 Koutsky LA, Ault KA, Wheeler CM, et al. A controlled trial of a human papillomavirus type 16 vaccine. N Engl J Med 2002;347:1645–51.

338 Harper DM, Franco EL, Wheeler C, et al. Efficacy of a bivalent L1 virus-like particle vaccine in prevention of infection with human papillomavirus types 16 and 18 in young women: a randomised controlled trial. Lancet 2004;364:1757–65.

339 Villa LL, Costa RL, Petta CA, et al. Prophylactic quadrivalent human papillomavirus (types 6, 11, 16, and 18) L1 virus-like particle vaccine in young women: a randomised double-blind placebo-controlled multicentre phase II efficacy trial. Lancet Oncol 2005;6:271–8.

340 Quadrivalent vaccine against human papillomavirus to prevent high-grade cervical lesions. N Engl J Med 2007;356:1915–27.

341 Paavonen J, Jenkins D, Bosch FX, et al. Efficacy of a prophylactic adjuvanted bivalent L1 virus-like-particle vaccine against infection with human papillomavirus types 16 and 18 in young women: an interim analysis of a phase III double-blind, randomised controlled trial. Lancet 2007;369:2161–70.

342 Garland SM, Hernandez-Avila M, Wheeler CM, et al. Quadrivalent vaccine against human papillomavirus to prevent anogenital diseases. N Engl J Med 2007;356:1928–43.

343 Joura EA, Leodolter S, Hernandez-Avila M, et al. Efficacy of a quadrivalent prophylactic human papillomavirus (types 6, 11, 16, and 18) L1 virus-like-particle vaccine against high-grade vulval and vaginal lesions: a combined analysis of three randomised clinical trials. Lancet 2007;369:1693–702.

344 Hildesheim A, Herrero R, Wacholder S, et al. Effect of human papillomavirus 16/18 L1 viruslike particle vaccine among young women with preexisting infection: a randomized trial. JAMA 2007;298:743–53.

345 Kim JJ, Goldie SJ. Health and economic implications of HPV vaccination in the United States. N Engl J Med 2008;359:821–32.

346 Stanberry L, Spruance S, Cunningham A, et al. Glycoprotein-d-adjuvant vaccine to prevent genital herpes. N Engl J Med 2002;347:1652–61.

347 Coutinho R, Lelie N, Albrecht-Van Lent P, et al. Efficacy of a heat inactivated hepatitis B vaccine in male homosexualys: outcome of a placebo controlled double blind trial. Br Med J (Clin Res Ed) 1983;286:1305–8.

348 Szmuness W, Stevens C, Harley E, et al. Hepatitis B vaccine: demonstration of efficacy in a controlled clinical trial in a high-risk population in the United States. N Engl J Med 1980;303:833–41.

349 Halliday M, Rankin J, Bristow N, Coates R, Corey P, Strickler A. A randomized double-blind clinical trial of a mammalian cell-derived recombinant DNA hepatitis B vaccine compared with a plasma-derived vaccine. Arch Intern Med 1990;150:1195–2000.

350 Sagliocca L, Amoroso P, Stroffolini T, et al. Efficacy of hepatitis A vaccine in prevention of secondary hepatitis A infection: a randomized trial. Lancet 353 1999;1139.

351 Innis BL, Snitbhan R, Kunasol P, et al. Protection against hepatitis A by an inactivated vaccine. JAMA 1994;271:1328–34.

352 Roumeliotou-Karayannis A, Papaevangelou G, Tassopoulos N, Richardson S, Krugman S. Post-exposure active immunoprophylaxis of spouses of acute viral hepatitis B patients. Vaccine 1985;3:31–4.

353 Turner CF, Rogers SM, Miller HG, et al. Untreated gonococcal and chlamydial infection in a probability sample of adults. JAMA 2002;287:726–33.

354 Ku L, St Louis M, Farshy C, et al. Risk behaviors, medical care, and chlamydial infection among young men in the United States. Am J Public Health 2002;92:1140–3.

355 Scholes D, Stergachis A, Heidrich FE, Andrilla H, Holmes KK, Stamm WE. Prevention of pelvic inflammatory disease by screening for cervical chlamydial infection. N Engl J Med 1996;334:1362–6.

356 Howell MR, Quinn TC, Gaydos CA. Screening for Chlamydia trachomatis in asymptomatic women attending family planning clinics. A cost-effectiveness analysis of three strategies. Ann Intern Med 1998;128:277–84.

357 Roberts TE, Robinson S, Barton P, Bryan S, Low N. Screening for Chlamydia trachomatis: a systematic review of the economic evaluations and modelling. Sex Transm Infect 2006;82:193–200.

358 Turner KM, Adams EJ, Lamontagne DS, Emmett L, Baster K, Edmunds WJ. Modelling the effectiveness of chlamydia screening in England. Sex Transm Infect 2006;82:496–502.

359 Gichangi PB, Ndinya-Achola JO, Ombete J, Nagelkerke NJ, Temmerman M. Antimicrobial prophylaxis in pregnancy: a randomized, placebo-controlled trial with cefetamet-pivoxil in pregnant women with a poor obstetric history. Am J Obstet Gynecol 1997;177:680–4.

360 Temmerman M, Njagi E, Nagelkerke N, Ndinya-Achola J, Plummer FA, Meheus A. Mass antimicrobial treatment in pregnancy. A randomized, placebo-controlled trial in a population with high rates of sexually transmitted diseases. J Reprod Med 1995;40:176–80.

361 Gray RH, Wabwire-Mangen F, Kigozi G, et al. Randomized trial of presumptive sexually transmitted disease therapy during pregnancy in Rakai, Uganda. Am J Obstet Gynecol 2001;185:1209–17.

362 Kaul R, Kimani J, Nagelkerke NJ, et al. Monthly antibiotic chemoprophylaxis and incidence of sexually transmitted infections and HIV-1 infection in Kenyan sex workers: a randomized controlled trial. JAMA 2004;291:2555–62.

363 Holmes KK, Johnson DW, Kvale PA, Halverson CW, Keys TF, Martin DH. Impact of a gonorrhea control program, including selective mass treatment, in female sex workers. J Infect Dis 1996;174 Suppl 2:S230-S239.

364 Rekart M, Patrick D, Chakraborty B, et al. Targeted mass treatment for syphilis with oral azithromycin. Lancet 2003;361:313–14.

365 Orroth KK, Korenromp EL, White RG, et al. Higher risk behaviour and rates of sexually transmitted diseases in Mwanza compared to Uganda may help explain HIV prevention trial outcomes. AIDS 2003;17:2653–60.

366 Celum C, Wald A, Hughes J, et al. Effect of aciclovir on HIV-1 acquisition in herpes simplex virus 2 seropositive women and men who have sex with men: a randomised, double-blind, placebo-controlled trial. Lancet 2008;371:2109–19.

367 Watson-Jones D, Weiss HA, Rusizoka M, et al. Effect of herpes simplex suppression on incidence of HIV among women in Tanzania. N Engl J Med 2008;358:1560–71.

368 Lin JS, Whitlock E, O'Connor E, Bauer V. Behavioral counseling to prevent sexually transmitted infections: a systematic review for the U.S. Preventive Services Task Force. Ann Intern Med 2008;149:497–9.

369 Kamb ML, Fishbein M, Douglas JM, Jr., et al. Efficacy of risk-reduction counseling to prevent human immunodeficiency virus and sexually transmitted diseases: a randomized controlled trial. Project RESPECT Study Group. JAMA 1998;280:1161–7.

370 Mayaud P, Changalucha J, Grosskurth H, et al. The value of urine specimens in screening for male urethritis and its microbial aetiologies in Tanzania. Genitourin Med 1992;68:361–5.

371 McNagny SE, Parker RM, Zenilman JM, Lewis JS. Urinary leukocyte esterase test: a screening method for the detection of asymptomatic chlamydial and gonococcal infections in men. J Infect Dis 1992;165:573–6.

372 Cacciatore B, Leminen A, Ingman-Friberg S, Ylostalo P, Paavonen J. Transvaginal sonographic findings in ambulatory patients with suspected pelvic inflammatory disease. Obstet Gynecol 1992;80:912–6.

373 Tukeva TA, Aronen HJ, Karjalainen PT, Molander P, Paavonen T, Paavonen J. MR imaging in pelvic inflammatory disease: comparison with laparoscopy and US. Radiology 1999;210:209–16.

374 Boardman LA, Peipert JF, Brody JM, Cooper AS, Sung J. Endovaginal sonography for the diagnosis of upper genital tract infection. Obstet Gynecol 1997;90:54–7.

375 Jue R, Puffer J, Wood RM, Schochet G, Smartt WH, Ketterer WA. Comparison of fluorescent and conventional darkfield methods for the detection of Treponema pallidum in syphilitic lesions. Tech Bull Regist Med Technol 1967;37:123–5.

376 Jethwa HS, Schmitz JL, Dallabetta G, et al. Comparison of molecular and microscopic techniques for detection of Treponema pallidum in genital ulcers. J Clin Microbiol 1995;33:180–3.

377 Leslie DE, Azzato F, Karapanagiotidis T, Leydon J, Fyfe J. Development of a real-time PCR assay to detect Treponema pallidum in clinical specimens and assessment of the assay's performance by comparison with serological testing. J Clin Microbiol 2007;45:93–6.

378 Palmer HM, Higgins SP, Herring AJ, Kingston MA. Use of PCR in the diagnosis of early syphilis in the United Kingdom. Sex Transm Infect 2003;79:479–83.

379 Koek AG, Bruisten SM, Dierdorp M, van Dam AP, Templeton K. Specific and sensitive diagnosis of syphilis using a real-time PCR for *Treponema pallidum*. Clin Microbiol Infect 2006;12:1233–6.

380 Larsen S, Hambie E, Pettit D, Perryman M, Kraus S. Specificity, sensitivity, and reproducibility among the fluorescent treponemal antibody-absorbtion test, the microhemagglutination assay for *Treponema pallidum* antibodies, and the hemagglutination treponemal test for syphilis. J Clin Microbiol 1981;14:441–5.

381 Huber T, Storms S, Young P, Phillips L, Rogers T, Moore D et al. Reactivity of microhemaagglutination, fluorescent treponemal antibody absorbtion, Venereal Disease Research Laboratory, and rapid plasma reagin tests in primary syphilis. J Clin Microbiol 1983;17:405–9.

382 Augenbraun M, Rolfs R, Johnson R, Joesoef R, Pope V. Treponemal specific tests for the serodiagnosis of syphilis. Sex Transm Dis 1998;25:549–52.

383 Rodriguez I, Alvarez E, Fernandez C, Miranda A. Comparison of a recombinant-antigen enzyme immunoassay with *Treponema pallidum* hemagglutination test for serological confirmation for serological confirmation of syphilis. Mem Inst Oswaldo Cruz 2002;97:347–9.

384 Sambri V, Marangoni A, Simone M, D'Antuono A, Negosanti M, Cevenini R. Evaluation of recomWell Treponema, a novel recombinant antigen-based enzyme-linked immunosorbent assay for the diagnosis of syphilis. Clin Microbiol Infect 2001;7:200–5.

385 Young H, Moyes A, Seagar L, McMillan A. Novel recombinant-antigen enzyme immunoassay for serological diagsnosis of syphilis. J Clin Microbiol 1998;36:913–7.

386 Farshy CE, Hunter EF, Helsel LO, Larsen SA. Four-step enzyme-linked immunosorbent assay for detection of *Treponema pallidum* antibody. J Clin Microbiol 1985;21:387–9.

387 Lefevre JC, Bertrand MA, Bauriaud R. Evaluation of the Captia enzyme immunoassays for detection of immunoglobulins G and M to *Treponema pallidum* in syphilis. J Clin Microbiol 1990;28:1704–7.

388 Backhouse J, Nesteroff S. *Treponema pallidum* Western blot: comparison with the FTA-ABS test as a confirmatory test for syphilis. Diagn Microbiol Infect Dis 2001;39:9–14.

389 Byrne RE, Laska S, Bell M, Larson D, Phillips J, Todd J. Evaluation of a *Treponema pallidum* Western immunoblot assay as a confirmatory test for syphilis. J Clin Microbiol 1992;30:115–22.

390 Sambri V, Marangoni A, Eyer C, et al. Western immunoblotting with five *Treponema pallidum* recombinant antigens for serologic diagnosis of syphilis. Clin Diagn Lab Immunol 2001;8:534–9.

391 Plummer F, Maggwa N, D'Costa L, et al. Cefotaxime treatment of *Haemophilus ducreyi* infection in Kenya. Sex Transm Dis 1984;11:304–7.

392 Bonnez W, Elswick RK, Jr., Bailey-Farchione A, et al. Efficacy and safety of 0.5% podofilox solution in the treatment and suppression of anogenital warts. Am J Med 1994;96:420–5.

393 von Krogh G, Szpak E, Andersson M, Bergelin I. Self-treatment using 0.25%–0.50% podophyllotoxin-ethanol solutions against penile condylomata acuminata: a placebo-controlled comparative study. Genitourin Med 1994;70:105–9.

394 Beutner K, Conant M, Friedman-Kien A, et al. Patient applied podfilox for treatment of genital warts. Lancet 1989;1:831–4.

395 Greenberg MD, Rutledge LH, Reid R, Berman NR, Precop SL, Elswick RK, Jr. A double-blind, randomized trial of 0.5% podofilox and placebo for the treatment of genital warts in women. Obstet Gynecol 1991;77:735–9.

396 Kirby P, Dunne A, King DH, Corey L. Double-blind randomized clinical trial of self-administered podofilox solution versus vehicle in the treatment of genital warts. Am J Med 1990;88:465–9.

397 Edwards L, Ferenczy A, Eron L, et al. Self-administered topical 5% imiquimod cream for external anogenital warts. HPV Study Group. Human PapillomaVirus. Arch Dermatol 1998;134:25–30.

398 Beutner K, Tyring S, Trofatter K, et al. Imiquimod, a patient-applied immune-response modifier for treatment of external genital warts. Antimicrob Agents Chemother 1998;42:789–94.

399 Syed TA, Ahmadpour OA, Ahmad SA, Ahmad SH. Management of female genital warts with an analog of imiquimod 2% in cream: a randomized, double-blind, placebo-controlled study. J Dermatol 1998;25:429–33.

400 Syed TA, Hadi SM, Qureshi ZA, Ali SM, Kwah MS. Treatment of external genital warts in men with imiquimod 2% in cream. A placebo-controlled, double-blind study. J Infect 2000;41:148–51.

401 Eron LJ, Judson F, Tucker S, et al. Interferon therapy for condylomata acuminata. N Engl J Med 1986;315:1059–64.

402 Friedman-Kien AE, Eron LJ, Conant M, et al. Natural interferon alfa for treatment of condylomata acuminata. JAMA 1988;259:533–8.

403 Reichman RC, Oakes D, Bonnez W, et al. Treatment of condyloma acuminatum with three different interferons administered intralesionally. A double-blind, placebo-controlled trial. Ann Intern Med 1988;108:675–9.

404 Vance JC, Bart BJ, Hansen RC, et al. Intralesional recombinant alpha-2 interferon for the treatment of patients with condyloma acuminatum or verruca plantaris. Arch Dermatol 1986;122:272–7.

405 Welander CE, Homesley HD, Smiles KA, Peets EA. Intralesional interferon alfa-2b for the treatment of genital warts. Am J Obstet Gynecol 1990;162:348–54.

CHAPTER 11

Human immunodeficiency virus

Ravindra K. Gupta & Brian J. Angus

Primary HIV infection

Case presentation 1

A 52-year-old homosexual man is feeling unwell with fever, malaise, a diffuse maculopapular rash and lymphadenopathy. He holidays regularly in Thailand and has had unprotected receptive anal sexual intercourse with a regular Thai partner as well as contact with five commercial sex workers in Bangkok. You suspect he has primary HIV infection and ask how best to make the diagnosis and whether he should be treated with antiretroviral drugs immediately.

Diagnostic confirmation

A study of 258 persons screened for primary HIV infection (PHI) compared the sensitivity and specificity of clinical symptoms, three HIV-1 RNA viral load assays, a p24 antigen enzyme immunoassay (EIA), and a third-generation enzyme immunoassay antibody test [1]. The symptoms most strongly associated with PHI in multivariate analysis were fever (odds ratio [OR] 5.2; 95% CI 2.3–11.7) and rash (OR 4.8; 95% CI 2.4–9.8). The sensitivity and specificity, respectively, for detecting pre-seroconversion HIV infection were: p24 antigen, 79% and 99%; third-generation EIA, 79% and 97%; HIV-1 RNA by branched chain DNA, 100% and 95%; HIV-1 RNA by polymerase chain reaction (PCR), 100% and 97%; HIV-1 RNA by transcription-mediated amplification

testing, 100% and 98%. False-positive HIV-1 RNA tests were not reproducible and had values <3000 copies/mL, while only one person with confirmed PHI was in this range. PCR is still relatively expensive with longer turnaround times than enzyme-linked tests. Some fourth-generation antibody tests combine the detection of HIV antibodies with that of viral p24 antigen and can detect infection as early as 6 weeks post-exposure. Qualitative detection of HIV-1 RNA in saliva (when plasma levels are >4000 copies/mL) is now possible [2]. This test may be useful in diagnosing acute infection in adults as well as vertical infection in infants.

A number of rapid HIV antibody tests are available, sometimes referred to as "point-of-care" [3]. One of these is suitable for oral fluids [4]. Sensitivity and specificity were compared with results of the EIA and Western blot. OraQuick™ sensitivity was 99.7% with whole blood and 99.1% with oral fluid from 327 persons who were HIV-antibody positive by the conventional algorithm. Specificity was 99.9% with whole blood and 99.6% with oral fluid from 12 010 HIV-negative persons; EIA specificity was 99.7%. These results suggest that the oral fluid antibody test is comparable to EIA tests and useful as a convenient screening tool.

Early treatment

In PHI there are no data on long-term clinical outcomes. Any perceived benefit comes from *in vitro* studies showing better immunologic responses [5,6]. There is one randomized study from 1993 of zidovudine monotherapy versus placebo for 6 months in 77 patients with PHI [7]. There was no difference in the mean duration of the retroviral syndrome. Minor opportunistic infections (oral candidiasis, herpes zoster,

Evidence-Based Infectious Diseases, 2nd edition. Edited by Mark Loeb, Fiona Smaill and Marek Smieja. © 2009 Wiley-Blackwell Publishing, ISBN: 978-1-4051-7026-0

and oral hairy leukoplakia) were less frequent in the zidovudine group (one infection) than in the placebo group (seven infections; $P = 0.009$ by the log-rank test). After adjustment for baseline CD4 cell count, the patients treated with zidovudine had an average gain of 8.9 CD4 cells/mm^3 per month (95% CI 1.4–19.1), whereas those receiving placebo had an average loss of 12.0 CD4 cells/mm^3 per month (95% CI 5.2–18.7), for a between-group difference of 20.9 CD4 cells/mm^3 per month (95% CI 8.5–33.2; $P < 0.001$). No long-term clinical benefits were found. The impact of short-term and longer-term treatment in PHI with highly active antiretroviral therapy (HAART) is currently being investigated by the international SPARTAC study.

Asymptomatic HIV infection

There is no good clinical evidence for when to start antiretroviral drug therapy in asymptomatic HIV-positive individuals. There is one Cochrane review (search date not stated, five randomized controlled trials [RCTs], 7722 people with asymptomatic HIV mainly with CD4 counts >200 cells/mm^3) comparing zidovudine given immediately versus zidovudine deferred until the early signs of AIDS [8]. It found that immediate versus deferred treatment significantly increased AIDS-free survival at 1 year (78/4431 [1.76%] with immediate zidovudine vs 131/3291 [3.98%] with deferred zidovudine; OR 0.52; 95% CI 0.39–0.68), but the difference was not significant at the end of the studies (median follow-up of 50 months; 1026/4431 [23.2%] with immediate zidovudine v 882/3291 [26.8%] with deferred zidovudine; OR 0.96; 95% CI 0.87–1.05). Overall survival was similar in the two groups at 1 year. The conclusion was that, although an initial effect was seen, this was not sustained. There is as yet no similar evidence for HAART. Results from treatment interruption studies (discussed later) have led some experts to recommend initiation of HAART at CD4 counts above 350 cells/mm^3, although there is at present no direct evidence on which to base this [9,10].

As far as harm from early zidovudine is concerned, in a metaanalysis of pooled toxicity data, early treatment in asymptomatic persons conferred a small but significant increase in the risk of anemia (relative risk [RR] of hemoglobin <8.0 g/dL, early vs deferred treatment 2.1; 95% CI 1.1–4.1; absolute risk [AR] 0.4 events per 100 person-years) [11]. There was also a small increase in risk of neutropenia with

early treatment (AR 1.1 events per 100 person-years; $P = 0.07$).

Epidemiology of drug resistance, baseline genotyping, and response to HAART

The prevalence of mutations associated with drug resistance in treatment-naive patients differs among demographic regions and likely reflects access to antiretroviral therapy. In a multicenter US study, 14% of 371 isolates from treatment-naive patients had at least one resistance mutation [12]. A European study known as CATCH assessed resistance in over 1630 newly infected people between 1996 and 2002 [13]. Overall, primary resistance mutations were detected in 10%. A larger European study named SPREAD (Strategy to Control Spread of HIV Drug Resistance) gathered resistance and clinical data from 2008 newly infected and ART-naive HIV patients [14]. Thirteen percent had nucleoside reverse transcriptase inhibitor (NRTI) mutations at the start of follow-up period, but this decreased by half over time; the frequency of non-nucleoside reverse transcriptase inhibitor (NNRTI) resistance mutations increased from 2.3% to 9.8%, and protease inhibitor (PI) resistance remained stable at 3–4%. An increase in resistance over time was also observed in non-B subtypes (from 2.0% in 1996–98 to 8.2% in 2000–01), reflecting increasing access to HAART in areas where non-B subtypes predominate. There have been recent data to suggest that the prevalence of resistance in the UK may be falling [15]. A peak in the number of individuals with transmitted drug resistance was observed in 2001–02, when one or more major resistance mutations were detected in 14% of all patients. By the end of 2004, however, only 8% of untreated individuals had resistance, a highly significant decline (P trend < 0.001). Among patients with recent infection, a similar pattern was detected, but the downward trend in the transmission of resistance occurred approximately 2 years earlier, from 2000 onwards (P trend = 0.002).

Transmission of drug-resistant virus

The clinical impact of acquiring a transmitted drug-resistant virus (TDR) in cohorts of seroconverters has been studied up to 1 year, and no significant difference was found between patients harboring TDR and those without on CD4 counts [16]. It is unclear whether unfit virus with a lower capacity to replicate will mean slower progression but the survey of 101 seroconverters found no evidence of a slower rate of disease progression, measured as time from estimated seroconversion date to a CD4 cell count of 350 cells/mm^3. Similar conclusions were reached in a 3-year follow-up of 46 Spanish seroconverters with available baseline genotypes [17]. However, San Francisco researchers have produced contradictory findings. They identified 130 seroconverters diagnosed since 1996, and found that those with genotypic evidence of drug resistance or virus with reduced replication capacity had significantly higher CD4 cell counts after controlling for duration of infection [18].

Transmitted primary resistance can persist for a long time. In the Spanish study, 10 patients with primary resistance mutations were followed over a median time of 41 months. In only one case was reversion to wild type observed after 7 years [17].

Transmitted resistance mutations can limit treatment options and reduce treatment response rates [19–23]. A retrospective study with 202 patients showed that, when initiating treatment without information on preexisting resistance, patients with preexisting mutations had a slower treatment response and a higher risk of treatment failure [20]. However, on careful consideration of any preexisting resistance, primary treatment success is often possible [24]. Most guidelines now recommend baseline genotyping in new patients to guide therapy [25,26] and it is considered to be cost-effective [27].

Transmission rates of resistant virus are possibly underestimated. Minority viral populations below 25% are not detected by standard sequencing techniques. Forty-nine virus isolates from acute seroconverters were tested for the presence of L90M, K103N, and M184V by quantitative realtime PCR using specific oligonucleotides for the three key resistance mutations [28]. In 10 out of 49 patients these mutants were detected. In 5 of these 10 patients the detected population represented a minor viral quasi-species and was not detected by direct sequencing.

Prognostic features for progression of disease

There is conflicting evidence about the value of viral load at baseline. Early studies suggested that high viral load was associated with an increased risk of death and it is associated with a more rapid fall in CD4 count [29]. However, an updated analysis of outcomes

for people starting HAART showed only a small effect of viral load influencing outcome [30]. During 61 798 person-years of follow-up, there were 1303 AIDS events and 1005 deaths. The risk of disease progression at 1 to 5 years after beginning treatment was calculated according to five key baseline variables: CD4 count, viral load, age, transmission category, and CDC stage. Overall, a CD4 count <200 cells/mm^3, viral load > 5 log (100 000 copies/mL), age > 50, being an injecting drug user, and being in CDC stage 3 predicted a poorer outcome. (There is a useful online risk calculator at http://www.art-cohort-collaboration.org)

Summary

Nucleic acid-based tests are sensitive and specific for the diagnosis of primary HIV infection. Newer methods may be available for rapid "near patient" testing. There are no published RCTs evaluating delayed versus early treatment with HAART, although most guidelines now suggest treatment for symptomatic early disease and CD4 counts of 350 cells/mm^3 and higher [10,31]. RCTs conducted when zidovudine was the only drug available found no significant difference between immediate versus delayed treatment in survival at 1 year despite early changes in surrogate markers. The increase in transmitted drug resistance means that baseline genotyping is recommended to guide therapy.

Case presentation 1 (continued)

The patient tests positive for HIV antibody on multiple ELISA tests. His CD4 count is 560 cells/mm^3 with a HIV viral load of 100 000 copies/mL by PCR which is Clade E and found to be wild type. He is HBV, HCV, and VDRL negative. He is offered treatment because he is symptomatic but declines it. He has a calculated risk of AIDS after starting HAART of 7.4% (95% CI 6.3–8.6) and of death of 3.2% (95% CI 2.5–3.9) at the end of year 3 of treatment.

Tuberculosis

Case presentation 2

A 38-year-old female asylum seeker from Ethiopia is admitted directly from an airport health screening

continued

Case presentation 2 (continued)

clinic. She has an abnormal chest radiograph with a cough, hemoptysis, and weight loss. On examination she has a fever with a temperature of 38.2°C, a pulse of 80 per minute, blood pressure 142/80 mmHg, and respiratory rate of 24 per minute. She looks pale and has widespread lymphadenopathy and hepatosplenomegaly. Her full blood count shows a hemoglobin of 8.4 g/dL, white cell count of 4.3×10^9/L, platelets of 166×10^9/L. Blood film is normochromic and normocytic and there are no malarial parasites seen on three occasions. Biochemistry is normal. Her chest radiograph shows left apical infiltration. She tests seropositive for HIV-1 infection, hepatitis B surface and core antibody positive, but she is HBV-antigen negative. She is hepatitis C seronegative and VDRL negative. CD4 count is 310 cells/mm³, viral load 70 000 copies/mL. You suspect she has *Mycobacterium tuberculosis* infection complicating HIV infection. She has evidence of previous hepatitis B infection. You question how best to confirm the diagnosis of tuberculosis (TB) and what your treatment options are.

The prevalence of *Mycobacterium tuberculosis*/HIV coinfection worldwide is 0.36% and 511 000 incident TB cases (9%) have HIV infection [32]. Of the estimated 33.2 million people currently living with HIV infection, 22.5 million of them are in Africa [33]. An estimated 1.84 million (1.59–2.22 million) people died of TB in 2000 of which 12% were attributable to HIV; in South Africa the attributable rate was 59%. The overall case fatality rate of HIV-infected TB cases has been estimated to be over 50%. Eighty percent of all incident TB cases have been found in 22 developing countries and nine of ten countries with the highest incidence rates per capita were in Africa.

Diagnosis

Significant clinical differences have been found between patients who are sputum-smear positive with acid-fast bacilli (AFB) and those who are smear negative with respect to cough, sputum production, and typical chest radiograph appearance (79%, 76%, and 79% sensitivity, respectively, for smear positive compared with 46%, 43%, and 40% for smear negative) [34]. In this study, there was no difference between HIV-positive and HIV-negative patients.

Sputum samples are just as likely to be AFB positive in HIV-positive as HIV-negative patients [35] and induced sputum may increase the yield [36]. Concentration methods of liquefied sputum in a large cohort of consecutive patients with suspected pulmonary TB showed that the overall sensitivity increased from 54.2% using conventional direct microscopy to 63.1% after concentration ($P = 0.015$) [37]. In HIV-positive patients, sensitivity increased from 38.5% to 50.0% ($P = 0.0034$).

Treatment

The efficacy of a 6-month short-course quadruple drug regimen of chemotherapy for pulmonary TB in the presence of HIV infection was confirmed in a study performed in Kinshasa, Zaire [38]. After 6 months, the rates of treatment failure between HIV-positive and HIV-negative participants were similar at 3.8% and 2.7%, respectively. At 24 months, the HIV-positive patients who received 6 months' extended treatment of rifampicin and isoniazid twice weekly had a relapse rate of 1.9%, as compared with 9% among the HIV-positive patients who received placebo for the second 6 months ($P = 0.01$). Extended treatment, however did not improve survival.

A prospective cohort study comparing a daily regimen of ethambutol, isoniazid, rifampicin, and pyrazinamide for 2 months, followed by ethambutol and isoniazid three times weekly for 6 months (2EHRZ/6E3H3); or the same initial intensive phase as the first regimen, followed by 4 months or 6 months of daily rifampicin and isoniazid (2EHRZ/4HR) and (2EHRZ/6HR) showed that the 2EHRZ/6E3H3 regimen was safe and effective but had a significant risk of relapse [39]. The relapse rate was 18.2 per 100 person-years observation (PYO) for the intermittent ethambutol arm compared to 9.7/100 PYO ($P = 0.0063$) and 4.8/100 PYO ($P = 0.0001$) in patients treated with 2 EHRZ/4HR or 2EHRZ/6HR, respectively.

A WHO-recommended 8-month regimen based on ethambutol and isoniazid was evaluated in a randomized clinical trial against a 6-month standard regimen in 1355 patients with newly diagnosed smear-positive pulmonary tuberculosis [40]. Subjects were assigned one of three regimens: daily ethambutol, isoniazid, rifampicin, and pyrazinamide for 2 months, followed by ethambutol and isoniazid for 6 months (2EHRZ/6HE); the same drugs but given three times weekly in the initial intensive phase (2[EHRZ]3/6HE); or the same initial intensive phase as the first regimen, followed by 4 months of daily rifampicin and isoniazid (2EHRZ/4HR). At 2 months, a significantly higher proportion of patients assigned the daily intensive phase than of those assigned the three-times-weekly regimen were culture negative (700/828 [85%] vs 333/433 [77%], $P = 0.001$). At 12 months after the end of chemotherapy, the proportions of unfavorable outcomes were 36 of 346 (10%) with 2EHRZ/6HE, 48 of 351 (14%) with 2(EHRZ)3/6HE, and 17 of 347 (5%) with 2EHRZ/4HR. Both 8-month regimens were significantly inferior to the control 6-month standard regimen (difference between control and 2EHRZ/6HE 5.5%, 95% CI 1.6–9.4; between control and 2(EHRZ)3/6HE 8.8%, 95% CI 4.5–13.0). Adverse effects leading to interruption of treatment for 7 days or longer occurred in 28 patients (12 2EHRZ/6HE, five 2[EHRZ]3/6HE, 11 2EHRZ/4HR).

Antituberoulosis prophylaxis

Without prophylaxis, people who are HIV-positive and tuberculin skin test-positive have a 50% or more lifetime risk of developing active TB compared with a 10% lifetime risk in people who are HIV-positive but tuberculin skin test-negative [41]. Two systematic reviews have found that anti-TB prophylaxis reduces the rate of developing active TB and death in the short term in people who are HIV-positive and tuberculin skin test-positive. A Cochrane review identified 11 well-conducted RCTs in 8130 HIV-positive adults from Haiti, Kenya, USA, Zambia, Spain, and Uganda [42]. All evaluated isoniazid (6–12 months) either compared with placebo or combination therapy (3 months). Mean follow-up was 2–3 years, and the main outcomes, stratified by tuberculin skin test positivity, were TB (either microbiologic or clinical) and death. Among tuberculin skin test-positive adults, anti-TB prophylaxis significantly reduced the incidence of TB (RR compared with placebo 0.38; 95% CI 0.25–0.57) and was associated with a trend towards reducing the risk of death (RR compared with placebo 0.80; 95% CI 0.63–1.02). Among tuberculin skin test-negative adults, there was no significant difference in risk of TB (RR compared with placebo 0.83; 95% CI 0.58–1.18) or death. There was a significant increase in adverse drug reactions requiring cessation

of treatment on treatment compared with placebo (RR 2.49; 95% CI 1.64–3.77).

The second review of seven trials with 4529 people compared isoniazid with placebo or no treatment [43]. Among tuberculin skin test-positive participants the incidence of TB was significantly reduced (RR compared with placebo 0.40; 95% CI 0.24–0.65), but this was not so among tuberculin skin test-negative participants (RR compared with placebo 0.84; 95% CI 0.54–1.30). This review found no evidence of any impact on mortality. In this analysis, the estimated RR of stopping treatment because of adverse reactions was 1.36 (95% CI 1.00–1.86) [43].

A metaanalysis concluded that RZ is equivalent to INH in terms of efficacy and mortality in the treatment of latent tuberculosis infection. However, this regimen increases the risk of severe adverse effects compared with INH in non-HIV-infected persons [44].

There is insufficient evidence about the long-term effects of prophylaxis on rates of TB and death, and recent studies have found no evidence of benefit in people who are HIV-positive but tuberculin skin test-negative [45].

Summary

TB remains one of the commonest causes of illness in the world both in HIV-infected and uninfected individuals. The diagnostic and therapeutic approach should be the same. Anti-TB chemoprophylaxis may be useful in HIV-positive people who are also tuberculin skin test-positive. However, in areas with constantly high rates of TB exposure, the impact of this is not clear.

> ### Case presentation 2 (continued)
>
> Her sputum is positive for acid-fast bacilli and she is commenced on rifampicin, isoniazid, pyrazinamide, and ethambutol orally for 6 months. Sputum culture is positive for *Mycobacterium tuberculosis* which is sensitive to rifampicin, pyrazinamide, and ethambutol but resistant to isoniazid and streptomycin.

The main concern in this patient is to treat her TB infection effectively. She is at some risk of hepatotoxicity (see later). Since this patient's CD4 count is adequate it would be prudent not to commence any other potentially hepatotoxic drugs or drugs that potentially may interact with her anti-TB therapy; starting HAART can probably be safely deferred. Careful consideration needs to be given to the risk of the patient having multidrug-resistant tuberculosis (MDR-TB). Previously in the UK the main risk was from people previously treated for TB, but nowadays travel is important. Twenty-nine papers were eligible for a metaanalysis [46]. The pooled risk of MDR-TB was 10.23 times higher in previously treated than in never-treated cases, with wide heterogeneity between studies. Study design and geographic area were associated with MDR-TB risk estimates in previously treated patients; the risk estimates were higher in cohort studies carried out in western Europe (RR 12.63; 95% CI 8.20–19.45) than in eastern Europe (RR 8.53; 95% CI 6.57–11.06). MDR-TB cases were more likely to be foreign born (OR 2.46; 95% CI 1.86–3.24), younger than 65 years (OR 2.53; 95% CI 1.74–4.83), male (OR 1.38; 95% CI 1.16–1.65), and HIV positive (OR 3.52; 95% CI 2.48–5.01).

Pneumocystis jiroveci (carinii) pneumonia

Case presentation 3

A 42-year-old Zimbabwean male nurse presents to the Accident and Emergency Department. He is short of breath on exertion and has a fever of 39°C, pulse 110 per minute, and a blood pressure of 110/76 mmHg. Pulse oximetry shows an oxygen saturation of 83% on room air. You suspect Pneumocystis jiroveci pneumonia (PCP) and wonder how best to investigate and manage him.

PCP remains the most common AIDS-related opportunistic infection (OI), usually occurring among those not receiving primary care [47].

Diagnosis

Kovacs et al. [48] described the differences between the clinical characteristics of PCP in 49 HIV-infected and in 39 HIV-negative persons. At presentation, patients with AIDS had a longer median duration of symptoms (28 vs 5 days) and higher median room air arterial oxygen tension (69 vs 52 mmHg, 9.2–6.9 kPa). In HIV-positive patients presenting with respiratory symptoms the sensitivity of induced sputum for the diagnosis of *P. carinii* was 13% and of BAL 77%. In the subgroup of patients with an adequate induced sputum sample, the sensitivity of induced sputum was 28% [49]. The sensitivities of different stains for detection of *P. carinii* in induced sputum were 92% with silver stain, 97% with direct immunofluorescent antibody (DFA), 97% with indirect immunofluorescent antibody (IFA), and 92% with Diff-Quik (DQ) (a modified Giemsa stain). The sensitivities for detection in bronchoalveolar lavage (BAL) were 86% with silver stain, 90% with DFA, 86% with IFA, and 81% with DQ [50]. PCR seems to be more sensitive than any of these methods [51] but newer molecular techniques are still not in routine clinical use [52,53].

Typical radiographic features of PCP are bilateral, symmetrical ground-glass opacities, but a wide variety of radiographic findings are observed. In 34 patients, high-resolution computed tomography of the lung showed ground-glass opacities sparing the lung periphery (41% of episodes) or displaying a mosaic pattern (29%), or being nearly homogeneous (24%), ground-glass opacities associated with air-space consolidation (21%), associated with cystic formation (21%), associated with linear-reticular opacities (18%), patchily and irregularly distributed (15%), associated with solitary or multiple nodules (9%), and associated with parenchymal cavity lesions (6%) [54].

Treatment

In the pre-AIDS era, co-trimoxazole (trimethoprim-sulfamethoxazole, TMP-SMX) was shown to be as effective as pentamidine in children with PCP and with fewer side effects [55]. In a study of PCP in HIV, 31 (86%) patients treated with co-trimoxazole and 20 (61%) with pentamidine survived and were without respiratory support at completion of treatment (95% CI for the difference in response, 5 to 45; $P = 0.03$) [56]. The arterial alveolar oxygen gradient ([A–a] DO$_2$) improved by greater than 1.3 kPa (10 mmHg) 8 days earlier for co-trimoxazole recipients (95% CI for the difference in response, −1 to 17; $P = 0.04$). Co-trimoxazole caused a rash (44%) and anemia (39%) more frequently ($P = 0.03$), whereas pentamidine caused nephrotoxicity (64%), hypotension (27%), or hypoglycemia (21%) more frequently ($P = 0.01$).

There is evidence from RCTs that corticosteroids are a useful adjunct to therapy in severe PCP. Six studies were included in a metaanalysis [57]. Risk ratios for overall mortality for adjunctive corticosteroids were 0.54 (95% CI 0.38–0.79) at 1 month and 0.67 (95% CI 0.49–0.93) at 3–4 months of follow-up. Numbers needed to treat, to prevent one death, are nine patients in a setting without highly active antiretroviral therapy (HAART) available and 22 patients with HAART available. Only the three largest trials provided data on the need for mechanical ventilation with a risk ratio of 0.37 (95% CI 0.20–0.70) in favor of adjunctive corticosteroids.

In mild disease (O_2 saturations >90% by pulse oximetry), early deterioration developed in 7/12 patients on placebo and 1/11 patients taking 60 mg per day oral prednisolone respectively ($P = 0.027$). Even though patients suffering early deterioration in the placebo group were switched to corticosteroids, significant differences between the groups remained at day 30 with regard to exercise tolerance [58].

Alternative treatments

The combination of clindamycin plus primaquine appears to be the most effective alternative treatment for patients with PCP who are unresponsive to first-line therapy [59]. In a metaanalysis of 27 published clinical drug trials, case series, and case reports 497 patients with microbiologically confirmed PCP (456 with HIV), whose initial antipneumocystis treatment had failed and who required alternative drug therapy, were reviewed. Efficacies of salvage regimens were as follows: clindamycin-primaquine 42–44 (88–92%) of 48 patients, $P < 0.001$; atovaquone 4/5 (80%); eflornithine hydrochloride 40/70 (57%), $P = 0.01$; co-trimoxazole 27/51 (53%), $P = 0.08$; pentamidine 64/164 (39%); and trimetrexate 47/159 (30%).

Summary

PCP remains the most common AIDS-related OI and there is good evidence supporting the use of co-trimoxazole and, if severe, steroids for its treatment.

Case presentation 3 (continued)

PCP is suspected on CXR and confirmed on silver staining of BAL fluid and he recovers well with intravenous co-trimoxazole therapy and steroids. He is continued on oral co-trimoxazole as secondary prophylaxis.

Antiretroviral regimen selection and adherence

Case presentation 4

A 28-year-old homeless, intravenous drug user is admitted with widespread psoriasis to the dermatology ward. He is found to have diffuse generalized lymphadenopathy and oral candidiasis. He is tested for HIV and found to be positive. His CD4 count is 120 cells/mm^3 and the viral load is >500 000 copies/mL. He is hepatitis C antibody-positive, HCV RNA-positive and hepatitis B surface antigen-negative. He wants to know what treatment you would recommend and you consider what might be useful in helping him to adhere to the treatment plan.

Which drugs to start?

Current first-line ART combination strategies are the result of historic developments in antiviral therapy, with the NRTIs being the first class to show clinical benefits. Therapy with a single NRTI followed by dual NRTIs however resulted in viral, immunologic, and clinical failure due to viral resistance, but with the use of three agents from two classes a sharp decline in AIDS morbidity and mortality was observed [60].

Number of drugs in first-line regimen

The question of which drugs to start in the treatment of naive patients is still unanswered [10] and unlikely to be addressed in a large enough trial; however, a large systematic review has provided evidence that three drugs are better than two, and two are better than monotherapy [61]. There were 20 404 patients included in the 54 RCTs with 66 comparison groups included in the analysis. For both the clinical outcomes and surrogate markers, combinations with up to, and including, three drugs (HAART) were progressively and significantly more effective. The odds ratio for disease progression or death for triple therapy compared with double therapy was 0.6 (95% CI 0.5–0.8). There was heterogeneity in effect sizes probably related to the different drugs used and differences in trial design.

A Cochrane review has shown that in HIV-infected adults who have responded to an initial three- or four-drug regimen, a two-drug maintenance regimen is associated with a higher risk of virologic failure compared with three or four drugs (OR 5.55; 95% CI 3.14–9.80) [62]. Other induction-maintenance regimens have been studied. The Forte trial compared induction with four drugs and maintenance with three drugs (two NRTIs, one NNRTI and one PI for 24 to 32 weeks, until viral load <50 copies/mL, followed by two NRTIs and one NNRTI compared with a standard dual NRTI and a single NNRTI regimen) [63]. More patients in the three-drug arm had virologic failure at 24 and 32 weeks. After 48 weeks, more patients in the induction/maintenance arm had viral loads below 50 copies/mL. There were no significant differences in the number of patients with serious adverse events or progression to AIDS or death between the two arms. In contrast, the TIME study did not provide support for a four-drug approach; patients were treated with AZT, 3TC, abacavir, and efavirenz for 48 weeks, then randomized to continue with the four-drug regimen or to drop efavirenz [64]. Despite low tolerability of the initial four-drug combination, intent-to-treat analysis revealed that the two approaches were equivalent at week 72. A similar approach was tested in the ESS40013 study, again with no significant differences in the proportions of patients with viral loads below 50 copies/mL and time to treatment failure between the two arms of the study 48 weeks after withdrawal of efavirenz from the maintenance arm [65].

Triple nucleoside vs dual nucleoside plus NNRTI

There are no data concerning which drugs have superior clinical outcomes. Recent studies looking at surrogate markers, in particular a drop in viral load to below a detectable level at 48 weeks seem to favor efavirenz-containing combinations. ACTG 5095 showed that efavirenz plus zidovudine-lamivudine with or without abacavir was virologically superior to the triple nucleoside combination of zidovudine-lamivudine-abacavir (Trizivir™) with 61% (95% CI 50–72%) having HIV-1 RNA <50 copies/mL at week 48 in the triple nucleoside group compared to 83% (95% CI 78–88%) in the combined efavirenz groups [66]. Triple nucleoside analogs alone are not recommended as standard therapy for this reason [10]. There was, however, no significant difference in CD4 count rise at the end of the follow-up period between groups.

Efavirenz vs nevirapine as NNRTI

Nevirapine may be as potent as efavirenz for up to 48 weeks. In a large international trial comparing these two NNRTIs 1216 antiretroviral-naive patients were randomized to receive nevirapine once daily, nevirapine twice daily, efavirenz, or a combination of efavirenz and nevirapine [67]. All patients took a background combination of lamivudine and stavudine. Viral suppression rates below the limit of detectability (<50 copies/mL) were as follows: 70.0% (95% CI 63.5–76.0) for nevirapine once daily, 65.4% (95% CI 60.4–70·1) for nevirapine twice daily, 70.0% (95% CI 65.2–74.5) for efavirenz, and 62.7% (95% CI 55.7–69.3) for nevirapine plus efavirenz. Overall, there were no significant differences in any of the four pairwise comparisons. These results, however relate to surrogate markers and not to clinical outcome; there was more hepatic toxicity in the nevirapine arms and adverse events were higher in the dual NNRTI arm.

NNRTI vs boosted PI as third agent

ACTG 5142 recruited 757 antiretroviral-naive people with a viral load >2000 copies/mL and any CD4 count (median 182 cells/mm^3) [68]. The open-label design randomized study participants to standard doses of efavirenz or lopinavir/ritonavir with lamivudine and a second NRTI, or to 533/133 mg of lopinavir/ritonavir twice daily plus standard-dose efavirenz. The primary endpoint was time to virologic failure; the median follow-up was 112 weeks. The time to virologic failure proved significantly faster in people who started lopinavir/ritonavir as the third agent rather than efavirenz ($P = 0.006$). However, people randomized to the boosted PI gained significantly more CD4 cells through 96 weeks than did people taking efavirenz.

The results of the 5-year FIRST trial CPCRA 058 that compared a PI plus NRTI versus NNRTI plus NRTI versus a three-class strategy support ACTG 5142 in finding a better virologic response to first-line NNRTIs than PIs [69]. However of the 1397 enrolled in FIRST, most randomized to NNRTI therapy took efavirenz, while 74% randomized to PIs used no ritonavir boost. The study found no difference between NNRTI and PI regimens in a composite endpoint including CD4 drop, progression to AIDS, and death (NNRTI versus PI hazard ratios [HRs] for the composite endpoint were 1.02 (95% CI

0.79–1.31), 1.07 (0.80–1.41), 0.95 (0.66–1.37), and 0.66 (0.56–0.78), respectively). 1196 patients were assessed for the three-class versus combined two-class primary endpoint. Mean change in CD4 cell count at or after 32 months was +234 cells/mm^3 and +227 cells/mm^3 for the three-class and the combined two-class strategies ($P = 0.62$), respectively. HRs (three-class vs combined two-class) for AIDS or death and virologic failure were 1.15 (0.91–1.45) and 0.87 (0.75–1.00), respectively. Better outcomes with an NNRTI compared with a PI may well be a class effect as similar findings were observed when ritonavir-boosted amprenavir was used as the PI [70].

Choice of NRTI

A large number of studies have been conducted to compare different NRTIs in combination with an NNRTI. None have shown differences in clinical endpoints, although 48-week virologic suppression rates have often favored newer agents such as abacavir and tenofovir. These differences are thought to be related to better tolerability/toxicity profiles rather than antiviral potency. Guidelines in well-resourced settings now recommend against stavudine and didanosine due to long-term toxicity concerns [10].

Side effects and drug–drug interactions associated with HAART

Aside from virologic and immunologic efficacy, there are other considerations when selecting combinations for individual patients. For example, the teratogenicity of efavirenz in animal studies makes it less attractive for women of childbearing age although recent data do not support substituting another drug for efavirenz in pregnancy [71]. Zidovudine is usually avoided in patients with anemia or when anemia can be predicted to occur with treatment such as with ribavirin for HCV [72] or chemotherapy for lymphoma. Nevirapine is more likely to cause severe rashes in women rather than men [73] and is also more likely to cause symptomatic liver function test derangement than efavirenz in women with CD4 counts above 250 cells/mm^3 and in men with CD4 counts above 400 cells/mm^3 [74]. Importantly, drug-drug interactions between rifampicin as part of antituberculosis therapy and nevirapine (a potent hepatic enzyme inducer) and boosted protease inhibitors are also key considerations in selecting regimens for TB/HIV-coinfected patients.

There are complex interactions between antiretroviral drugs and with other drugs. The website http://www.hiv-druginteractions.org/is a useful resource.

Pharmacogenomic screening for HLA-B*5701 is now being recommended, especially in white populations. In a double-blind, prospective randomized study of 1956 patients who had not previously received abacavir, the risk of an abacavir hypersensitivity reaction was reduced in patients who had prospective HLA-B*5701 screening (immunologically confirmed hypersensitivity reaction 0% vs 2.7% in the control group, $P < 0.001$) [75]. As well there was a significantly lower incidence of clinically diagnosed hypersensitivity reaction in the prospectively screened group (3.4%) than in the control group (7.8%) ($P < 0.001$).

The World Health Organization's HIV treatment guidelines panel (http://www.who.int/hiv/art/ART adultsaddendum.pdf) has concluded that the recommended adult dose of stavudine (d4T) should be reduced to 30 mg twice daily for adults weighing more than 60 kg, following a review of a metaanalysis of previously unpublished clinical trials. The analysis shows that a 30 mg dose is just as effective as a 40 mg dose, but carries less risk of side effects such as peripheral neuropathy [76].

Compliance/adherence

Compliance has been shown to be an important factor in the long-term outcome of treatment. It may be that the easiest drug combination to comply with will be the most effective irrespective of drug potency or resistance profile. Adherence to any long-term drug regimen is difficult; however, it is of particular importance in the treatment of HIV because of the propensity of the virus to mutate and escape drug control. Good adherence can predict for viral suppression [77] and the development of viral resistance is associated with low blood drug levels that are usually because of poor adherence [78,79]. Even a 10% increase in adherence can lead to a 20% reduction in disease progression [80]. After controlling for potential confounding variables, patients who were less than 95% adherent to medications were 3.5 times more likely to have treatment failure (HIV-1 RNA >50 copies/mL) than subjects with adherence rates of 95–100%. The strongest predictor of adherence was adverse clinical events (e.g., dermatologic, gastrointestinal symptoms): patients with adverse events were 12.8 times less likely to have 95–100% adherence [81].

To assess the effect of HAART adherence on survival in HIV-infected patients, a cohort study was performed on 1219 patients who began ART during the period 1990–99. In multivariate analysis, the variables that presented significant differences with respect to mortality were clinical stage at the beginning of treatment (AIDS: relative hazard [RH] = 2.97; 95% CI 2.14–4.13), CD4 cell count (<200 cells/mm³: RH = 5.89; 95% CI 3.44–10.10), type of treatment (monotherapy: RH = 9.76; 95% CI 4.56–20.9); two drugs (RH = 9.12; 95% CI 4.23–19.64), and adherence (nonadherence: RH = 3.87; 95% CI 1.77–8.46) [82]. A systematic review of 76 studies showed that once or twice a day was better than more frequent dosing (compliance with one dose = 79% ± 14%; two doses = 69% ± 15%; three doses = 65% ± 16%; four doses = 51% ± 20% ($P < 0.001$ among dose schedules, no significant difference between one and two doses) [83].

The principal factors associated with nonadherence for HAART appear to be mainly patient-related, including homelessness and substance and alcohol abuse, reflecting the types of individuals affected by HIV [84]. Other factors may also contribute, such as inconvenient dosing frequency, dietary restrictions, pill burden, side effects [85], patient healthcare provider relationships, and the system of care [86].

A systematic review on the effectiveness of patient support and education to improve adherence to HAART identified 19 RCTs involving 2159 participants [87]. Study interventions included cognitive behavioral therapy, motivational interviewing, medication management strategies, and interventions indirectly targeting adherence, such as programs to reduce risky sexual behaviors. There is evidence that interventions targeting practical medication management skills and those delivered over at least 12 weeks were associated with improved adherence. Interventions administered to individuals were more effective than group interventions. There was no evidence that interventions targeting women or patients with a history of alcoholic abuse were effective. Overall, effective adherence interventions have not been shown to be associated with improved virologic or immunologic outcomes.

Toxicity

Toxicity is also a determinant of a successful regimen both in terms of tolerability and adherence. Liver enzyme elevation (LEE) defined as transaminases greater than five times baseline or >100 IU/L is commonly observed after combination HAART is begun. Potential risk factors after treatment with ritonavir and saquinavir with or without stavudine were investigated in 208 HIV-infected patients, by use of the Cox proportional hazard model: 18 patients (9%) developed LEE during the 48-week follow-up. Multivariate analysis, adjusted for baseline levels of alanine aminotransferase (ALT) and aspartate aminotransferase (AST), showed that hepatitis B surface antigen (HBsAg) positivity (RR 8.8; 95% CI 3.3–23.1) and the use of stavudine (RR 4.9; 95% CI 1.5–16.0) were the only significant risk factors for developing LEE. After LEE occurred, ALT and AST concentrations decreased by >50% in 13 of 14 patients who continued antiretroviral treatment during LEE. Therefore, in this study, it appeared safe to continue treatment during LEE; however, more data from larger studies are required to confirm this finding [88].

In a retrospective study 65 patients taking HAART were evaluated and 24 were identified to have antiretroviral hepatotoxicity [89]. Patients older than 40 years had a 7-fold increased risk (RR 6.9; 95% CI 1.7–27.3) and those with an absolute CD4 count of <310 cells/mm³ had a 10-fold increased risk (RR 10.2; 95% CI 2.5–41.9) for antiretroviral hepatotoxicity, in comparison with those who were younger or who had a greater absolute CD4 count. Coexisting hepatitis C infection ($P = 0.035$) was significantly associated with hepatotoxicity; of the eight patients documented to have coexisting hepatitis C infection, six (75%) were in the antiretroviral hepatotoxicity group.

In another retrospective study of 394 patients 7% were HBsAg-positive and 14% were anti-HCV-positive [90]. Patients with chronic hepatitis had a higher risk for LEE compared with patients without coinfection: 37% versus 12% respectively. After adjustment for higher baseline transaminases, the presence of HBsAg or anti-HCV remained associated with an increased risk of LEE (RR 2.78; 95% CI 1.50–5.16 and RR 2.46; 95% CI 1.43–4.24, respectively). In patients with LEE, transaminases declined whether HAART was continued or modified. Of patients with chronic HBV infection 38% lost HBeAg or developed anti-HBe after initiation of HAART, and one seroconverted from HBsAg-positive to anti-HBs-positive. However, there was no clear relationship with LEE.

In the Swiss cohort, a prospective analysis revealed 1157 patients (37.2%) were coinfected with HCV, 1015 of whom (87.7%) had a history of intravenous drug use [91]. In multivariate Cox's regression, the probability of progression to a new AIDS-defining clinical event or to death was independently associated with HCV seropositivity (HR 1.7; 95% CI 1.26–2.30), and with active intravenous drug use (HR 1.38; 95% CI 1.02–1.88). Virologic response to HAART and the probability of treatment change were not associated with HCV serostatus. In contrast, HCV seropositivity was associated with a smaller CD4 cell recovery (HR for a CD4 cell count increase of at least 50 cells/mm^3 = 0.79; 95% CI 0.72–0.87).

There is a significantly elevated risk of severe liver disease in persons who are coinfected with HIV and HCV. A metaanalysis to quantify the effect of HIV coinfection on progressive liver disease in persons with HCV revealed eight studies that included outcomes of histologic cirrhosis or decompensated liver disease [92]. These studies yielded a combined adjusted RR of 2.92 (95% CI 1.70–5.01). Studies that examined decompensated liver disease had a combined RR of 6.14 (95% CI 2.86–13.20), whereas studies that examined histologic cirrhosis had a pooled RR of 2.07 (95% CI 1.40–3.07). The PRESCO study suggested that responses to therapy with pegylated interferon and high-dose (1000–1200 mg daily) ribavirin could approach those in non HIV-infected patients and, as had been previously observed, were dependent on HCV genotype [93,94].

Summary

There is no randomized trial evidence as to which drug regimen is most efficacious clinically. There is convincing evidence that three drugs are better than two or one. There has been considerable interest in the use of four drugs as part of an induction/maintenance approach but this has not been widely adopted. Potential increase in potency with four agents needs to be balanced against increased side effects, and there is no convincing body of evidence to support this approach at present. Dual nucleosides are the standard backbone in HAART. There seems to be little to choose between NNRTIs and boosted PIs when considering the third agent, although efavirenz seems to be better tolerated with more durable viral suppression than ritonavir-boosted lopinavir.

Adherence to HAART is critically important and, to facilitate this, drug regimens are becoming simpler, many with once-a-day drugs and no food or fluid restrictions. Once-a-day medications can be given as directly observed therapy combined, for example, with methadone [95] although there are important interactions with methadone and HAART [96]. There is still no consensus on how best to measure adherence. The studies to try to improve adherence through social means and education have been disappointing. Hepatotoxicity remains a challenge especially in the many patients who have coexisting liver disease and may be taking other hepatotoxic drugs. There is a high incidence of substance abuse and psychiatric illness amongst HIV-positive patients, which complicates the ability to take treatment [97].

Opportunistic infection prophylaxis

Although the risk of opportunistic infection has fallen in recent years it increases dramatically once a patient's CD4 count is less than 200 cells/mm^3 [47]. In the UK around 50% of patients present with a CD4 <350 cells/mm^3 and 30% with a CD4 <200 cells/mm^3 [98].

Prophylaxis for PCP

There have been two systematic reviews: Ioannidis et al. searching in 1995 and covering 35 RCTs [99] and Bucher et al. from 1997 [100] covering 22 trials. Both of these were before the widespread introduction of HAART. Since then the incidence of OIs in HIV patients has fallen so much that further studies are unlikely [101,102]. The main focus recently has been on stopping prophylaxis after immune restoration.

The first systematic review found that prophylaxis with co-trimoxazole or aerosolized pentamidine reduced the incidence of PCP more than placebo (RR 0.32; 95% CI 0.23–0.46) and that co-trimoxazole was more effective at preventing PCP than aerosolized pentamidine (RR 0.58; 95% CI 0.45–0.75) [99]. The second review found that co-trimoxazole was significantly more effective in preventing PCP than dapsone/pyrimethamine (RR 0.49; 95% CI 0.26–0.92) [100]. While the second review also showed that co-trimoxazole compared with dapsone (with or without pyrimethamine) was more effective, the result did not reach statistical significance (RR 0.61; 95% CI 0.34–1.10) [99].

There is no significant difference in the rate of PCP infection between lower dose (160/800 mg three times weekly or 80/400 mg daily) and higher dose (160/800 mg daily) co-trimoxazole although severe adverse effects (predominantly rash, fever, and hematologic effects leading to discontinuation within 1 year) occurred in more people taking higher doses of co-trimoxazole than lower doses (25% vs 15%) [99]. One subsequent RCT (2625 people) also found no significant difference in the rate of PCP infection in people receiving co-trimoxazole 160/800 mg daily compared with three times weekly (3.5 vs 4 per 100 person-years) [103]. Discontinuation because of adverse effects was significantly more common in people taking higher doses of co-trimoxazole (RR 2.14; $P < 0.001$).

One RCT of 545 people in sub-Saharan Africa with symptomatic disease (second or third clinical stage disease in the WHO staging system) regardless of CD4 cell count, comparing co-trimoxazole with placebo, found no significant difference in incidence of PCP or toxoplasmosis. Patients taking co-trimoxazole were less likely to suffer a serious event (death or hospital admission, irrespective of the cause) than those on placebo regardless of their initial CD4 cell count (84 vs 124; HR 0.57; 95% CI 0.43–0.75; $P < 0.001$). This implies that in Africa the effect of co-trimoxazole is on preventing bacterial infections, not PCP [104].

Summary
Systematic reviews have found that co-trimoxazole is the most effective prophylactic agent for PCP.

Adverse reactions

Case presentation 4 (continued)

He is started on co-trimoxazole initially. He develops a widespread maculopapular rash with nausea and vomiting. A diagnosis of co-trimoxazole hypersensitivity is made. What are the options for patients who cannot tolerate TMX/SMX?

The gradual initiation of co-trimoxazole may improve tolerance of the regimen (17% vs 33% at 12 weeks) [105]. Two RCTs (238 people; 50 people) found no significant benefit from acetylcysteine in preventing co-trimoxazole hypersensitivity reactions in HIV-infected people [106,107].

Atovaquone, dapsone and aerosolized pentamidine are effective in persons intolerant of co-trimoxazole. There is one RCT of atovaquone in 1057 people intolerant of co-trimoxazole, of whom 298 had a history of PCP [108]. When compared with dapsone there was no significant difference between atovaquone 1500 mg daily compared with dapsone 100 mg daily (15.7 vs 18.4 cases of PCP per 100 person-years; $P = 0.20$). The overall risk of stopping treatment because of adverse effects was similar in the two arms (RR 0.94; 95% CI 0.74–1.19). One RCT with 549 people intolerant of co-trimoxazole compared high-dose with low-dose atovaquone (1500 mg daily vs 750 mg daily) with monthly aerosolized pentamidine (300 mg). It found no significant difference between the groups in the incidence of PCP (26% vs 22% vs 17%) or mortality (20% vs 13% vs 18%) after a median follow-up of 11.3 months [109].

A metaanalysis of 16 trials with 4267 patients evaluating dapsone toxicity found no significant difference in mortality for dapsone (OR for mortality for dapsone vs other primary prophylaxis 1.11; 95% CI 0.96–1.29) [110,111]. Detels el al. found that adverse effects were dose-related for dapsone (low vs high dose: 29% vs 12%) [111].

Azithromycin, rifabutin, and both drugs in combination, added to standard PCP prophylaxis were compared in an RCT. Azithromycin, either alone or in combination with rifabutin, reduced the risk of developing PCP by 45% when compared with rifabutin alone ($P = 0.008$) [112]. Gastrointestinal side effects are common with azithromycin, but they are usually mild and do not lead to stopping treatment when used for mycobacterial infection. The addition of rifabutin significantly increased the risk of stopping treatment (RR 1.67; $P = 0.03$) [113].

Concomitant coverage for toxoplasmosis
Co-trimoxazole was more effective at preventing toxoplasmosis than aerosolized pentamidine (RR 0.78; 95% CI 0.55–1.11), but there was no significant difference between co-trimoxazole and dapsone/

pyrimethamine (RR 1.17; 95% CI 0.68–2.04) [100]. Toxoplasmosis risk is probably clinically meaningful only with CD4 < 100 cells/mm^3 and positive toxoplasma serology [114].

Case presentation 4 (continued)

The patient is commenced on dapsone and then 2 weeks later zidovudine, lamivudine, and efavirenz. His viral load falls to undetectable and CD4 count climbs to 320 cells/mm^3 within 6 months. He has some problems with recurrent cold sores. You wonder how to manage his herpes infection and when his PCP prophylaxis can be safely stopped.

Treatment of herpes simplex

Famciclovir and valacyclovir are effective for the suppression of herpes simplex virus (HSV) reactivation [115,116] and valacyclovir has been shown to be equivalent to acyclovir [117].

Stopping *Pneumocystis* prophylaxis

In the metaanalysis of 14 randomized and nonrandomized studies with 3584 subjects who had discontinued prophylaxis when their CD4 count was sustained >200 cells/mm^3 for 3 months, eight cases of PCP occurred during 3449 person-years (0.23 cases per 100 person-years; 95% CI 0.10–0.46) [118]. In the decision analysis, mortality and time spent alive without immunodeficiency in the modeled discontinuation strategy were similar to those in the continuation strategy. For patients who received primary prophylaxis, the discontinuation strategy led to slightly fewer episodes of PCP and fewer toxicity-related prophylaxis withdrawals (8.6 vs 34.5 cases per 100 patients during a 10-year period). Comparative results were similar for patients on secondary prophylaxis. The review found a low incidence of PCP in people discontinuing both primary and secondary prophylaxis after a mean of 1.5 years (7/3035 [0.23%] with discontinuing primary prophylaxis and 1/549 [0.18%] discontinuing secondary prophylaxis; mean annual incidence over 1.5 years 0.23%; 95% CI 0.10–0.46%; no statistical heterogeneity among studies). Neither of the two RCTs identified in the review found any cases of PCP after discontinuation [119,120]. A total of 146 patients were enrolled

in a randomized study of stopping secondary prophylaxis (77 in the treatment discontinuation arm). After >2 years, one definitive and one presumptive case of PCP were observed, both of which occurred in patients who discontinued therapy [121].

Prophylaxis for PCP was withdrawn in 524 patients (426 primary and 98 secondary prophylaxis), prophylaxis for *Mycobacterium avium* complex (MAC) was withdrawn in 28 patients (13 primary and 15 secondary), and prophylaxis for cytomegalovirus (CMV) retinitis was withdrawn in 10 patients [122]. CD4 counts were generally maintained above accepted prophylaxis threshold levels during the period of follow-up (95–98% of the time). Total follow-up to last report or reinitiation of prophylaxis was 680 and 144 person-years for patients discontinuing primary and secondary PCP prophylaxis, respectively. No cases of PCP were reported, giving incidence rates of 0.0 (upper 95% confidence limit 0.4) and 0.0 (2.1) per 100 person-years. No cases of MAC were reported, but one patient had a recurrence of CMV retinitis. PCP prophylaxis was restarted in 30 patients; no patients restarted MAC or CMV prophylaxis.

Nineteen patients with suppressed viral loads but CD4 counts below 200 cells/mm^3 were followed after prophylaxis was discontinued. Eleven had been taking daily TMP-SMX, seven were receiving monthly aerosolized pentamidine, and one patient never received any prophylaxis [123]. The median CD4 count at the time of discontinuation and at the most recent determination was 120 (range 34–184) and 138 (range 6–201) cells/mm^3 respectively. At the time of reporting, patients had been off PCP prophylaxis for a median of 9.0 (range 3–39) months (261 patient-months). No patient developed PCP. This is significantly different from the risk of developing PCP with a CD4 count of <200 cells/mm^3 in untreated HIV infection (rate difference 9.2%; 95% CI 5.7–12.8%; $P < 0.05$).

There is also no change in incidence of other bacterial infections after stopping prophylaxis [124].

Toxoplasmosis

There are three RCTs. The first, which was included in the systematic review, found no cases of toxoplasma encephalitis at 6 months in people discontinuing prophylaxis (see PCP above) [120]. The second RCT (302 people with a satisfactory response to HAART) compared discontinuation with continuation of toxoplasma prophylaxis [125]. After a median of 10 months it found no episodes of toxoplasma encephalitis in either group.

The efficacy of a thrice-weekly regimen was similar to that of a daily regimen in the prevention of relapses of toxoplasma encephalitis in a RCT in 124 Spanish patients. Administration of antiretroviral therapy was the only factor associated with a lower incidence of relapse [126].

Case presentation 4 (continued)

He returns after 6 months with CD4 now 400 cells/mm^3 and viral load undetectable. However after the death of a close friend it soon becomes apparent that he has developed a chaotic lifestyle, abusing substances, and has problems with taking regular medication. He decides not to attend the clinic for a while and is lost to follow-up. After 3 years he returns with a CD4 count of 50 cells/mm^3 and an increasing viral load. He has been intermittently attending another clinic and his current medication is stavudine, didanosine, abacavir, ritonavir, and fosamprenavir. Viral resistance testing, viral phenotyping, and therapeutic drug monitoring may be used to guide therapy in this circumstance but the situation is far from clear.

Genotypic resistance testing

There are three RCTs showing a benefit of genotypic resistance testing plus expert advice for patients failing HAART. A total of 326 HIV-1-infected patients on stable HAART with virologic failure were studied. The baseline CD4 cell count and plasma HIV-1 RNA were 387 ($\pm$224) cells/mm^3 and 4 ($\pm$1) log respectively. The proportion of patients with plasma HIV-1 RNA < 400 copies/mL at 24 weeks differed between genotyping and no genotyping arms (48.5 and 36.2%; P < 0.05). Factors associated with a higher probability of plasma HIV-1 RNA < 400 copies/mL were HIV-1 genotyping (OR 1.7; 95% CI 1.1–2.8; P = 0.016) and the expert advice in patients failing a second-line HAART (OR 3.2; 95% CI 1.2–8.3; P = 0.016) [127].

To compare standard care (control, n = 43) or treatment according to the resistance mutations in protease and reverse transcriptase genes (genotypic group, n = 65), 108 patients were enrolled in the VIRADAPT study [128]. At month 3, the mean change in HIV-1 RNA was −1.04 log in the study group compared with −0.46 log in the control group (mean difference 0.58 log; 95% CI 0.14–1.02; P = 0.01). At month 6, changes were 1.15 (0.15) log copies/mL, and 0.67 (0.19) log copies/mL in the genotypic group and the control group, respectively (mean difference 0.48 log; P = 0.05). At month 3, HIV-1 RNA was lower than detection level (200 copies/mL) in 29% (19/65) of patients in the genotypic group versus 14% (6/43) in the control group (P = 0.017). At month 6, the values were 32% (21/65) and 14% (6/43) (P = 0.067) for the genotypic group and the control group, respectively. Therapy was generally well tolerated, with 10 patients (six in the genotypic group, four in the control group) requiring toxic effect-related drug modification.

In the genotypic antiretroviral resistance testing (GART) study, 153 HIV-infected adults, with a 3-fold or greater rise in plasma HIV-1 RNA on at least 16 weeks of combination HAART, were randomized either to a GART group, where genotype interpretation and suggested regimens were provided to clinicians, or to a no-GART group, where treatment choices were made without such input [129]. HIV-1 RNA, averaged at 4 and 8 weeks following randomization, decreased by 1.19 log for the 78 GART patients and 0.61 log for the 75 no-GART patients (treatment difference: 0.53 log; 95% CI 0.77, 0.29; P = 0.00001). Overall, the best virologic responses occurred in patients who received three or more drugs to which their HIV-1 appeared to be susceptible. A note of caution is given here as discrepant results in "expert" interpretation of genotype resistance data have been shown [130].

In the CREST study 327 patients completing $\geqslant$1 month of follow-up were included in a randomized, open-label trial over 48 weeks to receive a genotype (group A) or genotype plus virtual phenotype (group B) prior to selection of their regimen [131]. At 48 weeks, there were no significant differences between the groups for mean change from baseline plasma HIV RNA (group A: 0.68 log copies/mL, group B: 0.58 log copies/mL; P = 0.23) and mean change from baseline CD4+ cell count (group A: 37 cells/mm^3, group B: 50 cells/mm^3; P = 0.28).

Viral phenotyping

A total of 272 subjects who failed to achieve or maintain virologic suppression (HIV-1 RNA plasma level

>2000 copies/mL) with previous exposure to two or more nucleoside reverse transcriptase inhibitors and one protease inhibitor were randomized to HAART guided by phenotyping or standard of care [132]. At week 16, using intent-to-treat (ITT) analysis, a greater proportion of subjects had HIV-1 RNA levels < 400 copies/mL in the phenotyping than in the standard-of-care arm ($P = 0.036$, ITT observed; $P = 0.079$, ITT missing equals failure). Subjects in the phenotyping arm had a significantly greater median reduction in HIV-1 RNA levels from baseline than the standard-of-care arm ($P = 0.005$ for 400 copies/mL; $P = 0.049$ for 50 copies/mL assay detection limit). Significantly more subjects in the phenotyping arm were treated with two or more "active" antiretroviral agents than in the standard-of-care arm ($P = 0.003$).

Therapeutic drug monitoring

There are no randomized controlled data to support therapeutic drug monitoring but, in a pharmacologic substudy of VIRADAPT, the impact of plasma protease inhibitor trough levels on changes in HIV RNA were assessed in 81 patients treated with genotypic-guided therapy [133]. Linear regression analysis showed a significant relationship between PI concentration and HIV RNA in the plasma. "Suboptimal" concentration (SOC) was defined as at least two PI plasma levels <2 times IC95 and patients were categorized into four groups: G1 (SOC/control), G2 (OC/control), G3 (SOC/genotype), and G4 (OC/genotype). OC and SOC were found in 67.9% (55/81) and 32.1% (26/81) of patients, respectively. Mean changes in HIV RNA from baseline at month 6 were: -0.23 ± 0.29 log copies/mL (G1); -0.97 ± 0.28 (G2); -0.68 ± 0.37 (G3); -1.38 ± 0.20 (G4). Multivariate analysis showed PI plasma concentrations to be an independent predictor of HIV-RNA evolution ($P = 0.017$).

Management of multiple resistance

The recent BHIVA guidelines addressing this question have three sections – continue, change, or interrupt – but there is no consensus at present [10]. There is evidence from recent trials of new agents that the more active drugs that are available to include in a new regimen in MDR-HIV the better [134,135]. There are an increasing number of new drugs and indeed new classes of drug which are active against MDR-HIV.

There is evidence of increasing accumulation of resistance mutations in continuing a failing regimen. In one study of patients with viral load >200 copies/mL, the average increase per year in the number of mutations was 0.5 for reverse transcriptase (RT) mutations, 0.2 for major PI mutations and 0.3 for minor PI mutations [136].

Structured treatment interruption

Small studies have shown conflicting results for structured treatment interruptions (STI) on surrogate markers, which may be explained by the length of the treatment interruption (on average 8–16 weeks) or on the number of drugs commenced after it (so called mega or giga HAART) [137–139]. There is a multinational clinical trial (OPTIMA) looking at the options in management with antiretrovirals in these so-called salvage therapy patients.

Other clinical trials have shown no benefit. A total of 147 patients were randomized in a Canadian study [140]: 79 to the immediate switch (IS) arm and 68 to the STI arm. Success was achieved by 64% in the IS arm and 51% in the STI arm (95% confidence interval for the difference from 5% in favor of STI to 30% in favor of IS). During the STI, the median decrease in CD4 count was 80 cells/mm and the increase in viral load was 0.8 $\log_{10}$ copies/mL. There were no differences in median CD4 cell counts or HIV RNA levels at week 60. Two unrelated deaths (one in each arm) and three AIDS-defining events (in the STI arm) occurred.

A metaanalysis of 17 studies confirmed a lack of benefit as far as virologic or immunologic endpoints were concerned [141]. There is evidence from the large EUROSIDA cohort that even at low CD4 counts there is a benefit from not stopping therapy [142] and the SMART study has highlighted the increased hazard associated with treatment interruption at any CD4 count [143].

As an interim measure, double boosted PIs have shown some promise in virologic improvement in selected patients [144] as has lamivudine monotherapy [145]. Nucleoside analogs often exert continued antiviral activity in the setting of drug-resistance mutations and both nucleoside analogs and PIs can select for drug-resistance mutations that reduce viral fitness [146]. These strategies need to be investigated further in clinical trials.

Summary

The strategy of treatment interruption is not recommended outside of the setting of a clinical trial. However there may be benefits for patients other than virologic improvement including quality of life and improved adherence with the next regimen, and there does not seem to be much harm to patients as long as they are closely monitored and given appropriate OI prophylaxis.

Treatment and prophylaxis of opportunistic infections (continued)

Case presentation 4 (continued)

The patient decides not to continue with therapy and is adamant that he no longer wants any in the future. He is admitted with increasing confusion, fever, and neck stiffness. Fundoscopy reveals CMV retinitis but no papilledema. His CD4 count is 10 cells/mm³. You consider the possible conditions he is at risk of and how best to manage him.

Table 11.1 lists the usual pathogens related to CD4 count.

Cryptococcal meningitis needs to be excluded by lumbar puncture and staining of cerebrospinal fluid (CSF) with Indian ink.

Case presentation 4 (continued)

The opening pressure is 30 mm of CSF, and CSF is positive for *Cryptococcus* with a white cell count of 115, mainly lymphocytes; a CSF protein of 2.4 g/dL (range −1.6 g/dL), and a glucose of 0.6 mmol/L. A diagnosis of cryptococcal meningitis is made.

Treatment of cryptococcal meningitis

In a double-blind multicenter study, patients with a first episode of AIDS-associated cryptococcal meningitis were randomly assigned to treatment with higher dose amphotericin B (0.7 mg/kg per day) with or without flucytosine (100 mg/kg per day) for

2 weeks (step 1), followed by 8 weeks of treatment with itraconazole (400 mg per day) or fluconazole (400 mg per day) (step 2) [147]. At 2 weeks, the CSF cultures were negative in 60% of the 202 patients receiving amphotericin B plus flucytosine and in 51% of the 179 receiving amphotericin B alone ($P = 0.06$). The clinical outcome did not differ significantly between the two groups. Overall mortality was 5.5% in the first 2 weeks and 3.9% in the next 8 weeks, with no significant difference between the groups. In a multivariate analysis, the addition of flucytosine during the initial 2 weeks and treatment with fluconazole for the next 8 weeks were independently associated with CSF sterilization. As a result standard guidelines for treatment of cryptococcal meningitis recommend 2 weeks of amphotericin B at a dose of 0.7 mg/kg per day (with flucytosine) followed by fluconazole at a dose of 400 mg per day for another 8 weeks.

There is one direct comparison between amphotericin B deoxycholate (0.7 mg/kg per day) and liposomal amphotericin (AmBisome) (4 mg/kg per day) in 27 patients showing that AmBisome therapy resulted in earlier negative CSF cultures [148]. The liposomal amphotericin was less nephrotoxic and this has been confirmed in other studies in HIV-positive patients [149].

In a randomized trial comparing amphotericin B and fluconazole, treatment was successful in 25 of the 63 amphotericin B recipients (40%; 95% CI 26–53) and in 44 of the 131 fluconazole recipients (34%; 95% CI 25–42%; $P = 0.40$) [150]. There was no significant difference between the groups in overall mortality owing to cryptococcosis (amphotericin vs fluconazole, 9 of 63 [4%] vs 24 of 131 [8%]; $P = 0.48$); however, mortality during the first 2 weeks of therapy was higher in the fluconazole group (15% vs 8%; $P = 0.25$). Multivariate analyses identified abnormal mental status (lethargy, somnolence, or obtundation) as the most important predictive factor of death during therapy ($P < 0.0001$). In Africa 30 patients were randomized to receive combination therapy with fluconazole, 200 mg once a day for 2 months, and flucytosine, 150 mg/kg per day) for the first 2 weeks, and 28 to receive fluconazole alone. Patients in both groups who survived for 2 months continued fluconazole as maintenance therapy at a dose of 200 mg three times per week for 4 months. The combination therapy prevented death within 2 weeks and significantly

Table 11.1 Pathogens related to CD4 counts

CD4 count	Infection	Noninfectious complications
>500	Acute HIV syndrome Candida vaginitis	Progressive generalized lymphadenopathy Polymyositis Aseptic meningitis Guillain–Barré syndrome
200–500	Pneumococcal and other bacterial pneumonia Pulmonary tuberculosis Kaposi sarcoma Herpes zoster Thrush Cryptosporidiosis, self-limiting Oral hairy leukoplakia	Carcinoma in situ Cervical cancer Lymphocytic interstitial pneumonitis Mononeuritis multiplex Anemia Idiopathic thrombocytopenia purpura
<200	*Pnemocystis carinii* pneumonia Candida esophagitis Disseminated/chronic herpes simplex Toxoplasmosis Cryptococcosis Disseminated histoplasmosis Disseminated coccidiomycosis Chronic cryptosporidiosis Progressive multifocal leukoencephalopathy (PMLE) Microsporidiosis Miliary/extrapulmonary tuberculosis	Wasting B-cell lymphoma Cardiomyopathy Peripheral neuropathy HIV-associated dementia CNS lymphoma HIV-associated nephropathy
<50	CMV disease Disseminated *Mycobacteruim avium* complex	

Reproduced by permission of Bartlett, JG, Gallant JE Medical Management of HIV Infection. Johns Hopkins University 2007

increased the survival rate among patients (32%) at 6 months over that among patients receiving monotherapy (12%) ($P = 0.022$) [151].

Oral itraconazole (200 mg twice a day) for 6 weeks was less effective than amphotericin B (0.3 mg/kg per day) plus flucytosine (150 mg/kg daily) in 28 patients [152].

The importance of controlling the raised intracranial pressure associated with cryptococcal meningitis by repeated lumbar puncture or CSF drainage was established in a retrospective analysis of 221 patients in the van der Horst study [147]. After receiving antifungal therapy, those patients whose CSF pressure was reduced by >10 mm or did not change had more frequent clinical response at 2 weeks than did those whose pressure increased >10 mm ($P = 0.001$). Patients with pretreatment opening pressure of <250 mm had increased short-term survival compared with those

with higher pressure [153]. This was confirmed in a small prospective study of 10 patients with raised ICP treated with CSF drainage [154].

Prophylaxis against fungal infection

Five studies were identified in a Cochrane review of interventions for the primary prevention of cryptococcal disease [155]. The authors concluded that prophylaxis with either itraconazole or fluconazole was effective (RR 0.21, 95% CI 0.09, 0.46 compared with placebo; $n = 1316$), however neither had a clear effect on overall mortality. One RCT found that itraconazole reduced relapses of successfully treated cryptococcal meningitis more than fluconazole (13/57 [23%] vs 2/51 [4%]; ARR 19%, 95% CI 6.2–31.7; RR 0.17, 95% CI 0.04–0.71; NNT 5, 95% CI 3–16). The trial was stopped early because of the higher rate of relapse with fluconazole [156].

A Cochrane review included 9 studies of interventions for the prevention of oropharyngeal candidiasis [157]. Fluconazole was effective in preventing clinical episodes compared with placebo (RR 0.61; 95% CI 0.5–0.74) and compared with no treatment (RR 0.16; 95% CI 0.08–0.34). In a RCT comparing dosing regimen, there was no difference in the rate of invasive fungal infections between fluconazole 200 mg daily with 400 mg once weekly over a follow-up of 74 weeks (8% vs 6%; ARR 2.2%, 95% CI −1.7% to 6.1) [158]. However, the incidence of candidiasis was twice as common in people taking the weekly dose.

In a RCT, fluconazole reduced the incidence of invasive fungal disease and mucocutaneous candidal infections compared with clotrimazole (4% vs 11%; RH 3.3; 95% CI 1.5–7.6) [159]. In HIV patients with candidiasis treated with itraconazole, relapse was reduced with itraconazole prophylaxis (5/24 [21%] with itraconazole vs 14/20 [70%] with placebo; ARR 49%, 95% CI 19–64; NNT 2, 95% CI 2–5), and the time interval before relapse occurred was increased (median time to relapse: itraconazole 8.0 weeks vs placebo 10.4 weeks, $P = 0.001$) [160].

There is one open-label uncontrolled study (44 people), which found that itraconazole may be effective in preventing the relapse of histoplasmosis [161].

Mycobacterium avium complex

Treatment

HIV-positive patients ($n = 246$) with disseminated *Mycobacterium avium* complex (MAC) received either azithromycin 250 mg every day, azithromycin 600 mg every day, or clarithromycin 500 mg twice a day, each combined with ethambutol, for 24 weeks. The azithromycin 250 mg arm of the study was dropped after an interim analysis showed a lower rate of clearance of bacteremia. At 24 weeks of therapy, the likelihood of patients developing two consecutive negative cultures (46% vs 56%; $P = 0.24$) or one negative culture (59% vs 61%; $P = 0.80$) was similar for azithromycin 600 mg ($n = 68$) and clarithromycin ($n = 57$), respectively. The likelihood of relapse was 39% versus 27% ($P = 0.21$) on azithromycin compared with clarithromycin, respectively. Of the six patients who experienced relapse, none of those randomized to receive azithromycin developed isolates resistant to macrolides, compared with two of three patients randomized to receive clarithromycin. Mortality was similar in patients comprising each arm of the study (69% vs 63%; HR 1.1, 95% CI 0.7–1.7) [162].

AIDS patients with disseminated MAC disease ($n = 85$) were randomized to receive a three-drug regimen of clarithromycin, rifabutin or clofazimine, and ethambutol. Two dosages of clarithromycin, 500 or 1000 mg twice daily, were compared [163]. After a mean follow-up of 4.5 months, 10 (22%) of 45 patients receiving clarithromycin at 500 mg twice daily had died (70 deaths per 100 person-years) compared with 17 (43%) of 40 patients receiving clarithromycin at 1000 mg twice daily (158 deaths per 100 person-years) (RR 2.43, 95% CI 1.11–5.34; $P = 0.02$). After 10.4 months, 20 (49%) of 41 patients receiving rifabutin had died (81 deaths per 100 person-years) compared with 23 (52%) of 44 patients receiving clofazimine (94 deaths per 100 person-years) (RR 1.20, 95% CI 0.65–2.19; $P = 0.56$). Bacteriologic outcomes were similar among treatment groups. In treating MAC disease in AIDS patients, the recommended maximum dose of clarithromycin is 500 mg twice daily.

The effect of two regimens for treatment of MAC bacteremia in an HIV-positive population on symptoms and health status outcomes were evaluated using a substudy of an open-label RCT comparing rifampin 600 mg plus ethambutol 15 mg/kg daily plus clofazimine 100 mg daily plus ciprofloxacin 750 mg twice daily (four-drug arm), with rifabutin 600 mg daily (amended to 300 mg daily in mid-trial) plus ethambutol 15 mg/kg daily plus clarithromycin 1000 mg twice daily (three-drug arm). The primary health status outcome was the change on the 8-item symptom subscale of the Medical Outcome Study (MOS)-HIV Health Survey adapted for MAC. Patients on the three-drug arm had better Karnofsky score at 16 weeks ($P = 0.001$) and better outcomes on the social function, mental health, energy/fatigue, health distress, and cognitive function subscales of the MOS-HIV. The three-drug arm was superior to the four-drug arm in terms of impact on MAC-associated symptoms, functional status, and other aspects of health status [164].

Prophylaxis

Prospective cohort studies have found that the risk of disseminated MAC disease increases substantially with a lower CD4 count but was clinically important only for CD4 <50 cells/mm³ [114].

Azithomycin and clarithromycin

There is one systematic review (search date 1997) of prophylaxis and treatment of MAC [165]. It identified one RCT (682 people with advanced AIDS) that found that clarithromycin compared with placebo significantly reduced the incidence of MAC (6% vs 16%; HR 0.31, 95% CI 0.18–0.53). It found no significant difference in the death rate (32% vs 41%; HR 0.75, $P = 0.026$). Adverse effects led to discontinuation of treatment in slightly more people taking clarithromycin than placebo (8% vs 6%; $P = 0.45$).

Azithromycin once weekly reduced the incidence of MAC more than placebo (11% vs 25%; $P = 0.004$). Gastrointestinal side effects were more likely with azithromycin than with placebo (71/90 [79%] vs 25/91 [28%]; number needed to harm [NNH] 2), but they were rarely severe enough to cause discontinuation of treatment (8% vs 2% in the two arms; $p = 0.14$) [166].

Other combinations

One RCT (1178 people with AIDS) compared rifabutin versus clarithromycin versus clarithromycin plus rifabutin [167]. The risk of MAC was significantly reduced in the clarithromycin alone group (relative risk reduction [RRR] 44% for clarithromycin vs rifabutin; $P = 0.005$) and the combination group when compared with rifabutin alone (RRR 57% for combination vs rifabutin; $P = 0.0003$). There was no significant difference in the risk of MAC between the combination and clarithromycin arms ($P = 0.36$).

The combination of azithromycin plus rifabutin versus azithromycin alone significantly reduced the incidence of MAC at 1 year (15.3% with rifabutin vs 7.6% for azithromycin vs 2.8% with rifabutin plus azithromycin; $P = 0.008$ for rifabutin vs azithromycin; $P = 0.03$ for combination vs azithromycin). Dose-limiting toxicity was more likely with azithromycin plus rifabutin than with azithromycin alone (HR 1.67; $P = 0.03$) [113].

Other combinations have been studied in RCTs. Clarithromycin (1000 mg daily), clofazimine, and ethambutol was associated with significantly fewer relapses of MAC than the combination of clarithromycin plus clofazimine without ethambutol (68% relapsed in the three-drug regimen vs 12% in the two-drug regimen at 36 weeks; $P = 0.004$) [168]. The addition of clofazimine to clarithromycin and ethambutol did not improve clinical response and was associated with higher mortality in the clofazimine arm (62% with clofazimine vs 38% without clofazimine; $P = 0.012$) [169]. Clarithromycin, rifabutin, and ethambutol reduced the relapse rate of MAC compared with clarithromycin plus clofazimine [170] but there was no significant difference in survival between people taking clarithromycin plus ethambutol and people taking clarithromycin plus ethambutol plus rifabutin [171].

Adverse events

Adverse events occurred in 31% of people receiving the combination of clarithromycin and rifabutin compared with 16% on clarithromycin alone and 18% on rifabutin alone ($P = 0.001$) [165]. Uveitis occurred in 42 people: 33 were on clarithromycin plus rifabutin, seven were on rifabutin alone, and two were on clarithromycin alone. In a review of 54 people with rifabutin-associated uveitis, uveitis was dose dependent, occurred from 2 weeks to more than 7 months after initiation of rifabutin treatment, and was more likely in people taking rifabutin and clarithromycin [172]. Combinations of drugs may lead to increased toxicity and mortality[163,169]. Optic neuropathy may occur with ethambutol, but has not been reported in RCTs in people with HIV where the dose and symptoms were carefully monitored.

Stopping prophylaxis

In 643 HIV-1-infected patients, with a previous CD4 cell count <50 cells/mm^3 and a sustained increase to >100 cells/mm^3 during HAART, given azithromycin 1200 mg once weekly ($n = 321$), or matching placebo ($n = 322$), there were two cases of MAC infection among the 321 patients assigned to placebo (incidence rate, 0.5 events per 100 person-years; 95% CI 0.06–1.83 events per 100 person-years) compared with no cases among the 322 patients assigned to azithromycin (95% CI 0–0.92 events per 100 person-years), resulting in a treatment difference of 0.5 events per 100 person-years (95% CI 0.20–1.21 events per 100 person-years) for placebo versus azithromycin. Both cases were atypical in that MAC was localized to the vertebral spine. Patients receiving azithromycin were more likely than those receiving placebo to discontinue treatment with the study drug permanently because of adverse events (8% vs 2%; HR 0.24, 95% CI 0.10–0.57) [173].

A second RCT compared azithromycin with placebo in 520 people without previous MAC disease with CD4 > 100 cells/mm^3 in response to HAART. There were no episodes of confirmed MAC disease in either group over a median follow-up of 12 months [174]. Again there were more adverse effects leading to discontinuation of treatment with azithromycin than with placebo (7% vs 1%; $P = 0.002$).

Summary

RCTs have found that clarithromycin and ethambutol, with or without rifabutin, reduce the incidence of MAC. Clofazimine and high-dose clarithromycin are associated with increased mortality. Clarithromycin alone and clarithromycin plus rifabutin both reduce the incidence of MAC compared with rifabutin alone. Azithromycin plus rifabutin reduces the incidence of MAC compared with azithromycin alone but is associated with more side effects.

Cytomegalovirus infection

Treatment of cytomegalovirus

Ganciclovir and foscarnet have been the mainstays of treatment of CMV disease [175]. With the availability of oral valganciclovir, this drug was compared with intravenous ganciclovir as induction therapy for newly diagnosed CMV retinitis in 160 patients with AIDS. After 4 weeks, all patients received valganciclovir as maintenance therapy. Of the patients who could be evaluated, seven of 70 assigned to intravenous ganciclovir (10.0%) and seven of 71 assigned to oral valganciclovir (9.9%) had progression of CMV retinitis during the first 4 weeks (difference in proportions, 0.1 percentage point; 95% CI −9.7 to 10·0); 47 of 61 patients (77.0%) assigned to intravenous ganciclovir and 46 of 64 (71.9%) assigned to valganciclovir had a satisfactory response to induction therapy (difference in proportions, 5.2 percentage points; 95% CI 20.4–10.1). The median times to progression of retinitis were 125 days in the group assigned to intravenous ganciclovir and 160 days in the group assigned to oral valganciclovir. The frequency and severity of adverse events were similar in the two treatment groups [176].

Prophylaxis for cytomegalovirus

One RCT (725 people with a median CD4 count of 22 cells/mm^3) found that oral ganciclovir halved the incidence of CMV compared with placebo (event rate 16% vs 30%; $P = 0.001$) but 25% of people who did not develop CMV developed severe neutropenia and were treated with granulocyte colony-stimulating factor [177]. A second RCT (994 HIV-1-infected people with CD4 < 100 cells/mm^3 and CMV seropositivity) found no difference in the rate of CMV in people taking oral ganciclovir compared with placebo (event rates 13.1 vs 14.6 per 100 person-years; HR 0.92, 95% CI 0.65–1.27) [178]. Neither RCT found a significant difference in overall mortality.

There is one systematic review of individual patient data (eight RCTs) in people with any stage of HIV infection or AIDS [179]. It found no difference in protection against CMV disease between acyclovir compared with no treatment or placebo. However, acyclovir significantly reduced overall mortality (RR 0.81; $P = 0.04$) and HSV and varicella zoster virus (VZV) infections ($P < 0.001$ for both). One RCT (1227 CMV seropositive people with CD4 < 100 cells/mm^3) compared valaciclovir, high-dose acyclovir, and low-dose acyclovir. It found increased mortality in the valaciclovir group, which did not reach statistical significance ($P = 0.06$) and 1-year discontinuation rates of 51% for valaciclovir, 46% for high-dose acyclovir, and 41% for low-dose acyclovir [180]. The CMV rate was lower in the valaciclovir group than in the acyclovir groups (12% vs 18%; $P = 0.03$).

Stopping CMV prophylaxis

There are no RCTs or reviews. There are several small case series [181–189]. The study with the longest follow-up (mean 20.4 months) found no relapses in 41 people discontinuing maintenance treatment [181]. However, another study with mean follow-up of 14.5 months found five (29%) relapses among 17 participants who withdrew from maintenance; all of them occurred after the CD4 cell count had dropped again to <50 cells/mm^3 (8 days/10 months after this event) [184]. In one observational series, 12/14 participants (86%) had evidence of immune reconstitution retinitis even before starting withdrawal of prophylaxis [183]. Worsening uveitis was associated with a substantial vision loss (>3 lines) in three participants. It is difficult to conduct a RCT of adequate sample size to exclude modest differences in relapse rates. The observational evidence suggests that withdrawal of CMV maintenance treatment may be considered in selected people in whom CMV disease is in remission, CD4 >100 cells/mm^3, and HIV replication remains suppressed. We found no clear evidence on whether quantification of CMV viremia should be considered in the decision to withdraw from maintenance. One small case series found that relapses were associated with a drop in the CD4 cell count [184]. However, we found no randomized or other reliable evidence of when CMV maintenance treatment should be reinstituted.

Case presentation 4 (continued)

The patient improves with amphotericin and is discharged home on oral fluconazole; however, he presents again 3 months later with increasing confusion. CT scan shows no focal lesions and CSF obtained by lumbar puncture shows neither evidence of cryptococcal infection nor any white cells. You review the causes of confusion in late HIV disease.

Other AIDS-related illness

Non-Hodgkin lymphoma

Patients with AIDS-associated lymphoma/leukemia historically have a poor prognosis and were frequently treated with low-intensity therapy. There is one RCT comparing reduced therapy with standard dose: 198 HIV-seropositive patients with previously untreated, aggressive non-Hodgkin lymphoma were randomly assigned to receive standard-dose therapy with methotrexate, bleomycin, doxorubicin, cyclophosphamide, vincristine, and dexamethasone (m-BACOD) along with granulocyte-macrophage colony-stimulating factor (GM-CSF; $n = 94$) or reduced-dose m-BACOD with GM-CSF administered only as indicated ($n = 98$) [190]. A complete response was achieved in 39 of the 94 assessable patients assigned to low-dose therapy (41%) and in 42 of the 81 assessable patients assigned to standard-dose therapy (52%, $P = 0.56$). There were no significant differences in overall or disease-free survival; median survival times were 35 weeks for patients receiving low-dose therapy and 31 weeks for those receiving standard-dose therapy (RR for death in the standard-dose group $= 1.17$; 95% CI 0.84–1.63, $P = 0.25$). Toxic effects of chemotherapy rated grade 3 or higher occurred in 66 of 94 patients assigned to standard-dose therapy (70%) and 50 of 98 patients assigned to low-dose treatment (51%; $P = 0.008$). Hematologic toxicity accounted for the difference. In a randomized trial of risk-adapted intensive chemotherapy for AIDS related lymphoma, 5-year overall survival was associated with HAART therapy (RR 1.6, $P < 0.001$), International Prognostic Index score (RR 1.5, $P < 0.001$), and stage of HIV but not with chemotherapy regimen [191].

AIDS dementia complex

A metaanalysis of 2411 patients in the ACTG 116A, ACTG116B/117, ACTG175, BMS010, and CTN002 trials had 21 documented cases of AIDS dementia complex (ADC) during the 15-month follow-up period. The rates per 100 person-years of follow-up were 0.70, 0.65, and 0.41 for the zidovudine, high-dose didanosine, and didanosine arms, respectively. There were no significant differences in risks of ADC between treatment arms (zidovudine vs high-dose didanosine: $P = 0.30$; zidovudine vs didanosine: $P = 0.97$; didanosine vs high-dose didanosine: $P = 0.41$) [192].

Progressive multifocal leukoencephalopathy

Progressive multifocal leukoencephalopathy (PMLE) affects about 4% of patients with AIDS, and survival after the diagnosis of leukoencephalopathy averages only about 3 months. JC virus PCR in blood has a poor positive predictive value (16%) but a good negative predictive value (96%) for PMLE [193]. However, in one study, PCR of CSF yielded sensitivity and specificity values of 100% and 90%, respectively [194].

Case presentation 4 (continued)

CSF samples are sent for JC virus PCR and this is positive. MRI scans show typical changes of PMLE. Lymph node biopsy does not show any evidence of lymphoma nor of Mycobacterium avium-intracellulare. He deteriorates further and dies in a hospice 2 months later.

In observational studies no benefit has been found using cidofovir [195] nor cytarabine administered either intravenously or intrathecally [196]. A small observational study in 27 patients found the use of cidofovir was independently associated with a reduced risk of death (HR 0.21; 95% CI 0.07–0.65, $P < 0.005$) [197].

Acknowledgments

The author is indebted to the work contained in Clinical Evidence in HIV (http://clinicalevidence.bmj.com/ceweb/conditions/hiv/0902/0902_contribdetails.jsp) by Professor Margaret Johnson, Professor David Wilkinson, and Professor Andrew Phillips, published by BMJ Publishing Group Ltd, as a basis for this work.

References

1 Hecht FM, Busch MP, Rawal B, et al. Use of laboratory tests and clinical symptoms for identification of primary HIV infection. AIDS 2002;16(8):1119–29.

2 Nugent C, Kolk D, Giachetti C, et al. Detection of HIV-1 in Saliva Using the APTIMA HIV-1 RNA Qualitative Assay. 14th Conference on Retroviruses and Opportunistic Infections 2007; Los Angeles, 2007. p. 679

3 Giles RE, Perry KR, Parry JV. Simple/rapid test devices for anti-HIV screening: do they come up to the mark? J Med Virol 1999;59(1):104–9.

4 Delaney KP, Branson BM, Uniyal A, et al. Performance of an oral fluid rapid HIV-1/2 test: experience from four CDC studies. AIDS 2006;20(12):1655–60.

5 Rosenberg ES, Altfeld M, Poon SH, et al. Immune control of HIV-1 after early treatment of acute infection. Nature 2000;407(6803):523–6.

6 Markowitz M, Vesanen M, Tenner-Racz K, et al. The effect of commencing combination antiretroviral therapy soon after human immunodeficiency virus type 1 infection on viral replication and antiviral immune responses. J Infect Dis 1999;179(3):527–37.

7 Kinloch-De Loes S, Hirschel BJ, Hoen B, et al. A controlled trial of zidovudine in primary human immunodeficiency virus infection. N Engl J Med 1995;333(7):408–13.

8 Darbyshire J, Foulkes M, Peto R, et al. Immediate versus deferred zidovudine (AZT) in asymptomatic or mildly symptomatic HIV infected adults. Cochrane Database Syst Rev 2000 (3), CD002039, DOI: 10.1002/14651858.

9 Phillips AN, Gazzard BG, Clumeck N, et al. When should antiretroviral therapy for HIV be started? BMJ 2007;334(7584):76–8.

10 Gazzard B, Bernard AJ, Boffito M, et al. British HIV Association (BHIVA) guidelines for the treatment of HIV-infected adults with antiretroviral therapy (2006). HIV Med 2006;7(8):487–503.

11 Ioannidis JP, Cappelleri JC, Lau J, et al. Early or deferred zidovudine therapy in HIV-infected patients without an AIDS-defining illness. Ann Intern Med 1995;122(11):856–66.

12 Ross LL, Lim ML, Liao Q, et al. Prevalence of antiretroviral drug resistance and resistance mutations in antiretroviral therapy (ART)-naïve HIV-infected individuals from 40 US cities during 2003. 44th Interscience Conference on Antimicrobial Agents and Chemotherapy 2004; Washington, USA; 2004. Abstract H-173.

13 Wensing AMJ, van der Vijver DA, Asjo B, et al. Analysis of more than 1600 newly diagnosed patients with HIV from 17 European countries shows that 10% of the patients carry primary drug resistance: The CATCH study. Second International AIDS Society Conference; 2003; Paris. 2003. p. 1.

14 Wensing AM, van de Vijver DA, Angarano G, et al. Prevalence of drug-resistant HIV-1 variants in untreated individuals in Europe: implications for clinical management. J Infect Dis 2005;192(6):958–66.

15 UK Collaborative Group on HIV Drug Resistance UCHCS, and UK Register of HIV Seroconverters. Evidence of a decline in transmitted HIV-1 drug resistance in the United Kingdom. AIDS 2007;21(8):1035–9.

16 Bhaskaran K, Pillay D, Walker AS, et al. Do patients who are infected with drug-resistant HIV have a different CD4 cell decline after seroconversion? An exploratory analysis in the UK Register of HIV Seroconverters. AIDS 2004;18(10):1471–3.

17 Mendoza CD, C R, A C. Long-term persistence of drug resistance mutations after HIV seroconversion. 10th European AIDS Conference (EACS); 2005; Dublin, Ireland; 2005. PE3.5/3.

18 Grant RM, Hecht FM, Warmerdam M, et al. Time trends in primary HIV-1 drug resistance among recently infected persons. JAMA 2002;288(2):181–8.

19 Harzic M, Pellegrin I, Deveau C, et al. Genotypic drug resistance during HIV-1 primary infection in France (1996–1999): frequency and response to treatment. AIDS 2002;16(5):793–6.

20 Little SJ, Holte S, Routy JP, et al. Antiretroviral-drug resistance among patients recently infected with HIV. N Engl J Med 2002;347(6):385–94.

21 Violin M, Forbici F, Cozzi-Lepri A, et al. Primary HIV-1 resistance in recently and chronically infected individuals of the Italian Cohort Naive for Antiretrovirals. J Biol Regul Homeost Agents 2002;16(1):37–43.

22 Hanna GJ, Caliendo AM. Testing for HIV-1 drug resistance. Mol Diagn 2001;6(4):253–63.

23 Balotta C, Berlusconi A, Pan A, et al. Prevalence of HIV-1 resistant strains in recent seroconverters. J Biol Regul Homeost Agents 2000;14(1):51–7.

24 Beerenwinkel N, Sing T, Lengauer T, et al. Computational methods for the design of effective therapies against drug resistant HIV strains. Bioinformatics 2005;21(21):3943–50.

25 Hirsch MS, Brun-Vezinet F, Clotet B, et al. Antiretroviral drug resistance testing in adults infected with human immunodeficiency virus type 1: 2003 recommendations of

an International AIDS Society-USA Panel. Clin Infect Dis 2003;37(1):113–28.

26 Hecht FM, Grant RM. Resistance testing in drug-naive HIV-infected patients: is it time? Clin Infect Dis 2005;41(9):1324–5.

27 Sax PE, Islam R, Walensky RP, et al. Should resistance testing be performed for treatment-naive HIV-infected patients? A cost-effectiveness analysis. Clin Infect Dis 2005;41(9):1316–23.

28 Metzner KJ, Rauch P, Walter H, et al. Detection of minor populations of drug-resistant HIV-1 in acute seroconverters. AIDS 2005;19(16):1819–25.

29 Mellors JW, Munoz A, Giorgi JV, et al. Plasma viral load and CD4+ lymphocytes as prognostic markers of HIV-1 infection. Ann Intern Med 1997;126(12):946–54.

30 May M, Sterne JA, Sabin C, et al. Prognosis of HIV-1-infected patients up to 5 years after initiation of HAART: collaborative analysis of prospective studies. AIDS 2007;21(9):1185–97.

31 Panel on Antiretroviral Guidelines for Adults and Adolescents. Guidelines for the use of antiretroviral agents in HIV-1-infected adults and adolescents. Department of Health and Human Services, USA; 3 November 2008. pp. 1–139. Available at http://www.aidsinfo.nih.gov/ContentFiles/AdultandAdolescentGL.pdf. Accessed 16 March 2009.

32 Corbett EL, Watt CJ, Walker N, et al. The growing burden of tuberculosis: global trends and interactions with the HIV epidemic. Arch Intern Med 2003;163(9):1009–21.

33 UNAIDS. AIDS epidemic update: December 2007. Available at http://www.data.unaids.org/pub/EPISlides/2007/2007_epiupdate_en.pdf. Accessed 13 March 2009.

34 Cohen R, Muzaffar S, Capellan J, et al. The validity of classic symptoms and chest radiographic configuration in predicting pulmonary tuberculosis. Chest 1996;109(2):420–3.

35 Long R, Scalcini M, Manfreda J, et al. The impact of HIV on the usefulness of sputum smears for the diagnosis of tuberculosis. Am J Public Health 1991;81(10):1326–8.

36 Parry CM, Kamoto O, Harries AD, et al. The use of sputum induction for establishing a diagnosis in patients with suspected pulmonary tuberculosis in Malawi. Tuber Lung Dis 1995;76(1):72–6.

37 Bruchfeld J, Aderaye G, Palme IB, et al. Sputum concentration improves diagnosis of tuberculosis in a setting with a high prevalence of HIV. Trans R Soc Trop Med Hyg 2000;94(6):677–80.

38 Perriens JH, St Louis ME, Mukadi YB, et al. Pulmonary tuberculosis in HIV-infected patients in Zaire. A controlled trial of treatment for either 6 or 12 months. N Engl J Med 1995;332(12):779–84.

39 Okwera A, Johnson JL, Luzze H, et al. Comparison of intermittent ethambutol with rifampicin-based regimens in HIV-infected adults with PTB, Kampala. Int J Tuberc Lung Dis 2006;10(1):39–44.

40 Jindani A, Nunn AJ, Enarson DA. Two 8-month regimens of chemotherapy for treatment of newly diagnosed pulmonary tuberculosis: international multicentre randomised trial. Lancet 2004;364(9441):1244–51.

41 Selwyn PA, Hartel D, Lewis VA, et al. A prospective study of the risk of tuberculosis among intravenous drug users with human immunodeficiency virus infection. N Engl J Med 1989;320(9):545–50.

42 Volmink J, Woldehanna S. Treatment of latent tuberculosis infection in HIV infected persons. Cochrane Database Syst Rev 2004 (1), CD000171, DOI: 10.1002/14651858.

43 Bucher HC, Griffith LE, Guyatt GH, et al. Isoniazid prophylaxis for tuberculosis in HIV infection: a meta-analysis of randomized controlled trials. AIDS 1999;13(4):501–7.

44 Gao XF, Wang L, Liu GJ, et al. Rifampicin plus pyrazinamide versus isoniazid for treating latent tuberculosis infection: a meta-analysis. Int J Tuberc Lung Dis 2006;10(10):1080–90.

45 Mohammed A, Myer L, Ehrlich R, et al. Randomised controlled trial of isoniazid preventive therapy in South African adults with advanced HIV disease. Int J Tuberc Lung Dis 2007;11(10):1114–20.

46 Faustini A, Hall AJ, Perucci CA. Risk factors for multidrug resistant tuberculosis in Europe: a systematic review. Thorax 2006;61(2):158–63.

47 Kaplan JE, Hanson D, Dworkin MS, et al. Epidemiology of human immunodeficiency virus-associated opportunistic infections in the United States in the era of highly active antiretroviral therapy. Clin Infect Dis 2000;30 Suppl 1:S5–14.

48 Kovacs JA, Hiemenz JW, Macher AM, et al. Pneumocystis carinii pneumonia: a comparison between patients with the acquired immunodeficiency syndrome and patients with other immunodeficiencies. Ann Intern Med 1984;100(5):663–71.

49 Miller RF, Kocjan G, Buckland J, et al. Sputum induction for the diagnosis of pulmonary disease in HIV positive patients. J Infect 1991;23(1):5–15.

50 Cregan P, Yamamoto A, Lum A, et al. Comparison of four methods for rapid detection of Pneumocystis carinii in respiratory specimens. J Clin Microbiol 1990;28(11):2432–6.

51 Ribes JA, Limper AH, Espy MJ, et al. PCR detection of Pneumocystis carinii in bronchoalveolar lavage specimens: analysis of sensitivity and specificity. J Clin Microbiol 1997;35(4):830–5.

52 Huggett JF, Taylor MS, Kocjan G, et al. Development and evaluation of a real-time PCR assay for detection of Pneumocystis jirovecii DNA in bronchoalveolar lavage fluid of HIV-infected patients. Thorax 2008;63(2):154–9.

53 de Oliveira A, Unnasch TR, Crothers K, et al. Performance of a molecular viability assay for the diagnosis of Pneumocystis pneumonia in HIV-infected patients. Diagn Microbiol Infect Dis 2007;57(2):169–76.

54 Fujii T, Nakamura T, Iwamoto A. Pneumocystis pneumonia in patients with HIV infection: clinical manifestations, laboratory findings, and radiological features. J Infect Chemother 2007;13(1):1–7.

55 Hughes WT, Feldman S, Chaudhary SC, et al. Comparison of pentamidine isethionate and trimethoprim-sulfamethoxazole in the treatment of Pneumocystis carinii pneumonia. J Pediatr 1978;92(2):285–91.

56 Sattler FR, Cowan R, Nielsen DM, et al. Trimethoprim-sulfamethoxazole compared with pentamidine for treatment

of *Pneumocystis carinii* pneumonia in the acquired immunodeficiency syndrome. A prospective, noncrossover study. Ann Intern Med 1988;109(4):280–7.

57 Briel M, Boscacci R, Furrer H, et al. Adjunctive corticosteroids for *Pneumocystis jiroveci* pneumonia in patients with HIV infection: a meta-analysis of randomised controlled trials. BMC Infect Dis 2005;5:101.

58 Montaner JS, Guillemi S, Quieffin J, et al. Oral corticosteroids in patients with mild *Pneumocystis carinii* pneumonia and the acquired immune deficiency syndrome (AIDS). Tuber Lung Dis 1993;74(3):173–9.

59 Smego RA, Jr., Nagar S, Maloba B, et al. A meta-analysis of salvage therapy for *Pneumocystis carinii* pneumonia. Arch Intern Med 2001;161(12):1529–33.

60 Palella FJ, Jr., Delaney KM, Moorman AC, et al. Declining morbidity and mortality among patients with advanced human immunodeficiency virus infection. HIV Outpatient Study Investigators. N Engl J Med 1998;338(13):853–60.

61 Jordan R, Gold L, Cummins C, et al. Systematic review and meta-analysis of evidence for increasing numbers of drugs in antiretroviral combination therapy. BMJ 2002;324(7340):757.

62 Rutherford GW, Sangani PR, Kennedy GE. Three- or four- versus two-drug antiretroviral maintenance regimens for HIV infection. Cochrane Database Syst Rev 2003 (4), CD002037, DOI: 10.1002/14651858.

63 Asboe D, Williams IG, Goodall RL, et al. A virological benefit from an induction/maintenance strategy: the Forte trial. Antivir Ther 2007;12(1):47–54.

64 Johnson M, S DW, B G. Induction therapy with Trizivir zidovudine/lamivudine/-abacavir) [TZV] plus efavirenz [EFV]: TIME Study (AZL30004) results at 24 weeks. 9th European AIDS Conference (EACS), 1st EACS Resistance & Pharmacology Workshop; 2003; Warsaw, Poland 2003. Abstract F1/4.

65 Markowitz M, Hill-Zabala C, Lang J, et al. Induction with abacavir/lamivudine/zidovudine plus efavirenz for 48 weeks followed by 48-week maintenance with abacavir/lamivudine/zidovudine alone in antiretroviral-naive HIV-1-infected patients. J Acquir Immune Defic Syndr 2005;39(3):257–64.

66 Gulick RM, Ribaudo HJ, Shikuma CM, et al. Three- vs four-drug antiretroviral regimens for the initial treatment of HIV-1 infection: a randomized controlled trial. JAMA 2006;296(7):769–81.

67 van Leth F, Phanuphak P, Ruxrungtham K, et al. Comparison of first-line antiretroviral therapy with regimens including nevirapine, efavirenz, or both drugs, plus stavudine and lamivudine: a randomised open-label trial, the 2NN Study. Lancet 2004;363(9417):1253–63.

68 Riddler SA, Haubrich R, DiRienzo AG, et al. Class-sparing regimens for initial treatment of HIV-1 infection. N Engl J Med 2008;358(20):2095–106.

69 MacArthur RD, Novak RM, Peng G, et al. A comparison of three highly active antiretroviral treatment strategies consisting of non-nucleoside reverse transcriptase inhibitors, protease inhibitors, or both in the presence of nucleoside

reverse transcriptase inhibitors as initial therapy (CPCRA 058 FIRST Study): a long-term randomised trial. Lancet 2006;368(9553):2125–35.

70 Bartlett JA, Johnson J, Herrera G, et al. Long-term results of initial therapy with abacavir and lamivudine combined with efavirenz, amprenavir/ritonavir, or stavudine. J Acquir Immune Defic Syndr 2006;43(3):284–92.

71 Chersich MF, Urban MF, Venter FW, et al. Efavirenz use during pregnancy and for women of child-bearing potential. AIDS Res Ther 2006;3:11.

72 Bani-Sadr F, Goderel I, Penalba C, et al. Risk factors for anaemia in human immunodeficiency virus/hepatitis C virus-coinfected patients treated with interferon plus ribavirin. J Viral Hepat 2007;14(9):639–44.

73 Bersoff-Matcha SJ, Miller WC, Aberg JA, et al. Sex differences in nevirapine rash. Clin Infect Dis 2001;32(1):124–9.

74 Leith J, Piliero P, Storfer S, et al. Appropriate use of nevirapine for long-term therapy. J Infect Dis 2005;192(3):545–6; author reply 6.

75 Mallal S, Phillips E, Carosi G, et al. HLA-B*5701 screening for hypersensitivity to abacavir. N Engl J Med 2008;358(6):568–79.

76 Hill A, Ruxrungtham K, Hanvanich M, et al. Systematic review of clinical trials evaluating low doses of stavudine as part of antiretroviral treatment. Exp Opin Pharmacother 2007;8(5):679–88.

77 Mannheimer S, Friedland G, Matts J, et al. The consistency of adherence to antiretroviral therapy predicts biologic outcomes for human immunodeficiency virus-infected persons in clinical trials. Clin Infect Dis 2002;34(8):1115–21.

78 Paterson DL, Swindells S, Mohr J, et al. Adherence to protease inhibitor therapy and outcomes in patients with HIV infection. Ann Intern Med 2000;133(1):21–30.

79 Nieuwkerk PT, Sprangers MA, Burger DM, et al. Limited patient adherence to highly active antiretroviral therapy for HIV-1 infection in an observational cohort study. Arch Intern Med 2001;161(16):1962–8.

80 Bangsberg D, Perry S, Charlesbois E. Adherence to HAART predicts progression to AIDS. 8th Conference on Retroviruses and Opportunistic Infections; Chicago; 2001.

81 Ickovics JR, Cameron A, Zackin R, et al. Consequences and determinants of adherence to antiretroviral medication: results from Adult AIDS Clinical Trials Group protocol 370. Antivir Ther 2002;7(3):185–93.

82 Garcia de Olalla P, Knobel H, Carmona A, et al. Impact of adherence and highly active antiretroviral therapy on survival in HIV-infected patients. J Acquir Immune Defic Syndr 2002;30(1):105–10.

83 Claxton AJ, Cramer J, Pierce C. A systematic review of the associations between dose regimens and medication compliance. Clin Ther 2001;23(8):1296–310.

84 Bamberger JD, Unick J, Klein P, et al. Helping the urban poor stay with antiretroviral HIV drug therapy. Am J Public Health 2000;90(5):699–701.

85 Nieuwkerk P, Gisolf E, Sprangers M, et al. Adherence over 48 weeks in an antiretroviral clinical trial: variable within patients, affected by toxicities and independently predictive of virological response. Antivir Ther 2001;6(2):97–103.

86 Chesney MA. Factors affecting adherence to antiretroviral therapy. Clin Infect Dis 2000;30 Suppl 2:S171–6.

87 Rueda S, Park-Wyllie LY, Bayoumi AM, et al. Patient support and education for promoting adherence to highly active antiretroviral therapy for HIV/AIDS. Cochrane Database Syst Rev 2006 (3), CD001442, DOI: 10.1002/14651858.

88 Gisolf EH, Dreezen C, Danner SA, et al. Risk factors for hepatotoxicity in HIV-1-infected patients receiving ritonavir and saquinavir with or without stavudine. Prometheus Study Group. Clin Infect Dis 2000;31(5):1234–9.

89 Hernandez LV, Gilson I, Jacobson J, et al. Antiretroviral hepatotoxicity in human immunodeficiency virus-infected patients. Aliment Pharmacol Ther 2001;15(10): 1627–32.

90 den Brinker M, Wit FW, Wertheim-van Dillen PM, et al. Hepatitis B and C virus co-infection and the risk for hepatotoxicity of highly active antiretroviral therapy in HIV-1 infection. AIDS 2000;14(18):2895–902.

91 Greub G, Ledergerber B, Battegay M, et al. Clinical progression, survival, and immune recovery during antiretroviral therapy in patients with HIV-1 and hepatitis C virus coinfection: the Swiss HIV Cohort Study. Lancet 2000;356(9244):1800–5.

92 Graham CS, Baden LR, Yu E, et al. Influence of human immunodeficiency virus infection on the course of hepatitis C virus infection: a meta-analysis. Clin Infect Dis 2001;33(4):562–9.

93 Nunez M, Miralles C, Berdun MA, et al. Role of weight-based ribavirin dosing and extended duration of therapy in chronic hepatitis C in HIV-infected patients: the PRESCO trial. AIDS Res Hum Retroviruses 2007;23(8):972–82.

94 Kim AI, Dorn A, Bouajram R, et al. The treatment of chronic hepatitis C in HIV-infected patients: a meta-analysis. HIV Med 2007;8(5):312–21.

95 Clarke S, Keenan E, Ryan M, et al. Directly observed antiretroviral therapy for injection drug users with HIV infection. AIDS Read 2002;12(7):305–7, 12–6.

96 Clarke SM, Mulcahy FM. Antiretroviral therapy for drug users. Int J STD AIDS 2000;11(10):627–31.

97 Chander G, Himelhoch S, Moore RD. Substance abuse and psychiatric disorders in HIV-positive patients: epidemiology and impact on antiretroviral therapy. Drugs 2006;66(6):769–89.

98 Gupta SB, Gilbert RL, Brady AR, et al. CD4 cell counts in adults with newly diagnosed HIV infection: results of surveillance in England and Wales, 1990–1998. CD4 Surveillance Scheme Advisory Group. AIDS 2000;14(7):853–61.

99 Ioannidis JP, Cappelleri JC, Skolnik PR, et al. A meta-analysis of the relative efficacy and toxicity of Pneumocystis carinii prophylactic regimens. Arch Intern Med 1996;156(2):177–88.

100 Bucher HC, Griffith L, Guyatt GH, et al. Meta-analysis of prophylactic treatments against Pneumocystis carinii pneumonia and toxoplasma encephalitis in HIV-infected patients. J Acquir Immune Defic Syndr Hum Retrovirol 1997;15(2):104–14.

101 Mocroft A, Monforte A, Kirk O, et al. Changes in hospital admissions across Europe: 1995–2003. Results from the EuroSIDA study. HIV Med 2004;5(6):437–47.

102 Mocroft A, Neaton J, Bebchuk J, et al. The feasibility of clinical endpoint trials in HIV infection in the highly active antiretroviral treatment (HAART) era. Clin Trials 2006;3(2):119–32.

103 El-Sadr WM, Luskin-Hawk R, Yurik TM, et al. A randomized trial of daily and thrice-weekly trimethoprim-sulfamethoxazole for the prevention of Pneumocystis carinii pneumonia in human immunodeficiency virus-infected persons. Terry Beirn Community Programs for Clinical Research on AIDS (CPCRA). Clin Infect Dis 1999;29(4):775–83.

104 Anglaret X, Chene G, Attia A, et al. Early chemoprophylaxis with trimethoprim-sulphamethoxazole for HIV-1-infected adults in Abidjan, Cote d'Ivoire: a randomised trial. Cotrimo- CI Study Group. Lancet 1999;353(9163): 1463–8.

105 Para MF, Finkelstein D, Becker S, et al. Reduced toxicity with gradual initiation of trimethoprim-sulfamethoxazole as primary prophylaxis for Pneumocystis carinii pneumonia: AIDS Clinical Trials Group 268. J Acquir Immune Defic Syndr 2000;24(4):337–43.

106 Walmsley SL, Khorasheh S, Singer J, et al. A randomized trial of N-acetylcysteine for prevention of trimethoprim- sulfamethoxazole hypersensitivity reactions in Pneumocystis carinii pneumonia prophylaxis (CTN 057). Canadian HIV Trials Network 057 Study Group. J Acquir Immune Defic Syndr Hum Retrovirol 1998;19(5): 498–505.

107 Akerlund B, Tynell E, Bratt G, et al. N-acetylcysteine treatment and the risk of toxic reactions to trimethoprim-sulphamethoxazole in primary Pneumocystis carinii prophylaxis in HIV-infected patients. J Infect 1997;35(2):143–7.

108 El-Sadr WM, Murphy RL, Yurik TM, et al. Atovaquone compared with dapsone for the prevention of Pneumocystis carinii pneumonia in patients with HIV infection who cannot tolerate trimethoprim, sulfonamides, or both. Community Program for Clinical Research on AIDS and the AIDS Clinical Trials Group. N Engl J Med 1998;339(26):1889–95.

109 Chan C, Montaner J, Lefebvre EA, et al. Atovaquone suspension compared with aerosolized pentamidine for prevention of Pneumocystis carinii pneumonia in human immunodeficiency virus-infected subjects intolerant of trimethoprim or sulfonamides. J Infect Dis 1999;180(2):369–76.

110 Saillourglenisson F, Chene G, Salmi LR, et al. [Effect of dapsone on survival in HIV infected patients: a meta-analysis of finished trials]. Rev Epidemiol Sante Publique 2000;48(1):17–30. Abstract.

111 Detels R, Tarwater P, Phair JP, et al. Effectiveness of potent antiretroviral therapies on the incidence of opportunistic infections before and after AIDS diagnosis. AIDS 2001;15(3):347–55.

112 Dunne MW, Bozzette S, McCutchan JA, et al. Efficacy of azithromycin in prevention of *Pneumocystis carinii* pneumonia: a randomised trial. California Collaborative Treatment Group. Lancet 1999;354(9182):891–5.

113 Havlir DV, Dubé MP, Sattler FR, et al. Prophylaxis against disseminated *Mycobacterium avium* complex with weekly azithromycin, daily rifabutin, or both. California Collaborative Treatment Group. N Engl J Med 1996;335(6):392–8.

114 Gallant JE, Moore RD, Chaisson RE. Prophylaxis for opportunistic infections in patients with HIV infection. Ann Intern Med 1994;120(11):932–44.

115 Schacker T, Hu HL, Koelle DM, et al. Famciclovir for the suppression of symptomatic and asymptomatic herpes simplex virus reactivation in HIV-infected persons. A double-blind, placebo-controlled trial. Ann Intern Med 1998;128(1):21–8.

116 Warren T, Harris J, Brennan CA. Efficacy and safety of valacyclovir for the suppression and episodic treatment of herpes simplex virus in patients with HIV. Clin Infect Dis 2004;39 Suppl 5:S258–66.

117 Conant MA, Schacker TW, Murphy RL, et al. Valaciclovir versus aciclovir for herpes simplex virus infection in HIV-infected individuals: two randomized trials. Int J STD AIDS 2002;13(1):12–21.

118 Trikalinos TA, Ioannidis JP. Discontinuation of *Pneumocystis carinii* prophylaxis in patients infected with human immunodeficiency virus: a meta-analysis and decision analysis. Clin Infect Dis 2001;33(11):1901–9.

119 Lopez Bernaldo de Quiros JC, Miro JM, Pena JM, et al. A randomized trial of the discontinuation of primary and secondary prophylaxis against *Pneumocystis carinii* pneumonia after highly active antiretroviral therapy in patients with HIV infection. Grupo de Estudio del SIDA 04/98. N Engl J Med 2001;344(3):159–67.

120 Mussini C, Pezzotti P, Govoni A, et al. Discontinuation of primary prophylaxis for *Pneumocystis carinii* pneumonia and toxoplasmic encephalitis in human immunodeficiency virus type I-infected patients: the changes in opportunistic prophylaxis study. J Infect Dis 2000;181(5):1635–42.

121 Mussini C, Pezzotti P, Antinori A, et al. Discontinuation of secondary prophylaxis for *Pneumocystis carinii* pneumonia in human immunodeficiency virus-infected patients: a randomized trial by the CIOP Study Group. Clin Infect Dis 2003;36(5):645–51.

122 Green H, Hay P, Dunn DT, et al. A prospective multicentre study of discontinuing prophylaxis for opportunistic infections after effective antiretroviral therapy. HIV Med 2004;5(4):278–83.

123 D'Egidio GE, Kravcik S, Cooper CL, et al. *Pneumocystis jiroveci* pneumonia prophylaxis is not required with a CD4+ T-cell count <200 cells/microl when viral replication is suppressed. AIDS 2007;21(13):1711–5.

124 Eigenmann C, Flepp M, Bernasconi E, et al. Low incidence of community-acquired pneumonia among human immunodeficiency virus-infected patients after interruption of *Pneumocystis carinii* pneumonia prophylaxis. Clin Infect Dis 2003;36(7):917–21.

125 Miro J, Lopez J, Podzamczer C, et al. Discontinuation of toxoplasmic encephalitis prophylaxis is safe in HIV-1 and T. gondii co-infected patients after immunological recovery with HAART. Preliminary results of the GESIDA 04/98B study. 7th Conference on Retroviruses and Opportunistic Infections; 2000; San Francisco. Foundation for Retrovirology and Human Health.

126 Podzamczer D, Miro JM, Ferrer E, et al. Thrice-weekly sulfadiazine-pyrimethamine for maintenance therapy of toxoplasmic encephalitis in HIV-infected patients. Spanish Toxoplasmosis Study Group. Eur J Clin Microbiol Infect Dis 2000;19(2):89–95.

127 Tural C, Ruiz L, Holtzer C, et al. Clinical utility of HIV-1 genotyping and expert advice: the Havana trial. AIDS 2002;16(2):209–18.

128 Durant J, Clevenbergh P, Halfon P, et al. Drug-resistance genotyping in HIV-1 therapy: the VIRADAPT randomised controlled trial. Lancet 1999;353(9171):2195–9.

129 Baxter JD, Mayers DL, Wentworth DN, et al. A randomized study of antiretroviral management based on plasma genotypic antiretroviral resistance testing in patients failing therapy. CPCRA 046 Study Team for the Terry Beirn Community Programs for Clinical Research on AIDS. AIDS 2000;14(9):F83–93.

130 Kijak G, AE R, SE P, et al. Discrepant results in the interpretation of HIV-1 drug resistance genotypic data among widely used algorithms. HIV Medicine 2003;4:72–8.

131 Hales G, Birch C, Crowe S, et al. A randomised trial comparing genotypic and virtual phenotypic interpretation of HIV drug resistance: the CREST study. PLoS Clin Trials 2006;1(3):e18.

132 Cohen CJ, Hunt S, Sension M, et al. A randomized trial assessing the impact of phenotypic resistance testing on antiretroviral therapy. AIDS 2002;16(4):579–88.

133 Durant J, Clevenbergh P, Garraffo R, et al. Importance of protease inhibitor plasma levels in HIV-infected patients treated with genotypic-guided therapy: pharmacological data from the Viradapt Study. AIDS 2000;14(10):1333–9.

134 Reynes J, Arasteh K, Clotet B, et al. TORO: ninety-six-week virologic and immunologic response and safety evaluation of enfuvirtide with an optimized background of antiretrovirals. AIDS Patient Care STDS 2007;21(8):533–43.

135 Molina JM, Cohen C, Katlama C, et al. Safety and efficacy of darunavir (TMC114) with low-dose ritonavir in treatment-experienced patients: 24-week results of POWER 3. J Acquir Immune Defic Syndr 2007;46(1):24–31.

136 Kristiansen TB, Pedersen AG, Eugen-Olsen J, et al. Genetic evolution of HIV in patients remaining on a stable HAART regimen despite insufficient viral suppression. Scand J Infect Dis 2005;37(11–12):890–901.

137 Ruiz L, Ribera E, Bonjoch A, et al. Virological and Immunological Benefit of a Salvage Therapy that Includes Kaletra plus Fortovase Preceded or not by Antiretroviral Therapy Interruption (TI) in Advanced HIV-Infected Patients (6-Month-Follow-up). 9th Conference on Retroviruses and Opportunistic Infections; 2002; Seattle.

138 Katlama C, Dominguez S, Duvivier C, et al. Benefits of Treatment Interruption (TI) in Patients with Multiple Therapy Failures, CD4 cells <200/mm³ and HIV RNA >50000 cp/ml (GIGHAART ANRS 097). Fourteenth International AIDS Conference; Barcelona; 2002.

139 Delaugerre C, Peytavin G, Dominguez S, et al. Virological and pharmacological factors associated with virological response to salvage therapy after an 8-week of treatment interruption in a context of very advanced HIV disease (GigHAART ANRS 097). J Med Virol 2005;77(3): 345–50.

140 Walmsley SL, Thorne A, Loutfy MR, et al. A prospective randomized controlled trial of structured treatment interruption in HIV-infected patients failing highly active antiretroviral therapy (Canadian HIV Trials Network Study 164). J Acquir Immune Defic Syndr 2007;45(4):418–25.

141 Pai NP, Lawrence J, Reingold AL, et al. Structured treatment interruptions (STI) in chronic unsuppressed HIV infection in adults. Cochrane Database Syst Rev 2006 (3), CD006148, DOI: 10.1002/14651858.

142 Lundgren JD, Vella S, Paddam L, ct al. Interruption/ Stopping Antiretroviral Therapy and the Risk of Clinical Disease: Results from the EuroSIDA Study. 9th Conference on Retroviruses and Opportunistic Infections; Seattle; 2002.

143 El-Sadr WM, Lundgren JD, Neaton JD, et al. CD4+ count-guided interruption of antiretroviral treatment. N Engl J Med 2006;355(22):2283–96.

144 Staszewski S, Babacan E, Stephan C, et al. The LOPSAQ study: 48 week analysis of a boosted double protease inhibitor regimen containing lopinavir/ritonavir plus saquinavir without additional antiretroviral therapy. J Antimicrob Chemother 2006;58(5):1024–30.

145 Castagna A, Danise A, Menzo S, et al. Lamivudine monotherapy in HIV-1-infected patients harbouring a lamivudine-resistant virus: a randomized pilot study (E-184V study). AIDS 2006;20(6):795–803.

146 Deeks SG, Hoh R, Neilands TB, et al. Interruption of treatment with individual therapeutic drug classes in adults with multidrug-resistant HIV-1 infection. J Infect Dis 2005;192(9):1537–44.

147 van der Horst CM, Saag MS, Cloud GA, et al. Treatment of cryptococcal meningitis associated with the acquired immunodeficiency syndrome. National Institute of Allergy and Infectious Diseases Mycoses Study Group and AIDS Clinical Trials Group. N Engl J Med 1997;337(1):15–21.

148 Leenders AC, Reiss P, Portegies P, et al. Liposomal amphotericin B (AmBisome) compared with amphotericin B both followed by oral fluconazole in the treatment of AIDS-associated cryptococcal meningitis. AIDS 1997;11(12):1463–71.

149 Coker RJ, Viviani M, Gazzard BG, et al. Treatment of cryptococcosis with liposomal amphotericin B (AmBisome) in 23 patients with AIDS. AIDS 1993;7(6):829–35.

150 Saag MS, Powderly WG, Cloud GA, et al. Comparison of amphotericin B with fluconazole in the treatment of acute AIDS-associated cryptococcal meningitis. The NIAID Mycoses Study Group and the AIDS Clinical Trials Group. N Engl J Med 1992;326(2):83–9.

151 Mayanja-Kizza H, Oishi K, Mitarai S, et al. Combination therapy with fluconazole and flucytosine for cryptococcal meningitis in Ugandan patients with AIDS. Clin Infect Dis 1998;26(6):1362–6.

152 de Gans J, Portegies P, Tiessens G, et al. Itraconazole compared with amphotericin B plus flucytosine in AIDS patients with cryptococcal meningitis. AIDS 1992;6(2): 185–90.

153 Graybill JR, Sobel J, Saag M, et al. Diagnosis and management of increased intracranial pressure in patients with AIDS and cryptococcal meningitis. The NIAID Mycoses Study Group and AIDS Cooperative Treatment Groups. Clin Infect Dis 2000;30(1):47–54.

154 Fessler RD, Sobel J, Guyot L, et al. Management of elevated intracranial pressure in patients with Cryptococcal meningitis. J Acquir Immune Defic Syndr Hum Retrovirol 1998;17(2):137–42.

155 Chang LW, Phipps WT, Kennedy GE, et al. Antifungal interventions for the primary prevention of cryptococcal disease in adults with HIV. Cochrane Database Syst Rev 2005 (3), CD004773, DOI: 10.1002/14651858.

156 Saag MS, Cloud GA, Graybill JR, et al. A comparison of itraconazole versus fluconazole as maintenance therapy for AIDS-associated cryptococcal meningitis. National Institute of Allergy and Infectious Diseases Mycoses Study Group. Clin Infect Dis 1999;28(2):291–6.

157 Pienaar ED, Young T, Holmes H. Interventions for the prevention and management of oropharyngeal candidiasis associated with HIV infection in adults and children. Cochrane Database Syst Rev 2006 (3), CD003940, DOI: 10.1002/14651858.

158 Havlir DV, Dubé MP, McCutchan JA, et al. Prophylaxis with weekly versus daily fluconazole for fungal infections in patients with AIDS. Clin Infect Dis 1998;27(6):1369–75.

159 Powderly WG, Finkelstein D, Feinberg J, et al. A randomized trial comparing fluconazole with clotrimazole troches for the prevention of fungal infections in patients with advanced human immunodeficiency virus infection. NIAID AIDS Clinical Trials Group. N Engl J Med 1995;332(11):700–5.

160 Smith D, Midgley J, Gazzard B. A randomised, double-blind study of itraconazole versus placebo in the treatment and prevention of oral or oesophageal candidosis in patients with HIV infection. Int J Clin Pract 1999;53(5):349–52.

161 Wheat J, Hafner R, Wulfsohn M, et al. Prevention of relapse of histoplasmosis with itraconazole in patients with the acquired immunodeficiency syndrome. The National Institute of Allergy and Infectious Diseases Clinical Trials and Mycoses Study Group Collaborators. Ann Intern Med 1993;118(8):610–6.

162 Dunne M, Fessel J, Kumar P, et al. A randomized, double-blind trial comparing azithromycin and clarithromycin in the treatment of disseminated Mycobacterium avium infection in patients with human immunodeficiency virus. Clin Infect Dis 2000;31(5):1245–52.

163 Cohn DL, Fisher EJ, Peng GT, et al. A prospective randomized trial of four three-drug regimens in the treatment of disseminated Mycobacterium avium complex disease in AIDS patients: excess mortality associated with high-dose clarithromycin. Terry Beirn Community Programs for Clinical Research on AIDS. Clin Infect Dis 1999;29(1):125–33.

164 Singer J, Thorne A, Khorasheh S, et al. Symptomatic and health status outcomes in the Canadian randomized MAC treatment trial (CTN010). Canadian HIV Trials Network Protocol 010 Study Group. Int J STD AIDS 2000;11(4):212–19.

165 Faris MA, Raasch RH, Hopfer RL, et al. Treatment and prophylaxis of disseminated *Mycobacterium avium* complex in HIV-infected individuals. Ann Pharmacother 1998;32(5):564–73.

166 Oldfield EC, 3rd, Fessel WJ, Dunne MW, et al. Once weekly azithromycin therapy for prevention of *Mycobacterium avium* complex infection in patients with AIDS: a randomized, double-blind, placebo-controlled multicenter trial. Clin Infect Dis 1998;26(3):611–9.

167 Benson CA, Williams PL, Cohn DL, et al. Clarithromycin or rifabutin alone or in combination for primary prophylaxis of *Mycobacterium avium* complex disease in patients with AIDS: A randomized, double-blind, placebo-controlled trial. The AIDS Clinical Trials Group 196/Terry Beirn Community Programs for Clinical Research on AIDS 009 Protocol Team. J Infect Dis 2000;181(4):1289–97.

168 Dubé MP, Sattler FR, Torriani FJ, et al. A randomized evaluation of ethambutol for prevention of relapse and drug resistance during treatment of *Mycobacterium avium* complex bacteremia with clarithromycin-based combination therapy. California Collaborative Treatment Group. J Infect Dis 1997;176(5):1225–32.

169 Chaisson RE, Keiser P, Pierce M, et al. Clarithromycin and ethambutol with or without clofazimine for the treatment of bacteremic *Mycobacterium avium* complex disease in patients with HIV infection. AIDS 1997;11(3):311–7.

170 May T, Brel F, Beuscart C, et al. Comparison of combination therapy regimens for treatment of human immunodeficiency virus-infected patients with disseminated bacteremia due to *Mycobacterium avium*. ANRS Trial 033 Curavium Group. Agence Nationale de Recherche sur le Sida. Clin Infect Dis 1997;25(3):621–9.

171 Gordin FM, Sullam PM, Shafran SD, et al. A randomized, placebo-controlled study of rifabutin added to a regimen of clarithromycin and ethambutol for treatment of disseminated infection with *Mycobacterium avium* complex. Clin Infect Dis 1999;28(5):1080–5.

172 Tseng AL, Walmsley SL. Rifabutin-associated uveitis. Ann Pharmacother 1995;29(11):1149–55.

173 Currier JS, Williams PL, Koletar SL, et al. Discontinuation of *Mycobacterium avium* complex prophylaxis in patients with antiretroviral therapy-induced increases in CD4+ cell count. A randomized, double-blind, placebo-controlled trial. AIDS Clinical Trials Group 362 Study Team. Ann Intern Med 2000;133(7):493–503.

174 El-Sadr WM, Burman WJ, Grant LB, et al. Discontinuation of prophylaxis for *Mycobacterium avium* complex disease in HIV-infected patients who have a response to antiretroviral therapy. Terry Beirn Community Programs for Clinical Research on AIDS. N Engl J Med 2000;342(15):1085–92.

175 Moyle G, Harman C, Mitchell S, et al. Foscarnet and ganciclovir in the treatment of CMV retinitis in AIDS patients: a randomised comparison. J Infect 1992;25(1):21–7.

176 Martin DF, Sierra-Madero J, Walmsley S, et al. A controlled trial of valganciclovir as induction therapy for cytomegalovirus retinitis. N Engl J Med 2002;346(15):1119–26.

177 Spector SA, McKinley GF, Lalezari JP, et al. Oral ganciclovir for the prevention of cytomegalovirus disease in persons with AIDS. Roche Cooperative Oral Ganciclovir Study Group. N Engl J Med 1996;334(23):1491–7.

178 Brosgart CL, Louis TA, Hillman DW, et al. A randomized, placebo-controlled trial of the safety and efficacy of oral ganciclovir for prophylaxis of cytomegalovirus disease in HIV- infected individuals. Terry Beirn Community Programs for Clinical Research on AIDS. Aids 1998;12(3):269–77.

179 Ioannidis JP, Collier AC, Cooper DA, et al. Clinical efficacy of high-dose acyclovir in patients with human immunodeficiency virus infection: a meta-analysis of randomized individual patient data. J Infect Dis 1998;178(2):349–59.

180 Feinberg JE, Hurwitz S, Cooper D, et al. A randomized, double-blind trial of valaciclovir prophylaxis for cytomegalovirus disease in patients with advanced human immunodeficiency virus infection. AIDS Clinical Trials Group Protocol 204/Glaxo Wellcome 123–014 International CMV Prophylaxis Study Group. J Infect Dis 1998;177(1):48–56.

181 Curi AL, Muralha A, Muralha L, et al. Suspension of anti-cytomegalovirus maintenance therapy following immune recovery due to highly active antiretroviral therapy. Br J Ophthalmol 2001;85(4):471–3.

182 Jouan M, Saves M, Tubiana R, et al. Discontinuation of maintenance therapy for cytomegalovirus retinitis in HIV-infected patients receiving highly active antiretroviral therapy. AIDS 2001;15(1):23–31.

183 Whitcup SM, Fortin E, Lindblad AS, et al. Discontinuation of anticytomegalovirus therapy in patients with HIV infection and cytomegalovirus retinitis. JAMA 1999;282(17):1633–7.

184 Torriani FJ, Freeman WR, Macdonald JC, et al. CMV retinitis recurs after stopping treatment in virological and immunological failures of potent antiretroviral therapy. AIDS 2000;14(2):173–80.

185 Postelmans L, Gerard M, Sommereijns B, et al. Discontinuation of maintenance therapy for CMV retinitis in AIDS patients on highly active antiretroviral therapy. Ocul Immunol Inflamm 1999;7(3–4):199–203.

186 Jabs DA, Bolton SG, Dunn JP, et al. Discontinuing anti-cytomegalovirus therapy in patients with immune reconstitution after combination antiretroviral therapy. Am J Ophthalmol 1998;126(6):817–22.

187 Vrabec TR, Baldassano VF, Whitcup SM. Discontinuation of maintenance therapy in patients with quiescent

cytomegalovirus retinitis and elevated CD4+ counts. Ophthalmology 1998;105(7):1259–64.

188 Macdonald JC, Torriani FJ, Morse LS, et al. Lack of reactivation of cytomegalovirus (CMV) retinitis after stopping CMV maintenance therapy in AIDS patients with sustained elevations in CD4 T cells in response to highly active antiretroviral therapy. J Infect Dis 1998;177(5):1182–7.

189 Tural C, Romeu J, Sirera G, et al. Long-lasting remission of cytomegalovirus retinitis without maintenance therapy in human immunodeficiency virus-infected patients. J Infect Dis 1998;177(4):1080–3.

190 Kaplan LD, Straus DJ, Testa MA, et al. Low-dose compared with standard-dose m-BACOD chemotherapy for non-Hodgkin's lymphoma associated with human immunodeficiency virus infection. National Institute of Allergy and Infectious Diseases AIDS Clinical Trials Group. N Engl J Med 1997;336(23):1641–8.

191 Mounier N, Spina M, Gabarre J, et al. AIDS-related non-Hodgkin lymphoma: final analysis of 485 patients treated with risk-adapted intensive chemotherapy. Blood 2006;107(10):3832 40.

192 Raboud JM, Montaner JS, Rae S, et al. Meta-analysis of five randomized controlled trials comparing continuation of zidovudine versus switching to didanosine in HIV-infected individuals. Antivir Ther 1997;2(4):237–47.

193 Andreoletti L, Lescieux A, Lambert V, et al. Semiquantitative detection of JCV-DNA in peripheral blood leukocytes from HIV-1-infected patients with or without progressive multifocal leukoencephalopathy. J Med Virol 2002;66(1):1–7.

194 Garcia de Viedma D, Alonso R, Miralles P, et al. Dual qualitative-quantitative nested PCR for detection of JC virus in cerebrospinal fluid: high potential for evaluation and monitoring of progressive multifocal leukoencephalopathy in AIDS patients receiving highly active antiretroviral therapy. J Clin Microbiol 1999;37(3):724–8.

195 Gasnault J, Kousignian P, Kahraman M, et al. Cidofovir in AIDS-associated progressive multifocal leukoencephalopathy: a monocenter observational study with clinical and JC virus load monitoring. J Neurovirol 2001;7(4):375–81.

196 Hall CD, Dafni U, Simpson D, et al. Failure of cytarabine in progressive multifocal leukoencephalopathy associated with human immunodeficiency virus infection. AIDS Clinical Trials Group 243 Team. N Engl J Med 1998;338(19):1345–51.

197 De Luca A, Giancola ML, Ammassari A, et al. Potent antiretroviral therapy with or without cidofovir for AIDS-associated progressive multifocal leukoencephalopathy: extended follow- up of an observational study. J Neurovirol 2001;7(4):364–8.

CHAPTER 12

Influenza

Ashley Roberts & Joanne M. Langley

Case presentation

A 66-year-old male with type 2 diabetes mellitus presents with a 2-day history of fever and cough during the month of January. He also complains of intermittent headaches, "aches and pains," and loss of appetite. He is having difficulty maintaining his usual tight glucose control during this illness. A retired schoolteacher, he just returned from a visit with his young grandchildren, all of whom had coughs, runny nose, and fever. He has no significant travel history or animal exposure. On examination, the patient looks uncomfortable and diaphoretic. His temperature is 38.5°C, respiratory rate 25, heart rate 90, and the O_2 saturation 98% on room air. There is mild increased work of breathing and crackles bilaterally at the lung bases. The rest of his examination is normal. The chest radiograph reveals nonspecific perihilar opacities and streaking bilaterally. There is no focal consolidation.

On further questioning, the patient remembers receiving "a vaccine for pneumonia" last year. He can't specifically remember getting the influenza vaccine this year. You recall getting an email from the public health authority about an influenza virus outbreak in a nearby nursing home, and wonder if you should institute a diagnostic test for influenza in this patient. You also wonder if antiviral treatment might help this patient.

Diagnosis

Influenza occurs in epidemics of variable severity every winter in temperate climates, affecting up to

Evidence-Based Infectious Diseases, 2nd edition. Edited by Mark Loeb, Fiona Smaill and Marek Smieja. © 2009 Wiley-Blackwell Publishing, ISBN: 978-1-4051-7026-0

20% of the general population [1]. In tropical and subtropical climates influenza occurs throughout the year with one or more peaks of activity. Pandemic outbreaks of influenza, related to major shifts in the viral hemagglutinin (H) or neuraminidase (N) antigens, may not have this seasonal pattern; this type of influenza is not discussed here. The seasonality of interpandemic influenza incidence affects the accuracy of diagnosis. The methods for diagnosis of influenza are clinical, laboratory testing of respiratory tract specimens or serum, and diagnostic imaging. Diagnostic accuracy is highest when influenza is circulating in the community, since the pretest likelihood will be higher due to increased disease prevalence. Laboratory confirmation of influenza virus infection remains the most accurate diagnostic tool.

Clinical diagnosis

Influenza is a viral infection of the respiratory tract, which is accompanied by nonspecific systemic symptoms. Generally of acute onset, the symptoms include systemic manifestations (fever, malaise, anorexia, chills, myalgia, headache) and those specific to the respiratory tract (cough, sore throat, rhinorrhea, tachypnea, sneezing). Two systematic reviews on the diagnosis of influenza were found that included primary prospective studies where clinical signs and symptoms were compared to a gold standard diagnosis using laboratory confirmation. A review by Ebell et al. found a positive likelihood ratio (LR) >2.0 for the following individual symptoms: rigors (7.2), sweating (2.86), confined to bed (2.4), and unable to cope with daily activities (2.3) [2]. A later review, which excluded studies based on quality criteria, included only three of the seven primary studies in Ebell's review and identified three other studies [3].

It concluded that no individual sign or symptom of influenza had a positive LR >2.0, that is, high enough to confirm influenza.

If the odds of laboratory-confirmed influenza in a patient without certain individual symptoms (i.e., negative LR) are <0.5 then it is likely that influenza can be ruled out [3]. In the first review [2] four individual symptoms had LR <0.50, indicating that one could quite accurately exclude a diagnosis of influenza if the symptom were absent: confined to bed (LR. 0.50), unable to cope with daily activities (LR, 0.39), any systemic symptom (LR, 0.36) and cough (LR, 0.38). Confidence intervals around these point estimates were not given. In the second review, three individual symptoms had LR <0.5, indicating that one could quite accurately exclude a diagnosis of influenza if these were absent [3]: fever ((LR 0.40, 95% CI 0.25–0.66), cough (LR 0.42, 95% CI 0.31–0.57), and nasal congestion (LR 0.49, 95% CI 0.42–0.59).

Two primary studies assessed a combination of symptoms, fever, and cough, in all ages [4] and in persons over 60 years of age [5]. These found positive LRs of 1.9 (95% 1.8–2.1) and 5.9 (95% CI 3.5–6.9) respectively during the winter months, suggesting that if influenza is present in the community the accuracy of a clinical diagnosis of influenza in a patient with fever and cough, especially in an older patient, is likely to be high.

Laboratory diagnosis

Influenza viruses are categorized into three antigenic types, A, B, and C, based on proteins in the nucleocapsid and matrix. Influenza A is further subtyped according to membrane glycoproteins H (hemagglutinin) and N (neuraminidase) [6]. There are 16 known H subtypes and nine N subtypes [6]. Influenza C is an uncommon cause of human infection. Influenza viruses undergo small antigenic changes or "drift" over time which results in yearly epidemics. Major antigenic changes, or "shift" in influenza A virus, with emergence of a new subtype that can be spread from human to human and causes clinically significant disease, result in influenza pandemics associated with worldwide morbidity and mortality, and are not discussed here.

Laboratory tests for the timely diagnosis of influenza are conducted on specimens procured from the respiratory tract obtained from nasal aspirate, swab or wash, or a throat swab or wash, or from serum (Table 12.1). Notably, sputum is not a useful specimen in the diagnosis of influenza and throat swabs are less sensitive than specimens from the nasopharynx. Influenza tests rely on detection of the virus, or the patient's immune response to the virus [7]. As seen in Table 12.1, the types of test available are viral culture, enzyme immunoassay, polymerase chain reaction (PCR), and serology. The usefulness of each test in altering decision-making (e.g., treatment, prophylaxis of contacts, outbreak management) is affected by the timeliness of results. As can be seen, only the respiratory tract specimens are available in a timeline that will be helpful to the clinician.

As with almost all microbiologic tests, accuracy of influenza testing is altered by the time specimens are taken in relation to disease onset and whether specimen procurement is done correctly. Viral shedding tends to be greatest earlier in influenza, and false-negative results may occur when testing is done after 3 days of symptoms since viral replication is decreasing or finished in the normal host. False-negative tests can also occur because of inappropriate specimen handling. False-positive tests are most commonly the result of laboratory error or test characteristics. A full discussion of the test characteristics is beyond the scope of this chapter; the reader is referred to comprehensive reviews which discuss test sensitivity, specificity, and technologic requirements and considerations [7,8].

Radiology

No systematic reviews on the accuracy of diagnosis of influenza-associated lower respiratory tract infection were found. The most commonly used diagnostic imaging test for pneumonia is the chest radiograph [9]. Although imaging can confirm involvement of the lungs, findings are too nonspecific to point to microbiologic etiology. Viral and bacterial pneumonias may have distinguishing features however. The radiologic pattern of viral pneumonia is usually less confluent and homogenous than bacterial pneumonia. The picture in viral infection may be one of air-space nodules (of 4–10 mm), patchy peribronchial ground glass opacity, or air-space consolidation [9]. Hyperinflation is more likely in viral than bacterial pneumonia because of the associated bronchiolitis [9].

Table 12.1 Options for laboratory confirmation of influenza virus infection

Source of specimen	Diagnostic test	Time to test result	Test characteristics
Respiratory tract (NP aspirate, NP swab/wash, throat swab)			
	Rapid antigen detection	<30 minutes	Less sensitive than other respiratory tract tests
	Immunofluorescence microscopy	~1–4 hours	Immunofluorescent antibody detection more sensitive but slower than direct fluorescent antibody detection
	Nucleic acid testing (e.g. RT-PCR)	4–6 hours	Most sensitive and specific tests for influenza
	Virus isolation – by shell vial culture – by conventional culture	18–48 hours 3–14 days	Shell vial method more sensitive
Serum	Neutralization test Hemagglutination-inhibition Enzyme immunoassay Complement fixation	Paired serum samples taken during acute and convalescent (2–3 weeks later) phases required	

Adapted from Petric M et al., Role of the laboratory in diagnosis of influenza during seasonal epidemics and potential pandemics [7] and Cox N et al., Manual of Clinical Microbiology [45].
NP, nasopharyngeal; RT-PCR, reverse-transcription polymerase chain reaction.

Treatment

Treatment of influenza includes specific antiviral therapies, alternative therapies, nonspecific supportive measures, and treatment of complications of influenza.

There are two classes of specific antiviral drugs that are available for treatment of influenza and have been shown to alter the natural history of uncomplicated symptomatic infection in randomized controlled blinded trials: M2 ion channel inhibitors (amantadine and rimantidine) and neuraminidase inhibitors (oseltamivir and zanamivir). Amantadine and rimantidine are active against influenza A only and interfere with viral replication by inhibiting the M2 ion channel, which is necessary to acidify the interior of the virus. The neuraminidase inhibitors interfere with the influenza viral enzyme neuraminidase, which cleaves terminal sialic acid from sialic-acid-containing cell surface glycoproteins during replication.

A systematic review of amantadine and/or rimantidine in the therapy of uncomplicated influenza A illness showed reduction in the duration of fever by about 1 day compared to placebo [10], but not a significant reduction in viral shedding from the upper airway. The adverse event profile was similar in placebo and antiviral agent groups [10]. Treatment must be initiated within 48 hours after symptom onset for greatest benefit. The most common adverse effect is central nervous system symptoms such as irritability, insomnia, agitation, and confusion.

Since 2001 an increasing incidence of amantadine- and rimantidine-resistant influenza viruses have been observed [11], leading public health authorities to recommend that this class of drugs not be used for treatment or prophylaxis [12]. Ongoing worldwide surveillance of influenza epidemiology and antiviral resistance will determine if this class of drugs will play a role in influenza management in the future.

Neuraminidase inhibitors prevent the replication of both type A and B influenza viruses by inhibiting influenza virus neuraminidase. Neuraminidase enables release of virions from infected cells by preventing them from self-aggregating and binding to the surface of infected cells. Oseltamivir is a neuraminidase inhibitor that is administered twice daily by mouth, while zanamivir is administered by inhalation.

Two systematic reviews of randomized controlled trials of oseltamivir and zanamivir in the treatment of influenza have shown that both reduce the duration of symptoms by 1 day, and reduce the time before normal activities are resumed by about half a day in healthy adults [13,14]. The most common adverse effect associated with oseltamivir use is gastrointestinal (nausea, vomiting). Zanamivir is not recommended in individuals with underlying airway disease (such as asthma or chronic obstructive pulmonary disease) because of the risk of airway irritation leading to bronchospasm.

A recent systematic review of randomized controlled trials of Chinese medicinal herbs for the treatment of influenza identified two studies with 1012 patients [15]; the evidence was considered insufficient to support or reject use of these products in influenza. Another systematic review of evidence for the effectiveness of a number of complementary therapies also concluded that there was insufficient evidence of therapeutic benefit [16]. A Cochrane review [17] of Oscillococcinum, a homeopathic product derived from duck liver and heart, reduced the length of influenza illness by 0.28 days (95% CI 0.50–0.06).

Supportive care for influenza consists of adequate hydration and symptomatic therapy for discomfort and fever with nonsteroidal inflammatory medications or acetaminophen. Patients who are unable to maintain fluid intake or develop respiratory distress may require care in the hospital setting.

In healthy people influenza is an acute febrile illness that lasts for about 1 week [18]. However, influenza can lead to serious complications including pneumonia (secondary bacterial or primary viral pneumonia) or exacerbation of preexisting lung, cardiac, or other chronic disease [19]. Other complications of influenza virus infection include myositis, encephalitis and other neurologic disorders, pericarditis, and myocarditis. Two recent studies, analyzing large health utilization databases with a combined population of over 80 000, indicate that persons diagnosed with influenza and to whom oseltamivir was prescribed had significant reductions in the risk of pneumonia [20] or respiratory disease [21], otitis media, and hospitalization [20,21]. An observational study of 77 adults admitted for influenza-associated illness found antiviral therapy was associated with a significant reduction in mortality (OR 0.21, 95% CI 0.06–0.80), but was not associated with length of stay [22].

Prognosis

In healthy persons influenza is associated with various combinations of fever, cough, rigors, myalgia, and headache of about 1 week's duration [16] often severe enough to result in workplace absenteeism [23–25]. Complicated influenza can occur in previously healthy persons, but is more likely to occur in persons with certain risk factors. The most striking risk factor for complicated influenza requiring hospital care or influenza-associated death is age. Children under 2 years of age and adults over 65 have admission rates to hospital near 100 per 100 000 age-specific population [26–28].

Certain chronic health conditions, in particular cardiac or pulmonary disease, diabetes and renal failure are associated with higher incidence of hospital admissions than occurs in healthy persons in the same age group [29]. Pregnant women with seasonal influenza are more likely than nonpregnant women to be admitted to hospital in several studies, but do not appear to be at increased risk of adverse fetal outcomes or maternal death [30]. Both age and the presence of the previously mentioned chronic health conditions increase risk of death associated with influenza [12,27,31]. In the US the average annual number of deaths attributable to influenza is 34 000 [12].

Prevention

Three categories of interventions exist for the prevention of influenza: vaccination, infection prevention and control measures, and antiviral drugs.

Immunization is the cornerstone of public health influenza control programs, and in almost all developed countries is recommended on an annual basis for persons at high risk of complicated influenza or of being hospitalized for care of influenza, such as persons over 65 years of age, and those with chronic health conditions such as cardiac or lung disease (Table 12.2). A second important component of influenza immunization is to vaccinate those who care for, or are in regular contact with, persons at high risk of influenza such as household contacts or healthcare providers. This strategy seeks to interrupt spread to vulnerable persons, especially those who cannot be immunized (e.g., children <6 months of age), or are

Table 12.2 Persons for whom annual influenza immunization is recommended because of increased risk of hospitalization, complicated influenza, or death

Children 6–23 months of age
Persons >65 years of age
Persons with immunosuppression, primary or secondary
Persons with chronic pulmonary (including asthma), cardiovascular, renal, metabolic or hematologic disorders
Residents of nursing homes or other chronic care facilities
Pregnant women

less likely to respond to the vaccine (e.g., elderly or immunocompromised people).

Commercial influenza vaccines were first introduced in 1945, and a number of vaccine types are available, namely, injectable inactivated or subunit vaccines, and nasally administered live attenuated products [32]. The strains to be used in each year's vaccine are chosen annually by the World Health Organization based on surveillance data gathered by participating laboratories worldwide.

The efficacy of influenza vaccines in preventing influenza has been evaluated in thousands of patients in randomized controlled clinical trials, and several systematic reviews summarizing these studies are available [1,33–38]. Estimates of influenza vaccine efficacy in a particular season vary according to the degree of match of the circulating strains with the vaccine strain, the age of the recipient and their previous experience with infection or immunization, and the type of influenza vaccine. Two types of outcome measures have been used to assess vaccine efficacy and effectiveness: clinical definitions of respiratory illness, and laboratory-confirmed influenza. Use of the latter more accurate outcome results in higher estimates of vaccine efficacy than does a measure of clinical outcome [1]. A number of different clinical definitions of influenza-like illness have been used, and this will affect the calculation of vaccine efficacy [39,40]. Clinical outcome measures capture non-influenza viral respiratory illness against which influenza vaccine is obviously not effective.

Randomized controlled trials of influenza vaccine demonstrate that influenza vaccine prevents laboratory-confirmed illness in 70–90% of in healthy persons when the circulating strain matches that in the vaccine [1,35]. Estimates of efficacy are lower when there is mismatch, estimated in a recent metaanalysis as 50% (95% CI 27–65) [35]. Randomized controlled trials of inactivated influenza vaccines also show reduction in exacerbations in adults with chronic obstructive pulmonary disease [36] and fewer deaths from pneumonia and overall deaths in elderly residents of nursing homes when their care-givers are immunized [41]. Other reviews have concluded that there is insufficient evidence that influenza immunization reduces asthma exacerbations [33], and that there is no evidence for or against the use of influenza vaccine to reduce pulmonary decline and respiratory exacerbations in patients with bronchiectasis [34].

Antiviral drugs have also been approved for the prevention of seasonal influenza as well as for treatment of established illness. Chemoprophylaxis can be considered in the following circumstances: to prevent infection in institutional settings (e.g., long-term care facility or hospital) once influenza is identified in the community or in the facility, or as post-exposure prophylaxis for high-risk persons in whom vaccine has not or cannot be administered or is not expected to be efficacious (e.g., immunocompromised people). Studies done prior to widespread adamantine resistance showed amantadine and rimantidine were effective in prevention of influenza A (60–70% reduction) [10] including in elderly persons [42]. This class of drugs is not recommended for prophylaxis at the time of writing because of high levels of resistance worldwide [43].

The neuraminidase inhibitors are effective in prevention of influenza subtypes A and B, and have been used as seasonal proprophylaxis (e.g. for 6 to 8 weeks when influenza is in the community) or as a post-exposure measure in household or other close contacts. Two metaanalyses had similar findings: one group found a relative reduction of 70–90% in the odds of developing influenza [14], and a second found an efficacy of 58–89% in healthy adults depending on the strategy of prophylaxis [13].

Infection prevention and control measures consist of behaviors and use of personal protective equipment that will interrupt transmission of influenza virus from infected persons or influenza-contaminated articles to susceptible persons. Influenza virus is transmitted predominantly through droplets from the respiratory tract which are expelled during coughing or sneezing, or transmitted during direct contact [44]. Hand hygiene using soap or antimicrobial agents (e.g., waterless handrubs, antimicrobial soap) is effective at eliminating virus from the hands. In addition to Standard Precautions, transmission-based Precautions are recommended for the care of a hospitalized patient with influenza. Placement in a single room is preferred and a standard surgical mask should be worn within 3 feet of the patient [45].

References

1 Langley JM, Faughnan ME. Prevention of influenza in the general population. CMAJ 2004;171(10):1213–22.

2 Ebell MH, White LL, Casault T. A systematic review of the history and physical examination to diagnose influenza. J Am Board Fam Pract 2004;17(1):1–5.

3 Call SA, Vollenweider MA, Hornung CA, Simel DL, McKinney WP. Does this patient have influenza? JAMA 2005;293(8):987–97.

4 Monto AS, Gravenstein S, Elliott M, Colopy M, Schweinle J. Clinical signs and symptoms predicting influenza infection. Arch Intern Med 2000;160(21):3243–7.

5 Govaert TM, Dinant GJ, Aretz K, Knottnerus JA. The predictive value of influenza symptomatology in elderly people. Fam Pract 1998;15(1):16–22.

6 Knipe DM, Howley PM (eds). Field's Virology. 5th ed. 2007, Wolters Kluwer. p. 3177.

7 Petric M, Comanor L, Petti CA. Role of the laboratory in diagnosis of influenza during seasonal epidemics and potential pandemics. J Infect Dis 2006;194 Suppl 2:S98–110.

8 World Health Organization. WHO recommendations on the use of rapid testing for influenza diagnosis. 2005 [cited 2008 20 July]; Available from: http://www.who.int/csr/disease/avian_influenza/guidelines/rapid_testing/en/.

9 Sharma S, Maycher B, Eschun G. Radiological imaging in pneumonia: recent innovations. Curr Opin Pulm Med 2007;13(3):159–69.

10 Jefferson T, Demicheli V, Di Pietrantonj C, Rivetti D. Amantadine and rimantadine for influenza A in adults. Cochrane Database Syst Rev 2006 (2), CD001169, DOI: 10.1002/14651858.

11 Deyde VM, Xu X, Bright RA, et al. Surveillance of resistance to adamantanes among influenza A(H3N2) and A(H1N1) viruses isolated worldwide. J Infect Dis 2007;196(2):249–57.

12 Fiore AE, Shay DK, Haber P, et al. Prevention and control of influenza. Recommendations of the Advisory Committee on Immunization Practices (ACIP), 2007. MMWR Recomm Rep 2007;56(RR-6):1–54.

13 Jefferson TO, Demicheli V, Di Pietrantonj C, Jones M, Rivetti D. Neuraminidase inhibitors for preventing and treating influenza in healthy adults. Cochrane Database Syst Rev 2006 (3), CD001265, DOI: 10.1002/14651858.

14 Cooper NJ, Sutton AJ, Abrams KR, Wailoo A, Turner D, Nicholson KG. Effectiveness of neuraminidase inhibitors in treatment and prevention of influenza A and B: systematic review and meta-analyses of randomised controlled trials. BMJ 2003;326(7401):1235.

15 Chen XY, Wu T, Liu G, et al. Chinese medicinal herbs for influenza. Cochrane Database Syst Rev 2007 (4), CD004559: DOI: 10.1002/14651858.

16 Guo R, Pittler MH, Ernst E. Complementary medicine for treating or preventing influenza or influenza-like illness. Am J Med 2007;120(11):923–929 e3.

17 Vickers AJ, Smith C. Homoeopathic Oscillococcinum for preventing and treating influenza and influenza-like syndromes. Cochrane Database Syst Rev 2006 (3), CD001957, DOI: 10.1002/14651858.

18 Nicholson KG, Human influenza, in Textbook of Influenza, KG Nicholson, RG Webster, AJ Hay (eds). 1998, Blackwell Sciences: Oxford. pp. 219–64.

19 Rothberg MB, Haessler SD, Brown RB. Complications of viral influenza. Am J Med 2008;121(4):258–64.

20 Gums JG, Pelletier EM, Blumentals WA. Oseltamivir and influenza-related complications, hospitalization and healthcare expenditure in healthy adults and children. Expert Opin Pharmacother 2008;9(2):151–61.

21 Blumentals WA, Schulman KL. Impact of oseltamivir on the incidence of secondary complications of influenza in adolescent and adult patients: results from a retrospective population-based study. Curr Med Res Opin 2007; 23(12):2961–70.

22 McGeer A, Green KA, Plevneshi A et al.; Toronto Invasive Bacterial Diseases Network. Antiviral therapy and outcomes of influenza requiring hospitalization in Ontario, Canada. Clin Infect Dis 2007;45(12):1568–75.

23 Nichol KL, Cost-benefit analysis of a strategy to vaccinate healthy working adults against influenza. Arch Intern Med 2001;161(5):749–59.

24 Nichol KL, D'Heilly S, Ehlinger E. Colds and influenza-like illnesses in university students: impact on health, academic and work performance, and health care use. Clin Infect Dis 2005;40(9):1263–70.

25 Nichol KL, Lind A, Margolis KL, et al. The effectiveness of vaccination against influenza in healthy, working adults. N Engl J Med 1995;333(14):889–93.

26 Thompson WW, Shay DK, Weintraub E, et al. Influenza-associated hospitalizations in the United States. JAMA 2004;292(11):1333–40.

27 Schanzer DL, Langley JM, Tam TW. Co-morbidities associated with influenza-attributed mortality, 1994–2000, Canada. Vaccine 2008;26(36):4697–703.

28 Schanzer DL, Langley JM, Tam TW. Hospitalization attributable to influenza and other viral respiratory illnesses in Canadian children. Pediatr Infect Dis J 2006;25(9):795–800.

29 Mullooly JP, Bridges CB, Thompson WW, et al. Influenza- and RSV-associated hospitalizations among adults. Vaccine 2007;25(5):846–55.

30 Mak TK, Mangtani P, Leese J, Watson JM, Pfeifer D. Influenza vaccination in pregnancy: current evidence and selected national policies. Lancet Infect Dis 2008;8(1):44–52.

31 Schanzer DL, Tam TW, Langley JM, Winchester BT. Influenza-attributable deaths, Canada 1990–1999. Epidemiol Infect 2007;135(7):1109–16.

32 Cox N, Bridges CB, Levandowski R, Katz J. Influenza vaccines (inactivated), in Vaccines, S. Plotkin, W. Orenstein, and P. Offit (eds). 2008, Saunders Elsevier.

33 Cates CJ, Jefferson T, Rowe BH. Vaccines for preventing influenza in people with asthma. Cochrane Database Syst Rev 2008 (2), CD000364, DOI: 10.1002/14651858.

34 Chang CC, Morris PS, Chang AB. Influenza vaccine for children and adults with bronchiectasis. Cochrane Database Syst Rev 2007 (3), CD006218, DOI: 10.1002/14651858.

35 Demicheli V, Di Pietrantonj C, Jefferson T, Rivetti A, Rivetti D. Vaccines for preventing influenza in healthy adults. Cochrane Database Syst Rev, 2007(2):CD001269, DOI: 10.1002/14651858..

36 Poole PJ, Chacko EE, Wood-Baker R, Cates CJ. Influenza vaccine for patients with chronic obstructive pulmonary disease. Cochrane Database Syst Rev 2006 (1), CD002733, DOI: 10.1002/14651858.

37 Rivetti D, Jefferson T, Thomas RE, et al. Vaccines for preventing influenza in the elderly. Cochrane Database Syst Rev 2006 (3), CD004876, DOI: 10.1002/14651858.

38 Tan A, Bhalla P, Smyth R. Vaccines for preventing influenza in people with cystic fibrosis. Cochrane Database Syst Rev 2000 (2), CD001753, DOI: 10.1002/14651858.

39 Beyer WE. Heterogeneity of case definitions used in vaccine effectiveness studies – and its impact on meta-analysis. Vaccine 2006;24(44–46):6602–4.

40 Nichol KL. Heterogeneity of influenza case definitions and implications for interpreting and comparing study results. Vaccine 2006;24(44–46):6726–8.

41 Thomas RE, Jefferson T, Demicheli V, Rivetti D. Influenza vaccination for healthcare workers who work with the elderly. Cochrane Database Syst Rev 2006 (3), CD005187, DOI: 10.1002/14651858.

42 Alves Galvao MG., Rocha Crispino Santos MA, Alves da Cunha AJ. Amantadine and rimantadine for influenza A in children and the elderly. Cochrane Database Syst Rev 2008 (1), CD002745, DOI: 10.1002/14651858.

43 Smith NM, Bresee JS, Shay DK, Uyeki TM, Cox NJ, Strikas RA. Prevention and Control of Influenza: recommendations of the Advisory Committee on Immunization Practices (ACIP). MMWR Recomm Rep 2006; 55(RR-10):1–42.

44 Siegel JD, Rhinehart E, Jackson M, Chiarello L; Health Care Infection Control Practices Advisory Committee. Guideline for isolation precautions: preventing transmission of infectious agents in health care settings. Am J Infect Control 2007;35(10 Suppl 2):S65–164.

45 Cox NJ, Ziegler T. Influenza viruses, in Manual of Clinical Microbiology, Murray PM et al. (eds), 2003. Washington DC: ASM Press.

CHAPTER 13

Critical care

Jocelyn A. Srigley & Maureen O. Meade

Infection represents a major source of morbidity and mortality in the intensive care unit (ICU). Whether infection is the principal cause of critical illness or a secondary complication, the prevention, surveillance, diagnosis, and treatment of infection in the ICU pose unique challenges and require vigilant care.

Case presentation

Mr KW is a 56-year-old obese male presenting to the emergency room feeling unwell. Three weeks ago he underwent an umbilical hernia repair including mesh placement. He now has fever, abdominal pain, and lightheadedness. His temperature is 39.4°Celsius. His heart rate is 128 bpm, supine blood pressure 88/60 mmHg, and respiratory rate 34 bpm. His abdominal incision is healed and nontender. His leukocyte count is 34 with toxic granulation. His chest radiograph shows patchy airspace disease, and a CT scan reveals an infected mesh.

Sepsis

Epidemiology

In the United States, the incidence of severe sepsis is estimated at 751 000 cases per year, with 2.26 cases for every 100 hospital discharges [1]. Estimates of the hospital mortality rate of sepsis range from 20% to 60% [2]. While hospital mortality rates from sepsis are declining in the US [3], survivors face an increased risk of death from nonseptic causes for up to 5 years [4].

Evidence-Based Infectious Diseases, 2nd edition. Edited by Mark Loeb, Fiona Smaill and Marek Smieja. © 2009 Wiley-Blackwell Publishing, ISBN: 978-1-4051-7026-0

Definitions

The pathophysiology of sepsis involves an uncontrolled inflammatory response. An initial hyperimmune state generally precedes immunosuppression [5]. Hemodynamic instability and dysregulation of coagulation and fibrinolysis are key contributors to tissue hypoxia and vital organ injury [6]. Multiple organ failure is a hallmark of severe sepsis and the most common cause of death.

In 1992, the American College of Chest Physicians and the Society of Critical Care Medicine published definitions of sepsis-related syndromes [7]. The cornerstone of these definitions was the systemic inflammatory response syndrome (SIRS), characterized by two or more of: hyper- or hypothermia, tachycardia, tachypnea, leukocytosis or leucopenia. Notably, SIRS may be precipitated by nonseptic events, including trauma, burn injury, and pancreatitis; therefore, the diagnosis of sepsis requires both SIRS and a confirmed or presumed source of infection. Severe sepsis refers to sepsis complicated by at least one major organ dysfunction. Septic shock includes persistent hypotension that is unresponsive to fluid resuscitation.

Revisions to these definitions in 2001 recognize alternative manifestations of SIRS including laboratory markers of inflammation, organ dysfunction, and other evidence of tissue hypoperfusion (Table 13.1) [8]. The revised criteria allow more room for clinical judgment, since missing the diagnosis can have catastrophic consequences.

Management

Management of the septic patient involves a multifaceted approach directed against the complex underlying pathophysiology. Early goal-directed resuscitation and prompt administration of antibiotics are crucial.

Table 13.1 Diagnostic criteria for sepsis

Infection,[a] documented or suspected, and some of the following:[b]
General variables
  Fever (core temperature >38.3°C)
  Hypothermia (core temperature <36°C)
  Heart rate >90 min^{-1} or >2 SD above the normal value for age
  Tachypnea
  Altered mental status
  Significant edema or positive fluid balance (>20 mL/kg over 24 h)
  Hyperglycemia (plasma glucose >120 mg/dL or 7.7 mmol/L) in the absence of diabetes
Inflammatory variables
  Leukocytosis (WBC count >12 000 μL^{-1})
  Leukopenia (WBC count <4000 μL^{-1})
  Normal WBC count with >10% immature forms
  Plasma C-reactive protein >2 SD above the normal value
  Plasma procalcitonin >2 SD above the normal value
Hemodynamic variables
  Arterial hypotension[b] (SBP <90 mmHg, MAP <70, or an SBP decrease >40 mmHg in adults or <2 SD below normal for age)
  SVo$_2$ >70%[b]
  Cardiac index >3.5 L min^{-1} M^{-} [23] [WU1]
Organ dysfunction variables
  Arterial hypoxemia (Pao$_2$/Flo$_2$ <300)
  Acute oliguria (urine output <0.5 mL kg^{-1} h^{-1} or 45 mmol/L for at least 2 h)
  Creatinine increase >0.5 mg/dL
  Coagulation abnormalities (INR >1.5 or aPTT >60 s)
  Ileus (absent bowel sounds)
  Thrombocytopenia (platelet count <100 000 μL^{-1})
  Hyperbilirubinemia (plasma total bilirubin >4 mg/dL or 70 mmol/L)
Tissue perfusion variables
  Hyperlactatemia (>1 mmol/L)
  Decreased capillary refill or mottling

WBC, white blood cell; SBP, systolic blood pressure; MAP, mean arterial blood pressure; SVo$_2$, mixed venous oxygen saturation; INR, international normalized ratio; aPTT, activated partial thromboplastin time.
[a]Infection defined as a pathologic process induced by a microorganism.
[b]SVo$_2$ sat >70% is normal in children (normally, 75–80%), and cardiac index 3.5–5.5 is normal in children; therefore, NEITHER should be used as signs of sepsis in newborns or children
Diagnostic criteria for sepsis in the pediatric population are signs and symptoms of inflammation plus infection with hyper- or hypothermia (rectal temperature >38.5°C or <35°C), tachycardia (may be absent in hypothermic patients), and at least one of the following indications of altered organ function: altered mental status, hypoxemia, increased serum lactate level, or bounding pulses.
Source: Levy MM, Fink MP, Marshall JC, et al. 2001 SCCM/ESICM/ACCP/ATS/SIS international sepsis definitions conference. Crit Care Med 2003;31:1250–6.

Thereafter, consideration of source control, activated protein C, and systemic corticosteroid therapy may be life-saving.

Early goal-directed therapy

The aim of goal-directed therapy in sepsis is the correction of hemodynamic disturbances that contribute to tissue hypoxia. Historically, goal-directed therapy referred to specific interventions aimed to achieve supraphysiologic values of cardiac index and oxygen delivery. A landmark trial of 762 septic patients showed no improvement in morbidity or mortality with this approach [9], and a later systematic review reinforced this finding [10]. However, the experimental interventions in these trials were generally initiated up to 48 hours after ICU admission.

Current evidence suggests that goal-directed resuscitation should be initiated earlier, before the onset of irreversible tissue damage, and should include more conservative physiologic goals. A recent innovative trial randomly allocated 263 septic patients, at the time of presentation to the emergency department, to 6 hours of early goal-directed therapy versus standard care prior to ICU admission [11]. The experimental intervention involved an iterative assessment of hemodynamic parameters with specific actions targeted to precise physiologic goals. First was the infusion of 500 mL of crystalloid solution every 30 minutes until central venous pressure (CVP) measurements ranged from 8 to 12 mmHg. At that point, vasopressor administration targeted a mean arterial pressure (MAP) of at least 65 mmHg. Thereafter, if central venous oxygen saturation was less than 70%, red blood cells were transfused to achieve a hematocrit of at least 30%. If central venous oxygen saturation remained below 70%, dobutamine was administered to achieve that goal. Antibiotics were given at the discretion of the treating physicians, and there were no significant differences between groups in terms of time to antibiotic administration or adequacy of antimicrobial coverage. With this multifaceted intervention, 28-day mortality rates decreased from 46.5% to 30.5%, corresponding to a relative risk of 0.58 (P = 0.009) and a number-needed-to-treat of 6. Early goal-directed therapy also reduced the duration of vasopressor therapy, mechanical ventilation, and hospital stay.

These findings popularized the notion that optimal sepsis management begins upon presentation to the emergency room. A subsequent synthesis of before-and-after studies evaluating comparable protocols for early goal-directed therapy in sepsis found a similar overall relative mortality risk of 0.54 [12]. Notwithstanding the selection bias and confounding factors that typically complicate before-and-after studies, this finding supported the feasibility of early goal-directed therapy in emergency departments and elsewhere in the hospital. Current guidelines, therefore, recommend early resuscitative efforts at the time of presentation, targeting a CVP of 8 to 12 mmHg, MAP not less than 65 mmHg, urine output exceeding 0.5 mL/kg/hour, and central or mixed venous oxygen saturation of at least 70% [13].

Antimicrobial therapy

Another pillar of sepsis management is the prompt administration of appropriate antimicrobial therapy. The importance of early antimicrobials was highlighted by a 5-year retrospective study of 2700 patients with septic shock [14]. Among patients who received antimicrobial therapy that was adequate to treat subsequently identified pathogens, delays in antimicrobial therapy clearly correlated with mortality

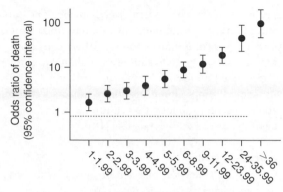

Time from hypotension onset (h)

Figure 13.1 Mortality risk (expressed as adjusted odds ratio of death) with increasing delays in initiation of effective antimicrobial therapy. Bars represent 95% confidence interval. An increased risk of death is already present by the second hour after hypotension onset (compared with the first hour after hypotension). The risk of death continues to climb, though, to > 36 h after hypotension onset. Reproduced from reference [14]: Kumar A, Roberts D, Wood KE, et al. Duration of hypotension before initiation of effective antimicrobial therapy is the critical determinant of survival in human septic shock. Crit Care Med 2006;34:1589–96.

(Fig. 13.1). Patients receiving appropriate coverage within the first hour of hypotension had a survival rate of 79.9%, and survival decreased by approximately 8% for each hour of delay.

The choice of empiric antimicrobial therapy is paramount. Among 655 critically ill patients with sepsis who ultimately had positive culture results, hospital mortality when initial antimicrobial therapy was inadequate to treat the pathogen was 52.1%, far exceeding the 12.2% mortality rate among patients receiving adequate antimicrobial therapy [15]. Regression modeling determined that inadequate antimicrobial treatment was the strongest determinant of hospital mortality, with an adjusted odds ratio of 4.27. Other studies reported similar findings [16,17].

Initial antimicrobial therapy depends on the presumed source of infection. Empiric therapy should cover any pathogens commonly associated with the particular infection, including resistant organisms for patients with known risk factors. An evidence-based review determined that acceptable empiric regimens in septic patients with an unclear source include a β-lactam in combination with an aminoglycoside, or monotherapy with a third- or fourth-generation cephalosporin, carbapenem, or extended-spectrum carboxypenicillin or, alternatively, ureidopenicillin with a β-lactamase inhibitor [18]. With the increasing prevalence of community-acquired MRSA, consideration may also be given to adding an antibiotic to cover MRSA based on local resistance patterns and clinical suspicion. Prompt administration of broad-spectrum empiric agents is followed by culture-directed tailoring of therapy as soon as possible [19].

Source control

A persisting collection of microorganisms will continue to trigger the inflammatory response of sepsis [20]. When a source of infection cannot be eradicated solely with antibiotics, one must consider source control [13,20]. Percutaneous or surgical drainage is indicated for infection within a closed space, including abscess, empyema, or cholangitis. Debridement involves the removal of infected or necrotic tissue, either surgically, with irrigation, or using wet-to-dry dressings. Device removal is important in patients with an infected foreign body, such as a central venous catheter, urinary catheter, or prosthetic joint. Other definitive source control measures include amputation of a gangrenous limb and resection of ischemic bowel.

Activated protein C

Among a host of immunomodulatory therapies proposed for the management of sepsis, drotrecogin alpha (activated), a recombinant human form of activated protein C (rhAPC), is currently the treatment with the strongest evidence for survival benefit.

Activated protein C is a naturally occurring inhibitor of both thrombosis and inflammation. The potential efficacy of rhAPC for severe sepsis was demonstrated in the original PROWESS trial where nearly 1700 patients with severe sepsis received either rhAPC or placebo infusion for 96 hours [21]. With rhAPC therapy, 28-day mortality fell from 30.8% to 24.7%, signifying a relative risk of 0.80 ($P = 0.005$). Patients receiving rhAPC, however, had a significantly higher rate of major bleeding events (3.5% versus 2.0%), and these occurred even more frequently (6.5%) in a subsequent open-label, single-arm study of over 2400 patients [22]. The open-label study also observed a significantly lower mortality rate among patients who received rhAPC within the first 24 hours of organ dysfunction (22.9% versus 27.4%).

Initial enthusiasm for rhAPC therapy in sepsis [13] has been tempered by less striking results of later trials in pediatrics [23] and in lower-risk [24], critically ill adults [25]. An additional trial is under way to clarify the role for early administration of rhAPC to patients who are most likely to respond. Meanwhile, current guidelines include a weak recommendation to administer rhAPC to patients with severe sepsis and APACHE II score greater than 25. Contraindications include active internal bleeding, hemorrhagic stroke within 3 months, neurosurgery or head trauma within 2 months, trauma with an increased risk of significant bleeding, epidural catheter, or intracranial mass lesion [13].

Corticosteroid therapy

The role for systemic corticosteroids in the management of sepsis is equally controversial. Known for their anti-inflammatory properties, steroid therapy did not live up to initial expectations: two metaanalyses including trials from 1966 to 1993 showed no evidence of a survival benefit [26,27]. However, early practice was to use short courses of high-dose corticosteroids. Current evidence suggests that sepsis is frequently complicated by adrenal insufficiency and glucocorticoid resistance [28]; therefore, longer treatment using smaller, physiologic doses of corticosteroids may be more appropriate. In a more recent systematic review [29], a subgroup analysis of five trials administering longer courses of low-dose corticosteroids (≥300 mg/day hydrocortisone or equivalent for at least 5 days) found a significant reduction in the relative risk of mortality at 0.80. Moreover, there was no apparent increase in the rate of adverse events.

A newly published trial was designed to retest the role for low-dose steroids in sepsis [30]. The largest trial to date, CORTICUS stopped early and was underpowered to detect a mortality effect. Of note, there was no apparent survival benefit even among patients found to be adrenally insufficient on corticotropin stimulation. Steroid therapy was associated with a shorter time to shock reversal; however, there was also an increased risk of complications. Since earlier trials had reasonably comparable methods, populations and therapeutic protocols, an update to the metaanalysis is prudent and will likely show a nonstatistically significant mortality reduction. For now, whether steroids benefit any critically ill septic patients remains uncertain. Refraining from steroid use altogether, administering only to the most ill, and administering to a wider group of septic patients all remain justifiable courses of action.

Case presentation (continued)

In the ER, Mr KW promptly receives intravenous piperacillin-tazobactam and the mesh is surgically removed that day. Postoperatively, he is transferred to the intensive care unit on vasopressors. His leukocyte count is 36, his lactate level 3.5. His chest radiograph reveals diffuse airspace disease.

Upon ICU admission, 2 L of intravenous crystalloid bring Mr KW's central venous pressure to 12 cmH$_2$O and his central venous oxygen saturation, measured through a right subclavian catheter, to 72%. He continues to require vasopressor support. Fluid collected during surgery shows gram-negative bacilli, as do two blood cultures. Later, *E. coli* sensitive to cephazolin is identified from all three cultures. The clinical team discontinues piperacillin-tazobactam and initiates cephazolin therapy. While his acute lung injury progresses, his blood pressure improves over 6 hours, though still requiring vasopressor support. With results from an ACTH stimulation test pending, Mr KW receives neither corticosteroid therapy nor rhAPC.

Later, off vasopressors and with his lung injury slowly resolving, Mr KW develops signs of a new infection: fever, tachycardia, increased respiratory rate, and recurrent leukocytosis with band cells.

Ventilator-associated pneumonia

Epidemiology

Ventilator-associated pneumonia (VAP) refers to pneumonia arising more than 48 hours after endotracheal intubation [31]. Incidence and mortality estimates vary depending on the population, diagnostic techniques, and other variables. A study of over 9000 ICU patients in the US found that VAP occurred in 9.3% [32]. Although the investigators detected no increase in mortality attributed to VAP, patients with VAP had prolonged mechanical ventilation, ICU stay, and hospitalization. Moreover, the

mean excess hospital costs attributable to each case of VAP exceeded \$40 000. A related study of patients in Canadian ICUs reported similar findings, with a trend towards higher mortality among patients with VAP (23.7% vs 17.9%), and ICU stays that were prolonged by an average of 4.3 days [33].

Pathophysiology and microbiology

Two main factors contribute to the development of VAP: bacterial colonization of the upper airways and aspiration [34,35]. Critically ill patients become colonized with a variety of organisms originating from their own gastrointestinal tract and from the hospital environment. This process is facilitated by patients' inability to clear their secretions and by numerous catheters that breach the skin and mucosal barriers. Colonizing bacteria infect the lower airways via aspiration of secretions from the upper respiratory tract.

The microbiology of VAP differs from community-acquired pneumonia, with gram-negative and drug-resistant organisms accounting for a significant proportion of cases. Gram-negative bacilli, including *Pseudomonas aeruginosa* and *Enterobacter* species, tend to be the most common organisms isolated. Gram-positive cocci are also a frequent cause, predominantly *Staphylococcus aureus*. Surveillance data from one American hospital revealed that 59% of VAP cases were caused by gram-negative bacilli, most commonly *P. aeruginosa*, *Stenotrophomonas maltophilia*, and *Acinetobacter* species. The most common gram-positive organism causing VAP was methicillin-resistant *S. aureus* (MRSA) [36]. Another American study similarly found that *P. aeruginosa* and *S. aureus* were the most common pathogens identified in the setting of VAP [37].

Prevention

Understandably, a great deal of research has focused on VAP prevention. Several preventive strategies are supported by current research evidence, including oral intubation, endotracheal tube care, patient positioning, oropharyngeal decontamination, and stress ulcer prophylaxis [35,38].

For patients requiring intubation, the oral route is preferred over the nasal route, which is associated with an increased incidence of maxillary sinusitis [39]. Sinusitis is associated with the development of VAP, presumably secondary to aspiration of infected nasal secretions into the lungs [35]. In a trial of 300 ICU patients randomized to either oral or nasal intubation, there were trends towards less sinusitis and pneumonia with orotracheal intubation [40].

Maintenance of the endotracheal tube can affect the incidence of VAP. Persistent endotracheal cuff pressures less than $20\,cmH_2O$ may increase the risk of VAP [41]. In addition, three trials have shown that aspiration of subglottic secretions can significantly reduce the incidence of VAP [42–44]. Both of these interventions help to prevent aspiration of secretions around the endotracheal tube and into the lungs. Interventions that appear to have no effect on the incidence of VAP include frequent changes of the ventilator circuit, suction catheter, or humidifier, and use of a closed suction system [35,38].

Patient positioning is another important consideration in VAP prevention. Nursing in the supine position facilitates aspiration of potentially infected secretions that lead to VAP [45]. A randomized trial to test this hypothesis stopped early after an interim analysis demonstrated a significantly reduced rate of VAP in patients nursed in a semirecumbent position compared to those who were supine (8% vs 34%, relative risk 0.24) [46].

Oropharyngeal decontamination may prevent VAP by reducing the amount of infected secretions in the oropharynx. A metaanalysis of eleven randomized trials found a statistically significant reduction in VAP rates with chlorhexidine mouthwash compared to placebo or standard care (relative risk 0.56; 95% CI 0.39–0.81), and a trend toward VAP reduction with oral decontamination using antibiotic agents [47]. This study did not detect an effect on mortality or duration of ICU stay.

The relationship between stress ulcer prophylaxis and VAP is controversial. Patients receiving mechanical ventilation and those with coagulopathy carry increased risk of gastrointestinal bleeding, and pharmacologic measures to reduce gastric acidity can reduce bleeding rates [48]. However, reducing gastric acidity also facilitates microbial colonization of the aerodigestive tract [45]. A multicentre trial that randomized 1200 mechanically ventilated patients to either ranitidine or sucralfate therapy found a lower rate of bleeding with ranitidine (RR 0.44, 95% CI 0.21–0.92), with no significant effect on VAP incidence. A subsequent metaanalysis confirmed that rates of pneumonia were similar between ranitidine and sucralfate, but also found that neither agent was significantly associated with increased pneumonia compared to placebo, and furthermore, neither differed from placebo with respect to bleeding rates [49]. After weighing all of the evidence, current guidelines recommend reserving stress ulcer prophylaxis for patients at high risk of gastrointestinal bleeding, and using histamine-receptor antagonists rather than sucralfate [35,38].

Diagnosis

The diagnosis of VAP presents unique challenges. Clinical manifestations typically consist of new or progressive infiltrates on chest radiography with purulent tracheal secretions, fever, and leukocytosis. However, a variety of alternative pathologies, alone or in combination, can lead to a similar constellation of findings, including acute lung injury, atelectasis, congestive heart failure, and nonpulmonary infections [50]. A study of 84 ICU patients with new infiltrates and purulent secretions demonstrated the limited utility of clinical features in the diagnosis of VAP [51]. A team of physicians predicted whether or not the patients had pneumonia based on all available clinical information, and the actual diagnosis was made based on histopathology, pleural fluid culture, or computed tomography criteria. Only 62% of patients with confirmed VAP were correctly diagnosed, as were 84% of patients without pneumonia.

The clinical pulmonary infection score (CPIS) was developed to improve the clinical diagnosis of VAP. The CPIS is a score of 0 to 12 based on temperature, leukocyte count, tracheal secretions, oxygenation, chest radiography, and microbiology findings, with scores greater than 6 suggestive of VAP [52]. A management strategy based on the CPIS was studied in 81 ICU patients with new pulmonary infiltrates [53]. Patients with a score of less than or equal to 6, who were considered to be at low likelihood of having VAP, were randomized to receive either standard VAP treatment or an experimental intervention that consisted of 3 days of antibiotic therapy followed by reevaluation of CPIS, at which time antibiotics would be discontinued if CPIS was still less than or equal to 6. The study found no difference between the two groups with respect to mortality or duration of ICU stay, though the experimental group had significantly lower rates of antimicrobial usage, antibiotic-resistant organisms, and superinfections. This suggested that the CPIS-based strategy may be a safe and cost-effective approach to the diagnosis and management of VAP. However, a subsequent study evaluating a modified version of the CPIS found that scores did not differ significantly between patients with and without confirmed pneumonia [54].

Since clinical criteria alone are insufficiently accurate to diagnose VAP, airway sampling for Gram stain and culture is often used to confirm the diagnosis. Samples may be obtained via endotracheal aspirate or, alternatively, during bronchoscopy using either a protected specimen brush (PSB) or bronchoalveolar lavage (BAL). Cultures with greater than 1000 colony-forming units (CFU)/mL from PSB sample or greater than 10000 CFU/mL for BAL specimens are generally considered diagnostic of VAP [55]. Both PSB and BAL samples for diagnosing VAP have been validated against postmortem lung examination [56]. On the other hand, bronchoscopy is an invasive and resource-intensive diagnostic technique, so many clinicians rely upon endotracheal aspiration. The utility of tracheal aspirates is limited by low specificity because the upper airways of ventilated patients are frequently colonized with bacteria that may not be infecting the lower airways [55].

Invasive and noninvasive diagnostic approaches have been compared, and a metaanalysis of randomized trials found significant heterogeneity among studies [57]. Overall there was no difference in mortality between the two techniques, although antibiotics were more likely to be changed among patients randomized to invasive diagnosis. A trial randomly assigning 740 patients with suspected VAP to undergo either BAL or endotracheal aspiration found no effect on mortality, duration of ICU or hospital stay, duration of mechanical ventilation, or antibiotic use [58]. Given that invasive diagnostic techniques have not been shown to improve clinical outcomes, noninvasive tracheal aspiration is an accepted method of airway sampling in patients with suspected VAP.

Management

Patients with suspected VAP require empiric antibiotic therapy to cover potential pathogens while awaiting the results of microbiologic testing. The initial choice of antibiotics will depend on the degree of risk of colonization with multidrug-resistant (MDR) organisms. Risk factors include duration of hospitalization 5 or more days, antimicrobial therapy within preceding 3 months, hospitalization within preceding 3 months, residence in a nursing home or other long-term

care facility, chronic dialysis, receiving home care for wounds or any intravenous therapy, immunosuppression, high rates of antibiotic resistance in the community or hospital, and household members known to have a MDR pathogen [31].

Patients with early-onset VAP (occurring in the first 4 days of hospitalization), in the absence of other risk factors, are more likely to have pneumonia caused by methicillin-sensitive *S. aureus* and antibiotic-sensitive *Enterobacteriaceae* [59]. Treatment options include a third-generation cephalosporin or a respiratory fluoroquinolone. Patients with late-onset VAP or other risk factors for MDR pathogens require combination therapy to cover MRSA and potentially drug-resistant gram-negative bacilli, in addition to the usual pathogens.

Prompt initiation of empiric antibiotic therapy is important. A study of 107 ICU patients with suspected VAP determined that a delay of greater than 24 hours was an independent risk factor for hospital mortality, with an adjusted odds ratio of 7.68 (95% CI 4.50–13.09, $P < 0.001$) [60]. The duration of antibiotic therapy can often be limited to 8 days based on the results of a multicenter trial of 401 ICU patients with VAP [61]. These patients were randomized to either 8-day or 15-day courses of antibiotics, and there was no significant mortality difference between the two groups. However, patients with pneumonia caused by nonfermenting gram-negative bacilli, including *P. aeruginosa*, were more likely to experience a relapse of their infection when treated for only 8 days and thus may require more prolonged therapy.

Case presentation (continued)

Investigating for a nosocomial infection, the clinical team performs a bronchoscopy (because there are scant secretions on endotracheal aspiration), a urine analysis (which is negative and not sent on for culture), and paired quantitative blood cultures. They remove the subclavian catheter that Mr KW no longer requires. Tenacious secretions are detected on bronchoscopy, and the chest radiograph shows a subtle new opacification in the right middle lobe; Mr KW is started empirically on piperacillin-tazobactam. However, 4 days later, with resolution of his fever and leukocytosis, no organisms cultured and persistent subtle opacification of the right middle lobe, empiric antibiotics are discontinued.

Catheter-related bloodstream infections

Epidemiology

ICU patients require various intravascular catheters for monitoring and treatment purposes, and catheter-related bloodstream infections (CRBSI) are one of the potential complications. Rates of CRBSI differ depending on the type of catheter and site of insertion [62]; however, a nationwide surveillance study in the US determined the overall incidence of CRBSI related to central venous catheters (CVCs) among ICU patients was 4% [63]. Estimates of the attributable mortality of CRBSI in ICU patients range from zero to 40%, but these studies consistently observed increased duration of ICU and hospital stay [64,65]. The mean excess costs associated with each CRBSI are estimated at US$30 000–40 000 [65,66].

Etiology

The pathogenesis of CRBSI involves bacterial colonization of the CVC, both in biofilms and in free forms [66]. Virtually all intravascular catheters become colonized, but the likelihood of developing a CRBSI is related to bacterial load, surface properties of the catheter, and host immunity. Colonizing organisms commonly originate from the skin and migrate along the extraluminal surface of the catheter into the bloodstream. Organisms may also enter the bloodstream intraluminally through the catheter hub, often via the hands of healthcare workers.

National surveillance in the US found the most common pathogens in CRBSI are coagulase-negative *Staphylococci* (35.9%), *S. aureus* (16.8%), *Candida* species (10.1%), and *Enterococcus* species (9.8%). These are followed by *P. aeruginosa* (4.7%) and other gram-negative bacilli [67].

Prevention

The risk of CRBSI is minimized with careful attention to the insertion site and technique, catheter care, and duration of use.

The site of catheter insertion is a significant determinant of infection risk. A prospective observational study of over 2000 patients found that the incidence rates of CRBSIs for subclavian, internal jugular, and femoral catheters were 0.97, 2.99, and 8.34 per 1000 catheter-days, respectively [68]. Increased infection risk with femoral catheters was confirmed in a trial of 289 ICU patients randomly assigned to femoral versus subclavian central venous catheterization [69]. Accordingly, current guidelines recommend avoiding femoral catheters and choosing the subclavian site whenever possible [70].

Use of sterile technique and full barrier precautions, including cap, mask, sterile gown and gloves, and large drape can reduce the risk of a CRBSI [70]. A randomized trial of 176 patients comparing maximum barrier precautions to limited barrier precautions with only sterile gowns and small drape observed significantly fewer CRBSIs with maximum barrier precautions (2.4% vs 7.2%, $P = 0.03$), and a nonsignificant reduction in the rate of sepsis [71].

Maintenance of the central catheter is another important consideration in preventing infection. Skin disinfection at the insertion site can reduce bacterial colonization of the skin. A metaanalysis of studies comparing chlorhexidine and povidone-iodine for catheter site care demonstrated a relative risk of 0.49 (95% CI 0.28–0.88) for CRBSI among patients treated with chlorhexidine-based solutions (Fig. 13.2) [72]. Catheter hubs should be cleaned with antiseptic prior to accessing the ports in order to reduce the risk of introducing microbes directly into the catheter lumen. Solutions containing 70% ethanol were more effective than chlorhexidine at reducing bacterial contamination of catheter hubs [73]. Finally, proper hand hygiene should be observed prior to catheter use or site care [70].

The risk of CRBSI increases over time, but prophylactic replacement of central venous catheters has not been found to reduce infection risk [74]. A systematic review of six trials comparing routine catheter changes (after 3 or 7 days) with catheter replacement on an "as needed" basis found no difference in CRBSI rates [75].

A multifaceted intervention to reduce CRBSI was evaluated in over 100 ICUs in the US [76]. The intervention consisted of five components: hand washing prior to any handling of the catheter, full barrier precautions during insertion, chlorhexidine for routine skin disinfection, avoidance of femoral catheterization whenever possible, and removal of unnecessary catheters. Measurement of CRBSI at baseline and at regular intervals for up to 18 months after implementation of the multifaceted intervention revealed a reduction in the mean infection rate from 7.7 per 1000 catheter-days at baseline to 1.4 per 1000 catheter-days during the

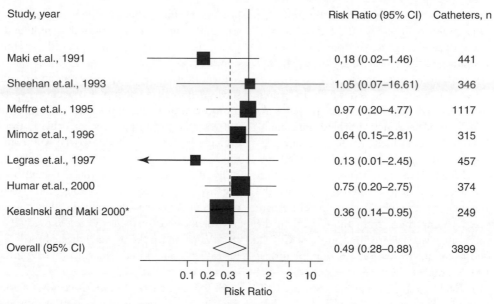

Study, year		Risk Ratio (95% CI)	Catheters, n
Maki et.al., 1991		0,18 (0.02–1.46)	441
Sheehan et.al., 1993		1.05 (0.07–16.61)	346
Meffre et.al., 1995		0.97 (0.20–4.77)	1117
Mimoz et.al., 1996		0.64 (0.15–2.81)	315
Legras et.al., 1997		0.13 (0.01–2.45)	457
Humar et.al., 2000		0.75 (0.20–2.75)	374
Keaslnski and Maki 2000*		0.36 (0.14–0.95)	249
Overall (95% CI)		0.49 (0.28–0.88)	3899

Figure 13.2 Analysis of catheter-related bloodstream infection in studies comparing chlorhexidine gluconate and povidone-iodine solutions for care of vascular catheter sites. The diamond indicates the summary risk ratio and 95% CI. Studies are ordered chronologically. The size of squares is proportional to the reciprocal of the variance of the studies. For the test for heterogeneity of treatment effect, P > 0.2. Reproduced from reference [72]: Chalyakunapruk N, Veenstra DL, Lipsky BA, Saint S. Chlorhexidine compared with povidone-iodine solution for vascular catheter-site care: a meta-analysis. Ann Intern Med 2002;136:792–801.

period of follow-up. This demonstrates that relatively simple measures can have a significant and prolonged effect on the prevention of CRBSI.

Diagnosis

The diagnosis of a primary bloodstream infection requires at least one of the following criteria: isolation of a pathogen from one or more blood cultures (not related to infection at any other site); isolation of a common skin contaminant from two or more blood cultures drawn on separate occasions with at least one systemic manifestation of infection (fever, chills, hypotension) and no other suspected source of infection; or a positive antigen test (e.g., *Streptococcus pneumoniae*, group B streptococcus, *Haemophilus influenzae*, or *Neisseria meningitides*) in the setting of systemic manifestation of infection, with no other apparent source. CRBSI is present if a patient with a primary bloodstream infection has had a central venous catheter in use during the 48 hours prior to the onset of infection [70].

Most patients with CRBSI develop a fever and they may have other features of SIRS. However, these findings are not specific for CRBSI [77]. Further, prospective evaluation suggests that signs of inflammation at the catheter insertion site, including pain, swelling, erythema, and purulence, are present in only 10% of patients with CRBSI. These features have high specificity (94 to 99%) but low sensitivity (0 to 3%) [78].

Clinical features suggestive of infection in a patient with an intravascular catheter should prompt further microbiologic evaluation. Two samples of blood should be cultured with at least one taken from a peripheral venipuncture site [77]. Positive blood cultures drawn from a CVC can be difficult to interpret because they may represent catheter colonization rather than bloodstream infection. A retrospective study of 271 ICU patients compared the utility of blood cultures drawn from central venous catheters and peripheral venipuncture [79]. Negative predictive values were similar (97% and 95%, respectively); however, positive predictive values were higher for peripheral samples (82%) than central catheters (61%), and the difference was statistically significant. Therefore a positive culture from a peripheral sample is helpful in differentiating true CRBSI from colonization of a central venous catheter.

Once bacteremia is established, or whenever a CRBSI is suspected, several techniques may help to determine whether an intravascular catheter is the source. One option is to remove the catheter and to culture it either semiquantitatively or quantitatively. The disadvantage of this approach is that it may lead to unnecessary removal of catheters [77].

Alternative diagnostic approaches include "paired quantitative blood cultures" and "differential time to positivity" [80]. The principle behind both methods is that the bacterial load will be inversely proportional to the distance from an infected catheter. The first technique involves obtaining two quantitative blood cultures drawn simultaneously from the central venous catheter and a peripheral vein. A five times greater colony count from the CVC than the peripheral sample is considered diagnostic of CRBSI. The second technique involves comparing the time it takes for each sample to become positive. A diagnosis of CRBSI is established if the culture from the CVC becomes positive at least 2 hours before the peripheral sample.

A metaanalysis of 51 studies compared the diagnostic properties of qualitative, semiquantitative, and quantitative catheter cultures, qualitative and quantitative catheter-drawn cultures, paired quantitative cultures, differential time to positivity, and a rapid diagnostic test called acridine orange leukocyte cytospin [81]. Paired quantitative blood culture was most accurate, with an overall sensitivity of 89% and specificity of 98%.

Case presentation (continued)

Among the investigations for nosocomial infection, the blood culture from Mr KW's central venous catheter identified coagulase-negative staphylococci and the peripheral blood culture was negative, consistent with contamination of the central catheter specimen or colonization of the catheter itself.

Management

Management of suspected CRBSI includes antimicrobial therapy and consideration of catheter removal. Vancomycin is a common choice for empiric therapy that will cover the most common pathogens, coagulase-negative staphylococci and *S. aureus*. Empiric gram-negative and *P. aeruginosa* coverage may be prudent if the patient is demonstrating signs of sepsis. Prompt catheter removal is indicated if the patient is septic or has signs of infection at the insertion site [77].

Identification of the causative organism will guide subsequent management. For coagulase-negative staphylococcal infection, immediate catheter removal is not essential for all patients, particularly those with difficult venous access or those who will require central access for a short period of time. A retrospective study of 70 patients with catheter-related coagulase-negative staphylococcal infection found recurrence in 20% of patients with retained catheters versus 3% of patients whose catheters were removed ($P < 0.05$) [82]. Vancomycin therapy is indicated for 5–7 days if the catheter is removed, versus 10–14 days if the catheter remains in place [77].

CRBSI caused by *S. aureus* requires removal of the catheter; failure to do so significantly increases the risk for infection recurrence and mortality [83]. *S. aureus* bacteremia is also commonly associated with metastatic infections, including infective endocarditis; therefore, transesophageal echocardiography (TEE) should be considered to identify cases of *S. aureus* endocarditis, which requires prolonged antibiotic therapy [77,84]. If the *S. aureus* is susceptible, β-lactam antibiotics or a first-generation cephalosporin are appropriate as first-line therapy. The recommended duration of therapy for patients with no evidence of infective endocarditis is 14 days [77].

CRBSI due to gram-negative bacilli are less common, but a small retrospective study found that catheter removal significantly reduced the likelihood of recurrence (odds ratio 0.13, 95% CI 0.02–0.75) [85]. Catheter removal is followed by a 14-day course of antibiotic therapy [77].

Catheter removal is also essential in CRBSI caused by *Candida* species. A prospective study of 145 patients with catheter-related candidemia found that failure to remove the catheter was significantly associated with mortality (OR 4.81) [86]. Options for empiric antifungal therapy include amphotericin B, an echinocandin, or fluconazole; the choice may depend upon the local incidence of fluconazole-resistant *C. glabrata* and *C. krusei* [80]. Blood cultures should be repeated routinely, and the recommended duration of treatment is 14 days after the last positive blood culture [87].

References

1 Angus DC, Linde-Zwirble WT, Lidicker J, et al. Epidemiology of severe sepsis in the United States: analysis of incidence, outcome, and associated costs of care. Crit Care Med 2001;29:1303–10.

2 Linde-Zwirble WT, Angus DC. Severe sepsis epidemiology: sampling, selection, and society. Crit Care Med 2004;8:222–6.

3 Martin GS, Mannino DM, Eaton S, Moss M. The epidemiology of sepsis in the United States from 1979 through 2000. N Engl J Med 2003;348:1546–54.

4 Quartin AA, Schein RM, Kett DH, Peduzzi PN. Magnitude and duration of the effect of sepsis on survival. JAMA 1997;277:1058–63.

5 Hotchkiss RS, Karl IE. The pathophysiology and treatment of sepsis. N Engl J Med 2003;348:138–50.

6 Beal AL, Cerra FB. Multiple organ failure syndrome in the 1990s: systemic inflammatory response and organ dysfunction. JAMA 1994;271:226–33.

7 Bone RC, Balk RA, Cerra FB, et al. American College of Chest Physicians/Society of Critical Care Medicine Consensus Conference: definitions for sepsis and organ failure and guidelines for the use of innovative therapies in sepsis. Crit Care Med 1992;20:864–74.

8 Levy MM, Fink MP, Marshall JC, et al. 2001 SCCM/ESICM/ACCP/ATS/SIS international sepsis definitions conference. Crit Care Med 2003;31:1250–6.

9 Gattinoni L, Brazzi L, Pelosi, P, et al. A trial of goal-oriented hemodynamic therapy in critically ill patients. N Engl J Med 1995;333:1025–32.

10 Heyland DK, Cook DJ, King D, Kernerman P, Brun-Buisson C. Maximizing oxygen delivery in critically ill patients: a methodologic appraisal of the evidence. Crit Care Med 1996; 24:517–524.

11 Rivers E, Nguyen B, Havstad S, et al. Early goal-directed therapy in the treatment of severe sepsis and septic shock. N Engl J Med 2001;345:1368–77.

12 Otero RM, Nguyen HB, Huang DT, et al. Early goal-directed therapy in severe sepsis and septic shock: concepts, controversies, and contemporary findings. Chest 2006;130:1579–95.

13 Dellinger RP, Carlet JM, Masur H, et al. Surviving Sepsis Campaign guidelines for management of severe sepsis and septic shock. Crit Care Med 2004;32:858–73.

14 Kumar A, Roberts D, Wood KE, et al. Duration of hypotension before initiation of effective antimicrobial therapy is the critical determinant of survival in human septic shock. Crit Care Med 2006;34:1589–96.

15 Kollef MH, Sherman G, Ward S, Fraser VJ. Inadequate antimicrobial treatment of infections: a risk factor for hospital mortality among critically ill patients. Chest 1999;115:462–74.

16 Valles J, Rello J, Ochagavia A, et al. Community-acquired bloodstream infection in critically ill adult patients: impact of shock and inappropriate antibiotic therapy on survival. Chest 2003;123:1615–24.

17 MacArthur RD, Miller M, Albertson T, et al. Adequacy of early empiric antibiotic treatment and survival in severe sepsis: experience from the MONARCS trial. Clin Infect Dis 2004;38:284–8.

18 Bochud PY, Bonten M, Marchetti O, Calandra T. Antimicrobial therapy for patients with severe sepsis and septic shock: an evidence-based review. Crit Care Med 2004;32:S495–512.

19 Rivers EP, McIntyre L, Morro DC, Rivers KK. Early and innovative interventions for severe sepsis and septic shock: taking advantage of a window of opportunity. Can Med Assoc J 2005;173:1054–65.

20 Marshall JC, Maier RV, Jiminez M, Dellinger EP. Source control in the management of severe sepsis and septic shock: an evidence-based review. Crit Care Med 2004;32:S513–26.

21 Bernard GR, Vincent JL, Laterre PF, et al. Efficacy and safety of recombinant human activated protein C for severe sepsis. N Engl J Med 2001;344:699–709.

22 Vincent JL, Bernard GR, Beale R, et al. Drotrecogin alfa (activated) treatment in severe sepsis from the global open-label trial ENHANCE: further evidence for survival and safety and implications for early treatment. Crit Care Med 2005;33:2266–77.

23 Nadel S, Goldstein B, Williams MD, et al for the REsearching severe Sepsis and Organ dysfunction in children: a gLobal perspective (RESOLVE) study group. Drotrecogin alfa (activated) in children with severe sepsis: a multicentre phase III randomised controlled trial. Lancet 2007;369:836–843.

24 Abraham E, Laterre PF, Garg R, et al. Drotrecogin alfa (activated) for adults with severe sepsis and a low risk of death. N Engl J Med 2005;353:1332–41.

25 Friedrich JO, Adhikari NKJ, Meade MO. Drotrecogin alfa (activated) in patients with severe sepsis and a high risk of death. Crit Care 2006;10(6):427.

26 Lefering R, Neugebauer EAM. Steroid controversy in sepsis and septic shock: a metaanalysis. Crit Care Med 1995;23:1294–303.

27 Cronin L, Cook DJ, Carlet J, et al. Corticosteroid treatment for sepsis: a critical appraisal and meta-analysis of the literature. Crit Care Med 1995;23:1430–9.

28 Annane D. Corticosteroids for septic shock. Crit Care Med 2001;29:S117–20.

29 Annane D, Bellissant E, Bollaert PE, et al. Corticosteroids for severe sepsis and septic shock: a systematic review and meta-analysis. Brit Med J 2004;329:480–8.

30 Sprung CL, Annane D, Keh D, et al. Hydrocortisone therapy for patients with septic shock. N Engl J Med 2008;358:111–24.

31 Guidelines for the management of adults with hospital-acquired, ventilator-associated, and healthcare-associated pneumonia. Am J Respir Crit Care Med 2005;171:388–416.

32 Rello J, Ollendorf DA, Oster G, et al. Epidemiology and outcomes of ventilator-associated pneumonia in a large US database. Chest 2002;122:2115–21.

33 Heyland DK, Cook DJ, Griffith L, et al. The attributable morbidity and mortality of ventilator-associated pneumonia in the critically ill patient. Am J Respir Crit Care Med 1999;159:1249–56.

34 Craven DE, Steger KA. Epidemiology of nosocomial pneumonia: new perspectives on an old disease. Chest 1995;108: S1–16.

35 Kollef MH. The prevention of ventilator-associated pneumonia. New Engl J Med 1999;340:627–34.

36 Weber DJ, Rutala WA, Sickbert-Bennett EE, et al. Microbiology of ventilator-associated pneumonia compared with that of hospital-acquired pneumonia. Infect Control Hosp Epidemiol 2007;28:825–31.

37 Ibrahim EH, Ward S, Sherman G, Kollef MH. A comparative analysis of patients with early-onset vs late-onset nosocomial pneumonia in the ICU setting. Chest 2000;117:1434–42.

38 Dodek P, Keenan S, Cook D, et al. Evidence-based clinical practice guideline for the prevention of ventilator-associated pneumonia. Ann Int Med 2004;141:305–313.

39 Rouby JJ, Laurent P, Gosnach M, et al. Risk factors and clinical relevance of nosocomial maxillary sinusitis in the critically ill. Am J Respir Crit Care Med 1994;150:776–83.

40 Holzapfel L, Chevret S, Madinier G, et al. Influence of long-term oro- or nasotracheal intubation on nosocomial maxillary sinusitis and pneumonia: results of a prospective, randomized, clinical trial. Crit Care Med 1993;21:1132–8.

41 Rello J, Sonora R, Jubert P, et al. Pneumonia in intubated patients: role of respiratory airway care. Am J Respir Crit Care Med 1996;154:111–5.

42 Valles J, Artigas A, Rello J, et al. Continuous aspiration of subglottic secretions in preventing ventilator-associated pneumonia. Ann Intern Med 1995;122:179–86.

43 Kollef MH, Skubas NJ, Sundt TM. A randomized clinical trial of continuous aspiration of subglottic secretions in cardiac surgery patients. Chest 1999;116:1339–46.

44 Smulders K, van der Hoeven H, Weers-Pothoff I, Vandenbroucke-Grauls C. A randomized clinical trial of intermittent subglottic drainage in patients receiving mechanical ventilation. Chest 2002;121:858–62.

45 Bonten MJM, Kollef MH, Hall JB. Risk factors for ventilator-associated pneumonia: from epidemiology to patient management. Clin Infect Dis 2004;38:1141–9.

46 Drakulovic MB, Torres A, Bauer TT, et al. Supine body position as a risk factor for nosocomial pneumonia in mechanically ventilated patients: a randomised trial. Lancet 1999;354:1851–8.

47 Chan EY, Ruest A, Meade MO, Cook DJ. Oral decontamination for prevention of pneumonia in mechanically ventilated adults: systematic review and meta-analysis. Brit Med J 2007;334:889–99.

48 Cook DJ, Fuller HD, Guyatt GH, et al. Risk factors for gastrointestinal bleeding in critically ill patients. New Engl J Med 1994;330:377–81.

49 Messori A, Trippoli S, Vaiani M, et al. Bleeding and pneumonia in intensive care patients given ranitidine and sucralfate for prevention of stress ulcer: meta-analysis of randomized controlled trials. BMJ 2000;321:1103–10.

50 Meduri GU, Mauldin GL, Wunderink RG, et al. Causes of fever and pulmonary densities in patients with clinical manifestations of ventilator-associated pneumonia. Chest 1994;106:221–35.

51 Fagon JY, Chastre J, Hance AJ, et al. Evaluation of clinical judgement in the identification and treatment of nosocomial pneumonia in ventilated patients. Chest 1993;103:547–53.

52 Pugin J, Auckenthaler R, Mili N, et al. Diagnosis of ventilator-associated pneumonia by bacteriologic analysis of bronchoscopic and nonbronchoscopic "blind" bronchoalveolar lavage fluid. Am Rev Respir Dis 1991;143:1121–9.

53 Singh N, Rogers P, Atwood CW, et al. Short-course empiric antibiotic therapy for patients with pulmonary infiltrates in the intensive care unit: a proposed solution for indiscriminate antibiotic prescription. Am J Respir Crit Care Med 2000;162:505–11.

54 Fartoukh M, Maitre B, Honore S, et al. Diagnosing pneumonia during mechanical ventilation: the clinical pulmonary infection score revisited. Am J Respir Crit Care Med 2003:168:173–9.

55 Baselski VS, el-Torky M, Coalson JJ, Griffin JP. The standardization of criteria for processing and interpreting laboratory specimens in patients with suspected ventilator-associated pneumonia. Chest 1992;102:571S-9S.

56 Chastre J, Fagon JY, Bornet-Lesco M, et al. Evaluation of bronchoscopic techniques for the diagnosis of nosocomial pneumonia. Am J Respir Crit Care Med 1995;152:231–40.

57 Shorr AF, Sherner JH, Jackson WL, Kollef MH. Invasive approaches to the diagnosis of ventilator-associated pneumonia: a meta-analysis. Crit Care Med 2005;33:46–53.

58 The Canadian Critical Care Trials Group. A randomized trial of diagnostic techniques for ventilator-associated pneumonia. New Engl J Med 2006:355:2619–30.

59 Trouillet JL, Chastre J, Vuagnat A, et al. Ventilator-associated pneumonia caused by potentially drug-resistant bacteria. Am J Respir Crit Care Med 1998;157:531–9.

60 Iregui M, Ward S, Sherman G, et al. Clinical importance of delays in the initiation of appropriate antibiotic treatment for ventilator-associated pneumonia. Chest 2002;122:262–8.

61 Chastre J, Wolff M, Fagon JY, et al. Comparison of 8 vs 15 days of antibiotic therapy for ventilator-associated pneumonia in adults. J Am Med Assoc 2003;290:2588–98.

62 Maki DG, Kluger DM, Crnich CJ. The risk of bloodstream infection in adults with different intravascular devices: a systematic review of 200 published prospective studies. Mayo Clin Proc 2006;81:1151–79.

63 Warren DK, Zack JE, Elward AM, et al. Nosocomial primary bloodstream infections in intensive care unit patients in a nonteaching community medical center: a 21-month prospective study. Clin Infect Dis 2001;33:1329–35.

64 Pittet D, Tarara D, Wenzel RP. Nosocomial bloodstream infection in critically ill patients: excess length of stay, extra costs, and attributable mortality. J Am Med Assoc 1994;271:1598–1601.

65 DiGiovine B, Chenoweth C, Watts C, Higgins M. The attributable mortality and costs of primary nosocomial bloodstream infections in the intensive care unit. Am J Respir Crit Care Med 1999;160:976–81.

66 Raad I. Intravascular-catheter-related infections. Lancet 1998;351:893–8.

67 Wisplinghoff H, Bischoff T, Tallent SM, et al. Nosocomial bloodstream infections in US hospitals: analysis of 24,179 cases from a prospective nationwide surveillance study. Clin Infect Dis 2004;39:309–17.

68 Lorente L, Henry C, Martin MM, et al. Central venous catheter-related infection in a prospective and observational study of 2,595 catheters. Crit Care 2005;9:R631–5.

69 Merrer J, De Jonghe B, Golliot F, et al. Complications of femoral and subclavian venous catheterization in critically ill patients: a randomized controlled trial. J Am Med Assoc 2001;286:700–7.

70 O'Grady NP, Alexander M, Dellinger EP, et al. Guidelines for the prevention of intravascular catheter-related infections. Clin Infect Dis 2002;35:1281–307.

71 Raad II, Hohn DC, Gilbreath BJ, et al. Prevention of central venous catheter-related infections by using maximal sterile barrier precautions during insertion. Infect Control Hosp Epidemiol 1994;15:231–8.

72 Chalyakunapruk N, Veenstra DL, Lipsky BA, Saint S. Chlorhexidine compared with povidone-iodine solution for vascular catheter-site care: a meta-analysis. Ann Intern Med 2002;136:792–801.

73 Salzman MB, Isenberg HD, Rubin LG. Use of disinfectants to reduce microbial contamination of hubs of vascular catheters. J Clin Microbiol 1993;31:475–9.

74 McGee DC, Gould MK. Preventing complications of central venous catheterization. New Engl J Med 2003;348:1123–33.

75 Cook D, Randolph A, Kernerman P, et al. Central venous catheter replacement strategies: a systematic review of the literature. Crit Care Med 1997;25:1417–24.

76 Pronovost P, Needham D, Berenholtz S, et al. An intervention to decrease catheter-related bloodstream infections in the ICU. N Engl J Med 2006;355:2725–32.

77 Mermel LA, Farr BM, Sherertz RJ, et al. Guidelines for the management of intravascular catheter-related infections. Clin Infect Dis 2001;32:1249–72.

78 Safdar N, Maki DG. Inflammation at the insertion site is not predictive of catheter-related bloodstream infection with short-term, noncuffed central venous catheters. Crit Care Med 2002;30:2632–5.

79 Martinez JA, DesJardin JA, Aronoff M, et al. Clinical utility of blood cultures drawn from central venous or arterial catheters in critically ill surgical patients. Crit Care Med 2002;30:7–13.

80 Raad I, Hanna H, Maki D. Intravascular catheter-related infections: advances in diagnosis, prevention, and management. Lancet Infect Dis 2007;645–57.

81 Safdar N, Fine JP, Maki DG. Meta-analysis: methods for diagnosing intravascular device-related bloodstream infection. Ann Intern Med 2005;142:451–66.

82 Raad I, Davis S, Khan A, et al. Impact of central venous catheter removal on the recurrence of catheter-related coagulase-negative staphylococcal bacteremia. Infect Control Hosp Epidemiol 1992;13:215–21.

83 Fowler VG, Sanders LL, Sexton DJ, et al. Outcome of Staphylococcus aureus bacteremia according to compliance with recommendations of infectious disease specialists: experience with 244 patients. Clin Infect Dis 1998;27:478–86.

84 Fowler VG, Li J, Corey R, et al. Role of echocardiography in evaluation of patients with Staphylococcus aureus bacteremia: experience in 103 patients. J Am Coll Cardiol 1997;30:1072–8.

85 Hanna H, Afif C, Alakech B, et al. Central venous catheter-related bacteremia due to gram-negative bacilli: significance of catheter removal in preventing relapse. Infect Control Hosp Epidemiol 2004;24:646–9.

86 Nucci M, Colombo AL, Silveira F, et al. Risk factors for death in patients with candidemia. Infect Control Hosp Epidemiol 1998;19:846–50.

87 Pappas PG, Rex JH, Sobel JD, et al. Guidelines for treatment of candidiasis. Clin Infect Dis 2004;38:161–89.

PART 2
Special populations

CHAPTER 14

Infection control

Graham M. Snyder, Eli N. Perencevich & Anthony D. Harris

Surgical site infections

> ### Case presentation 1
>
> A new chief of surgery, who happens to be a cardiothoracic surgeon, arrives at your hospital. She calls you and says that she is concerned that the risk-adjusted surgical site infection rates at her new hospital might be higher than the rates at her previous hospital. She wants to set up a meeting with you to discuss ways to minimize the risk of surgical site infection in her patients.

Burden of illness, cost, and relevance to clinical practice

Surgical site infections (SSIs) are defined as either incisional or organ/organ space infections. Incisional SSIs are then divided into superficial, involving the skin and subcutaneous tissue, and deep, involving the muscle and fascia [1]. Typically an infection is considered an SSI if it occurs within 30 days of the operation. SSI rates vary by procedure with rates being highest with cardiac surgery (2.5 infections per 100 patient discharges) [2]. As estimated by the US National Nosocomial Infections Surveillance System, there are approximately 1.7 million heathcare-associated infections annually in US hospitals, of which approximately 22% are SSIs – second only to urinary tract infections [3]. This totals nearly 300 000 surgical site

Evidence-Based Infectious Diseases, 2nd edition. Edited by Mark Loeb, Fiona Smaill and Marek Smieja. © 2009 Wiley-Blackwell Publishing, ISBN: 978-1-4051-7026-0

infections yearly (about two SSIs per 100 procedures) and an estimated 8205 excess attributable deaths [3]. Of all those that died with an SSI, 77% were found to have the infection causally related to their deaths [4].

It is recognized that a cost analysis for a medical intervention (e.g., an intervention to reduce SSI) is complex in its method of analysis and determination of outcome, and may not be accurately reported in the literature [5]. Nevertheless, there are many studies attempting to evaluate the cost of SSIs, and recent significant studies are summarized in Table 14.1. Reviews of the cost of SSIs have also been published by Yasunaga et al. [6] and Urban [7].

Risk factors

The incidence of SSIs varies depending on the surgeon, the hospital, procedure type, and individual patient risk factors. The fact that confounding factors such as procedure type, duration of procedure, comorbid conditions, and baseline severity of illness of patients can impact surgical infection occurrence necessitates the risk adjustment of SSI rates for fair comparison between surgeons and hospitals. Determination of risk factors is most useful when identified risk factors are modifiable. Therefore, factors such as specific hospital and procedure type may be interesting to note, but their identification as risk factors does not help surgeons, anesthesiologists, and infection control personnel prevent SSIs. In fact, duration of surgery, age, obesity, and underlying disease are some of the most commonly noted risk factors for development of SSI, yet they are fixed parameters from the perspective of the infection control practitioner. While it may seem that identifying an individual surgeon as a risk factor could be more disruptive than helpful, it has been shown that one of the most successful ways to reduce

Table 14.1 Cost of surgical site infections by various estimates

Source reference	Subjects, no. (SSI/non-SSI)	Surgical procedure	Costs evaluated: type of SSI	Cost analysis	Cost
Olsen et al., 2008 [160]	888 (50/838)	Mastectomy, breast reconstruction	In-hospital, LOS Various	Crude cost	$4091
Jenney et al., 2001 [161]	216 (108/108)	CABG	In-hospital, LOS, antibiotic use Superficial, deep	Crude cost	$12 419 (AU)
Hollenbeak et al., 2000 [162]	201 (41/160)	CABG	In-hospital, total cost, LOS Deep	Crude cost	$18 938
Hall et al., 1997 [163]	6791 (176/6615)	CABG	In-hospital, total cost Unspecified	Crude cost	$23 200 (adjusted for variables)
Coskun et al., 2005 [164]	176 (88/88, 52 deep SSI, 36 superficial SSI)	CABG	In-hospital, LOS, antibiotic use, testing Superficial, deep	Crude cost	$6851 (deep) $3741 (superficial)
Whitehouse et al., 2002 [165]	62 (31/31): university 46 (23/23): community	Orthopedic	In hospital; variable, fixed and indirect costs Superficial, deep	Crude cost (median)	$38 640 (SSI) $10 671 (controls)
Perencevich et al., 2003 [166]	267 (89/178)	Various	Insurance provider database, all costs within 8 weeks post-discharge Unspecified	Crude cost	$5155 (SSI) $1773 (controls)
Kirkland et al., 1999 [167]	510 (255/255)	Various	In hospital, readmission within 30 days Superficial, deep	Crude cost	$8864 (SSI) $4391 (controls)
Herwaldt et al., 2006 [168]	3864 (438/3425, 438 nosocomial infections, 316 of which were SSIs)	Various: general surgical (2408), neurosurgical (732), cardiothoracic (724)	In hospital, 30 days postoperative Not described	Crude cost	$6364 (SSI only) $3343 (without infection)
Reilly et al., 2001 [169]	2202 (220/1982)	Various	In hospital, LOS, outpatient, home services Not described	Crude cost	£87 276
McGarry et al., 2004 [170]	286 (96/190, controls included 59 uninfected elderly and 131 younger patients with *Staphylococcus aureus* SSI)	Various	Hospital charges within 90 days postoperative Superficial, deep (post-cardiothoracic superficial SSIs excluded), due to *Staphylococcus aureus*	Crude cost	$41 117 (attributable cost compared with uninfected elderly) $2746 (attributable cost compared with younger patients with SSI)

(continued)

Source reference	Subjects, no. (SSI/non-SSI)	Surgical procedure	Costs evaluated: type of SSI	Cost analysis	Cost
Coello et al., 2005 [171]	67410 (2832/64578)	Various	Charge from prior study, adjusted for inflation, LOS Superficial, deep	Crude cost	£959-£6103 (depending on procedure) £814-£6161 (superficial) £1947-£6626 (deep)
Kasatpibal et al., 2005 [172]	280 (140/140)	Various	Hospital charge Not described	Crude cost	43658 baht
Dimick et al., 2004 [173]	1008 (75/933)	Various	In-hospital cost Superficial, deep, sepsis, wound dehiscence	Crude cost	$1398 (adjusted for variables)
Engermann et al., 2003 [174]	479 (186/193, 165 patients with MSSA SSI, 121 patients with MRSA SSI)	Various	In-hospital cost Superficial, deep	Crude cost (median)	$92363 (MRSA SSI) $52791 (MSSA SSI) $29455 (controls)

SSIs is proper surveillance of infection rates and feedback of rates to individual surgeons [8]. Throughout the rest of this section we will describe the evidence that supports specific risk factors for SSI with a particular focus on modifiable risk factors and randomized controlled clinical trials demonstrating improved outcomes with their modification.

Glucose control

Diabetes is known to increase the risk of developing a SSI. Unlike other comorbidities, such as obesity, there is a potential for lowering the risk of SSI through perioperative glucose control. One proposed mechanism includes improved neutrophil phagocytic function (but not antibody-dependent cell cytotoxicity), as demonstrated in a randomized trial of patients receiving either intensive or standard insulin treatment during surgery [9]. Furthermore, a recent review of the impact of hyperglycemia on the immune system suggests that despite limitations to the breadth of research, there is good evidence that the immune system is impaired with short-term hyperglycemia [10].

As a recent review of hyperglycemia and SSIs in cardiothoracic surgical cases points out, there is ample evidence to demonstrate an association between perioperative hyperglycemia and SSI risk [11]. In one study of cardiothoracic surgery patients, a postoperative glucose level greater than 200 mg/dL within 48 hours after surgery was shown to increase the odds of developing

an SSI by 86% in known diabetic patients and by 114% in patients with no history of diabetes, and these results were largely unchanged with multivariable analysis [12]. Similarly, among 260 patients undergoing mastectomy (50 SSIs were observed; 37 superficial, 13 deep), the presence of any perioperative glucose value ≥150 mg/dL increased the risk of SSI three-fold, even after correction for the presence of diabetes [13].

Another group found that an elevated average blood glucose over the 48-hour postoperative period was the strongest predictor of deep sternal wound infection in diabetic patients undergoing open-heart procedures [14]. Additionally, they performed a quasi-experimental trial in which historical controls, who had perioperative blood glucose controlled with subcutaneous insulin injections, were compared to a later group who had continuous insulin infusions and found that continuous insulin infusion was associated with a two-third reduction in the risk of deep sternal wound infection [15]. Trials that use historical controls, however, are limited by the fact that additional changes may occur through time, which cannot be controlled for in the quasi-experimental design and could explain or partially explain the reduced infection rates.

Perioperative warming

Hypothermia is thought to increase a patient's risk of developing a SSI through thermoregulatory vasoconstriction and resultant reduced tissue oxygen levels, and impairment immune function including T-cell-mediated antibody production and oxidative neutrophilic bacterial killing [16]. Unwarmed patients in surgery lose heat until their core temperature falls about 2°C, after which core temperature is stabilized by peripheral vasoconstriction and altered heat distribution [17,18].

Several limited studies have demonstrated an indeterminate relationship between perioperative warming and surgical site infections. A prospective cohort study of 290 patients undergoing laparoscopic cholecystectomies demonstrated that patients with mild perioperative hypothermia (156 with hypothermia, 105 without hypothermia) were more likely to have SSIs (18 in the hypothermic group, two in the normothermic group), but were also more likely to have a longer surgery. The role of age, diabetes mellitus, and prophylactic antibiotic use cannot be excluded as confounding difference, however [19]. A retrospective cohort study of 150 consecutive patients undergoing colectomy (101 normothermic patients and 49 patients with intraoperative temperature less than 95.5°F) found similar postoperative infection rates and postoperative length of stay between the two groups [20]. A relatively small case–control study among patients who underwent cesarean section with 18 cases who developed SSI compared to 18 controls found intraoperative temperature to not be a significant risk factor for the development of SSI [21]. In a small randomized controlled trial of 173 patients undergoing intracranial surgery in Japan, four of 122 patients (3.3%) randomized to intentional mild hypothermia (goal temperature 34.5°C) developed SSI, compared with none of the 51 patients randomized to normothermia [22].

Two randomized controlled trials, however, provide a clearer picture of SSI rates with control of perioperative temperature. In a randomized controlled trial in patients undergoing colorectal surgery, Kurz et al. demonstrated an approximately three-fold reduction in SSI rates in patients actively warmed approximately 2°C to the desired temperature of 36.6°C by intravenous fluid warming and forced-air warming in the intraoperative period [23]. The same study also found that patients who were in the hypothermic arm of the study had 20% longer hospital stay. In a randomized controlled trial of patients undergoing breast, varicose vein, or hernia surgery, Melling et al. found that warming patients before surgery reduced postoperative SSIs. Patients were randomized to one of the following: systemic warming (whole-body warming by blanket and forced air in the 30-minute preoperative period), localized warming (30 minutes of preoperative warming localized to the planned wound area), and nonwarming standard care [24]. The study found that both systemic warming (absolute risk reduction 7.9%, 95% CI 1.0–14.8) and local warming (ARR 10.1%, 95% CI 3.6–16.6) were associated with reduced SSIs compared to standard nonwarmed treatment. The study was not powered to find a difference between the systemic and local warming groups.

A broad recommendation across all types of surgery cannot be given since patients who undergo certain procedures actually benefit from hypothermia. Mild hypothermia has a documented cerebro-protective effect in neurosurgery patients [25], which would likely outweigh their very low risk of SSI [26]. In addition, core temperatures are lowered in cardiac surgery to protect the myocardium and central nervous system [18].

Supplemental oxygen

Neutrophilic bactericidal activity is mediated by superoxide radical-dependent oxidative killing, which is linked to the partial pressure of oxygen in the tissue [27]. A cohort study of patients at high risk for SSI found that the oxygen tension of the subcutaneous tissue measured perioperatively was a very strong predictor of subsequent development of SSI [28]. The infection rate was 43% (6 of 14 patients) in those with maximum oxygen tension between 40 and 50 mmHg and 0% (0 of 15 patients) in those with maximum oxygen tension above 90 mmHg. The wound hypoxia has been correlated with reduced leukocyte killing from depressed oxygen consumption and superoxide formation [29].

Greif et al. performed a randomized controlled trial in patients undergoing colorectal surgery compared patients who received 30% inspired oxygen to those receiving 80% inspired oxygen [27]. The oxygen was given intraoperatively and in the 2 hours after surgery. Even though arterial oxygen saturation was normal in both groups, the subcutaneous partial pressure of oxygen was significantly higher in those who received 80% inspired oxygen. Importantly the infection rate was only 5.2% in the 80% inspired oxygen group compared to an infection rate of 11.2% in the 30% inspired oxygen group (ARR 6.0%, 95% CI 7.3–15.1%). The duration of hospitalization was the same in both groups. The study was ended early because of the significant benefit from supplemental perioperative oxygen. A subgroup analysis found that higher oxygen was not associated with any additional risk for radiologically confirmed pulmonary atelectasis [27].

Subsequently, a double-blind, randomized controlled trial among 165 patients undergoing major intraabdominal surgery compared SSIs within 14 days of surgery among 80 patients receiving 80% inspired oxygen (85 initially randomized) and 80 patients receiving 35% inspired oxygen (80 initially randomized) intraoperatively and 2 hours postoperatively [30]. Perhaps significantly, rates of obesity were higher in the 80% inspired oxygen group and rates of COPD were higher in the 35% inspired oxygen group, rates of blood loss and fluid resuscitation were higher and operation length were longer in the 80% inspired oxygen group, and the 80% inspired oxygen group were more likely to require postoperative intubation. Twenty patients in the 80% inspired oxygen group (25%) and nine patients in the 35% inspired oxygen group (11.3%) had SSIs ($P = 0.02$). Hospitalization duration and reoperation rates were higher in the 80% inspired oxygen group, though not statistically significant. Infection depth/location was not significantly different between the two groups. Significant limitations to this study include small sample size, analysis of infection rates by retrospective chart review, inadequate assessment of tissue perfusion and possibly oxygenation, and the above-mentioned differences in study groups [30].

Prompted by the discrepancy between these two trials, a randomized controlled trial similar in methodology to Greif et al. [27] also compared rates of SSI in 291 patients undergoing elective colorectal resection who received either 30% or 80% inspired oxygen intraoperatively and 6 hours postoperatively [31]. Other than measurements of FiO_2 and PaO_2, the 143 patients in the 30% inspired oxygen and the 148 patients in the 80% inspired oxygen groups were similar. Perioperative use of 80% inspired oxygen was associated with a significant protective effect of postoperative SSI; among patients receiving 30% inspired oxygen, 35 (24.4%) had an SSI within a 15-day

postoperative period, while 22 (14.9%) of those in the 80% inspired oxygen group had an SSI (RR 0.61, 95% CI 0.38–0.98). In multivariate analysis, only 30% inspired oxygen and coexisting respiratory disease significantly increased risk of SSI [31].

One potential risk of high oxygen concentrations during the perioperative period is the theoretical risk of atelectasis and subsequent pneumonia [30], although two studies addressing the issue of oxygen concentration, atelectasis, and lung function suggest that any difference may be negligible [32,33]. The studies by Grief and Belda provide methodologically sound evidence of postoperative benefit from perioperative supplemental oxygen. While oxygen supplementation is increasingly recommended for its apparent benefits and minimal risk [34], the best data to date is in the limited operative subset of colorectal surgeries, although these are at higher risk of infection than many other types of surgery [8].

Hair removal

Hair removal as part of the preparation of the surgical site has long been a practice of surgeons to improve exposure to the incision site and subsequent wound, facilitate wound closure and dressing, and has been thought to prevent SSIs. Three methods of hair removal are commonly practiced: shaving, clipping, and depilatory creams. It is now suspected that shaving changes the normal flora, removes the hairs' natural protective effect, and causes minor trauma which may allow for an entry site for bacteria or produce exudates that support bacterial growth; all of these factors when combined may increase the risk of infection [35].

The most comprehensive and recent review of the evidence for hair removal in reducing SSI rates is the Cochrane review on the topic published in 2008 [36]. After evaluating 11 randomized controlled trials, the authors concluded that hair removal prior to surgery did not affect SSI rates, although removing hair using a razor increased rates of SSIs compared with clipping or depilatory cream [36]. Two randomized controlled trials involving 358 adults undergoing abdominal surgery compared preoperative hair removal with no hair removal, each finding an absence of statistical difference between SSI rates. Pooled, 9.6% (17/177) of people who underwent shaving prior to surgery developed an SSI compared with 6.1% (11/181) of those with intact hair (RR 1.59, 95% CI 0.77–3.27) [37,38]. Court Brown also investigated depilatory cream compared with no hair removal, and found SSI rates of 7.9% (10/126) and 7.8% (11/141) among patients receiving depilatory cream and no hair removal, respectively (RR 1.02, 95% CI 0.45–2.31) [37]. In three trials investigating shaving versus clipping [39–41], statistically higher rates of SSI were observed in the shaving group (2.8% [46/1627] vs 1.4% [21/1566], RR 2.02, 95% CI 1.21–3.36), although all studies had methodological limitations [36]. Seven trials among 1213 patients receiving varied types of surgeries compared hair removal with depilatory cream versus razor use [37,42–47]. Again, methodological variations and limitations are significant, however, pooled data demonstrates 7% (38/543) of patients receiving depilatory cream versus 10% (65/670) of patients who were shaved had postoperative courses complicated by SSI (RR 1.54, 95% CI 1.05–2.24) [36].

It appears that hair removal should be limited to situations where it will impede the operation and if necessary hair should be removed with clippers or depilatory cream and not a razor. Issues without definitive data include optimal timing of hair removal in proximity to surgery and optimal location to perform hair removal (i.e., ward, preoperative suite, or operating room) [36].

Smoking cessation

Rates of tobacco use in the United States remain above 20% of adults despite a slowed but continued decrease in rates in the last 50 years [48]. The causal association of tobacco use (smoking) and postoperative complications – including pulmonary and wound healing – is well-studied [49]. Smoking likely affects postoperative risk of SSI in mechanisms similar to hypoxia, including inhibiting immune response [50], promoting peripheral vasoconstriction, disruption of endothelial function, and superoxide radical ion production [51].

Several cohort studies have demonstrated a positive association between smoking and SSI, including a four-fold increased risk of SSI among 1505 Veterans Administration patients undergoing ventral hernia repair [52], a 1.8-fold increased risk of superficial (though not deep) sternal wound infection among 4004 patients undergoing coronary artery bypass grafting [53], a 1.75-fold increased risk of SSI among 4855 patients undergoing open gastrointestinal

surgery [54], and a 3- to 3.5-fold risk among patients undergoing breast cancer or reconstructive breast surgery [55,56]. Two smaller studies designed to analyze the risk of wound infections among smokers versus nonsmokers have also demonstrated significantly increased risk of SSI among smokers, in a populations of patients undergoing postbariatric abdominoplasty [57] and ambulatory surgery [58].

Although one small study of 60 patients undergoing elective colorectal surgery who were randomized to either short-term preoperative smoking cessation (2–3 week preoperative intervention) or continuation of habit demonstrated no significant difference in postoperative complications including wound infection [59], two randomized controlled trials have demonstrated a significant increase in postoperative wound infections in smokers. Sorensen et al. investigated an intervention of smoking cessation in reducing postoperative SSI risk among incisional wounds created by a punch biopsy [60]. In 48 healthy smokers, sutured incisional wounds were made to excise the previously made 5-mm full-thickness punch biopsy wounds at weeks 1, 4, 8, and 12 of the study; among 30 healthy never-smokers, identical wounds were made in six, and a one-time wound was made in the other 24 subjects. After the first week of the study, smokers were randomized to continuous smoking, smoking abstinence with transdermal nicotine patch, or smoking abstinence with placebo patch (each subgroup with eight men and eight women). At 1, 4, 8, and 12 weeks, continuous smokers had significantly more wound infections (total of 10 infections in 12 patients) than either abstinent smokers (one infection) or never-smokers (one infection).

Three Danish hospitals participated in a randomized controlled trial of 120 patients undergoing elective knee or hip arthroplasty. Sixty patients were randomly assigned 6–8 weeks prior to surgery to either a smoking cessation intervention with counseling and nicotine replacement or standard care. Among the 56 patients in the intervention group that completed the study, 36 stopped smoking, 14 decreased tobacco use, and six continued smoking; among the 52 patients in the control group completing the study, four stopped smoking and 48 continued smoking. Cardiovascular complications, repeat surgery, and wound-related complications were higher among the control group. Twelve patients (23%) had "positive culture" wound infections from the control group, compared with only two patients (4%) from the intervention group ($P < 0.05$).

While the magnitude of effect and optimal time for cessation is not fully characterized, there is strong evidence that smoking contributes to SSI risk and that cessation prior to surgery decreases this risk. Due to SSI and other perioperative risk, as well as nonsurgical, noninfectious health risks, it is highly advisable to counsel patients to quit smoking prior to surgery.

Staphylococcus aureus elimination with mupirocin ointment and chlorhexidine scrub

Staphylococcus aureus is a frequent cause of SSIs, and data has suggested that nasal carriers of *S. aureus* may be at higher risk than noncarriers for SSIs [61]. Mupirocin ointment may be successful in eliminating nasal carriage of *S. aureus*. A large cohort study of cardiothoracic surgery patients using both concurrent and historical controls found between a 4.5% and 5.8% reduction in SSIs in patients treated with nasal mupirocin ointment started on the day prior and continued for 4 days after surgery [62]. An analysis using this same data found that perioperative mupirocin was cost-effective and in most settings would be cost-saving [63]. A second prospective cohort study among open-heart surgery patients (992 control patients and 854 patients receiving intranasal mupirocin the day prior surgery, the day of surgery, and 5 days postoperatively) found a 1.8% absolute risk reduction in SSIs (2.7% vs 0.9%) with mupirocin use, a significant difference that was sustained among diabetic patients, nondiabetic patients, and among deep and superficial surgical wounds [64]. In a study among orthopedic patients, perioperative mupirocin in addition to preoperative triclosan wash was found to decrease the rate of MRSA SSIs and nasal *S. aureus* carriage compared with the pre-intervention period. Among 420 cases pre-intervention, and 1758 case with intervention, the rate of MRSA SSIs decreased from 2.3% to 0.3–0.4%, without change in the rate of MSSA SSIs (1.6% to 1.4–2.0%) [65]. In the other orthopedic study to date, Gernaat-van der Sluis et al. compared 1260 historical controls with 1044 patients treated with muprocin perioperatively and found a statistically significant decrease in SSIs from 2.7% to 1.3%. Although the rate of *S. aureus* SSIs decreased from 1.1% to 0.7%, this difference was not statistically significant [66].

Four randomized clinical trials have been conducted to evaluate the role of mupirocin in reducing SSIs [67–70]. In a randomized, double-blind placebo-controlled trial published in 2002 by Perl et al. [69] among 3864 patients undergoing various surgeries, there was no significant difference between SSI rates among patients receiving mupirocin (152/1933, 7.9%) and those receiving placebo (164/1931, 8.5%) and there was no significant difference in *S. aureus* SSIs between both groups (2.3% vs 2.4%, respectively). For *S. aureus* carriers randomized to both groups, mupirocin resulted in a significant reduction in *S. aureus* carriage in the mupirocin group and not the placebo group. Nevertheless, despite a trend in decreased rates of nosocomial infections (total and *S. aureus* specific) and SSIs (total and *S. aureus* specific) between *S. aureus* carriers receiving mupirocin and placebo, this difference was only significant for nosocomial *S. aureus* infections. In a double-blind, randomized, placebo-controlled trial among 263 patients with nasal *S. aureus* carriage undergoing elective cardiac surgery in Toronto, patients randomized to mupirocin use demonstrated slightly higher – though not significant – rates of total, sternal, and leg infections (13.8% vs 8.6%, 5.4% vs 4.7%, and 8.5% vs 3.9%, respectively) [68]. There was a significantly higher rate of *S. aureus* nasal colonization carriage rates among patients receiving mupirocin versus those receiving placebo. Kalmeijer et al. [67] studied preoperative mupirocin versus placebo in 315 and 299 patients, respectively, undergoing orthopedic surgeries. SSIs were similar among patients receiving mupirocin (12/315, 3.8%) and placebo (14/299, 4.7%), including when analyzed by deep and superficial SSIs as well as *S. aureus* and endogenous *S. aureus* SSIs. Rates of nasal carriage eradication were significantly higher among mupirocin-treated patients than placebo-treated patients. Lastly, in a trial among 395 patients undergoing abdominal digestive surgery, 193 patients were randomized to receive mupirocin 3 days preoperatively and 202 patients were randomized to no treatment [70]. Although limited by the absence of reporting of *S. aureus* carriage and the predominance of gram-negative over gram-positive or mixed bacteria causing superficial and deep SSIs, there was no significant difference in the rate of SSIs among the two studied groups.

Taking the data in its entirety, there appears to be a suggestion that mupirocin may reduce SSI rates in cohort studies that is not borne out in clinical trials,

3

despite large studies and subgroup analysis. A recent review [71] and metanalysis [72] have a similar summary of the data. Though some authors argue that mupirocin use may be cost-effective [63,73], this analysis cannot be made prior to establishing its efficacy, and subsequently the risk of inducing mupirocin resistance [74]. Further studies may establish a clear benefit in populations of S. aureus carriers or specific surgeries.

Bathing with chlorhexidine or similar antimicrobial agent prior to surgery is an alternative and complementary strategy to minimize SSI, and has been demonstrated to reduce bacterial burden on the skin [75,76]. The most definitive summary of evidence to date is a Cochrane systematic review [77] investigating bathing or showering with skin antiseptics prior to surgery. The review identified six randomized controlled trials of over 10 000 patients, three of which (7691 patients) compared 4% chlorhexidine ("Hibiscrub" or "Hibiclens") with placebo scrub and three of which (1443 patients) compared bar soap with chlorhexidine and (in the case of two of these three trials) chlorhexidine with no washing. Although one of the trials comparing chlorhexidine with bar soap found a statistically significant difference in SSI [78], there are methodological concerns with the trial, and when combined with two other trials, found no significant difference [77]. Similarly, of the two trials comparing chlorhexidine scrub with no washing, there were methodological differences compared to each other and compared to present-day practice; one study found no significant difference in SSI rates [79] while the second study found a 2.9% absolute risk reduction with chlorhexidine use [80]. The remainder of the studies failed to show a statistically significant benefit in SSI rates after chlorhexidine use. Taken together, these studies do not produce conclusive evidence that preoperative chlorhexidine scrubs reduce SSI rates. Consideration for the use of preoperative chlorhexidine warrants further evaluation, balancing the generally low risk to the patient, but an as yet poorly defined risk of developing antimicrobial resistance, including possible promotion of Acinetobacter infections [81].

Perioperative antimicrobial prophylaxis

Not all surgeries require antibiotic prophylaxis. The initial step in deciding whether antimicrobial prophylaxis is indicated in a particular surgery is to determine which type of procedure will be performed.

Table 14.2 Surgical wound classification

Class I/Clean: Uninfected operative wound with no inflammation and the respiratory, alimentary, genital, or uninfected urinary tract is not entered. Cleans wounds are primarily closed and necessary drains are closed.

Class II/Clean-Contaminated: Operative wound with controlled entry into the respiratory, alimentary, genital, or urinary tract. Specifically, operations of the biliary tract, appendix, vagina, and oropharynx are included if no evidence of infection or break in sterile technique.

Class III/Contaminated: Open, fresh accidental wounds or ones with breaks in sterile technique, gastrointestinal spillage, or incisions in which nonpurulent inflammation is encountered are contaminated.

Class IV/Dirty-Infected: Presence of old traumatic wounds with devitalized tissue or ones with existing clinical infection or perforated viscera suggesting preexisting organisms prior to the operation.

Source: Mangram et al. [1].

Table 14.2 lists the surgical wound classification scheme, which is by definition a postoperative assessment of intraoperative wound contamination, since breaks in sterile technique and other intraoperative findings cannot be predicted preoperatively. This classification allows the surgeon to estimate preoperatively the wound class of a given operation. Antimicrobial prophylaxis is indicated for clean-contaminated wounds (class II), which is separate from the practice of bowel decontamination, and in clean wounds (class I) if the SSI might be a clinical catastrophe as would be the case in intravascular or joint prosthesis implantations [1]. Antimicrobial prophylaxis is not indicated in class III or IV operations since these would involve specific antimicrobial treatment and would not be prophylaxis.

There are several issues surrounding the use of prophylactic antibiotics during the perioperative period including the timing of antibiotic initiation and the duration of dosing in the postoperative period. Classen et al. in a large prospective cohort study determined the effect of prophylactic antibiotic timing on the rate of SSI in 2847 patients who had clean (class I) or clean-contaminated (class II) operations [82]. Patients who received antibiotics preoperatively, defined as zero to 2 hours prior to incision, had the lowest rate of SSI (0.6%). Higher rates of SSI were seen for perioperative administration, within 3 hours after incision (1.4%),and in those that received antibiotics more than 2 hours before (3.8% SSI rate) and more than 3 hours after (3.3% SSI rate) the incision. A logistic-regression analysis confirmed that timing of antimicrobial prophylaxis within 2 hours prior to incision was associated with the lowest odds of developing an SSI. The authors estimated that 27 SSIs would have been prevented in the 1-year study period if optimal timing of antimicrobial prophylaxis within 2 hours prior to incision was completely adhered to [82]. More recently, a study investigating the timing of antibiotic prophylaxis in patients undergoing total hip arthroplasty confirmed the goal of administering antibiotics within an hour prior to incision [83]. It requires a great deal of institutional effort to insure that antimicrobial prophylaxis is appropriately timed. At one medical center a random sample retrospective chart review found that after shifting responsibility of antibiotic dosing to the anesthesiologist with assistance of the pharmacy personnel in selecting patients for prophylaxis, the percent of patients receiving antimicrobial prophylaxis within 1 hour prior to surgery rose from 38% to 88% [84].

Increasingly, it is demonstrated and recommended not only that antibiotics should be given within 60 minutes of the surgical incision, but also that the postoperative duration of antimicrobial prophylaxis should be less than 24 hours [85]. A metaanalysis of 28 randomized trials with 9478 patients compared single versus multiple dose antimicrobial prophylaxis in a broad range of surgical procedure types and found no difference between the two groups; random effects model (OR 1.04, 95% CI 0.86–1.25) [86]. Another metaanalysis of 25 randomized trials found that prophylactic antibiotics are effective in reducing SSIs in patients undergoing total hip and total knee replacement surgeries (RR 0.24, 95% CI (0.14–0.43), NNT = 30), but found no benefit for prophylaxis extended beyond 1 day postoperatively [87]. A recent cohort study of 2641 patients undergoing coronary artery bypass graft surgery determined that prolonged antibiotic prophylaxis (greater than 48 hours after surgery) was not significantly associated with less risk of SSI compared to shorter duration (<48 hours) antibiotic prophylaxis [88]. Interestingly, this study found that prolonged antibiotic prophylaxis beyond 48 hours after surgery was significantly associated with an increased risk of acquiring a clinical culture growing either cephalosporin-resistant enterobacteriaceae or vancomycin-resistant enterococci when compared to shorter-duration prophylaxis.

These findings support the current Centers for Disease Control and Prevention (CDC) guidelines for SSI prevention that suggest that a full therapeutic dose of a bactericidal agent be given early enough so that peak levels are present at the time of the incision (e.g., 1–2 g cefazolin no more than 30 minutes prior to incision) and that therapeutic levels be continued throughout the operation and for no more than a few hours after incisional closure [1]. Exceptions mentioned within these guidelines state that higher antibiotic doses should be used in obese patients and that initial doses of antibiotics in cesarean section should be given immediately after umbilical cord clamping.

Comprehensive interventions

Ultimately, no single method should be used to reduce SSI rates. A comprehensive infection control program that utilizes many of the above strategies mentioned will have the greatest benefit through additive independent mechanisms and a combined effect. A 4-year observational study of a cardiothoracic surgery service after the initiation of a comprehensive infection control program that included surveillance, feedback to the surgeons, chlorhexidine showers the night before and morning of surgery, hair clipping if necessary, antibiotic prophylaxis in the holding area 30–120 minutes prior to surgery, and elimination of iced cardioplegia solution along with other changes was found to significantly reduce the rate of SSIs (OR = 0.37; 95% CI 0.22–0.63). In addition there were trends toward reduced rates of deep chest infection and mortality [2]. As part of a 56-hospital National Surgical Infection Prevention Collaborative, 44 hospitals presented data on 35 543 surgical cases over a 12-month period during which a comprehensive plan to reduce SSIs was implemented [89]. Interventions included antibiotic timing within 1 hour of surgery, appropriate antibiotic selection, discontinuation of antibiotic within 24 hours of surgery, normothermia (intraoperative temperature >36°C), avoiding shaving surgical site, hyperoxia (FIO_2 >80%), and glucose control (≤200 mg/dL) and all interventions showed statistically significant improvement during the four 3-month periods evaluated. The overall SSI rate fell from 2.28% in the first quarter to

1.65% in the final quarter (statistically significant by Wilcoxon rank sum), though the month-to-month trend was not significant by Poisson regression analysis. Subsequently, the University of Virginia joined the initiative, and implemented the above interventions during colorectal surgeries except avoiding preoperative shaving (and also included the placement of Penrose drains in the subcutaneous space of patients with a body mass index $\geqslant$25). While comparing 132 patients during the study period with 175 historical controls, compliance with antibiotic guidelines showed statistically significant improvement and rates of normothermia and perioperative glucose values demonstrated nonsignificant improvement. SSI rates decreased from 26% to 16% ($P = 0.04$), as did mean length of stay [90]. Lastly, in a single-site study investigating effect of a protocol including appropriate antibiotic use (selection, administration pre- and postoperatively as above), normothermia (>36°C), and glucose control (<200 mg/dL), 379 patients undergoing intra-abdominal surgical procedures during the first four months of the protocol were compared with 390 patients followed during the last 4 months of the 11-month study period. There was statistically significant improvement in antibiotic selection and timeliness of administration, while cessation of antibiotic postoperatively remained above 90% and the incidence of hypothermia fell a nonsignificant 15% to 10%. The 30-day incidence of SSI decreased from 9.2% to 5.6% ($P = 0.07$) [91].

In conclusion, an optimal infection control program to limit SSIs in surgical patients should include surveillance for SSIs in the inpatient setting and if possible tracking of SSIs that manifest after hospital discharge, and the SSI rates should be fed back to individual surgeons. Evidence supports the use of preoperative smoking cessation, perioperative glucose monitoring and control, perioperative warming as feasible by procedure, supplemental oxygen intraoperatively and for several hours after surgery, hair removal if necessary by clipping, perioperative antimicrobial prophylaxis with dosing that allows peak levels to be achieved prior to incision (cefazolin about 30 minutes prior and vancomycin about 1 hour prior), and repeat dosing if necessary to maintain levels during the procedure, and discontinuation of antibiotic prophylaxis within a few hours after completion of surgery. Whether or not attempted eradication of potential pathogenic organisms with intranasal mupirocin or whole-body chlorhexidine wash decreases SSI risk is not fully established, and warrants further investigation.

Methicillin-resistant bacteria

Case presentation 2

A 45-year-old male with type 1 diabetes is admitted with a soft-tissue infection of the left foot. You are called by the patient's attending physician when wound cultures are positive for MRSA and *Pseudomonas aeruginosa*. The patient is being treated with vancomycin and piperacillin-tazobactam. The current plan for the patient is a course of antibiotics. No immediate surgery is planned although the patient may require arterial bypass surgery at some point. The attending physician asks you the following questions:

1. What should I do to prevent other patients from acquiring this patient's MRSA?
2. What is this patient's risk in terms of morbidity and mortality?
3. What is the role for decolonization in this patient?

As hospital epidemiologist, you decide to put the patient on contact precautions involving the use of gloves and gowns. You explain to the physician that the patient is at risk for an increased hospital length of stay. The patient is also at risk of increased mortality if he develops an MRSA bacteremia. You advise against decolonization in this patient and in this setting.

Carriage, colonization and infection: clinical presentation of MRSA

Staphylococci are gram-positive bacteria that are normal skin flora and MRSA, like MSSA, primarily colonizes and is most readily cultured from the nares but may also colonize adjacent structures, such as the perineum, wounds, burns, respiratory secretions (including among intubated patients), urine, and feces [92].

Carriers of *S. aureus* are classified as: (1) persistent carriers, (2) intermittent carriers, or (3) noncarriers [93,94]. Approximately 10–35% of healthy people are persistent carriers, 20–75% are intermittent carriers and 5–50% are noncarriers; persistent carriers are less likely to have variation in *S. aureus* strains than intermittent carriers [93,94]. While cross-sectional studies demonstrate an approximately 35% carriage rate in the general hospitalized population, certain populations have increased rates of carriage, particularly those undergoing renal replacement therapy, those with insulin-dependent diabetes mellitus, those with HIV infection, and patients receiving repeat injections for allergies 93,94]. Among patients colonized with MRSA, long-term carriage rate seems to vary between 30% and 60% depending upon the patient population [95]. The prevalence of MRSA carriage in the general community has been harder to estimate, and is likely much lower than that among hospitalized populations. A metaanalysis of 10 studies performing surveillance cultures (among a total of 8350 persons) demonstrated a pooled prevalence of MRSA colonization of 1.3%. When studies were clustered by the risk-level study participants represent, the pooled prevalence ranged from 0.2% in the lowest risk populations to 5.4% in populations with MRSA-contacts or at-risk environments [96]. More recently, one study demonstrated a 1.0% prevalence of MRSA colonization in a random sample of 295 healthy subjects in four non-healthcare locations [97]. In a larger study of 9622 persons as part of the National Health and Nutrition Examination Survey (2001–02), *S. aureus* was identified in 32.4% of persons, and MRSA colonization among 0.8% of persons [98]. Lastly, it should be mentioned that, while the majority of studies investigate MSSA/MRSA colonization by surveying nasal carriage, there is evidence that solely sampling the nares may inadequately capture all carriers. In one study among 5041 hospitalized patients, healthcare workers, and blood donors, 37.1% had nasal carriage of *S. aureus* (with or without throat carriage), and 12.8% had throat colonization alone (representing 25.7% of all *S. aureus* carriers) [99]. Although few other recent data is available investigating this issue, it is suggestive that a strategy of culturing areas other than the nares (forehead, axilla, groin, rectum) might be more sensitive for detection of MRSA carriers [99–102].

Colonization with MRSA usually precedes infection with the organism and, as an example, *S. aureus* nasal carriage has been strongly associated with increased risk of developing a surgical site infection [61,93,94]. However, although it is thought that relatively few individuals colonized with MRSA spontaneously develop infections, this relationship has mainly been studied in a clinical population (not a general asymptomatic one) and many questions remain regarding the relationship between colonization and infection [103,104]. There is some data to suggest that colonization with MRSA on admission or during hospital admission increases the risk of MRSA infection [105,106].

MRSA causes a very broad range of infections, although the vast majority are skin and soft-tissue infections. Skin and soft-tissue infections may vary from cellulitis and SSIs to abscess, necrotizing fasciitis, and myositis. Infections may also be associated with indwelling catheters, including urinary catheters, intravenous catheters and central nervous system shunts, as well as surgical prostheses and implants. MRSA may also cause pulmonary infections including pneumonia with or without abscess or necrosis, empyema and ventilator-associated pneumonia, as well as endovascular infections and intraabdominal or renal abscesses.

Burden of illness of MRSA

The CDC's National Nosocomial Infections Surveillance (NNIS) system found that the percentage of inpatient MRSA isolates among *S. aureus* isolates rose from 2.4% in 1975 to 29% in 1991 [107]. The same reporting system found that, in 2003, there was an 11% increase in MRSA infections in ICU patients compared with the period from 1998 through 2002, with resistance rates of 59.5% among 4100 isolates. MRSA was found to be prevalent in all healthcare settings: median rates of MRSA isolates among *S. aureus* isolates among 157 intensive care units, 56 nonintensive care inpatient units, and 49 outpatient areas were 48.1%, 44.9%, and 24.6%, respectively [108]. The significance of high prevalence is not limited to the US. In a survey of bloodstream isolates from over 15 000 patients in the US, Canada, Latin America, Europe, and the western Pacific during the period 1997–99, MRSA prevalence ranged from 5.7% (Canada) to 46% (western Pacific region). Prevalence for specific countries ranged from less than 2% in the Netherlands and Switzerland to more than 70% in Japan and Hong Kong [109].

Death rates attributable to MRSA infections have been estimated to be 2.5 times higher than that attributable to MSSA [110]. In one study, the mean cost attributable to MRSA infection was US$9275 [111]. MRSA infections have been shown to increase hospital length of stay by 4 days [111]. A metaanalysis was performed to assess the impact of methicillin resistance on mortality in *Staphylococcus aureus* bacteremia. Thirty-one cohort studies were included, 24 of which found no significant difference in mortality and seven of which found a significant difference. When results were pooled using a random-effects model, a significant increase in mortality due to MRSA bacteremia was evident (OR 1.93, 95% CI 1.54–2.42, $P < 0.001$). It should be noted that significant statistical hetereogeneity existed among the studies [112].

A recently published study demonstrated a notably high incidence rate of 31.8 invasive MRSA infections per 100 000 persons [113]. Among 8987 observed cases from the geographically and demographically varied Active Bacterial Core Surveillance/Emerging Infections Program Network in the US, collected from July 2004 through December 2005, 58.4% were community-onset healthcare-associated, 26.6% were hospital-onset heathcare-associated, and 13.7% were community-associated. Most significantly, the 988 deaths among 5287 hospitalized patients with MRSA infection reported in the study extrapolates to a nationwide death rate due to MRSA exceeding many other significant infectious causes.

The cost of MRSA-associated morbidity and mortality has likely not been fully estimated, although the difficulty and complexity of estimating the significance of antimicrobial resistance has been described [114]. It appears clear from available data that – whether due to confounding factors, strain differences, or treatment differences – MRSA takes a higher morbidity and mortality toll than MSSA, is a burden to the healthcare system in addition to (and not in replacement of) MSSA, and presents a patient and financial cost burden for many disease states beyond bacteremia [115].

Community-associated and healthcare-associated MRSA

Although MRSA had been identified in the community as early as the 1980s, these cases were strongly associated with populations such as intravenous drug abusers and residents of long-term care facilities who are frequently hospitalized. More substantial trends

Table 14.3 Clinical characteristics of community-associated MRSA infection

Develops within 48 hours of hospitalization
No history of MRSA colonization or infection
No indwelling medical device (including intravenous catheter) present at the time of isolation
No history of hospitalization, surgery, or hemodialysis within 1 year

in community-associated MRSA (CA-MRSA) were reported by the mid- to late-1990s throughout the US [116] and elsewhere [117], and began to include case reports in the absence of predisposing risk factors [118,119]. CA-MRSA is defined by the characteristics in Table 14.3. CA-MRSA strains are currently classified by pulsed-field electrophoretic patterns (described as strains USA100 through USA1200), and currently USA300 is the major circulating strain.

Distinctions between HA-MRSA and CA-MRSA lie in the distinct spectrum of disease; resistance characteristics, and toxins expressed by each [116,119]. Two population-based studies in particular demonstrate these distinctions. In one prospective cohort study from 12 regionally varied laboratories in Minnesota in 2000 [116], 1100 MRSA isolates were identified as either CA-MRSA (131, 12%) or HA-MRSA (937, 85%) and compared for type of clinical infection, microbiologic characteristics, and exotoxin production; 3% could not be classified as either CA-MRSA or HA-MRSA. In this population, 25% (range from individual sites, 10–49%) of *S. aureus* isolates were methicillin-resistant. CA-MRSA patients were younger (median age 23 years vs 68 years), more likely to involve skin and soft-tissue infections (75% vs 37%), and were less likely to have respiratory or urinary tract infections than HA-MRSA patients. Among a representative sample, CA-MRSA isolates were generally susceptible to antimicrobials other than β-lactams and were more likely to be susceptible to multiple agents. Antibiotics which CA-MRSA was more likely to be susceptible to than HA-MRSA at a statistically significant rate were: ciprofloxacin (79% vs 16%), clindamycin (83% vs 21%), erythromycin (44% vs 9%), and gentamicin (94% vs 80%). Compared to HA-MRSA, CA-MRSA isolates were more likely to have distinct molecular features based on pulsed-field gel electrophoresis (clonality) and had a higher prevalence of PVL genes (77% vs 4%). Although all isolates carried the *mecA* gene conferring methicillin resistance, SCC*mec* IV allele and *agr* 3 allele were more associated with CA-MRSA whereas SCC*mec* II and *agr* 2 were more commonly associated with HA-MRSA.

A study among 283 isolates in a California teaching hospital performed from December 2003 through May 2004 demonstrated similar results [119]: CA-MRSA most commonly caused skin and soft-tissue infections (86% of CA-MRSA isolates vs 42% of HA-MRSA isolates), CA-MRSA isolates were less likely than HA-MRSA isolates to cause urinary or respiratory infections; CA-MRSA isolates were more likely to be susceptible to ciprofloxacin and clindamycin (although neither CA-MRSA nor HA-MRSA were likely to be susceptible to erythromycin, and both were highly susceptible to gentamicin). This study is also notable for documenting high rates of USA300 clone (87% of CA-MRSA isolates, 33% of HA-MRSA isolates), a clone that is rapidly becoming ubiquitous. Very similar trends regarding spectrum of disease, microbiologic characteristics, and increasing prevalence rates have also been found in pediatric populations [120].

While not commonly evaluated, the distinction between HA-MRSA and CA-MRSA may prove significant in recognizing patterns of disease, transmission risk, and antibiotic selection. Further studies investigating these differences are warranted.

Risk factors for MRSA

The early literature on the topic identified risk factors for colonization or infection with MRSA including prior hospitalization, intravenous drug use, and comorbid conditions [121–130]. Numerous studies have demonstrated these categories as risk factors but unfortunately very few have concurred on common risk factors. Differences have arisen due to differences in study design/epidemiologic methodology [131,132].

A more recent trend developing through the 1990s to the present is the acquisition of MRSA (particularly CA-MRSA) in settings of close contacts and in populations with few to absent risk factors, although there is some data to suggest that the prevalence of MRSA among people who are truly without risk factors may

be low [96,133,134]. Notable cases include transmission documented among a professional American football team [135], demonstrating the role of close contact and hygiene, and more recently, the emergence of a multidrug-resistant USA300 strain among men who have sex with men [136]. This latter case is of particular concern as CA-MRSA has traditionally had a more limited range of antibiotic resistance characteristics than HA-MRSA. The close contact among military recruits, incarcerated persons, and athletes has also proven to be a risk factor for transmission [135,137–141].

The relative causal component of risk factors for MRSA is still uncertain. In general, it is felt that MRSA incidence increases due to patient-to-patient transmission, with possible contributions from antibiotic use.

Preventive measures aimed at decreasing MRSA incidence

Hand disinfection and contact precautions

There is data that suggests that increased compliance with hand disinfection can reduce MRSA. A study by Pittet et al. demonstrated that institution of a whole hand hygiene program that included the institution of an alcohol-based hand disinfectant, compliance with hand disinfection increased from 48% to 66% and was associated with a decrease in the incidence of MRSA infections from 2.16 to 0.93 episodes per 10 000 patient-days. A limitation of this study is that it was a multifaceted intervention that included active surveillance, implementation of prevention guidelines, and the use of an alcohol-based hand disinfectant so it was difficult to determine the magnitude of benefit that was directly attributable to hand disinfection alone [142]. More recently, in a 2-year prospective study in the intensive care unit setting, investigators observed 17 994 minutes and 3678 hand hygiene opportunities in a crossover trial of alcohol-based hand gel [143]. Although rates of adherence to hand gel use improved markedly in both arms of the trial, there was no change in the rates of device-associated infection or infection with multidrug-resistant pathogens. This study throws into question the efficacy of alcohol-based hand gels as a *single* intervention in preventing transmission of multidrug-resistant organisms.

In the nosocomial setting, isolation or cohorting of patients identified as MRSA carriers or MRSA-infected and the use of contact precautions – disposable gown and gloves – is increasingly used to limit the spread of MRSA. Several studies have demonstrated the efficacy of isolation procedures and contact precautions in reducing rates of antibiotic-resistant organisms among hospitalized patients during outbreak investigations [144–149], but the mechanisms for this benefit are not well understood. One systematic review of studies evaluating isolation measures and the incidence of MRSA colonization and infection was published in 2004 [150]. The authors reviewed 46 studies, including 18 among isolation wards, 9 with nurse cohorting, and 19 involving other policies such as single bedded rooms, cohorting of patients, and barrier precautions. Shortcomings of the studies abound, including absent randomization (39 studies), significant differences in care for patients (e.g., differences in antibiotic use, lengths of stay; 31 and 29 studies, respectively), and lack of follow-up after discharge from hospital to reevaluate colonization or infection (all studies). Fourteen studies lack data warranting conclusions. In the six strongest studies, four demonstrated interventions (single room isolation, nurse cohorting, isolation ward) demonstrated control of major outbreaks, one demonstrated failure to control the epidemic, and one demonstrated initial success with eventual failure. Of the remaining studies, most demonstrated evidence of control, with some descriptions of failure. The CDC recommend contact precautions for healthcare workers caring for hospitalized patients with MRSA [151].

Active surveillance

Currently, there is ongoing debate about the benefit of active (or universal) surveillance as a strategy to reduce MRSA transmission and disease. The Dutch method of "search and destroy" – an aggressive and comprehensive surveillance program in addition to mandatory decolonization – has as evidence of efficacy the remarkably low rates of MRSA in that country [152,153].

While several studies have investigated a policy of universal screening in the ICU setting with mixed results, two recent studies investigate the value of universal screening in addition to a decolonization regimen for MRSA The first study, by Harbarth et al. [154], does not demonstrate a benefit to MRSA infection rates after implementation of universal screening and decolonization. In this study, surgical units at one major teaching hospital were divided into two groups, and using a control-intervention crossover design, implemented rapid MRSA screening of the nares, perineal region, and other sites ("when clinically indicated"). Both control and intervention arms underwent standard infection control measures and identified carriers underwent mupirocin and chlorhexidine decolonization. Among 10910 control patients, 76 (0.7%) had identified MRSA infections, versus 93 of 10844 (0.9%) during the intervention periods (incidence rate ration 1.2 per 1000 patient-days, 95% CI 0.9–1.7). There was no statistical difference in the rates of MRSA SSIs or in the incidence of nosocomial MRSA acquisition. Limitations to this study include a purely surgical setting and low rates of MRSA SSIs and infections.

In the second study, by Robicsek et al. [155], investigators followed a baseline year of routine surveillance with 1 year of nasal surveillance for all ICU admissions and subsequently 1 year of nasal surveillance for all hospital admissions; there were 39521, 40392, and 73427 hospitalized patients during each period, respectively. Colonized patients were placed on contact isolation and were treated at the discretion of the treating physician with a 5-day decolonization regimen with mupirocin topical twice daily to the nares and a chlorhexidine wash every 2 days (during the third portion of the study only). The primary outcome – aggregate MRSA infection rate including bloodstream, respiratory, urinary tract, and surgical site infections within 48 hours of admission through 30 days post-discharge – demonstrated a 70% reduction in HA-MRSA in the intervention periods. However, several limitations include a quasi-experimental design, increasing adherence rates during the study periods, more rapid detection (PCR) during the universal period than the ICU period, and the uncontrolled addition of other interventions, including decolonization and isolation.

Decolonization

Many decolonization regimens have been used for MRSA, but typically employed regimens include the topical and systemic agents mupirocin, chlorhexidine, and rifampin. A good review on the topic has been published by Boyce et al. [156]. In one of the very few prospective randomized controlled trials performed, Simor et al evaluated the efficacy of chlorhexidine, mupirocin, rifampin and doxycycline versus no treatment for the eradication of MRSA [157]. Among 146 patients from 8 hospitals identified as colonized (on admission or as part of an outbreak investigation) but not infected, 111 were randomized to study treatment and 35 were randomized to no treatment; at the primary outcome of 3-month follow-up, 87 patients and 25 patients could be evaluated in each group, respectively. Cultures were obtained from the nares, perineum, skin lesions, and catheter or medical device exit sites at study onset, weekly for 4 weeks, and monthly for an additional 7 months. Patients randomized to treatment received a 7-day regimen of 2% chlorhexidine gluconate washing daily, 2% mupirocin ointment to both nares three times daily, rifampin 300 mg twice daily and doxycycline 100 mg twice daily. At 3-month follow-up 74% (64 of 87) of those treated and 32% (8 of 25) of untreated patients remained culture-negative for MRSA (relative risk 1.55, 95%CI 1.17–2.04). At the end of the 7-day decolonization regimen, 92% of patients cleared MRSA from all sites; at eight months, 54% of 48 patients available for follow-up remained negative for MRSA. After multivariate logistic regression analysis, mupirocin-resistant MRSA at baseline was independently associated with recolonization with MRSA at 3 months, while functional status, presence of skin lesions, presence of a medical device and MRSA recovered from more than one body site were not associated with recolonization. Of significance, among 61 treated study participants with mupirocin-susceptible MRSA isolates at baseline, three (5%) had MRSA isolates with high-level mupirocin resistance in follow-up.

Prior to the Simor study, a Cochrane review of antimicrobial drugs for treating MRSA colonization summarized the six randomized controlled trials (384 non-healthcare worker participants) performed to date, and found "insufficient evidence to support use of topical or systemic antimicrobial therapy for eradicating MRSA" [158]. The six trials investigated: fusidic acid vs no therapy; mupirocin twice daily for 5 days vs placebo ointment; rifampin 600 mg orally twice daily vs minocycline 100 mg orally twice daily vs minocycline and rifampin (all for 5 days); mupirocin three times daily vs fusidic acid three times daily vs oral trimethoprim-sulfamethoxazole (TMP-SMX, DS) daily; ciprofloxacin 750 mg orally twice daily and rifampin 300 mg orally

twice daily vs oral TMP-SMX (DS) twice daily (both for 14 days); novobiocin 500 mg orally twice daily and rifampin 300 mg orally twice daily vs. oral TMP-SMX (DS) twice daily and rifampin 300 mg orally twice daily (both regimens for 7 days). Outcomes of MRSA colonization (and in one case, infection) were reported at time points ranging from 12 to 180 days (typically 14). None of the trial endpoints demonstrated significant efficacy of any trial agents.

Guidelines

Recent Society for Healthcare Epidemiology of America (SHEA) [159] and Healthcare Infection Control Practices Advisory Committee (HICPAC) [151] guidelines outline recommendations for the prevention of the spread and infection due to antibiotic-resistant organisms. Together, they each emphasize hand hygiene, environmental cleaning measures, and contact precautions for carriers, but diverge in their recommendations regarding active surveillance. SHEA recommendations advocate surveillance in high-risk populations while HICPAC recommends selective populations for surveillance.

In summary, active surveillance for MRSA in addition to strict isolation precautions and decolonization may help reduce transmission, however the process has neither been definitely proven nor disproven. Improving adherence to hand disinfection and investigating further the role of screening are worthwhile strategies.

References

1 Mangram AJ, Horan TC, Pearson ML, Silver LC, Jarvis WR. Guideline for prevention of surgical site infection, 1999. Hospital Infection Control Practices Advisory Committee. Infect Control Hosp Epidemiol 1999;20(4):250–78; quiz 279–80.

2 McConkey SJ, L'Ecuyer PB, Murphy DM, Leet TL, Sundt TM, Fraser VJ. Results of a comprehensive infection control program for reducing surgical-site infections in coronary artery bypass surgery. Infect Control Hosp Epidemiol 1999;20(8):533–8.

3 Klevens RM, Edwards JR, Richards CL, Jr., et al. Estimating health care-associated infections and deaths in US hospitals, 2002. Public Health Rep 2007;122(2):160–6.

4 Smyth ET, Emmerson AM. Surgical site infection surveillance. J Hosp Infect 2000;45(3):173–84.

5 Perencevich EN, Stone PW, Wright SB, Carmeli Y, Fisman DN, Cosgrove SE. Raising standards while watching the bottom line: making a business case for infection control. *Infect Control Hosp Epidemiol* 2007;28(10):1121–33.

6 Yasunaga H, Ide H, Imamura T, Ohe K. Accuracy of economic studies on surgical site infection. J Hosp Infect 2007;65(2):102–7.

7 Urban JA. Cost analysis of surgical site infections. Surg Infect (Larchmt) 2006;7 Suppl 1:S19–22.

8 Gaynes RP, Culver DH, Horan TC, Edwards JR, Richards C, Tolson JS. Surgical site infection (SSI) rates in the United States, 1992–1998: the National Nosocomial Infections Surveillance System basic SSI risk index. Clin Infect Dis 2001;33 Suppl 2:S69–77.

9 Rassias AJ, Marrin CA, Arruda J, Whalen PK, Beach M, Yeager MP. Insulin infusion improves neutrophil function in diabetic cardiac surgery patients. Anesth Analg 1999;88(5):1011–16.

10 Turina M, Fry DE, Polk HC, Jr. Acute hyperglycemia and the innate immune system: clinical, cellular, and molecular aspects. Crit Care Med 2005;33(7):1624–33.

11 Talbot TR. Diabetes mellitus and cardiothoracic surgical site infections. Am J Infect Control 2005;33(6):353–9.

12 Latham R, Lancaster AD, Covington JF, Pirolo JS, Thomas CS. The association of diabetes and glucose control with surgical-site infections among cardiothoracic surgery patients. Infect Control Hosp Epidemiol 2001;22(10):607–12.

13 Vilar-Compte D, Alvarez de Iturbe I, Martin-Onraet A, Perez-Amador M, Sanchez-Hernandez C, Volkow P. Hyperglycemia as a risk factor for surgical site infections in patients undergoing mastectomy. Am J Infect Control 2008;36(3):192–8.

14 Zerr KJ, Furnary AP, Grunkemeier GL, Bookin S, Kanhere V, Starr A. Glucose control lowers the risk of wound infection in diabetics after open heart operations. Ann Thorac Surg 1997;63(2):356–61.

15 Furnary AP, Zerr KJ, Grunkemeier GL, Starr A. Continuous intravenous insulin infusion reduces the incidence of deep sternal wound infection in diabetic patients after cardiac surgical procedures. Ann Thorac Surg 1999;67(2):352–60; discussion 360–2.

16 Sessler DI. Non-pharmacologic prevention of surgical wound infection. Anesthesiol Clin 2006;24(2):279–97.

17 Kurz A, Sessler DI, Christensen R, Dechert M. Heat balance and distribution during the core-temperature plateau in anesthetized humans. Anesthesiology 1995;83(3):491–9.

18 Sessler DI. Mild perioperative hypothermia. N Engl J Med 1997;336(24):1730–7.

19 Flores-Maldonado A, Medina-Escobedo CE, Rios-Rodriguez HM, Fernandez-Dominguez R. Mild perioperative hypothermia and the risk of wound infection. *Arch Med Res* 2001;32(3):227–31.

20 Barone JE, Tucker JB, Cecere J, et al. Hypothermia does not result in more complications after colon surgery. Am Surg 1999;65(4):356–9.

21 Munn MB, Rouse DJ, Owen J. Intraoperative hypothermia and post-cesarean wound infection. Obstet Gynecol 1998;91(4):582–4.

22 Kawaraguchi Y, Kawaguchi M, Inoue S, et al. [Effect of deliberate mild hypothermia on the incidence of surgical-wound infection and duration of hospitalization in neurosurgical patients]. Masui 1999;48(3):232–7.

23 Kurz A, Sessler DI, Lenhardt R. Perioperative normothermia to reduce the incidence of surgical-wound infection and shorten hospitalization. Study of Wound Infection and Temperature Group. N Engl J Med 1996;334(19):1209–15.

24 Melling AC, Ali B, Scott EM, Leaper DJ. Effects of preoperative warming on the incidence of wound infection after clean surgery: a randomised controlled trial. Lancet 2001;358(9285):876–80.

25 Ginsberg MD, Sternau LL, Globus MY, Dietrich WD, Busto R. Therapeutic modulation of brain temperature: relevance to ischemic brain injury. Cerebrovasc Brain Metab Rev 1992;4(3):189–225.

26 Winfree CH, Baker KZ, Connollly ES. Perioperative normothermia and surgical-wound infection. N Engl J Med 1996;335(10):749; author reply 749–50.

27 Greif R, Akca O, Horn EP, Kurz A, Sessler DI. Supplemental perioperative oxygen to reduce the incidence of surgical-wound infection. Outcomes Research Group. N Engl J Med 2000;342(3):161–7.

28 Hopf HW, Hunt TK, West JM, et al. Wound tissue oxygen tension predicts the risk of wound infection in surgical patients. Arch Surg 1997;132(9):997–1004; discussion 1005.

29 Allen DB, Maguire JJ, Mahdavian M, et al. Wound hypoxia and acidosis limit neutrophil bacterial killing mechanisms. Arch Surg 1997;132(9):991–6.

30 Pryor KO, Fahey TJ, 3rd, Lien CA, Goldstein PA. Surgical site infection and the routine use of perioperative hyperoxia in a general surgical population: a randomized controlled trial. JAMA 2004;291(1):79–87.

31 Belda FJ, Aguilera L, Garcia de la Asuncion J, et al. Supplemental perioperative oxygen and the risk of surgical wound infection: a randomized controlled trial. JAMA 2005;294(16):2035–42.

32 Akca O, Podolsky A, Eisenhuber E, et al. Comparable postoperative pulmonary atelectasis in patients given 30% or 80% oxygen during and 2 hours after colon resection. Anesthesiology 1999;91(4):991–8.

33 Edmark L, Kostova-Aherdan K, Enlund M, Hedenstierna G. Optimal oxygen concentration during induction of general anesthesia. Anesthesiology 2003;98(1):28–33.

34 Dellinger EP. Increasing inspired oxygen to decrease surgical site infection: time to shift the quality improvement research paradigm. JAMA 2005;294(16):2091–2.

35 Bekar A, Korfali E, Dogan S, Yilmazlar S, Baskan Z, Aksoy K. The effect of hair on infection after cranial surgery. Acta Neurochir (Wien) 2001;143(6):533–6; discussion 537.

36 Tanner J, Woodings D, Moncaster K. Preoperative hair removal to reduce surgical site infection. Cochrane Database Syst Rev 2006 (3), CD004122, DOI: 10.1002/14651858.

37 Court-Brown CM. Preoperative skin depilation and its effect on postoperative wound infections. J R Coll Surg Edinb 1981;26(4):238–41.

38 Rojanapirom S, Danchaivijitr S. Pre-operative shaving and wound infection in appendectomy. J Med Assoc Thai 1992;75 Suppl 2:20–3.

39 Alexander JW, Fischer JE, Boyajian M, Palmquist J, Morris MJ. The influence of hair-removal methods on wound infections. Arch Surg 1983;118(3):347–52.

40 Balthazar ER, Colt JD, Nichols RL. Preoperative hair removal: a random prospective study of shaving versus clipping. South Med J 1982;75(7):799–801.

41 Ko W, Lazenby WD, Zelano JA, Isom OW, Krieger KH. Effects of shaving methods and intraoperative irrigation on suppurative mediastinitis after bypass operations. Ann Thorac Surg 1992;53(2):301–5.

42 Breiting V, Hellberg S. [Chemical depilation as an alternative to shaving. A comparative study of preoperative skin preparation]. Ugeskr Laeger 1981;143(26):1646–7.

43 Goeau-Brissonniere O, Coignard S, Merao AP, Haicault G, Sasako M, Patel JC. [Preoperative skin preparation. A prospective study comparing a depilatory agent in shaving]. Presse Med 1987;16(31):1517–9.

44 Powis SJ, Waterworth TA, Arkell DG. Preoperative skin preparation: clinical evaluation of depilatory cream. Br Med J 1976;2(6045):1166–8.

45 Seropian R, Reynolds BM. Wound infections after preoperative depilatory versus razor preparation. Am J Surg 1971;121(3):251–4.

46 Thorup J, Fischer A, Lindenberg S, Schjorring-Thyssen U, Jensen J, Burcharth F. [Chemical depilation versus shaving. A controlled clinical trial of self-depilation in ambulatory surgery]. Ugeskr Laeger 1985;147(13):1108–10.

47 Thur de Koos P, McComas B. Shaving versus skin depilatory cream for preoperative skin preparation. A prospective study of wound infection rates. Am J Surg 1983;145(3):377–8.

48 Cigarette smoking among adults – United States, 2006. MMWR Morb Mortal Wkly Rep 2007;56(44):1157–61.

49 Theadom A, Cropley M. Effects of preoperative smoking cessation on the incidence and risk of intraoperative and postoperative complications in adult smokers: a systematic review. Tob Control 2006;15(5):352–8.

50 Sopori M. Effects of cigarette smoke on the immune system. Nat Rev Immunol 2002;2(5):372–7.

51 Rejali M RA, Zhang L, Yang S. Effects of nicotine on the cardiovascular system. Vasc Dis Preven 2005;2:135–144.

52 Finan KR, Vick CC, Kiefe CI, Neumayer L, Hawn MT. Predictors of wound infection in ventral hernia repair. Am J Surg 2005;190(5):676–81.

53 Crabtree TD, Codd JE, Fraser VJ, Bailey MS, Olsen MA, Damiano RJ, Jr. Multivariate analysis of risk factors for deep and superficial sternal infection after coronary artery bypass grafting at a tertiary care medical center. Semin Thorac Cardiovasc Surg 2004;16(1):53–61.

54 Sorensen LT, Hemmingsen U, Kallehave F, et al. Risk factors for tissue and wound complications in gastrointestinal surgery. Ann Surg 2005;241(4):654–8.

55 Sorensen LT, Horby J, Friis E, Pilsgaard B, Jorgensen T. Smoking as a risk factor for wound healing and infection in breast cancer surgery. Eur J Surg Oncol 2002;28(8):815–20.

56 Goodwin SJ, McCarthy CM, Pusic AL, et al. Complications in smokers after postmastectomy tissue expander/implant breast reconstruction. Ann Plast Surg 2005;55(1):16–19; discussion 19–20.

57 Gravante G, Araco A, Sorge R, Araco F, Delogu D, Cervelli V. Wound infections in post-bariatric patients undergoing body contouring abdominoplasty: the role of smoking. Obes Surg 2007;17(10):1325–31.

58 Myles PS, Iacono GA, Hunt JO, et al. Risk of respiratory complications and wound infection in patients undergoing ambulatory surgery: smokers versus nonsmokers. Anesthesiology 2002;97(4):842–7.

59 Sorensen LT, Jorgensen T. Short-term pre-operative smoking cessation intervention does not affect postoperative complications in colorectal surgery: a randomized clinical trial. Colorectal Dis 2003;5(4):347–52.

60 Sorensen LT, Karlsmark T, Gottrup F. Abstinence from smoking reduces incisional wound infection: a randomized controlled trial. Ann Surg 2003;238(1):1–5.

61 Wenzel RP, Perl TM. The significance of nasal carriage of Staphylococcus aureus and the incidence of postoperative wound infection. J Hosp Infect 1995;31(1):13–24.

62 Kluytmans JA, Mouton JW, VandenBergh MF, et al. Reduction of surgical-site infections in cardiothoracic surgery by elimination of nasal carriage of Staphylococcus aureus. Infect Control Hosp Epidemiol 1996;17(12):780–5.

63 VandenBergh MF, Kluytmans JA, van Hout BA, et al. Cost-effectiveness of perioperative mupirocin nasal ointment in cardiothoracic surgery. Infect Control Hosp Epidemiol 1996;17(12):786–92.

64 Cimochowski GE, Harostock MD, Brown R, Bernardi M, Alonzo N, Coyle K. Intranasal mupirocin reduces sternal wound infection after open heart surgery in diabetics and nondiabetics. Ann Thorac Surg 2001;71(5):1572–8; discussion 1578–9.

65 Wilcox MH, Hall J, Pike H, et al. Use of perioperative mupirocin to prevent methicillin-resistant Staphylococcus aureus (MRSA) orthopaedic surgical site infections. J Hosp Infect 2003;54(3):196–201.

66 Gernaat-van der Sluis AJ, Hoogenboom-Verdegaal AM, Edixhoven PJ, Spies-van Rooijen NH. Prophylactic mupirocin could reduce orthopedic wound infections. 1,044 patients treated with mupirocin compared with 1,260 historical controls. Acta Orthop Scand 1998;69(4):412–14.

67 Kalmeijer MD, Coertjens H, van Nieuwland-Bollen PM, et al. Surgical site infections in orthopedic surgery: the effect of mupirocin nasal ointment in a double-blind, randomized, placebo-controlled study. Clin Infect Dis 2002;35(4):353–8.

68 Konvalinka A, Errett L, Fong IW. Impact of treating Staphylococcus aureus nasal carriers on wound infections in cardiac surgery. J Hosp Infect 2006;64(2):162–8.

69 Perl TM, Cullen JJ, Wenzel RP, et al. Intranasal mupirocin to prevent postoperative Staphylococcus aureus infections. N Engl J Med 2002;346(24):1871–7.

70 Suzuki Y, Kamigaki T, Fujino Y, Tominaga M, Ku Y, Kuroda Y. Randomized clinical trial of preoperative intranasal mupirocin to reduce surgical-site infection after digestive surgery. Br J Surg 2003;90(9):1072–5.

71 Trautmann M, Stecher J, Hemmer W, Luz K, Panknin HT. Intranasal mupirocin prophylaxis in elective surgery. A review of published studies. Chemotherapy 2008;54(1):9–16.

72 Kallen AJ, Wilson CT, Larson RJ. Perioperative intranasal mupirocin for the prevention of surgical-site infections: systematic review of the literature and meta-analysis. Infect Control Hosp Epidemiol 2005;26(12):916–22.

73 Young LS, Winston LG. Preoperative use of mupirocin for the prevention of healthcare-associated *Staphylococcus aureus* infections: a cost-effectiveness analysis. Infect Control Hosp Epidemiol 2006;27(12):1304–12.

74 Perl TM. Prevention of *Staphylococcus aureus* infections among surgical patients: beyond traditional perioperative prophylaxis. Surgery 2003;134(5 Suppl):S10–7.

75 Kaiser AB, Kernodle DS, Barg NL, Petracek MR. Influence of preoperative showers on staphylococcal skin colonization: a comparative trial of antiseptic skin cleansers. Ann Thorac Surg 1988;45(1):35–8.

76 Paulson DS. Efficacy evaluation of a 4% chlorhexidine gluconate as a full-body shower wash. Am J Infect *Control* 1993;21(4):205–9.

77 Webster J, Osborne S. Preoperative bathing or showering with skin antiseptics to prevent surgical site infection. Cochrane Database Syst Rev 2007 (2), CD004985, DOI: 10.1002/14651858.

78 Hayek LJ, Emerson JM. Preoperative whole body disinfection – a controlled clinical study. J Hosp Infect 1988;11 Suppl B:15–9.

79 Randall PE, Ganguli L, Marcuson RW. Wound infection following vasectomy. Br J Urol 1983;55(5):564–7.

80 Wihlborg O. The effect of washing with chlorhexidine soap on wound infection rate in general surgery. A controlled clinical study. Ann Chir Gynaecol 1987;76(5):263–5.

81 Milstone AM, Passaretti CL, Perl TM. Chlorhexidine: expanding the armamentarium for infection control and prevention. Clin Infect Dis 2008;46(2):274–81.

82 Classen DC, Evans RS, Pestotnik SL, Horn SD, Menlove RL, Burke JP. The timing of prophylactic administration of antibiotics and the risk of surgical-wound infection. N Engl J Med 1992;326(5):281–6.

83 van Kasteren ME, Mannien J, Ott A, Kullberg BJ, de Boer AS, Gyssens IC. Antibiotic prophylaxis and the risk of surgical site infections following total hip arthroplasty: timely administration is the most important factor. Clin Infect Dis 2007;44(7):921–7.

84 Matuschka PR, Cheadle WG, Burke JD, Garrison RN. A new standard of care: administration of preoperative antibiotics in the operating room. Am Surg 1997;63(6):500–3.

85 Bratzler DW, Houck PM. Antimicrobial prophylaxis for surgery: an advisory statement from the National Surgical Infection Prevention Project. Am J Surg 2005;189(4):395–404.

86 McDonald M, Grabsch E, Marshall C, Forbes A. Single-versus multiple-dose antimicrobial prophylaxis for major surgery: a systematic review. Aust N Z J Surg 1998;68(6):388–96.

87 Glenny A, Song F. Antimicrobial prophylaxis in total hip replacement: a systematic review. Health Technol Assess 1999;3(21):1–57.

88 Harbarth S, Samore MH, Lichtenberg D, Carmeli Y. Prolonged antibiotic prophylaxis after cardiovascular surgery and its effect on surgical site infections and antimicrobial resistance. Circulation 2000;101(25):2916–21.

89 Dellinger EP, Hausmann SM, Bratzler DW, et al. Hospitals collaborate to decrease surgical site infections. Am J Surg 2005;190(1):9–15.

90 Hedrick TL, Heckman JA, Smith RL, Sawyer RG, Friel CM, Foley EF. Efficacy of protocol implementation on incidence of wound infection in colorectal operations. J Am Coll Surg 2007;205(3):432–8.

91 Hedrick TL, Turrentine FE, Smith RL, et al. Single-institutional experience with the surgical infection prevention project in intra-abdominal surgery. Surg Infect (Larchmt) 2007;8(4):425–35.

92 Cunha BA. Methicillin-resistant *Staphylococcus aureus*: clinical manifestations and antimicrobial therapy. Clin Microbiol Infect 2005;11 Suppl 4:33–42.

93 Kluytmans JA, Wertheim HF. Nasal carriage of *Staphylococcus aureus* and prevention of nosocomial infections. Infection 2005;33(1):3–8.

94 Vandenbergh MF, Verbrugh HA. Carriage of *Staphylococcus aureus*: epidemiology and clinical relevance. J Lab Clin Med 1999;133(6):525–34.

95 Rampling A, Wiseman S, Davis L, et al. Evidence that hospital hygiene is important in the control of methicillin-resistant *Staphylococcus aureus*. J Hosp Infect 2001;49(2):109–16.

96 Salgado CD, Farr BM, Calfee DP. Community-acquired methicillin-resistant *Staphylococcus aureus*: a meta-analysis of prevalence and risk factors. Clin Infect Dis 2003;36(2):131–9.

97 Rim JY, Bacon AE, 3rd. Prevalence of community-acquired methicillin-resistant *Staphylococcus aureus* colonization in a random sample of healthy individuals. Infect Control Hosp Epidemiol 2007;28(9):1044–6.

98 Kuehnert MJ, Kruszon-Moran D, Hill HA, et al. Prevalence of *Staphylococcus aureus* nasal colonization in the United States, 2001–2002. J Infect Dis 2006;193(2):172–9.

99 Mertz D, Frei R, Jaussi B, et al. Throat swabs are necessary to reliably detect carriers of *Staphylococcus aureus*. Clin Infect Dis 2007;45(4):475–7.

100 Rohr U, Wilhelm M, Muhr G, Gatermann S. Qualitative and (semi)quantitative characterization of nasal and skin methicillin-resistant *Staphylococcus aureus* carriage of hospitalized patients. Int J Hyg Environ Health 2004;207(1):51–5.

101 Eveillard M, de Lassence A, Lancien E, Barnaud G, Ricard JD, Joly-Guillou ML. Evaluation of a strategy of screening multiple anatomical sites for methicillin-resistant *Staphylococcus aureus* at admission to a teaching hospital. Infect Control Hosp Epidemiol 2006;27(2):181–4.

102 Meurman O, Routamaa M, Peltonen R. Screening for methicillin-resistant *Staphylococcus aureus*: which anatomical sites to culture? J Hosp Infect 2005;61(4):351–3.

103 Creech CB, 2nd, Talbot TR, Schaffner W. Community-associated methicillin-resistant *Staphylococcus aureus*: the way to the wound is through the nose. J Infect Dis 2006;193(2):169–71.

104 Ellis MW, Hospenthal DR, Dooley DP, Gray PJ, Murray CK. Natural history of community-acquired methicillin-resistant *Staphylococcus aureus* colonization and infection in soldiers. Clin Infect Dis 2004;39(7):971–9.

105 Pujol M, Pena C, Pallares R, et al. Nosocomial *Staphylococcus aureus* bacteremia among nasal carriers of methicillin-resistant and methicillin-susceptible strains. Am J Med 1996;100(5):509–16.

106 Davis KA, Stewart JJ, Crouch HK, Florez CE, Hospenthal DR. Methicillin-resistant *Staphylococcus aureus* (MRSA) nares colonization at hospital admission and its effect on subsequent MRSA infection. Clin Infect Dis 2004;39(6):776–82.

107 Panlilio AL, Culver DH, Gaynes RP, et al. Methicillin-resistant *Staphylococcus aureus* in US hospitals, 1975–1991. Infect Control Hosp Epidemiol 1992;13(10):582–6.

108 National Nosocomial Infections Surveillance (NNIS) System Report, data summary from January 1992 through June 2004, issued October 2004. Am J Infect Control 2004;32(8):470–85.

109 Diekema DJ, Pfaller MA, Schmitz FJ, et al. Survey of infections due to *Staphylococcus* species: frequency of occurrence and antimicrobial susceptibility of isolates collected in the United States, Canada, Latin America, Europe, and the Western Pacific region for the SENTRY Antimicrobial Surveillance Program, 1997–1999. Clin Infect Dis 2001;32 Suppl 2:S114–32.

110 Rubin RJ, Harrington CA, Poon A, Dietrich K, Greene JA, Moiduddin A. The economic impact of *Staphylococcus aureus* infection in New York City hospitals. Emerg Infect Dis 1999;5(1):9–17.

111 Chaix C, Durand-Zaleski I, Alberti C, Brun-Buisson C. Control of endemic methicillin-resistant *Staphylococcus aureus*: a cost-benefit analysis in an intensive care unit. JAMA 1999;282(18):1745–51.

112 Cosgrove SE, Sakoulas G, Perencevich EN, Schwaber MJ, Karchmer AW, Carmeli Y. Comparison of mortality associated with methicillin-resistant and methicillin-susceptible *Staphylococcus aureus* bacteremia: a meta-analysis. Clin Infect Dis 2003;36(1):53–9.

113 Klevens RM, Morrison MA, Nadle J, et al. Invasive methicillin-resistant *Staphylococcus aureus* infections in the United States. JAMA 2007;298(15):1763–71.

114 Cosgrove SE, Carmeli Y. The impact of antimicrobial resistance on health and economic outcomes. Clin Infect Dis 2003;36(11):1433–7.

115 Gould IM. Costs of hospital-acquired methicillin-resistant *Staphylococcus aureus* (MRSA) and its control. Int J Antimicrob Agents 2006;28(5):379–84.

116 Naimi TS, LeDell KH, Como-Sabetti K, et al. Comparison of community- and health care-associated methicillin-resistant *Staphylococcus aureus* infection. JAMA 2003;290(22):2976–84.

117 Dufour P, Gillet Y, Bes M, et al. Community-acquired methicillin-resistant *Staphylococcus aureus* infections in France: emergence of a single clone that produces Panton-Valentine leukocidin. Clin Infect Dis 2002;35(7):819–24.

118 Herold BC, Immergluck LC, Maranan MC, et al. Community-acquired methicillin-resistant *Staphylococcus aureus* in children with no identified predisposing risk. JAMA 1998;279(8):593–8.

119 Huang H, Flynn NM, King JH, Monchaud C, Morita M, Cohen SH. Comparisons of community-associated methicillin-resistant *Staphylococcus aureus* (MRSA) and hospital-associated MSRA infections in Sacramento, California. J Clin Microbiol 2006;44(7):2423–7.

120 Dietrich DW, Auld DB, Mermel LA. Community-acquired methicillin-resistant *Staphylococcus aureus* in southern New England children. Pediatrics 2004;113(4):e347–52.

121 Boyce JM. Methicillin-resistant *Staphylococcus aureus*. Detection, epidemiology, and control measures. Infect Dis Clin North Am 1989;3(4):901–13.

122 Brumfitt W, Hamilton-Miller J. Methicillin-resistant *Staphylococcus aureus*. N Engl J Med 1989;320(18): 1188–96.

123 Lowy FD. *Staphylococcus aureus* infections. N Engl J Med 1998;339(8):520–32.

124 Thompson RL, Cabezudo I, Wenzel RP. Epidemiology of nosocomial infections caused by methicillin-resistant *Staphylococcus aureus*. Ann Intern Med 1982;97(3): 309–17.

125 Craven DE, Rixinger AI, Goularte TA, McCabe WR. Methicillin-resistant *Staphylococcus aureus* bacteremia linked to intravenous drug abusers using a "shooting gallery." Am J Med 1986;80(5):770–6.

126 Berman DS, Schaefler S, Simberkoff MS, Rahal JJ. *Staphylococcus aureus* colonization in intravenous drug abusers, dialysis patients, and diabetics. J Infect Dis 1987;155(4):829–31.

127 Saravolatz LD, Markowitz N, Arking L, Pohlod D, Fisher E. Methicillin-resistant *Staphylococcus aureus*: Epidemiologic observations during a community-acquired outbreak. Ann Intern Med 1982;96(1):11–6.

128 Solberg CO. Spread of *Staphylococcus aureus* in hospitals: causes and prevention. Scand J Infect Dis 2000;32(6):587–95.

129 Graffunder EM, Venezia RA. Risk factors associated with nosocomial methicillin-resistant *Staphylococcus aureus* (MRSA) infection including previous use of antimicrobials. J Antimicrob Chemother 2002;49(6):999–1005.

130 Herwaldt LA. Control of methicillin-resistant *Staphylococcus aureus* in the hospital setting. Am J Med 1999;106(5A):11S–18S; discussion 48S–52S.

131 Harris AD, Karchmer TB, Carmeli Y, Samore MH. Methodological principles of case-control studies that analyzed risk factors for antibiotic resistance: a systematic review. Clin Infect Dis 2001;32(7):1055–61.

132 Harris AD, Samore MH, Carmeli Y. Control group selection is an important but neglected issue in studies of antibiotic resistance. Ann Intern Med 2000;133(2):159.

133 Bancroft EA. Antimicrobial resistance: it's not just for hospitals. JAMA 2007;298(15):1803–4.

134 Daum RS. Clinical practice. Skin and soft-tissue infections caused by methicillin-resistant *Staphylococcus aureus*. |N Engl J Med 2007;357(4):380–90.

135 Kazakova SV, Hageman JC, Matava M, et al. A clone of methicillin-resistant *Staphylococcus aureus* among professional football players. N Engl J Med 2005;352(5):468–75.

136 Diep BA, Chambers HF, Graber CJ, et al. Emergence of multidrug-resistant, community-associated, methicillin-resistant *Staphylococcus aureus* clone USA300 in men who have sex with men. Ann Intern Med 2008;148(4):249–57.

137 Zinderman CE, Conner B, Malakooti MA, LaMar JE, Armstrong A, Bohnker BK. Community-acquired methicillin-resistant *Staphylococcus aureus* among military recruits. Emerg Infect Dis 2004;10(5):941–4.

138 Campbell KM, Vaughn AF, Russell KL, et al. Risk factors for community-associated methicillin-resistant *Staphylococcus aureus* infections in an outbreak of disease among military trainees in San Diego, California, in 2002. J Clin Microbiol 2004;42(9):4050–3.

139 Methicillin-resistant *Staphylococcus aureus* infections in correctional facilities – -Georgia, California, and Texas, 2001–2003. MMWR Morb Mortal Wkly Rep 2003;52(41):992–6.

140 Begier EM, Frenette K, Barrett NL, et al. A high-morbidity outbreak of methicillin-resistant *Staphylococcus aureus* among players on a college football team, facilitated by cosmetic body shaving and turf burns. Clin Infect Dis 2004;39(10):1446–53.

141 Lindenmayer JM, Schoenfeld S, O'Grady R, Carney JK. Methicillin-resistant *Staphylococcus aureus* in a high school wrestling team and the surrounding community. Arch Intern Med 1998;158(8):895–9.

142 Pittet D, Hugonnet S, Harbarth S, et al. Effectiveness of a hospital-wide programme to improve compliance with hand hygiene. Infection Control Programme. Lancet 2000;356(9238):1307–12.

143 Rupp ME, Fitzgerald T, Puumala S, et al. Prospective, controlled, cross-over trial of alcohol-based hand gel in critical care units. Infect Control Hosp Epidemiol 2008;29(1):8–15.

144 Jernigan JA, Titus MG, Groschel DH, Getchell-White S, Farr BM. Effectiveness of contact isolation during a hospital outbreak of methicillin-resistant *Staphylococcus aureus*. Am J Epidemiol 1996;143(5):496–504.

145 Montecalvo MA, Jarvis WR, Uman J, et al. Infection-control measures reduce transmission of vancomycin-resistant enterococci in an endemic setting. Ann Intern Med 1999;131(4):269–72.

146 Puzniak LA, Leet T, Mayfield J, Kollef M, Mundy LM. To gown or not to gown: the effect on acquisition of vancomycin-resistant enterococci. Clin Infect Dis 2002;35(1):18–25.

147 Srinivasan A, Song X, Ross T, Merz W, Brower R, Perl TM. A prospective study to determine whether cover gowns in addition to gloves decrease nosocomial transmission of vancomycin-resistant enterococci in an intensive care unit. Infect Control Hosp Epidemiol 2002;23(8):424–8.

148 Tenorio AR, Badri SM, Sahgal NB, et al. Effectiveness of gloves in the prevention of hand carriage of vancomycin-resistant enterococcus species by health care workers after patient care. Clin Infect Dis 2001;32(5):826–9.

149 McBryde ES, Bradley LC, Whitby M, McElwain DL. An investigation of contact transmission of methicillin-resistant *Staphylococcus aureus*. J Hosp Infect 2004;58(2):104–8.

150 Cooper BS, Stone SP, Kibbler CC, et al. Isolation measures in the hospital management of methicillin resistant *Staphylococcus aureus* (MRSA): systematic review of the literature. BMJ 2004;329(7465):533.

151 Siegel JD, Rhinehart E, Jackson M, Chiarello L. Management of multidrug-resistant organisms in health care settings, 2006. Am J Infect Control 2007;35(10 Suppl 2):S165–93.

152 Vos MC, Ott A, Verbrugh HA. Successful search-and-destroy policy for methicillin-resistant *Staphylococcus aureus* in The Netherlands. J Clin Microbiol 2005;43(4):2034; author reply 2034–5.

153 Wannet WJ, Spalburg E, Heck ME, Pluister GN, Willems RJ, De Neeling AJ. Widespread dissemination in The Netherlands of the epidemic berlin methicillin-resistant *Staphylococcus aureus* clone with low-level resistance to oxacillin. J Clin Microbiol 2004;42(7):3077–82.

154 Harbarth S, Fankhauser C, Schrenzel J, et al. Universal screening for methicillin-resistant *Staphylococcus aureus* at hospital admission and nosocomial infection in surgical patients. JAMA 2008;299(10):1149–57.

155 Robicsek A, Beaumont JL, Paule SM, et al. Universal surveillance for methicillin-resistant *Staphylococcus aureus* in 3 affiliated hospitals. Ann Intern Med 2008;148(6):409–18.

156 Boyce JM. MRSA patients: proven methods to treat colonization and infection. J Hosp Infect 2001;48 Suppl A:S9–14.

157 Simor AE, Phillips E, McGeer A, et al. Randomized controlled trial of chlorhexidine gluconate for washing, intranasal mupirocin, and rifampin and doxycycline versus no treatment for the eradication of methicillin-resistant *Staphylococcus aureus* colonization. Clin Infect Dis 2007;44(2):178–85.

158 Loeb M, Main C, Walker-Dilks C, Eady A. Antimicrobial drugs for treating methicillin-resistant *Staphylococcus aureus* colonization. Cochrane Database Syst Rev 2003 (4), CD003340, DOI: 10.1002/14651858.

159 Muto CA, Jernigan JA, Ostrowsky BE, et al. SHEA guideline for preventing nosocomial transmission of multidrug-resistant strains of *Staphylococcus aureus* and enterococcus. Infect Control Hosp Epidemiol 2003;24(5):362–86.

160 Olsen MA, Chu-Ongasakul S, Brandt KE, Dietz JR, Mayfield J, Fraser VJ. Hospital-associated costs due to surgical site infection after breast surgery. Arch Surg 2008;143(1):53–60.

161 Jenney AWJ, Harrington GA, Russo PL, Spelman DW. Cost of surgical site infections following coronary artery bypass surgery. ANZ J Surg 2001;71:662–4.

162 Hollenbeak CS, Murphy DM, Koenig S, Woodward RS, Dunagan WC, Fraser VJ. The clinical and economic impact of deep chest surgical site infections following coronary artery bypass graft surgery. Chest 2000;118:397–402.

163 Hall RE, Ash AS, Ghali WA, Moskowitz MA. Hospital cost of complications associated with coronary artery bypass graft surgery. Am J Cardiol 1997;79:1680–2.

164 Coskun D, Aytac J, Aydinli A, Bayer A. Mortality rate, length of stay and extra cost or sternal surgical site infections following coronary artery bypass grafting in a private medical centre in Turkey. J Hosp Infect 2005;60:176–9.

165 Whitehouse JD, Friedman ND, Kirkland KB, Richardson WJ, Sexton DJ. The impact of surgical-site infections following orthopedic surgery at a community hospital and a university hospital: adverse quality of life, excess length of stay, and extra cost. Infect Control Hosp Epidemiol 2002;23:183–9.

166 Perencevich EN, Sands KE, Cosgrove SE, Guadagnoli E, Meara E, Platt R. Health and economic impact of surgical site infections diagnosed after hospital discharge. Emerg Infect Dis 2003;9:196–203.

167 Kirkland KB, Briggs JP, Trivette SL, Wilkinson WE, Sexton DJ. The impact of surgical-site infections in the 1990s: attributable mortality, excess length of hospitalization, and extra costs. Infect Control Hosp Epidemiol 1999;20(11):725–730.

168 Herwaldt LA, Cullen JJ, Scholz D, French P, Zimmerman MB, Pfaller MA, Wenzel RP, Perl TM. A prospective study of outcomes, healthcare resource utilization, and costs associated with postoperative nosocomial infections. Infect Control Hosp Epidemiol 2006;27:1291–8.

169 Reilly J, Twaddle S, McIntosh J, Kean L. An economic analysis of surgical wound infection. J Hosp Infect 2001;49:245–9.

170 McGarry SA, Engemann JJ, Schmader K, Sexton DJ, Kaye KS. Surgical site infection due to *Staphylococcus aureus* among elderly patients: mortality, duration of hospitalization, and cost. Infect Control Hosp Epidemiol 2004;25:461–467.

171 Coello R, Charlett A, Wilson J, Ward V, Pearson A, Borriello P. Adverse impact of surgical site infections in English hospitals. J Hosp Infect 2005;60:93–103.

172 Kasatpibal N, Thongpiyapoom S, Narong MN, Suwalak N, Jamulitrat S. Extra charge and extra length of postoperative stay attributable to surgical site infection in six selected operations. J Med Assoc Thai 2005;88:1083–91. [abstract]

173 Dimick JB, Chen SL, Taheri PA, Henderson WG, Khuri SF, Campbell Jr DA. Hospital costs associated with surgical complications: a report from the private-sector National Surgical Quality Improvement Program. J Am Coll Surg 2004;199:531–7.

174 Engermann JJ, Carmeli Y, Cosgrove SE, Fowler VG, Bronstein MZ, Trivette SL, Briggs JP, Sexton DJ, Kaye KS. Adverse clinical and economic outcomes attributable to methicillin resistance among patients with *Staphylococcus aureus* surgical site infection. Clin Infect Dis 2003;36:592–8.

CHAPTER 15
Infections in neutropenic hosts

Stuart J. Rosser & Eric J. Bow

Case presentation

A 34-year-old male was admitted complaining of fever, generalized malaise, and increasing fatigue over the preceding 4 weeks. On examination, he was pale; his blood pressure was 122/78 mmHg; oral temperature 38.2°C, and pulse 110 per minute. His liver had a 14-cm span in the midclavicular line and the spleen tip was 10 cm below the left costal margin. Petechiae were present in the skin of the lower limbs. A complete blood count revealed a total leukocyte count of 35×10^9/L, an absolute neutrophil count (ANC) of 0.824×10^9/L, an absolute lymphocyte count (ALC) of 0.4×10^9/L, an absolute monocyte count (AMC) of 0.2×10^9/L, and a circulating blast count of 33×10^9/L. His serum uric acid was elevated at 590 μmol/L and his serum lactate dehydrogenase was 1890 IU/L. A chest roentgenogram was normal. A bone marrow examination revealed a hypercellular marrow specimen 90% infiltrated by blast cells, some of which contained Auer rods. Acute myeloid leukemia (AML) (French–American–British classification, M2) was diagnosed. A typical AML remission-induction regimen was administered, consisting of a 7-day continuous infusion of cytarabine plus an anthracycline, idarubicin, administered daily on days 1, 2, and 3. Beginning on day + 1 of cytotoxic therapy, ciprofloxacin 500 mg every 12 hours and oral acyclovir 800 mg every 12 hours were administered to prevent aerobic gram-negative bacterial infections and mucositis due to reactivation of herpes simplex virus respectively. Oral fluconazole 400 mg daily was administered to prevent superficial and invasive fungal infection due to *Candida albicans*. The blood cultures obtained at the time of hospital admission remained sterile and the fever resolved as the cytotoxic therapy was administered. The ANC fell to $<0.5 \times 10^9$/L on day + 3 of induction therapy and to $<0.1 \times 10^9$/L on day + 5.

Acute leukemia is a rapidly progressive disease. In the untreated patient, it results in early death owing to hemorrhage or infection – the consequences, respectively, of thrombocytopenia and neutropenia from marrow failure. Historically, infection has been the major contributor to mortality and has been designated as the primary cause of death in over one-third of acute leukemia cases. Notwithstanding advances in cytotoxic chemotherapy for the underlying malignancy and in the use of marrow-stimulating growth factors and antimicrobials to support individuals through their disease- and treatment-related marrow insufficiency, infection remains the major contributor to 66% of deaths in patients treated for acute myeloid leukemia (AML) [1]. The early recognition and appropriate treatment of infection remains a priority in the care of these profoundly immunocompromised individuals.

Case presentation (continued)

A detailed physical examination as well as diagnostic and microbiologic testing suggested no obvious infection, and the fever was subsequently felt to be disease-related.

Evidence-Based Infectious Diseases, 2nd edition. Edited by Mark Loeb, Fiona Smaill and Marek Smieja. © 2009 Wiley-Blackwell Publishing, ISBN: 978-1-4051-7026-0

Neutrophils are the principal mediators of nonspecific (innate) cellular immunity. A deficiency in either the number or function of neutrophils can predispose an individual to infection. Diminished numbers of neutrophils, as opposed to qualitative defects in granulocyte function, are the more common cause of granulocytic immunodeficiency. While a total neutrophil count of $<1.0 \times 10^9$/L of blood defines neutropenia, the risk of bacterial and fungal sepsis rises exponentially below a level of 0.5×10^9/L. This profound degree of neutropenia occasionally results from an underlying inflammatory, infectious, or malignant condition, but is more often a consequence of the treatment of these diseases. In particular, the treatment of hematological and other malignancies with certain cytotoxic regimens will reliably induce profound and protracted neutropenia. Much of the data regarding the epidemiology, microbiology, diagnosis, and treatment of neutropenic sepsis is derived from studies of leukemia and bone marrow transplant patients. While there may be subtle differences in the characteristics of neutropenia-related sepsis arising from one disease state to the next, most of what we have learned from the hematology and oncology studies can be generalized to other conditions producing neutropenia of similar magnitude and duration.

The febrile neutropenic episode

Cytotoxic therapy for acute myeloid leukemia will predictably result in neutropenia, with absolute neutrophil counts of $<0.5 \times 10^9$/L for 10–14 days, or longer. While a patient may become febrile at any point during the course of treatment, the median time to first fever is typically 14 days from the first chemotherapy day [2], but may develop as early as day 9 (or about 3 days following the onset of neutropenia) [3]. The designation of a "febrile neutropenic episode" (FNE) applies when a neutropenic patient's oral temperature exceeds 38°C for at least 1 hour [4–6]. The fever itself arises from the production of proinflammatory cytokines (interleukin-1α, IL-1β, IL-4, IL-6, and tumor necrosis factor-α) [7], most often in response to either infection- or therapy-related cell membrane damage [8–12]. While fever is generally the first, and frequently the only sign of infection, not all febrile episodes will be the result of infection. The Infectious Diseases Society of America (IDSA) and the

National Comprehensive Cancer Network (NCCN) define fever due to an infection as an episode associated with an oral temperature above 38.3°C (101°F) in the absence of noninfectious causes [4,6]. Some of the common noninfectious causes of fever in populations being treated for malignancies are outlined in Box 15.1. Febrile neutropenic episodes associated with infection may be further classified as microbiologically documented (either bacteremic or nonbacteremic) or clinically documented, where a site of infection is identified without a pathogen or where fever occurs without an alternate explanation. While a diligent search for infection may result in as few as 8% of febrile episodes being classified as "unexplained" [13], contemporary studies suggest that the actual proportion for which no infectious cause can be found may be as high as 35–60% [14–16].

> **Box 15.1 Fever in the neutropenic cancer patient: non-infectious causes**
>
> - Underlying malignancy
> - Infusion of blood products
> - Drugs: cytarabine, cyclophosphamide, hydroxyurea, polyenes (e.g., amphotericin B deoxycholate)
> - Noninfectious inflammatory conditions: phlebltis, hematomas, thromboembolic disease

Measures to prevent infection in the neutropenic host

Protected environments

Non-antimicrobial measures aimed at preventing infections in patients with established or anticipated neutropenia have included: the placement of patients in a single room; the use of gowns, gloves, and masks by hospital personnel when entering patients' rooms; positive pressure ventilation in patients' rooms; and high efficiency particulate air (HEPA) filtration, with or without laminar (unidirectional) flow. A number of recommendations and guidelines regarding protected environments for high-risk patient populations have been published [17–23]. Most of the infections that occur during the pre-engraftment neutropenic period, however, represent reactivation of latent infection such as herpes simplex virus, or translocation of bacteria or opportunistic yeasts colonizing mucosal surfaces damaged by cytotoxic therapies. The risk of airborne transmission of mold conidia has been shown to be reduced by HEPA-based protected environments [24,25]. A case-controlled, registry-based analysis among European patients undergoing allogeneic hematopoietic stem cell transplantation [26] and a retrospective analysis of the outcomes among transplant patients in Seattle [27] have suggested a survival benefit with the use of HEPA filtration. Despite these observations, prospective randomized studies have not been able to demonstrate an effect on the rates of invasive bacterial or fungal infections [26,28]. Although a systematic review of nonrandomized trials suggested a protective effect against invasive aspergillosis [29], no single study has been powered sufficiently to detect an effect of HEPA filtration on this relatively rare condition given event rates <10% in most neutropenic patient populations at risk [30,31]. It may be prudent to consider HEPA filtering with or without laminar flow for the protection of high-risk inpatients managed under circumstances where the invasive mold infection risk exceeds 6–8%, and where azole-based mold-active prophylaxis is not employed (see below). Such environments may include those in close proximity to hospital construction and maintenance projects [32]. As part of routine care, placement of patients in a single room and diligent hand washing on the part of healthcare workers and visitors are to be encouraged, while other protective measures should be reserved for high-risk patients (see Risk assessment, below).

Prophylactic antimicrobials

Antibacterial agents

The pathogens most commonly implicated in neutropenic sepsis are gram-positive and gram-negative bacteria derived from colonized skin and mucosal surfaces [33,34]. With this in mind, investigators have sought to prevent infections by reducing the burden of potential pathogens with antimicrobials. Initial efforts with oral, nonabsorbable agents had equivocal effects on infection-related outcomes in the neutropenic host [35–42] and had several economic and logistic drawbacks. Early studies using trimethoprim-sulfamethoxazole (TMP-SMX) showed reductions in bloodstream [43,44], microbiologically documented

[43,45], and overall infections [45]. However, subsequent metaanalyses of studies comparing fluoroquinolone-based prophylaxis with TMP-SMX or with "no prophylaxis" showed that the risk of infection-related morbidity and mortality in TMP-SMX-treated populations was not significantly lower than for the groups receiving no prophylactic agent [46]. The latter finding may relate to the increasing prevalence over the past two decades of TMP-SMX resistance among aerobic gram-negative bacteria causing neutropenic sepsis [47,48].

Fluoroquinolones (principally ciprofloxacin and levofloxacin) have predominated as the agents of choice for antibacterial prophylaxis in the treatment of hematological malignancies since the mid-1990s. Multiple systematic reviews and metaanalyses have been published examining the role of systemic antibacterial prophylaxis in general, and of fluoroquinolone-based prophylaxis in particular, in neutropenic populations [46,49–55]. Protective treatment effects have been demonstrated for a number of clinically important outcomes including the frequency of febrile episodes, clinically and microbiologically documented infections, bloodstream infections, and gram-negative infections. Recent analyses have demonstrated a reduction not only for infection-related mortality, but for all-cause mortality, on the order of 33% [51,53]. Based on a pooled estimate of 6% all-cause mortality in groups treated without prophylaxis, the authors of these reviews estimate that prophylactic fluoroquinolone administration to 50 individuals would be required to prevent one death among patients with chemotherapy-induced neutropenia. Importantly, these studies have not identified an increased risk of infections with antibiotic-resistant organisms such as *Clostridium difficile*-associated diarrheal (CDAD) illness [52], notwithstanding evidence linking CDAD to fluoroquinolone use [56].

The benefits of fluoroquinolone prophylaxis are not restricted to those groups at highest risk for prolonged and severe neutropenia, such as the leukemic and stem cell transplantation populations mentioned above. A recent study from the United Kingdom evaluated levofloxacin-based prophylaxis in solid tumor and lymphoma outpatients at lower risk for neutropenic fevers [57]. The results demonstrated a significant reduction in febrile episodes attributable to infection and in hospitalizations for suspected infection by 29%

and 27%, respectively [57]. The majority of febrile episodes occurred during the first cycle of chemotherapy [58], as has been observed by others [59]. The risk for hospitalization for suspected infection was greatest for patients receiving chemotherapy for testicular cancers and small cell lung cancer, and among those with a poor baseline performance status [58]. The authors concluded that patients at risk should receive prophylaxis during cycle 1 of chemotherapy, but not during subsequent cycles unless a previous episode of febrile neutropenia had occurred. The reported all-cause mortality among low-risk recipients of fluoroquinolone *prophylaxis* compared to placebo has been 1.4% and 2.7%, respectively [53]. The all-cause mortality among low-risk patients receiving oral fluoroquinolones as part of empirical antibacterial *therapy* for neutropenic fever has been 1.7% and 2.5%, respectively [60]. The survival benefit appears to be in the use of fluoroquinolone therapy per se, rather than in the timing of that use, and there would seem to be no advantage to applying fluoroquinolone-based prophylaxis strategies among the low-risk patients with solid tumors and lymphoma, as compared to reserving those drugs for the ambulatory treatment of febrile neutropenic episodes in this population.

Based on the available evidence, the Infectious Diseases Working Party of the European Blood and Marrow Transplant Group, the European Leukemia Net, the Infectious Diseases Group of the European Organisation for Research and Treatment of Cancer, and the International Immunocompromised Host Society have endorsed the use of fluoroquinolone-based antibacterial prophylaxis in neutropenic patients undergoing induction therapy for acute leukemia or myeloablative hematopoietic stem cell transplantation [61]. The strongest endorsements were for ciprofloxacin (AI) and levofloxacin (AI). Further, the recommendations called for prophylaxis to begin with cytotoxic therapy and end with myeloid reconstitution or onset of a febrile neutropenic episode (AII). The National Comprehensive Cancer Network (NCCN) recently published recommendations for antibacterial prophylaxis based upon risk assessment [6]. The NCCN panel has not recommended prophylaxis for low-risk patients, defined as those for whom the expectation of the duration of cytotoxic therapy-induced neutropenia (ANC $< 0.5 \times 10^9$/L) is less than 7 days. In contrast, prophylaxis might be considered

for intermediate-risk patients: that is, those undergoing autologous hematopoietic stem cell transplantation, those receiving purine analog therapy, and those being treated with intensive therapy for lymphoreticular malignancies where the expected duration of neutropenia is 7–10 days. The panel continues to recommend prophylaxis for high-risk patients undergoing allogeneic stem cell transplantation, and those receiving intensive cytotoxic therapy for acute leukemia or myelodysplastic syndromes. In contrast, the German guidelines have endorsed prophylaxis for those undergoing allogeneic hematopoietic stem cell transplant [62], underscoring a lack of consensus based on the available evidence. Overall, the weight of opinion favors applying fluoroquinolone-based prophylaxis predominantly to those patients classified to be at high risk for neutropenic fevers.

The general enthusiasm for fluoroquinolone prophylaxis has been tempered by concern over colonization with, and subsequent infection by, fluoroquinolone-resistant gram-negative rods and gram-positive organisms against which the most frequently used fluoroquinolones have limited activity. Increases in the proportion of *E. coli* isolates resistant to fluoroquinolones within hematology-oncology populations have been widely recognized [63–65], notwithstanding a general decline in gram-negative bacteremic episodes among febrile neutropenics [66]. Analyses of the relevant trials [67] showed no significant increase in either colonization or infection with quinolone-resistant organisms when fluoroquinolone prophylaxis was compared to placebo ($RR_{Infection}$ 1.04; 95% CI 0.73–1.5); they showed a *reduced* risk of colonization or infection with resistant organisms when fluoroquinolones and TMP-SMX were compared ($RR_{Infection}$ 0.45; 95% CI 0.27–0.74, favoring quinolone prophylaxis) [52]. A similar reduced risk of bacteremic and other infections with gram-positive organisms has been noted (RR 0.44; 95% CI 0.38–0.51, for bacteremia), with no significant difference between fluoroquinolone and TMP-SMX-based regimens with regard to infection by gram-positive organisms. In consecutive two-period design studies at a single European centre [63,68], the suspension of routine fluoroquinolone prophylaxis for patients with chemotherapy-induced neutropenia resulted in an excess of bacteremic episodes involving fluoroquinolone-susceptible gram-negative organisms, and (in one study period) an excess mortality [68], prompting early discontinuation of the study protocol. These studies attest to the efficacy of fluoroquinolone prophylaxis, even in settings where there is a moderate degree of preexisting fluoroquinolone resistance. While the available evidence supports the continued use of fluoroquinolones as antibacterial prophylaxis in the context of chemotherapy-related neutropenia, the generalizability of these findings to populations other than those with hematologic malignancies (studies of which comprised the bulk of the recent systematic review) is limited. Fluoroquinolone prophylaxis should continue to be reserved for those high-risk individuals whose duration of neutropenia is anticipated to be >10 days; whose neutropenia is expected to be profound (ANC <0.1 × 10^9/L); and who are receiving treatment at institutions where the prevalence of quinolone resistance among facultatively anaerobic gram-negative bacilli is less than 15–20% [14]. In practice, the majority of these patients will be undergoing treatment for acute leukemia, myelodysplastic syndromes, or undergoing hematopoietic stem cell transplant.

Antifungal agents

Myeloablative conditioning regimens for hematopoietic stem cell transplantation and intensive cytotoxic therapies for acute leukemia predictably produce severe neutropenia (ANC < 0.5 × 10^9/L) with durations of greater than 10 to 14 days [2,69]. Studies of antifungal chemoprophylaxis have traditionally focused on high-risk patients with acute leukemia (see discussion of Risk assessment, below), principally with regard to preventing infections due to yeasts. However, the incidence of invasive mold infection, predominantly due to *Aspergillus* spp. (in 90% of cases), has been increasing [70,71], making the prevention of these infections a higher priority. Filamentous fungi such as *Aspergillus* spp. are generally acquired through inhalation of conidia, which subsequently germinate to produce tissue-invasive disease. As such, they have been considered targets for environmental control measures (see discussion of Protected Environments, above) or mold-active antifungal chemoprophylaxis. Yeasts, on the other hand, colonize the mucosal surfaces of chemotherapy-treated patients, and are more prone to translocate across damaged epithelial surfaces, with subsequent invasive infections in the neutropenic host. These characteristics make yeasts an appealing target for orally administered prophylactic antifungal strategies.

A number of systematic reviews and metaanalyses of randomized-controlled trials on anti-fungal chemoprophylaxis have been published [72–76]. These analyses demonstrate that, in principle, antifungal chemoprophylaxis may improve important outcomes with respect to: invasive fungal infections (particularly where the baseline event rate for invasive candidiasis is >15% [74]); superficial fungal infections; attributable mortality due to fungal infection [73,75,77]; and even all-cause mortality, by almost 50% [77]. A reduction in all-cause mortality has only been demonstrated among the highest-risk patients, such as those with durations of severe neutropenia of >15 days [75] and those undergoing acute leukemia therapy or hematopoietic stem cell transplantation [77]. With regard to specific agents, systematic analysis has not demonstrated an advantage for itraconazole over that of fluconazole for invasive fungal infection overall [76], despite the anti-mold activity of the former agent. The formulation of itraconazole is an important confounding variable: the oral solution has better bioavailability than the capsules [73]. Moreover, daily dosing of >200 mg for fluconazole [75] or itraconazole solution [73] is required for maximum benefit.

Infections with filamentous fungi such as *Aspergillus* species, many of which will have their origin in a chemotherapy-induced neutropenic episode, are a major issue in the care of hematopoietic stem cell transplant recipients. Incidence rates for invasive aspergillosis among allogeneic stem cell recipients in the literature range from 2.9% to 16% (median 8.1%) [71], with attributable mortalities ranging from 36% to 87% (median 57.5%) [71]. Newer mold-active azole antifungals with significant activity against *Aspergillus* species have been evaluated in the context of chemotherapy-induced neutropenia, among them voriconazole and posaconazole. The data on voriconazole as a *prophylactic* agent in high-risk patients are sparse [78,79], and its utility in this setting has not been defined. Posaconazole has been compared to fluconazole and itraconazole in a prospective randomized clinical trial of prophylaxis for invasive fungal infections in patients undergoing remission-induction chemotherapy for acute myelogenous leukemia [30]: using standard definitions for *proven*, *probable*, and *possible* invasive fungal infection [80], its performance was superior to the two comparators with regard to preventing *Aspergillus* infections. This benefit was attributed to an excess of *probable*, not *proven* infections in the fluconazole and itraconazole groups [30]. A second trial evaluated the prophylactic efficacy of posaconazole compared to fluconazole in allogeneic hematopoietic stem cell transplant recipients with acute or chronic graft-versus-host disease [31]. Similar protective benefits were observed among the posaconazole recipients, with a reduction of 68% in the risk for invasive aspergillosis. The number of patients requiring treatment to prevent one case of invasive aspergillosis was 19 [31]. The relative merits of prophylaxis with an expanded-spectrum azole such as posaconazole, versus a preemptive strategy of fluconazole prophylaxis and close serologic/radiographic monitoring have been reviewed elsewhere [30,81–83].

Recently published European guidelines advocate the use of fluconazole or posaconazole for the prevention of opportunistic yeast infections in patients undergoing hematopoietic stem cell transplantation (AI) [84]. Itraconazole (BI), the echinocandin micafungin (CI), and amphotericin B (CI) may be considered as alternatives. For acute leukemia patients undergoing induction or reinduction therapy posaconazole was favored (AI) over fluconazole or itraconazole (CI). The German guidelines are similar [85]. In contrast, the 2007 NCCN Guidelines endorse only fluconazole for the prevention of invasive candidiasis in acute lymphoblastic leukemia patients, arguing cytochrome P450 enzyme inhibition caused by agents such as itraconazole, voriconazole, and posaconazole may enhance the toxicity of the vinca alkaloids [6]. The NCCN panel recommended posaconazole or voriconazole prophylaxis for AML and MDS patients receiving intensive induction therapy, to be administered through myeloid reconstitution. Fluconazole or micafungin was recommended for autologous HSCT patients with mucositis. Antifungal prophylaxis with any of fluconazole, itraconazole, micafungin, voriconazole, or posaconazole should be considered for allogeneic HSCT recipients, and administered until at least day 75 after transplantation [6].

Adjuvant therapies

The association of infection-related morbidity with treatment-emergent neutropenia in oncology populations has spurred interest in the use of colony stimulating factors (CSFs) to decrease the incidence of febrile neutropenic episodes and their infectious complications. Six systematic reviews with metaanalyses evaluating the roles of CSFs have been published [86–91]. Primary prophylaxis – that is, the administration of colony stimulating factors following the administration of the cyototoxic therapy with each cycle, prior to a neutropenic event – has been shown to reduce the risk of febrile neutropenic episodes and infection-related mortality in general oncology populations [90], with a recent metaanalysis implying a substantial benefit with respect to early all-cause mortality (RR 0.599, 95% CI 0.433–0.830, favors CSFs) [92]. Despite these positive observations, another review of CSFs in malignant lymphoma patients failed to demonstrate a treatment effect for infection-related mortality (RR 1.37, 95%CI 0.66–2.82) [91], suggesting that efficacy differences may exist within subpopulations of cancer patients. Hematological malignancies by their very nature are not amenable to primary prophylaxis with CSFs, and aggressive secondary prophylaxis has generally been avoided in this context, in part because of lack of proven benefit, and in part because one retrospective study found that allogeneic hematopoietic stem cell recipients who received GCSF within the first 14 days after transplantation had both higher rates of acute and chronic graft-versus-host disease, and greater transplant-related mortality [69]. Two subsequent systematic reviews evaluating the use of granulocyte colony stimulating factor (GCSF) and granulocyte-monocyte colony stimulating factor (GMCSF) in hematopoietic stem cell transplant [87] and mixed hematology-oncology populations [93] have shown no increased risk of GVHD in the former group [87], and have demonstrated reductions in hospital length of stay [87,93], time to neutrophil recovery [93], and number of febrile days [87] with the use of CSFs. Borderline effects on both documented infections and infection-related mortality were also noted (upper limit of 95% CI = 1.0 for both). Given an estimated cost of US$20 400 per episode of febrile neutropenia complicating the treatment of a hematologic malignancy [94], the minor clinical benefits described above could have a significant cost benefit. The American Society of Clinical Oncology [95] acknowledged this potential impact in the most recent iteration of its guidelines for the use of colony-stimulating factors, recommending CSF administration in post-remission consolidation therapy for acute myeloid leukemia, and for established febrile neutropenic episodes with high-risk indicators (see Risk assessment, below).

Case presentation (continued)

By day + 9, the patient complained of pain with swallowing. On day + 12, he complained of chills, muscle aches, headache, and abdominal discomfort. His oral temperature was 39.2°C, respiratory rate 26 per minute, pulse 100 per minute, and blood pressure 122/72 mmHg lying down and 98/60 mmHg standing. The oropharynx was diffusely erythematous with ulcerations over the hard palate and right buccal margin. There was no lymphadenopathy. The chest examination revealed inspiratory râles over the right medial basal segment. The abdominal examination revealed normal bowel sounds, but focal tenderness over the right lower quadrant was noted with light palpation. The ANC and AMC were 0, the ALC 0.3 × 10^9/L, and the platelet count was 12 × 10^9/L. A chest roentgenogram was unremarkable. Blood cultures were obtained from each lumen of the central venous catheter and from a peripheral site. Intravenous fluids, and empirical antibacterial therapy with a third-generation cephalosporin, ceftazidime, were administered; 24 hours later the blood cultures from all catheter lumens were reported as growing gram-positive cocci in chains. The patient remained febrile. Further blood cultures were obtained and vancomycin was empirically added to the ceftazidime.

Assessment and management of the febrile neutropenic episode

Most neutropenic patients with infections present with fever, whether or not a definable clinical focus of infection can be identified. Accordingly, the most important component of the clinical assessment of these patients is having an index of suspicion. The time course for a neutropenic episode is referenced from the first day of the current cycle upon which the patient received cytotoxic therapy. Most neutropenic fevers occur after the first week [3] at a median of day +14, and coincide with the time of maximal cytotoxic therapy-induced intestinal mucosal damage [2,96].

When a patient with an absolute neutrophil count of <0.5 × 10^9/L meets the temperature criteria for a febrile neutropenic episode, vigorous attempts to document a source and/or to isolate a potential pathogen must be made. This requires a focused physical examination, and a minimum laboratory evaluation consisting of a full blood count, creatinine, liver enzyme tests, a chest radiographic examination; cultures of urine and sputum if urinary or respiratory symptoms are present; and cultures of blood drawn from each of two sites including each lumen of any indwelling venous catheter, as well as blood from at least one peripheral site. The latter recommendation derives from a study of neutropenic cancer patients [97], in which a negative culture from either a central or peripheral site had a predictive value for the absence of "true bacteremia" of 98–99%. A positive culture at either site had a predictive value for the presence of "true bacteremia" that was substantially lower (63% for the central venous catheter, 73% for the peripheral site). Overall, single negative cultures from the central or peripheral sites are more helpful in ruling out a true bacteremia than single positive cultures are at ruling it in. The high negative predictive values were not sensitive to changes in overall prevalence of true bloodstream infection.

If infection is suspected, empirical therapy with broad-spectrum antimicrobial agents should be instituted. Consensus recommendations also advise that any neutropenic individual with a clinically suspected infection should receive treatment, even in the absence of fever [4]. The choice of empiric therapy will be influenced by the results of the physical examination and key laboratory tests, by whether or not the individual's circumstances suggest a low risk for serious infection (see below), and by an understanding of which endogenous microflora cause infections most often in this population.

Physical examination

The salient features of a focused history and physical examination, as they pertain to the evaluation of a febrile neutropenic patient, are summarized in Table 15.1. The classic signs of inflammation associated with pyogenic infection in an immunocompetent individual may be absent or diminished in the context of absolute neutropenia. A seminal descriptive analysis of presenting signs and symptoms for

Table 15.1 Physical examination of the febrile neutropenic patient

Region	Examine for
Head and neck	
– fundi	Retinal hemorrhages (bleeding diatheses)
	Retinal exudates (disseminated fungal infection)
– auditory canals/tympanic membranes	Erythema (otitis externa/media; viral upper respiratory infection)
	Vesicles (herpetic infection)
– anterior nasal mucosa	Ulcerations/vesicular lesions (fungal disease, herpetic infection)
– oropharynx	Mucositis (predisposition to bacteremias/fungemias)
	Ulcerative gingivo-stomatitis (anaerobic bacteria)
	Pseudomembranous pharyngitis (thrush, a risk for candidemia)
Chest	Râles (more consistent than cough/sputum in diagnosis of pneumonia)
	Edema, pain, erythema around central venous catheter tunnel and exit sites
Abdomen	Localized tenderness (right lower quadrant: typhlitis; right upper quadrant: hepatobiliary infection; perianal tissues [not a digital rectal examination]: cellulitis, abscess or fistula)
Skin	Tenderness, erythema, swelling around intravenous sites
	Ulcerative or necrotic lesions (*Pseudomonas aeruginosa, Staphylococcus aureus*)
	Diffuse pustular/erythematous lesions (metastatic seeding with *Candida* spp.)
	Vesicular lesions (herpes simplex/zoster)
	Hypersensitivity reactions

neutropenic versus non-neutropenic hosts [98] showed that, with regard to skin and soft-tissue infections, edema was reduced in neutropenic patients (73% of neutropenic vs 100% of non-neutropenic individuals, $P = 0.02$), while fluctuance and exudation were for the most part absent (5% vs 50%; $P = 0.003$; and 5% vs 92%; $P < 0.001$, respectively) [98]. Where pneumonia was ultimately diagnosed, cough and sputum production were less frequent among neutropenic patients (67% vs 93%, $P = 0.002$; and 58% vs 85%, $P = 0.003$, respectively), but bacteremia was more common (55% vs 17%; $P < 0.001$) [98]. This effect of neutropenia on the presentation of bacterial sepsis must be taken into account in the evaluation of the patient. The basic vital signs including the temperature, heart rate, and respiratory rate, together with the neutropenic state can be used to estimate a SIRS (systemic inflammatory response syndrome) score which may correlate with the risk for bloodstream infection or progression to more severe sepsis syndromes [99,100].

Risk assessment

"Risk" in neutropenic patients may be defined differently, depending upon circumstances. The Infectious Diseases Working Party of the German Society of Hematology and Oncology defines risk in terms of the *likelihood of developing* a febrile neutropenic episode [5]. The European Organisation for Research and Treatment of Cancer defines risk in terms of *failing to respond* to initial treatment of a febrile neutropenic episode, and of *complications* arising from the neutropenic episode that necessitate or prolong hospitalization, all in the context of clinical trials of empirical antibacterial therapy.

An individual's estimated risk for developing serious complications related to infection during a febrile neutropenic episode will have a bearing on the type of empiric antimicrobial therapy that is recommended and the setting in which it is administered. The concept of infection risk in this population has been more extensively reviewed elsewhere [101–103]. Patients may be conveniently divided into low, intermediate, and high-risk groups.

Low-risk individuals are those for whom the duration of neutropenia is expected to be short (3–5 days), who are clinically stable and without significant comorbidities, and who are ambulatory. These individuals may be treated empirically with oral antibacterial agents during their febrile neutropenic episodes, where the following circumstances apply:

- the individual is judged to be compliant
- immediate access to medical care is available in the event of deterioration
- a caretaker is present to monitor the patient.

Intermediate-risk patients are those with solid tumors or lymphoproliferative malignancies who are undergoing stem cell transplantation and who may therefore be expected to have a more prolonged period of neutropenia (8–13 days). By definition they should have minimal comorbidity and be clinically stable. They are treated initially with inpatient intravenous therapy and, if an early response is achieved, they may be "stepped down" to complete a course of further intravenous or oral therapy as an outpatient. High-risk patients are those receiving treatment for hematological malignancies (cytotoxic chemotherapy and/or stem cell allografting) for whom the duration of severe neutropenia will be protracted (>14 days), who may have significant comorbidities, or who are unstable (hemodynamically). These patients are much more likely to develop medical complications or to die [104], and should be treated as inpatients with intravenous antibiotics until their febrile neutropenic episode resolves.

The dichotomization of febrile neutropenic patients into only low-risk and high-risk categories with regard to recommendations for empiric antimicrobial therapy has also been advocated [4]. Here, the assessment of risk relies on a validated scoring system developed by a multinational collaborative group, in which treatment for a solid tumor, young age, outpatient status, and the absence of hypotension, symptoms, or significant comorbidity result in higher point scores: achieving a higher total point score (≥21) defines an individual as being at "low risk" for complications, and warrants the management outlined above for low-risk patients [105,106]. The positive predictive value of this point score (that is, the likelihood that an individual with a score of ≥21 will not experience a complication) is estimated to be 90–98% [103,106]. When used to inform decisions regarding the disposition of 383 first febrile neutropenic episodes at a single institution, the scoring system performed well, with only 4% of those patients discharged at less than 48 hours requiring readmission [107]. However, 38% of "low-risk" individuals in that study who could have been discharged but who remained in hospital had no objective medical reason for doing so, suggesting that the outpatient management of febrile neutropenic episodes was not universally endorsed [107].

Spectrum of bacterial infections in neutropenic cancer patients

In previous decades more than 75% of the systemic infections in patients dying with acute leukemia were due to enterobacteriaceae (*Escherichia coli*, *Klebsiella pneumoniae*), *Pseudomonas aeruginosa,* or *Staphylococcus aureus* [108,109]. More recently, grampositive organisms have come to predominate as the etiologic agents of bacteremic infections. This shift may be related to several factors, including:

- the widespread use of central venous access catheters [110], which predictably results in a greater incidence of bacteremia with gram-positive skin colonizers such as the coagulase-negative staphylococci
- more intensive chemotherapeutic regimens, with greater toxicity to the gastrointestinal mucosa [111–113] and easier access to the bloodstream for viridans group streptococci and enterococci
- fluoroquinolone chemoprophylaxis, which suppresses the aerobic gram-negative bacilli colonizing the gut epithelium, but not the coexistent microaerophilic streptococci or coagulase-negative staphylococci.

It is therefore prudent to ensure adequate coverage for gram-positive pathogens in any empiric antibacterial regimen, particularly if the individual has received fluoroquinolone chemoprophylaxis. However, the risk of infection-related mortality is still highest for aerobic gram-negative bacteremic infections, particularly when *P. aeruginosa* is the causative agent [114], and recommended empiric antibacterial regimens include specific coverage for the latter organism.

Choice and duration of empirical antibacterial therapy

Table 15.2 lists a range of single-agent and combination antimicrobial regimens that have been used successfully in the management of fever from suspected infection in the neutropenic host. Low-risk patients

Table 15.2 Empirical antibacterial regimens for the management of febrile neutropenic episodes

Regimen type	Antimicrobial type	Examples
Monotherapy	Anti-pseudomonal penicillin+	Piperacillin/tazobactam
	β-lactamase inhibitor	Ticarcillin/clavulanate
	Carbapenem	Imipenem/cilastatin, meropenem
	Fluoroquinolone*	Ciprofloxacin, levofloxacin, moxifloxacin
	3rd or 4th generation cephalosporin	Ceftazidime, cefepime, ceftriaxone,** cefixime**
Combination therapy	Antipseudomonal β-lactam +	Piperacillin, carbapenem, or antipseudomonal cephalosporin
	Aminoglycoside	Gentamicin, tobramycin, amikacin, netilmicin
	or	
	Fluoroquinolone	Ciprofloxacin, levofloxacin

* Outpatient therapy in low-risk patients not receiving fluoroquinolone-based antibacterial chemoprophylaxis.
** Outpatient therapy in low-risk patients.

for whom oral therapy is deemed appropriate may be treated with ciprofloxacin and amoxicillin-clavulanate, if the former drug has not been administered as part of a prophylactic regimen. Vancomycin may be added to an empiric regimen at the start of treatment if infection of an intravascular device is suspected (and coagulase-negative staphylococci are therefore implicated), or if the individual is known to be colonized with a β-lactam resistant gram-positive pathogen [115] such as methicillin-resistant *S. aureus*. Alternatively, it may be added to a regimen between days 3 and 5 of antimicrobial treatment, if the patient remains febrile, and if the chosen empirical regimen is judged to have suboptimal coverage for *S. aureus* and streptococci (e.g., ceftazidime monotherapy). However, given that 40% of patients with gram-positive bacteremias may respond to these regimens (i.e., ceftazidime alone) [116–118]; that vancomycin use has been associated with an increased risk of colonization and infection with glycopeptide-resistant enterococci [119–121]; and that the early/immediate addition of a glycopeptide provides no advantage in terms of mortality or time-to-resolution of the febrile episode [122], the routine use of vancomycin in empiric regimens is not recommended. A recent systematic review [123] suggests that β-lactam monotherapy options are equivalent to dual-therapy regimens in terms of both mortality and other less rigorous endpoints, with two possible exceptions: cefepime monotherapy has been associated with higher all-cause mortality in both the review

(RR 1.44, 95% CI 1.06–1.94) [123] and a subsequent randomized controlled trial [15]; and the carbapenems (principally imipenem/cilastatin) have been associated with a greater risk of *C. difficile* toxin-mediated diarrhea (RR 1.94, 95% CI 1.24–3.04) [123]. Notwithstanding these distinctions, and acknowledging that individual patient factors (renal impairment, allergy) may also influence the choice of antibacterial agents, the selection of any particular regimen will depend more on institutional practice and local antimicrobial resistance patterns than on a proven survival benefit for any single drug or combination therapy.

Patients who are profoundly neutropenic, who remain febrile (without a documented source of infection) despite 5–7 days of empirical antibacterial therapy, and for whom neutrophil counts are not expected to recover in the short term are at high risk (approximately 20%) for invasive fungal infections [4,124]. Empirical antifungal therapy is felt to reduce the risk of invasive fungal infection in these patients by anywhere from 50% to 80%, and to reduce mortality from fungal infections by 23–45% [116–118]. Early studies of empiric amphotericin B therapy in febrile neutropenic cancer patients – where amphotericin B was added to background antibacterial therapy, at doses of 0.5–0.7 mg/kg/day – showed a trend towards reduced morbidity and mortality attributable to fungal infections, particularly in the highest-risk subgroups [125]. Overall, the available data justified a BII recommendation (B – should usually be offered;

II – based on clinical trials, with [at least] laboratory endpoints; United States Public Health Service/ Infectious Diseases Society of America rating scheme) for the use of amphotericin B deoxycholate, or any antifungal agent in the neutropenic patient who remains febrile on broad-spectrum antibacterials for >3 days, if the neutrophil counts are not expected to recover in the ensuing 5–7 days. Other antifungal agents, such as the lipid-based formulations of amphotericin B [126–129], intravenous itraconazole [130], voriconazole [131], and the echinocandin caspofungin [132] appear to have equivalent efficacy to amphotericin B deoxycholate as empirical antifungal therapy in neutropenic hosts. Toxicity and pharmacoeconomic considerations may lead to the eventual replacement of conventional amphotericin B deoxycholate therapy with one or more of these newer options.

The decision to modify or discontinue empirical antibacterial or antifungal therapy will be influenced by several factors. If a specific microbe is isolated and implicated as the cause of the febrile episode, the spectrum of antimicrobial therapy can be narrowed to cover that organism (or group of organisms), and an appropriate course of therapy should then be undertaken for the organism and anatomic site involved. Other decisions regarding continued antimicrobial therapy will depend on the resolution of the febrile episode, and the recovery of the neutrophil count to $>0.5 \times 10^9$/L.

The median time to defervescence for low-risk patients is 2–3 days [133,134], while for high-risk patients it is 4–6 days [13,117,135,136]. Given these parameters, and in the absence of a positive culture, a documented source of infection, or clinical deterioration, changes to the empirical regimen are generally not warranted for the first 5 days of the febrile episode. Otherwise, expert opinion suggests the following guidelines [4]:

- Patients who defervesce within the first 5 days of empirical therapy should have their treatment continued for a total of at least 7 days; low-risk patients may step down to oral therapy; high-risk patients should continue on their intravenous medications.
- Patients who remain febrile, in the absence of an identifiable source of infection, should have their antimicrobial agents continued until 4 or 5 days after their neutrophil counts rise to $>0.5 \times 10^9$/L, or, if the counts do not recover, to a total of 2 weeks'

treatment; the patient must be in stable condition prior to stopping the antimicrobials, and the need for further antimicrobials should be assessed on an ongoing basis, until the neutrophil count recovers.

Case presentation (continued)

The patient remained febrile over the first 5 days of antibacterial therapy. The gram-positive organism in the blood cultures was identified as a viridans group streptococcus (*S. mitis*). By day + 17 of induction therapy (day +5 of antibacterial therapy), the patient remained febrile with oral temperatures peaking daily between 38.5°C and 39°C and continued to complain of right lower quadrant pain, now associated with diarrhea and signs of peritoneal irritation. Stool cultures grew no pathogenic bacteria or yeasts, and a test for *Clostridium difficile* toxin A and B in the liquid stool was negative. Repeated blood cultures and chest roentgenogram were ultimately nondiagnostic. A computer tomographic examination of the abdomen identified cecal and ascending colonic wall thickening, with additional thickening of the ileal wall and the sigmoid colonic wall, consistent with neutropenic enterocolitis. The patient was treated with metronidazole intravenously. Over the course of the next 72 hours (until day + 20 of induction), the fever persisted; however, the patient's condition stabilized. The volume of diarrhea decreased and the abdominal pain, while still present, began to subside. The ANC and AMC were 0.001 and 0.2 × 10⁹/L, respectively. By day +22, the ANC, AMC, and platelet count were 0.186, 0.8, and 37 × 10⁹/L, respectively, consistent with marrow regeneration. The fever had abated, and the diarrhea resolved.

Selected infectious problems in the neutropenic host

Some infections in the neutropenic host may be anticipated. For example, in the clinical example above, a viridans streptococcal bacteremia in the context of mucositis with ciprofloxacin prophylaxis and empiric therapy with ceftazidime – neither of which affords reliable coverage for gram-positive organisms – is not unexpected. Certain other infectious syndromes are relatively common in the neutropenic host, and deserve specific attention.

Neutropenic enterocolitis

Neutropenic enterocolitis presents with a clinical triad of persistent fever, abdominal pain, and diarrhea. The spectrum of pathology ranges from mild mucosal inflammation to transmural necrosis. In a pooled analysis of case series and cohort studies evaluating individuals treated for acute leukemias, the incidence rate was estimated to be 5.6% (95% CI 4.6–6.9%) [137]. The likelihood of developing neutropenic enterocolits depends not only on the intensity of the chemotherapeutic regimen [138], but the type of chemotherapy, e.g., taxane-based therapy for solid tumors [139,140]. Onset of the first sign of neutropenic enterocolitis, diarrhea, occurs at a median of 9–10 days from the start of chemotherapy [141,142] and the syndrome is diagnosed at a median of 15 days from the start of chemotherapy [141]. The condition must be differentiated from other common causes of diarrhea in neutropenic cancer patients, including *Clostridium difficile* toxin-mediated diarrhea, and the direct effects of antimicrobial and cytotoxic agents. Abdominal computed tomography or ultrasound examination will typically show thickening of the bowel mucosa [143,144], with more frequent involvement of the cecum: a bowel wall thickness of >4 mm is considered suggestive, if not diagnostic [144]. The condition is associated with a high risk for translocation of, and subsequent bloodstream infection with, bacteria and yeasts.

Treatment is supportive, with fluids, blood products, analgesics, parenteral nutrition, and broad-spectrum antimicrobial therapy, including specific coverage for anaerobic bacteria. It is not uncommon for the fever associated with this condition to persist until resolution of the neutropenic episode, as in the case above: the addition of empirical amphotericin B therapy to this patient's antimicrobial regimen in the context of continued fever on broad-spectrum antibacterials was not considered necessary, given the diagnosis of neutropenic enterocolitis. Surgery is reserved for cases with perforation or refractory bleeding, and most patients can be managed medically [143].

Infections of intravascular devices

Central venous catheters are commonly implanted in patients undergoing protracted courses of chemotherapy, both for the administration of medications and for blood sampling. These catheters have up to a 20-fold increased risk of infection compared with peripheral devices [145]. Infection may occur at any point along the length of the device and, epidemiologically, these infections may be categorized [146] as:

- exit site infections, with <2 cm of inflammation at the site where the catheter leaves the skin
- tunnel infections, with >2 cm of inflammation, extending proximally from the exit site
- port pocket infections, where inflammation with or without fluctuance overlies the buried access bulb of a completely implanted system
- a catheter-related bloodstream infection, where blood cultures drawn from the device lumen(s) are positive.

Tunnel infections account for up to 50% of line-related infections; exit sites for 25%; febrile bacteremias (bloodstream infection) for 19%; and septic thrombophlebitis for 6% [147]. A bloodstream infection is generally attributed to an intravenous catheter if positive blood cultures are obtained from the catheter port or lumen, and no other source of infection (e.g., pneumonia, translocation of bowel microflora) is suspected. Quantitative blood cultures showing higher colony counts from a catheter lumen than from peripheral sites, or isolation of >15 colony forming units on the tip of a removed catheter by the semiquantitative roll-plate technique [148] would also implicate an intravascular device as the source of bacteremia. The use of antimicrobial-impregnated catheters for short-term venous access (mean 17 days) in patients with hematological malignancies has been associated with lower rates of line colonization and catheter-related bloodstream infection [149], but these data cannot be generalized to the longer-term, tunneled catheters favored for induction-remission chemotherapy in the setting of acute leukemia and marrow transplantation.

Central venous line removal is not required for all cases of catheter-associated bacteremia. Infections due to coagulase-negative staphylococci can be treated with the catheter left in place [150,151], although there is a greater potential for bacteremic relapse with this practice (20% vs 3% with catheter removal) [152,153]. The majority of exit site infections not due to *Pseudomonas* spp. may also be treated with the catheter in situ [150]. In other circumstances where the intravenous device is implicated in the febrile neutropenic episode, it should be removed.

Most febrile neutropenic episodes and bacteremias, for which a source other than the intravascular device itself is suspected, can be managed without catheter removal [154]. If blood cultures remain persistently positive after 48 hours of effective therapy, removal of the catheter may be warranted [151].

Case presentation (continued)

On day + 32, just prior to planned hospital discharge, the patient was noted to have a low-grade fever (oral temperature 38°C) and to be complaining of right upper quadrant discomfort. An examination revealed a liver span of 14 cm. A liver function profile demonstrated a total bilirubin of 24 μmol/L, an aspartate transaminase (AST) of 34 IU/L, alanine transferase (ALT) of 54 IU/L, lactate dehydrogenase (LDH) of 203 IU/L, alkaline phosphatase (ALP) of 267 IU/L, and gamma glutamyl transferase (GGT) of 376 IU/L consistent with a cholestatic enzymopathy. A repeat infused CT scan of the abdomen demonstrated multiple radiolucencies present in the parenchyma of the liver and the spleen. A diagnosis of hepatosplenic fungal infection was suspected. Further blood cultures grew no pathogens and a chest CT demonstrated no evidence of nodular lesions or consolidation. Culture of an open biopsy of the liver failed to grow any microorganisms; however, a silver methenamine-stained preparation demonstrated the presence of budding yeasts consistent with invasive candidiasis. On the basis of this information, a diagnosis of chronic disseminated candidiasis infection – presumed to have developed while the patient was receiving fluconazole antifungal prophylaxis – was established.

Chronic disseminated candidiasis

Chronic disseminated candidiasis (CDC) manifests as a persistent or recrudescent febrile illness in an individual who has received broad-spectrum antibacterial therapy for a febrile neutropenic episode, and whose neutrophil count has recovered [155–158]. Colonization of the gastrointestinal tract by yeasts [9,159,160], and chemotherapy with high-dose cytarabine (with associated oral and gastrointestinal mucositis) [158, 161] were the earliest identified risk factors; prolonged neutropenia (>15 days), younger age, and fluoroquinolone prophylaxis are likely contributing

factors [162]. Fluconazole prophylaxis, outside of the marrow transplant population, has no apparent impact on the risk for development of CDC [74,162]. There is often an associated fungemic episode, the median time to which is day + 15 [9] or later [162,163]; the median time to recognition of disseminated infection is day + 40, at which time the neutrophil counts have recovered [9]. The pathogenesis is presumed to involve translocation of opportunistic yeasts across a damaged gut epithelium [9,161], with seeding of the liver and spleen. Most of the cases are accounted for by *Candida* spp, with the relative proportions of *C. albicans* and non-albicans yeasts varying with the uptake of fluconazole prophylaxis [71,163,164].

The presenting signs and symptoms of chronic disseminated candidiasis include fever in 85% and abdominal pain in over 50% of cases, with a cholestatic enzymopathy (elevated serum ALP and GGT) [165]. The total bilirubin may also be elevated. Abdominal computed tomography remains the diagnostic modality of choice at many centers: a scan showing multiple hypodense lesions in the liver and spleen, some of which may have a "bull's eye" appearance [166], reinforces the presumptive diagnosis. Magnetic resonance imaging of the liver has demonstrated improved sensitivity, negative predictive value, and overall diagnostic accuracy for CDC when compared to CT scanning or ultrasonography [167,168], showing typical, round, well-demarcated lesions early on that are hyperintense on T2 imaging, and a characteristic evolution of those lesions over several weeks of effective therapy. Histopathologic examination of a liver biopsy remains the reference standard for diagnosis, and will show typical granulomatous changes, with fungal elements on methenamine silver or PAS staining. Cultures of the biopsy specimen are most often negative [162,169], but the combination of an appropriate history with suggestive laboratory, imaging, and histology results should be sufficient to make the diagnosis.

There are no prospective studies comparing response rates among the different regimens used to treat CDC. Amphotericin B deoxycholate, at a dose of 0.6 mg/kg per day, for a total dose of 1.5–2.0 g, is considered the mainstay of therapy. Approximately half of the members of an expert panel recommended adding flucytosine to the amphotericin B regimen [170] for the treatment of patients who are acutely ill with their CDC, notwithstanding the increased risk of flucytosine-related marrow toxicity in this population. Based on case-report and case-series data, [171–173] it has been suggested [124] that patients who are stable, and who have not been heavily colonized or fungemic with a fluconazole-resistant species of *Candida* (*C. glabrata*, *C. krusei*), can be treated successfully with that triazole antifungal at doses of 6 mg/kg per day (approximately 400 mg per day in an average sized adult). The lipid-based formulations of amphotericin B [174,175], voriconazole [176], caspofungin [177], are also effective in the treatment of CDC. It is recommended that any treatment be continued until symptoms, laboratory and imaging markers have resolved, or the lesions have calcified, and that patients continue to receive antifungal therapy during subsequent antileukemic therapy [178]. For individuals with refractory disease, adjunctive therapy with gamma-interferon and granulocyte-macrophage colony stimulating factor may be of some benefit [179].

References

1 Hann I, Viscli C, Paesmans M, et al. A comparison of outcome from febrile neutropenic episodes in children compared with adults: results from four EORTC studies. International Antimicrobial Therapy Cooperative Group (IATCG) of the European Organization for Research and Treatment of Cancer (EORTC). Br J Haematol 1997;99(3):580–8.

2 Bow EJ, Meddings JB. Intestinal mucosal dysfunction and infection during remission-induction therapy for acute myeloid leukaemia. Leukemia 2006;20(12):2087–92.

3 Laverdiere M, Rotstein C, Bow EJ, et al. Impact of fluconazole prophylaxis on fungal colonization and infection rates in neutropenic patients. The Canadian Fluconazole Study. J Antimicrob Chemother 2000;46(6):1001–8.

4 Hughes WT, Armstrong D, Bodey GP, et al. 2002 guidelines for the use of antimicrobial agents in neutropenic patients with cancer. Clin Infect Dis 2002;34(6):730–51.

5 Link H, Bohme A, Cornely OA, et al. Antimicrobial therapy of unexplained fever in neutropenic patients – guidelines of the Infectious Diseases Working Party (AGIHO) of the German Society of Hematology and Oncology (DGHO), Study Group Interventional Therapy of Unexplained Fever, Arbeitsgemeinschaft Supportivmassnahmen in der Onkologie (ASO) of the Deutsche Krebsgesellschaft (DKG-German Cancer Society). Ann Hematol 2003;82 Suppl 2:S105–17.

6 Freifeld A, Segal B, Baden LR, et al. Prevention and treatment of cancer-related infections. National Comprehensive Cancer Network – Clinical practice guidelines in Oncology v2. 4-9-2007. Electronic Citation. 2007.

7 Mackowiak PA, Bartlett JG, Borden EC, et al. Concepts of fever: recent advances and lingering dogma. Clin Infect Dis 1997;25(1):119–38.

8 Antin JH, Ferrara JL. Cytokine dysregulation and acute graft-versus-host disease. Blood 1992;80(12):2964–8.

9 Bow EJ, Loewen R, Cheang MS, et al. Cytotoxic therapy-induced D-xylose malabsorption and invasive infection during remission-induction therapy for acute myeloid leukemia in adults. J Clin Oncol 1997;15(6):2254–61.

10 Ferrara JL. Cytokines other than growth factors in bone marrow transplantation. Curr Opin Oncol 1994;6(2):127–34.

11 Krenger W, Ferrara JL. Graft-versus-host disease and the Th1/Th2 paradigm. Immunol Res 1996;15(1):50–73.

12 Sonis ST, Oster G, Fuchs H, et al. Oral mucositis and the clinical and economic outcomes of hematopoietic stem-cell transplantation. J Clin Oncol 2001;19(8):2201–5.

13 Peacock JE, Herrington DA, Wade JC, et al. Ciprofloxacin plus piperacillin compared with tobramycin plus piperacillin as empirical therapy in febrile neutropenic patients. A randomized, double-blind trial. Ann Intern Med 2002;137(2):77–87.

14 Bucaneve G, Micozzi A, Menichetti F, et al. Levofloxacin to prevent bacterial infection in patients with cancer and neutropenia. N Engl J Med 2005;353(10):977–87.

15 Bow EJ, Rotstein C, Noskin GA, et al. A randomized, open-label, multicenter comparative study of the efficacy and safety of piperacillin-tazobactam and cefepime for the empirical treatment of febrile neutropenic episodes in patients with hematologic malignancies. Clin Infect Dis 2006;43(4):447–59.

16 Cordonnier C, Buzyn A, Leverger G, et al. Epidemiology and risk factors for gram-positive coccal infections in neutropenia: toward a more targeted antibiotic strategy. Clin Infect Dis 2003;36(2):149–58.

17 Guidelines for preventing opportunistic infections among hematopoietic stem cell transplant recipients. Biol Blood Marrow Transplant 2000;6(6a):659–713; 5; 7–27; quiz 29–33.

18 Guidelines for prevention of nosocomial pneumonia. Centers for Disease Control and Prevention. MMWR Recomm Rep 1997;46(RR-1):1–79.

19 Dykewicz CA. Hospital infection control in hematopoietic stem cell transplant recipients. Emerg Infect Dis 2001;7(2):263–7.

20 Dykewicz CA. Summary of the Guidelines for Preventing Opportunistic Infections among Hematopoietic Stem Cell Transplant Recipients. Clin Infect Dis 2001;33(2):139–44.

21 Sehulster L, Chinn RY. Guidelines for environmental infection control in health-care facilities. Recommendations of CDC and the Healthcare Infection Control Practices Advisory Committee (HICPAC). MMWR Recomm Rep 2003;52(RR-10):1–42.

22 Tablan OC, Anderson LJ, Besser R, et al. Guidelines for preventing health-care – associated pneumonia, 2003: recommendations of CDC and the Healthcare Infection Control Practices Advisory Committee. MMWR Recomm Rep 2004;53(RR-3):1–36.

23 Sullivan KM, Dykewicz CA, Longworth DL, et al. Preventing opportunistic infections after hematopoietic stem cell

transplantation: the Centers for Disease Control and Prevention, Infectious Diseases Society of America, and American Society for Blood and Marrow Transplantation Practice Guidelines and beyond. Hematology Am Soc Hematol Educ Program 2001:392–421.

24 Sherertz RJ, Belani A, Kramer BS, et al. Impact of air filtration on nosocomial *Aspergillus* infections. Unique risk of bone marrow transplant recipients. Am J Med 1987;83(4):709–18.

25 Cornet M, Levy V, Fleury L, et al. Efficacy of prevention by high-efficiency particulate air filtration or laminar airflow against *Aspergillus* airborne contamination during hospital renovation. Infect Control Hosp Epidemiol 1999;20(7):508–13.

26 Passweg JR, Rowlings PA, Atkinson KA, et al. Influence of protective isolation on outcome of allogeneic bone marrow transplantation for leukemia. Bone Marrow Transplant 1998;21(12):1231–8.

27 Wald A, Leisenring W, van Burik JA, et al. Epidemiology of *Aspergillus* infections in a large cohort of patients undergoing bone marrow transplantation. J Infect Dis 1997;175(6):1459–66.

28 Nauseef WM, Maki DG. A study of the value of simple protective isolation in patients with granulocytopenia. N Engl J Med 1981;304(8):448–53.

29 Eckmanns T, Ruden H, Gastmeier P. The influence of high-efficiency particulate air filtration on mortality and fungal infection among highly immunosuppressed patients: a systematic review. J Infect Dis 2006;193(10):1408–18.

30 Cornely OA, Maertens J, Winston DJ, et al. Posaconazole vs. fluconazole or itraconazole prophylaxis in patients with neutropenia. N Engl J Med 2007;356(4):348–59.

31 Ullmann AJ, Lipton JH, Vesole DH, et al. Posaconazole or fluconazole for prophylaxis in severe graft-versus-host disease. N Engl J Med 2007;356(4):335–47.

32 Loo VG, Bertrand C, Dixon C, et al. Control of construction-associated nosocomial aspergillosis in an antiquated hematology unit. Infect Control Hosp Epidemiol 1996;17(6):360–4.

33 Bodey GP, Rodriguez V, Chang HY, et al. Fever and infection in leukemic patients: a study of 494 consecutive patients. Cancer 1978;41(4):1610–22.

34 Schimpff SC, Young VM, Greene WH, et al. Origin of infection in acute nonlymphocytic leukemia. Significance of hospital acquisition of potential pathogens. Ann Intern Med 1972;77(5):707–14.

35 Dietrich M, Gaus W, Vossen J, et al. Protective isolation and antimicrobial decontamination in patients with high susceptibility to infection. A prospective cooperative study of gnotobiotic care in acute leukemia patients. I: clinical results. Infection 1977;5(2):107–14.

36 Dietrich M, Rasche H, Rommel K, et al. Antimicrobial therapy as a part of the decontamination procedures for patients with acute leukemia. Eur J Cancer 1973;9(6):443–7.

37 Levi JA, Vincent PC, Jennis F, et al. Prophylactic oral antibiotics in the management of acute leukaemia. Med J Aust 1973;1(21):1025–9.

38 Levine AS, Siegel SE, Schreiber AD, et al. Protected environments and prophylactic antibiotics. A prospective controlled study of their utility in the therapy of acute leukemia. N Engl J Med 1973;288(10):477–83.

39 Preisler HD, Goldstein IM, Henderson ES. Gastrointestinal "sterilization" in the treatment of patients with acute leukemia. Cancer 1970;26(5):1076–81.

40 Rodriguez V, Bodey GP, Freireich EJ, et al. Randomized trial of protected environment – prophylactic antibiotics in 145 adults with acute leukemia. Medicine (Baltimore) 1978;57(3):253–66.

41 Schimpff SC, Greene WH, Young VM, et al. Infection prevention in acute nonlymphocytic leukemia. Laminar air flow room reverse isolation with oral, nonabsorbable antibiotic prophylaxis. Ann Intern Med 1975;82(3): 351–8.

42 Yates JW, Holland JF. A controlled study of isolation and endogenous microbial suppression in acute myelocytic leukemia patients. Cancer 1973;32(6):1490–8.

43 Gualtieri RJ, Donowitz GR, Kaiser DL, et al. Double-blind randomized study of prophylactic trimethoprim/sulfamethoxazole in granulocytopenic patients with hematologic malignancies. Am J Med 1983;74(6):934–40.

44 Gurwith MJ, Brunton JL, Lank BA, et al. A prospective controlled investigation of prophylactic trimethoprim/sulfamethoxazole in hospitalized granulocytopenic patients. Am J Med 1979;66(2):248–56.

45 Dekker AW, Rozenberg-Arska M, Sixma JJ, et al. Prevention of infection by trimethoprim-sulfamethoxazole plus amphotericin B in patients with acute nonlymphocytic leukaemia. Ann Intern Med 1981;95(5):555–9.

46 Engels EA, Lau J, Barza M. Efficacy of quinolone prophylaxis in neutropenic cancer patients: a meta-analysis. J Clin Oncol 1998;16(3):1179–87.

47 Bow EJ, Rayner E, Louie TJ. Comparison of norfloxacin with cotrimoxazole for infection prophylaxis in acute leukemia. The trade-off for reduced gram-negative sepsis. Am J Med 1988;84(5):847–54.

48 Lew MA, Kehoe K, Ritz J, et al. Ciprofloxacin versus trimethoprim/sulfamethoxazole for prophylaxis of bacterial infections in bone marrow transplant recipients: a randomized, controlled trial. J Clin Oncol 1995;13(1):239–50.

49 Cruciani M, Rampazzo R, Malena M, et al. Prophylaxis with fluoroquinolones for bacterial infections in neutropenic patients: a meta-analysis. Clin Infect Dis 1996; 23(4):795–805.

50 Cruciani M, Malena M, Bosco O, et al. Reappraisal with meta-analysis of the addition of Gram-positive prophylaxis to fluoroquinolone in neutropenic patients. J Clin Oncol 2003;21(22):4127–37.

51 Gafter-Gvili A, Fraser A, Paul M, et al. Meta-analysis: antibiotic prophylaxis reduces mortality in neutropenic patients. Ann Intern Med 2005;142(12 Pt 1):979–95.

52 Gafter-Gvili A, Paul M, Fraser A, et al. Effect of quinolone prophylaxis in afebrile neutropenic patients on microbial resistance: systematic review and meta-analysis. J Antimicrob Chemother 2007;59(1):5–22.

53 Leibovici L, Paul M, Cullen M, et al. Antibiotic prophylaxis in neutropenic patients: new evidence, practical decisions. Cancer 2006;107(8):1743–51.

54 van de Wetering MD, de Witte MA, Kremer LC, et al. Efficacy of oral prophylactic antibiotics in neutropenic afebrile oncology patients: a systematic review of randomised controlled trials. Eur J Cancer 2005;41(10):1372–82.

55 Imran H, Tleyjeh IM, Arndt CA, et al. Fluoroquinolone prophylaxis in patients with neutropenia: a meta-analysis of randomized placebo-controlled trials. Eur J Clin Microbiol Infect Dis 2008;27(1):53–63.

56 Pepin J, Saheb N, Coulombe MA, et al. Emergence of fluoroquinolones as the predominant risk factor for Clostridium difficile-associated diarrhea: a cohort study during an epidemic in Quebec. Clin Infect Dis 2005;41(9):1254–60.

57 Cullen M, Steven N, Billingham L, et al. Antibacterial prophylaxis after chemotherapy for solid tumors and lymphomas. N Engl J Med 2005 8;353(10):988–98.

58 Cullen MH, Billingham LJ, Gaunt CH, et al. Rational selection of patients for antibacterial prophylaxis after chemotherapy. J Clin Oncol 2007;25(30):4821–8.

59 Lyman GH, Delgado DJ. Risk and timing of hospitalization for febrile neutropenia in patients receiving CHOP, CHOP-R, or CNOP chemotherapy for intermediate-grade non-Hodgkin lymphoma. Cancer 2003;98(11):2402–9.

60 Vidal L, Paul M, Ben dor I, et al. Oral versus intravenous antibiotic treatment for febrile neutropenia in cancer patients: a systematic review and meta-analysis of randomized trials. J Antimicrob Chemother 2004;54(1):29–37.

61 Bucaneve G, Castagnola E, Viscoli C, et al. Quinolone prophylaxis for bacterial infections in afebrile high risk neutropenic patients. Eur J Cancer Supp 2007;5(2):5–12.

62 Kruger WH, Bohlius J, Cornely OA, et al. Antimicrobial prophylaxis in allogeneic bone marrow transplantation. Guidelines of the infectious diseases working party (AGIHO) of the german society of haematology and oncology. Ann Oncol 2005;16(8):1381–90.

63 Kern WV, Klose K, Jellen-Ritter AS, et al. Fluoroquinolone resistance of Escherichia coli at a cancer center: epidemiologic evolution and effects of discontinuing prophylactic fluoroquinolone use in neutropenic patients with leukemia. Eur J Clin Microbiol Infect Dis 2005;24(2):111–8.

64 Cometta A, Calandra T, Bille J, et al. Escherichia coli resistant to fluoroquinolones in patients with cancer and neutropenia. N Engl J Med 1994;330(17):1240–1.

65 Kern WV, Andriof E, Oethinger M, et al. Emergence of fluoroquinolone-resistant Escherichia coli at a cancer center. Antimicrob Agents Chemother 1994;38(4):681–7.

66 Viscoli C, Varnier O, Machetti M. Infections in patients with febrile neutropenia: epidemiology, microbiology, and risk stratification. Clin Infect Dis 2005;40 Suppl 4:S240–5.

67 Gafter-Gvili A, Fraser A, Paul M, et al. Antibiotic prophylaxis for bacterial infections in afebrile neutropenic patients following chemotherapy. Cochrane Database Syst Rev 2005 (4), CD004386, DOI: 10.1002/14651858.

68 Reuter S, Kern WV, Sigge A, et al. Impact of fluoroquinolone prophylaxis on reduced infection-related mortality among patients with neutropenia and hematologic malignancies. Clin Infect Dis 2005;40(8):1087–93.

69 Ringden O, Labopin M, Gorin NC, et al. Treatment with granulocyte colony-stimulating factor after allogeneic bone marrow transplantation for acute leukemia increases the risk of graft-versus-host disease and death: a study from the Acute Leukemia Working Party of the European Group for Blood and Marrow Transplantation. J Clin Oncol 2004;22(3):416–23.

70 Pagano L, Caira M, Candoni A, et al. The epidemiology of fungal infections in patients with hematologic malignancies: the SEIFEM-2004 study. Haematologica 2006;91(8):1068–75.

71 Pagano L, Caira M, Nosari A, et al. Fungal infections in recipients of hematopoietic stem cell transplants: results of the SEIFEM B-2004 study – Sorveglianza Epidemiologica Infezioni Fungine Nelle Emopatie Maligne. Clin Infect Dis 2007;45(9):1161–70.

72 Cornely OA, Ullmann AJ, Karthaus M. Evidence-based assessment of primary antifungal prophylaxis in patients with hematologic malignancies. Blood 2003;101(9):3365–72.

73 Glasmacher A, Prentice A, Gorschluter M, et al. Itraconazole prevents invasive fungal infections in neutropenic patients treated for hematologic malignancies: evidence from a meta-analysis of 3,597 patients. J Clin Oncol 2003;21(24):4615–26.

74 Kanda Y, Yamamoto R, Chizuka A, et al. Prophylactic action of oral fluconazole against fungal infection in neutropenic patients. A meta-analysis of 16 randomized, controlled trials. Cancer 2000;89(7):1611–25.

75 Bow EJ, Laverdiere M, Lussier N, et al. Antifungal prophylaxis for severely neutropenic chemotherapy recipients: a meta analysis of randomized-controlled clinical trials. Cancer 2002;94(12):3230–46.

76 Vardakas KZ, Michalopoulos A, Falagas ME. Fluconazole versus itraconazole for antifungal prophylaxis in neutropenic patients with haematological malignancies: a meta-analysis of randomised-controlled trials. Br J Haematol 2005;131(1):22–8.

77 Robenshtok E, Gafter-Gvili A, Goldberg E, et al. Antifungal prophylaxis in cancer patients after chemotherapy or hematopoietic stem-cell transplantation: systematic review and meta-analysis. J Clin Oncol 2007;25(34):5471–89.

78 Vehreschild JJ, Bohme A, Buchheidt D, et al. A double-blind trial on prophylactic voriconazole (VRC) or placebo during induction chemotherapy for acute myelogenous leukaemia (AML). J Infect 2007;55(5):445–9.

79 Wingard J, Carter C, Walsh TJ, et al. Results of a randomized, double-blind trial of fluconazole (FLU) vs. voriconazole (VORI) for the prevention of invasive fungal infections (IFI) in 600 allogeneic blood and marrow transplant (BMT) patients (Abstract #163). Blood 2007;110(11):55a.

80 Ascioglu S, Rex JH, de Pauw B, et al. Defining opportunistic invasive fungal infections in immunocompromised patients with cancer and hematopoietic stem cell transplants: an international consensus. Clin Infect Dis 2002;34(1):7–14.

81 De Pauw BE, Donnelly JP. Prophylaxis and aspergillosis – has the principle been proven? N Engl J Med 2007; 356(4):409–11.

82 De Pauw BE. Between over- and undertreatment of invasive fungal disease. Clin Infect Dis 2005;41(9): 1251–3.

83 Maertens J, Theunissen K, Verhoef G, et al. Galactomannan and computed tomography-based preemptive antifungal therapy in neutropenic patients at high risk for invasive fungal infection: a prospective feasibility study. Clin Infect Dis 2005;41(9):1242–50.

84 Maertens J, Frere P, Lass-Florl C, et al. Primary antifungal prophylaxis in leukaemia patients. Eur J Cancer Suppl 2007;5(2):43–8.

85 Cornely OA, Bohme A, Buchheidt D, et al. Prophylaxis of invasive fungal infections in patients with hematological malignancies and solid tumors – guidelines of the Infectious Diseases Working Party (AGIHO) of the German Society of Hematology and Oncology (DGHO). Ann Hematol 2003;82 Suppl 2:S186–200.

86 Wittman B, Horan J, Lyman GH. Prophylactic colony-stimulating factors in children receiving myelosuppressive chemotherapy: a meta-analysis of randomized controlled trials. Cancer Treat Rev 2006;32(4):289–303.

87 Dekker A, Bulley S, Beyene J, et al. Meta-analysis of randomized controlled trials of prophylactic granulocyte colony-stimulating factor and granulocyte-macrophage colony-stimulating factor after autologous and allogeneic stem cell transplantation. J Clin Oncol 2006;24(33):5207–15.

88 Sung L, Nathan PC, Lange B, et al. Prophylactic granulocyte colony-stimulating factor and granulocyte-macrophage colony-stimulating factor decrease febrile neutropenia after chemotherapy in children with cancer: a meta-analysis of randomized controlled trials. J Clin Oncol 2004;22(16):3350–6.

89 Lyman GH, Kuderer NM. The economics of the colony-stimulating factors in the prevention and treatment of febrile neutropenia. Crit Rev Oncol Hematol 2004;50(2):129–46.

90 Lyman GH, Kuderer NM, Djulbegovic B. Prophylactic granulocyte colony-stimulating factor in patients receiving dose-intensive cancer chemotherapy: a meta-analysis. Am J Med 2002;112(5):406–11.

91 Bohlius J, Reiser M, Schwarzer G, et al. Granulopoiesis-stimulating factors to prevent adverse effects in the treatment of malignant lymphoma. Cochrane Database Syst Rev 2004 (3), CD003189\, DOI: 10.1002/14651858.

92 Kuderer NM, Dale DC, Crawford J, et al. Impact of primary prophylaxis with granulocyte colony-stimulating factor on febrile neutropenia and mortality in adult cancer patients receiving chemotherapy: a systematic review. J Clin Oncol 2007;25(21):3158–67.

93 Clark OA, Lyman GH, Castro AA, et al. Colony-stimulating factors for chemotherapy-induced febrile neutropenia: a meta-analysis of randomized controlled trials. J Clin Oncol 2005;23(18):4198–214.

94 Caggiano V, Weiss RV, Rickert TS, et al. Incidence, cost, and mortality of neutropenia hospitalization associated with chemotherapy. Cancer 2005;103(9):1916–24.

95 Smith TJ, Khatcheressian J, Lyman GH, et al. 2006 update of recommendations for the use of white blood cell growth factors: an evidence-based clinical practice guideline. J Clin Oncol 2006;24(19):3187–205.

96 Spielberger R, Stiff P, Bensinger W, et al. Palifermin for oral mucositis after intensive therapy for hematologic cancers. N Engl J Med 2004;351(25):2590–8.

97 DesJardin JA, Falagas ME, Ruthazer R, et al. Clinical utility of blood cultures drawn from indwelling central venous catheters in hospitalized patients with cancer. Ann Intern Med 1999;131(9):641–7.

98 Sickles EA, Greene WH, Wiernik PH. Clinical presentation of infection in granulocytopenic patients. Arch Intern Med 1975;135(5):715–9.

99 Rangel-Frausto MS, Pittet D, Costigan M, et al. The natural history of the systemic inflammatory response syndrome (SIRS). A prospective study. JAMA 1995;273(2):117–23.

100 Regazzoni CJ, Khoury M, Irrazabal C, et al. Neutropenia and the development of the systemic inflammatory response syndrome. Intensive Care Med 2003;29(1):135–8.

101 Rolston KV. New trends in patient management: risk-based therapy for febrile patients with neutropenia. Clin Infect Dis 1999;29(3):515–21.

102 Rolston KV, Rubenstein EB, Freifeld A. Early empiric antibiotic therapy for febrile neutropenia patients at low risk. Infect Dis Clin North Am 1996;10(2):223–37.

103 Kern WV. Risk assessment and treatment of low-risk patients with febrile neutropenia. Clin Infect Dis 2006;42(4):533–40.

104 Talcott JA, Siegel RD, Finberg R, et al. Risk assessment in cancer patients with fever and neutropenia: a prospective, two-center validation of a prediction rule. J Clin Oncol 1992;10(2):316–22.

105 Klastersky J, Paesmans M, Rubenstein EB, et al. The Multinational Association for Supportive Care in Cancer risk index: A multinational scoring system for identifying low-risk febrile neutropenic cancer patients. J Clin Oncol 2000;18(16):3038–51.

106 Uys A, Rapoport BL, Anderson R. Febrile neutropenia: a prospective study to validate the Multinational Association of Supportive Care of Cancer (MASCC) risk-index score. Support Care Cancer 2004;12(8):555–60.

107 Klastersky J, Paesmans M, Georgala A, et al. Outpatient oral antibiotics for febrile neutropenic cancer patients using a score predictive for complications. J Clin Oncol 2006;24(25):4129–34.

108 Chang HY, Rodriguez V, Narboni G, et al. Causes of death in adults with acute leukemia. Medicine (Baltimore) 1976;55(3):259–68.

109 Hersh EM, Bodey GP, Nies BA, et al. Causes of Death in Acute Leukemia: a Ten-Year Study of 414 Patients from 1954–1963. JAMA 1965;193:105–9.

110 Lowder JN, Lazarus HM, Herzig RH. Bacteremias and fungemias in oncologic patients with central venous

catheters: changing spectrum of infection. Arch Intern Med 1982;142(8):1456–9.

111 Bishop JF, Lowenthal RM, Joshua D, et al. Etoposide in acute nonlymphocytic leukemia. Australian Leukemia Study Group. Blood 1990;75(1):27–32.

112 Bochud PY, Eggiman P, Calandra T, et al. Bacteremia due to viridans streptococcus in neutropenic patients with cancer: clinical spectrum and risk factors. Clin Infect Dis 1994;18(1):25–31.

113 Weisman SJ, Scoopo FJ, Johnson GM, et al. Septicemia in pediatric oncology patients: the significance of viridans streptococcal infections. J Clin Oncol 1990;8(3):453–9.

114 Schimpff S, Satterlee W, Young VM, et al. Empiric therapy with carbenicillin and gentamicin for febrile patients with cancer and granulocytopenia. N Engl J Med 1971;284(19):1061–5.

115 Feld R. Vancomycin as part of initial empirical antibiotic therapy for febrile neutropenia in patients with cancer: pros and cons. Clin Infect Dis 1999;29(3):503–7.

116 The EORTC International Antimicrobial Therapy Cooperative Group. Ceftazidime combined with a short or long course of amikacin for empirical therapy of gram-negative bacteremia in cancer patients with granulocytopenia. N Engl J Med 1987;317(27):1692–8.

117 Vancomycin added to empirical combination antibiotic therapy for fever in granulocytopenic cancer patients. European Organization for Research and Treatment of Cancer (EORTC) International Antimicrobial Therapy Cooperative Group and the National Cancer Institute of Canada-Clinical Trials Group. J Infect Dis 1991;163(5):951–8.

118 The International Antimicrobial Therapy Cooperative Group of the European Organization for Research and Treatment of Cancer. Efficacy and toxicity of single daily doses of amikacin and ceftriaxone versus multiple daily doses of amikacin and ceftazidime for infection in patients with cancer and granulocytopenia. Ann Intern Med 1993;119(7 Pt 1):584–93.

119 Edmond MB, Ober JF, Weinbaum DL, et al. Vancomycin-resistant Enterococcus faecium bacteremia: risk factors for infection. Clin Infect Dis 1995;20(5):1126–33.

120 Morris JG, Jr., Shay DK, Hebden JN, et al. Enterococci resistant to multiple antimicrobial agents, including vancomycin. Establishment of endemicity in a university medical center. Ann Intern Med 1995;123(4):250–9.

121 Shay DK, Maloney SA, Montecalvo M, et al. Epidemiology and mortality risk of vancomycin-resistant enterococcal bloodstream infections. J Infect Dis 1995;172(4):993–1000.

122 Paul M, Borok S, Fraser A, et al. Additional anti-Gram-positive antibiotic treatment for febrile neutropenic cancer patients. Cochrane Database Syst Rev 2005 (3), CD003914, DOI: 10.1002/14651858.

123 Paul M, Yahav D, Fraser A, et al. Empirical antibiotic monotherapy for febrile neutropenia: systematic review and meta-analysis of randomized controlled trials. J Antimicrob Chemother 2006;57(2):176–89.

124 Rex JH, Walsh TJ, Sobel JD, et al. Practice guidelines for the treatment of candidiasis. Infectious Diseases Society of America. Clin Infect Dis 2000;30(4):662–78.

125 EORTC International Antimicrobial Therapy Cooperative Group. Empiric antifungal therapy in febrile granulocytopenic patients. Am J Med 1989;86(6 Pt 1):668–72.

126 Leenders AC, Daenen S, Jansen RL, et al. Liposomal amphotericin B compared with amphotericin B deoxycholate in the treatment of documented and suspected neutropenia-associated invasive fungal infections. Br J Haematol 1998;103(1):205–12.

127 Prentice HG, Hann IM, Herbrecht R, et al. A randomized comparison of liposomal versus conventional amphotericin B for the treatment of pyrexia of unknown origin in neutropenic patients. Br J Haematol 1997;98(3):711–8.

128 Walsh TJ, Finberg RW, Arndt C, et al. Liposomal amphotericin B for empirical therapy in patients with persistent fever and neutropenia. National Institute of Allergy and Infectious Diseases Mycoses Study Group. N Engl J Med 1999;340(10):764–71.

129 White MH, Bowden RA, Sandler ES, et al. Randomized, double-blind clinical trial of amphotericin B colloidal dispersion vs. amphotericin B in the empirical treatment of fever and neutropenia. Clin Infect Dis 1998;27(2):296–302.

130 Boogaerts M, Winston DJ, Bow EJ, et al. Intravenous and oral itraconazole versus intravenous amphotericin B deoxycholate as empirical antifungal therapy for persistent fever in neutropenic patients with cancer who are receiving broad-spectrum antibacterial therapy. A randomized, controlled trial. Ann Intern Med 2001;135(6):412–22.

131 Walsh TJ, Pappas P, Winston DJ, et al. Voriconazole compared with liposomal amphotericin B for empirical antifungal therapy in patients with neutropenia and persistent fever. N Engl J Med 2002;346(4):225–34.

132 Walsh TJ, Teppler H, Donowitz GR, et al. Caspofungin versus liposomal amphotericin B for empirical antifungal therapy in patients with persistent fever and neutropenia. N Engl J Med 2004;351(14):1391–402.

133 Kern WV, Cometta A, De Bock R, et al. Oral versus intravenous empirical antimicrobial therapy for fever in patients with granulocytopenia who are receiving cancer chemotherapy. International Antimicrobial Therapy Cooperative Group of the European Organization for Research and Treatment of Cancer. N Engl J Med 1999;341(5):312–8.

134 Maher DW, Lieschke GJ, Green M, et al. Filgrastim in patients with chemotherapy-induced febrile neutropenia. A double-blind, placebo-controlled trial. Ann Intern Med 1994;121(7):492–501.

135 Cometta A, Calandra T, Gaya H, et al. Monotherapy with meropenem versus combination therapy with ceftazidime plus amikacin as empiric therapy for fever in granulocytopenic patients with cancer. The International Antimicrobial Therapy Cooperative Group of the European Organization for Research and Treatment of Cancer and the Gruppo Italiano Malattie Ematologiche Maligne dell'Adulto Infection Program. Antimicrob Agents Chemother 1996;40(5):1108–15.

136 De Pauw BE, Deresinski SC, Feld R, et al. Ceftazidime compared with piperacillin and tobramycin for the empiric treatment of fever in neutropenic patients with cancer. A multicenter randomized trial. The Intercontinental Antimicrobial Study Group. Ann Intern Med 1994;120(10):834–44.

137 Gorschluter M, Mey U, Strehl J, et al. Neutropenic enterocolitis in adults: systematic analysis of evidence quality. Eur J Haematol 2005;75(1):1–13.

138 Yates J, Glidewell O, Wiernik P, et al. Cytosine arabinoside with daunorubicin or adriamycin for therapy of acute myelocytic leukemia: a CALGB study. Blood 1982;60(2):454–62.

139 Bremer CT, Monahan BP. Necrotizing enterocolitis in neutropenia and chemotherapy: a clinical update and old lessons relearned. Curr Gastroenterol Rep 2006; 8(4):333–41.

140 Kouroussis C, Samonis G, Androulakis N, et al. Successful conservative treatment of neutropenic enterocolitis complicating taxane-based chemotherapy: a report of five cases. Am J Clin Oncol 2000;23(3):309–13.

141 Kasper K, Loewen R, Bow E. Neutropenic enterocolitis (NEC) in adult leukemia (AL) patients (pts) in Manitoba. Clin Infect Dis 1996;23(2):866.

142 Wade DS, Nava HR, Douglass HO, Jr. Neutropenic enterocolitis. Clinical diagnosis and treatment. Cancer 1992;69(1):17–23.

143 Gomez L, Martino R, Rolston KV. Neutropenic enterocolitis: spectrum of the disease and comparison of definite and possible cases. Clin Infect Dis 1998;27(4):695–9.

144 Gorschluter M, Marklein G, Hofling K, et al. Abdominal infections in patients with acute leukaemia: a prospective study applying ultrasonography and microbiology. Br J Haematol 2002;117(2):351–8.

145 Maki DG. Reactions associated with midline catheters for intravenous access. Ann Intern Med 1995;123(11):884–6.

146 Greene JN. Catheter-related complications of cancer therapy. Infect Dis Clin North Am 1996;10(2):255–95.

147 Press OW, Ramsey PG, Larson EB, et al. Hickman catheter infections in patients with malignancies. Medicine (Baltimore) 1984;63(4):189–200.

148 Maki DG, Weise CE, Sarafin HW. A semiquantitative culture method for identifying intravenous-catheter-related infection. N Engl J Med 1977;296(23):1305–9.

149 Jaeger K, Zenz S, Juttner B, et al. Reduction of catheter-related infections in neutropenic patients: a prospective controlled randomized trial using a chlorhexidine and silver sulfadiazine-impregnated central venous catheter. Ann Hematol 2005;84(4):258–62.

150 Benezra D, Kiehn TE, Gold JW, et al. Prospective study of infections in indwelling central venous catheters using quantitative blood cultures. Am J Med 1988;85(4):495–8.

151 Hiemenz J, Skelton J, Pizzo PA. Perspective on the management of catheter-related infections in cancer patients. Pediatr Infect Dis 1986;5(1):6–11.

152 Raad, II, Bodey GP. Infectious complications of indwelling vascular catheters. Clin Infect Dis 1992;15(2):197–208.

153 Raad I, Davis S, Khan A, et al. Impact of central venous catheter removal on the recurrence of catheter-related coagulase-negative staphylococcal bacteremia. Infect Control Hosp Epidemiol 1992;13(4):215–21.

154 Raaf JH. Results from use of 826 vascular access devices in cancer patients. Cancer 1985;55(6):1312–21.

155 Fleece DM, Faerber EN, de Chadarevian JP. Pathological case of the month. Hepatosplenic candidiasis in a patient with leukemia. Arch Pediatr Adolesc Med 1998;152(10):1033–4.

156 Ong ST, Kueh YK. Hepatic candidiasis: persistent pyrexia in a patient with acute myeloid leukaemia after recovery from consolidation therapy-induced neutropenia. Ann Acad Med Singapore 1993;22(2):257–60.

157 Verdeguer A, Fernandez JM, Esquembre C, et al. Hepatosplenic candidiasis in children with acute leukemia. Cancer 1990;65(4):874–7.

158 Woolley I, Curtis D, Szer J, et al. High dose cytosine arabinoside is a major risk factor for the development of hepatosplenic candidiasis in patients with leukemia. Leuk Lymphoma 1997;27(5–6):469–74.

159 Chubachi A, Miura I, Ohshima A, et al. Risk factors for hepatosplenic abscesses in patients with acute leukemia receiving empiric azole treatment. Am J Med Sci 1994;308(6):309–12.

160 Rotstein C, Bow EJ, Laverdiere M, et al. Randomized placebo-controlled trial of fluconazole prophylaxis for neutropenic cancer patients: benefit based on purpose and intensity of cytotoxic therapy. The Canadian Fluconazole Prophylaxis Study Group. Clin Infect Dis 1999;28(2):331–40.

161 Bow EJ, Loewen R, Cheang MS, et al. Invasive fungal disease in adults undergoing remission-induction therapy for acute myeloid leukemia: the pathogenetic role of the anti-leukemic regimen. Clin Infect Dis 1995;21(2):361–9.

162 Sallah S, Wan JY, Nguyen NP, et al. Analysis of factors related to the occurrence of chronic disseminated candidiasis in patients with acute leukemia in a non-bone marrow transplant setting: a follow-up study. Cancer 2001;92(6):1349–53.

163 Marr KA, Seidel K, White TC, et al. Candidemia in allogeneic blood and marrow transplant recipients: evolution of risk factors after the adoption of prophylactic fluconazole. J Infect Dis 2000;181(1):309–16.

164 Viscoli C, Girmenia C, Marinus A, et al. Candidemia in cancer patients: a prospective, multicenter surveillance study by the Invasive Fungal Infection Group (IFIG) of the European Organization for Research and Treatment of Cancer (EORTC). Clin Infect Dis 1999;28(5):1071–9.

165 Masood A, Sallah S. Chronic disseminated candidiasis in patients with acute leukemia: emphasis on diagnostic definition and treatment. Leuk Res 2005;29(5):493–501.

166 von Eiff M, Fahrenkamp A, Roos N, et al. Hepatosplenic candidosis – a late manifestation of Candida septicemia. Mycoses 1990;33(6):283–90.

167 Semelka RC, Kelekis NL, Sallah S, et al. Hepatosplenic fungal disease: diagnostic accuracy and spectrum of appearances on MR imaging. AJR Am J Roentgenol 1997;169(5):1311–6.

168 Anttila VJ, Lamminen AE, Bondestam S, et al. Magnetic resonance imaging is superior to computed tomography and ultrasonography in imaging infectious liver foci in acute leukaemia. Eur J Haematol 1996;56(1–2):82–7.

169 Anttila VJ, Ruutu P, Bondestam S, et al. Hepatosplenic yeast infection in patients with acute leukemia: a diagnostic problem. Clin Infect Dis 1994;18(6):979–81.

170 Edwards JE, Jr., Bodey GP, Bowden RA, et al. International Conference for the Development of a Consensus on the Management and Prevention of Severe Candidal Infections. Clin Infect Dis 1997;25(1):43–59.

171 Anaissie E, Bodey GP, Kantarjian H, et al. Fluconazole therapy for chronic disseminated candidiasis in patients with leukemia and prior amphotericin B therapy. Am J Med 1991;91(2):142–50.

172 Flannery MT, Simmons DB, Saba H, et al. Fluconazole in the treatment of hepatosplenic candidiasis. Arch Intern Med 1992;152(2):406–8.

173 Kauffman CA, Bradley SF, Ross SC, et al. Hepatosplenic candidiasis: successful treatment with fluconazole. Am J Med 1991;91(2):137–41.

174 Sharland M, Hay RJ, Davies e.g. Liposomal amphotericin B in hepatic candidosis. Arch Dis Child. 1994 Jun;70(6):546–7.

175 Lopez-Berestein G, Bodey GP, Frankel LS, et al. Treatment of hepatosplenic candidiasis with liposomal-amphotericin B. J Clin Oncol 1987;5(2):310–7.

176 Perfect JR, Marr KA, Walsh TJ, et al. Voriconazole treatment for less-common, emerging, or refractory fungal infections. Clin Infect Dis 2003;36(9):1122–31.

177 Cornely OA, Lasso M, Betts R, et al. Caspofungin for the treatment of less common forms of invasive candidiasis. J Antimicrob Chemother 2007;60(2):363–9.

178 Walsh TJ, Whitcomb PO, Revankar SG, et al. Successful treatment of hepatosplenic candidiasis through repeated cycles of chemotherapy and neutropenia. Cancer 1995;76(11):2357–62.

179 Poynton CH, Barnes RA, Rees J. Interferon gamma and granulocyte-macrophage colony-stimulating factor for the treatment of hepatosplenic candidosis in patients with acute leukemia. Clin Infect Dis 1998;26(1):239–40.

CHAPTER 16

Infections in general surgery

Christine H. Lee

Surgical site infections

Case presentation 1

A previously healthy 17-year-old male underwent emergency appendectomy for perforated appendicitis. Perioperatively, he received intravenous gentamicin and metronidazole. Within 24 hours of surgery, he developed progressively severe, generalized abdominal and right flank pain. This was associated with nausea, anorexia, and diaphoresis. On examination, he appeared flushed. The heart rate was 140 per minute; blood pressure 100/40; respiratory rate 26 per minute; temperature 39.4°C. Abdomen was diffusely tender. Surgical wound site revealed areas of dusky discoloration, purulent discharge, and foul odor.

Postoperative site soft-tissue infections

It is estimated more than 40 million surgeries are performed each year in the United States [1]. Surgical site infections (SSI) are one of the most common types of infections among surgical patients and occur following 2–17.9% of operations [2,3]. This, however, is likely an underestimation as the postoperative length of hospital stay has decreased significantly over the past decade and several studies indicate that 50–84% of SSIs occur after hospital discharge [3–6].

SSIs are subclassified into *superficial incisional*, involving the skin and subcutaneous tissues; *deep incisional*, affecting the fascial and muscle layers of the incision, and *organ space*, which describes infections in any part of the organs or spaces other than the incision that was exposed during the procedure. Organ space infections include postoperative intraabdominal abscesses, empyema, or mediastinitis [7]. Management of organ space infections is predominantly surgical and is beyond the scope of this review. The SSI risk factors, burden on healthcare costs, associated morbidity, mortality, and preventive measures are well described in the literature.

Evaluation of postoperative patients with suspected infection

Fever is the most common symptom of postoperative infection. Fever occurs in approximately 30–40% of patients after a major operative procedure [8,9]. Fever during the first 3 days of the postoperative period is often due to a noninfectious cause: medications, atelectases, deep vein thrombosis, or injury to tissue [10]. In a retrospective review of patients undergoing major gynecologic surgery, Fanning et al. identified that 84% of patients, who were discharged despite experiencing fever of ≥38.0°C, did not have a documented infectious etiology for the fever [8]. Presence of fever alone is not an indication for initiation of antibiotic therapy.

A postoperative patient with fever requires a systematic, complete evaluation. This includes careful, repeat history, complete physical examination, along with supportive laboratory tests, if indicated: complete blood count with differential, urinalysis, bacteriologic cultures of blood, tissue/aspirated fluid from surgical site. Selective imaging studies, particularly computed tomography of the abdomen and pelvis, may be useful in evaluating a patient with late-onset, postoperative fever, after an abdominal surgery,

Evidence-Based Infectious Diseases, 2nd edition. Edited by Mark Loeb, Fiona Smaill and Marek Smieja. © 2009 Wiley-Blackwell Publishing, ISBN: 978-1-4051-7026-0

without an apparent source, in localizing occult infection or intraabdominal abscess. The common causes of nonsurgical site-related, postoperative infections and fever, which include urinary, respiratory tracts, and catheter-related infections can be readily delineated by meticulous assessment of the patient. The majority of SSIs occur 5 or more days after surgery but necrotizing soft tissue infections, particularly due to clostridial species or Group A streptococci can manifest within 36 hours after an operation [11].

If the clinical assessment establishes the diagnosis of surgical site infection, as indicated by presence of purulent discharge from the wound, then the treatment is to open the wound for drainage. To date, there are no RCTs which have compared drainage to conservative management. The next step is to determine whether further operative intervention is necessary. SSIs, with the exception of uncomplicated cellulitis, require mechanical procedures to open an infected wound, drain abscesses, and remove devitalized tissues. An empiric antibiotic therapy is warranted along with exploration of the wound if there is painful spreading erythema over the surgical incision site, suggestive of cellulitis, or accompanying fever of ≥38.0°C, tenderness, edema, and an extending margin of erythema at or around the surgical incision site.

A number of factors will influence the choice of empiric antimicrobial agent(s). These include patient-associated factors, including host immunity, presence of diabetes mellitus, and length of preoperative hospital stay; procedure-associated factors such as the type and duration of perioperative antimicrobial prophylaxis, and the duration of operation, class of surgical site [12]; and institution-specific factors such as the hospital's microbial antibiogram (antibiotic susceptibility profile). Many SSIs are polymicrobial, often including microbes resistant to antibiotics. *Staphylococcus aureus* is the most commonly isolated organism from SSIs, followed by *Streptococcus pyogenes*, *Escherichia coli*, other enterobacteriaceae and anaerobes [13,14]. Based on these data, the responsible pathogens and the antibiotic susceptibility can be postulated and appropriate antibiotic can be instituted until the culture results are available.

Diagnostic work-up recommendations include obtaining aerobic and anaerobic cultures from the site of infection prior to initiating antibiotic treatment. The rationale for obtaining culture is to identify the bacteria involved in the infection and to institute appropriate antibiotic therapy [15]. Cultures should be transported at room temperature to the laboratory in appropriate aerobic and anaerobic transport media within 2 hours of specimen collection. Deep aspirates or tissue cultures are superior to swab samples in providing clinically relevant results [16]. The results of culture and antibiotic susceptibility can aid in modifying the antibiotic regimen as treatment failure can occur in the presence of resistant organisms [17,18].

Postoperative necrotizing fasciitis

Case presentation 1 (continued)

The wound was completely exposed and packed with sterile dressings. The infectious diseases service was consulted. Recommendation was made to surgically explore the wound to rule out possible necrotizing fasciitis and the addition of intravenous cefazolin to the existing antibiotic regimen of gentamicin and metronidazole. Surgical exploration revealed infection tracking into transversalis fascia and internal oblique. Portions of the transversalis fascia were necrotic. Infected and necrotic materials were completely evacuated. A Jackson-Pratt drain was placed in the pelvis. Histopathology confirmed the diagnosis of necrotizing fasciitls. Culture of the tissue grew mixed facultative anaerobic and anaerobic intestinal organisms.

Necrotizing fasciitis is a rare but potentially life-threatening, soft-tissue infection and it encompasses two types based on the bacteriologic entities [19]. Type I is caused by anaerobic species, especially *B. fragilis* in combination with one or more facultative anaerobic organisms other than Group A streptococci. Type II is caused by Group A streptococci, alone or in combination with other bacteria, most commonly *Staphylococcus aureus*. It is useful to distinguish the two types of necrotizing fasciitis as the medical management of type II differs from type I, although there is no difference in surgical management between the two types. Postoperative necrotizing fasciitis, as with other necrotizing fasciitis, is usually an acute, rapidly extensive inflammatory process [20]. The affected area is initially exquisitely painful and tender and this is associated with rapidly progressive erythema, and poorly demarcated edema. The course is followed by fever, hemodynamic instability, skin discoloration from erythema to violaceous-gray, bullae formation and crepitation may be present. By day 4 and 5 of onset, frank cutaneous gangrene develops. Owing to associated morbidity and mortality with delay in diagnosis and management, it is paramount to recognize and institute immediate operative intervention when necrotizing fasciitis is clinically suspected [21,22].

During the early stage, it may be difficult to clinically distinguish necrotizing fasciitis from cellulitis as the local features of the affected area can be nonspecific. Presence of severe systemic toxicity and fever while the cutaneous appearance is innocuous should alert the clinician of possible underlying necrotizing fasciitis. The diagnosis of necrotizing fasciitis is made at surgery and it is essential to extensively excise the affected skin and subcutaneous tissues beyond healthy fascia [20,22]. Post debridement, a patient with necrotizing fasciitis usually requires critical care support and at times repeated surgical debridement.

Empiric antibiotic therapy and intravenous fluid must be promptly administered as soon as the diagnosis of invasive soft-tissue infection is considered. Initially, the antimicrobial therapy should consist of a regimen which reliably targets streptococci, *S. aureus*, enterobacteriaceae, and anaerobic organisms. For type I necrotizing fasciitis, broad-spectrum antibiotic is continued as it is an infection due to mixed organisms. In type II necrotizing fasciitis, confirmed by detection of Group A streptococci, a combination of high-dose intravenous penicillin G and clindamycin is the treatment of choice [23–25]. Necrotizing fasciitis may be accompanied by streptococcal toxic shock syndrome (STSS), as evidenced by a blood pressure of 90mmHg systolic or below and evidence of end-organ damage, including renal, liver, pulmonary (adult respiratory distress syndrome) impairment in addition to rash or necrosis. A comparative observational study by Kaul et al. [26] showed that intravenous immunoglobulin (IVIG) administration for STSS was associated with an increase in 30-day survival. Others have also described the successful use of IVIG in patients with STSS [27,28].

In summary, despite advances in surgical techniques and infection control practices SSIs continue to be common nosocomial infections. The basic principle of management of SSIs is to open the infected site and allow it to drain. Antibiotics have an adjunct role only when there is invasive infection. There is no guideline or study which specifically addresses the duration of antibiotic therapy for SSIs. The patient's overall clinical response to surgical and adjunct pharmacologic interventions should guide the duration and the route of antibiotic administration.

Mesh infections after incisional hernia repair

Case presentation 2

A 59-year-old woman presents with a 4-day history of purulent discharge from a previous abdominal surgical site, fever, and malaise. One month prior to this presentation, she underwent abdominal wall sarcoma resection, followed by insertion of polytetrafluoroethylene mesh and reconstruction of the abdominal wall. She has a temperature of 37.6°C, a blood pressure of 128/82 mmHg, a respiratory rate of 20 breaths per minute, a heart rate of 90 beats per minute, and oxygen saturation of 96% while breathing ambient air. Abdominal examination revealed erythema and induration over the right, lateral aspect of the abdomen. There were three small areas of opening with thick, purulent yellow secretion at the right lateral corner of the graft. The white blood cell count was 14.3×10^9/L. The skin and subcutaneous tissues are opened and the mesh was exposed. The patient was managed with surgical debridement and irrigation of the wound.

The culture of the wound grew Staphylococcus aureus, sensitive to methicillin. Intravenous cloxacillin 2g was started and the surgeon sought your advice for further management of this patient.

Following an elective laparotomy, between 10% and 20% of patients develop incisional hernia [29]. Without prompt reduction and repair, there maybe serious complications, such as incarceration and strangulation of the small bowel [29–31]. The major risk factors for developing incisional hernia are obesity, malnutrition, wound infection, and reopened incisions [32]. After a primary repair, several studies have found high rates of recurrent hernia, from 24% to 54%. A number of studies [33,34], including a multicenter randomized trial [29], indicated reduced relapse rates using prosthetic biomaterials compared to suture repair of the hernia.

Evidence to guide management of mesh infections is based on biologic principles and animal studies, as there are no cohort or randomized controlled trials. Polypropylene (Marlex, Bard Inc.) and polytetrafluoroethylene (Gore-Tex, WL Gore and Assoc. Inc.) are the most commonly used prosthetic biomaterials for ventral hernia repairs [34]. Compared to polypropylene mesh (PPM), polytetrafluoroethylene (PTFE) possesses significantly superior mechanical properties, which facilitate incorporation of the mesh into fibrocollagenous tissue and at the same time prevent permeation of water. PPM has been shown to cause extensive visceral adhesions and erosion of the skin or intestines with long-term use [35–37]. Two small animal studies addressed the role of PPM and PTFE use in repair of contaminated abdominal wall defects. Bleichrodt et al. [35] from the Netherlands studied 42 rats; PTFE patch were used on 21 rats to repair abdominal wall defects contaminated with bacteria and, similarly, 21 other rats received PPM mesh. Wound infection occurred in 16/21 rats in the PTFE and in 14/21 rats in the PPM group. Two rats in each group died as a result of ileus (1/4) or peritonitis (3/4). In contrast, Brown et al. [36] reported significantly fewer bacteria ($P < 0.05$) adhered to PTFE compared to PPM, in an experimental model using 100 guinea pigs with simulated abdominal wall defects in the presence of *Staphylococcus aureus*-related intraabdominal infection. Based on the above results and paucity of human studies, it appears that there is a lack of distinction between the two prosthetic biomaterials in repair of contaminated abdominal wall defects.

Contrary to common perception, there are no data to suggest that infection occurs more commonly with the use of mesh insertion, compared with conventional suture repair. The reported infection rates related to mesh use is 0.03–0.8%, and that of suture repair is 1.0–1.2% [38–41].

The immediate host response to mesh implantation is recruitment and infiltration of inflammatory cells. In an ideal milieu, acute inflammation is replaced by fibroblasts, multinucleated giant cells, leading to complete incorporation of deposited mesh into the neighboring tissues and induction of collagen synthesis [42,43]. When the inserted mesh is not properly taken up, complications such as accumulation of seromas (an excellent medium for bacterial growth), chronic sinus formation, fecal fistula, or mesh extrusion may occur [32,44–47]. In a study by Amid et al. [48] the majority of these complications were attributable to errors in surgical techniques, for example improper positioning of the mesh, inadequate fixation and use of unabsorbable sutures.

Surgical site infections occurring early in the postoperative phase are usually independent of mesh utilization. These infections are primarily limited to the skin or subcutaenous layers and do not appear to interfere with proper mesh incorporation into host tissues [32,43]. With administration of appropriate antibiotics, proper drainage, and debridement, it is rarely imperative to remove the mesh to eradicate the infection [40].

Deep prosthetic-related infections, on the other hand, usually occur several weeks to months after surgery and occur infrequently at a rate of 0.03–0.8% [38].

Mesh-related infections result in cardinal symptoms of inflammation with a wide spectrum of severity. The factors that determine clinical presentation include: virulence of the infecting pathogen, the nature of the host tissue and its ability to support microbial growth, and the host response to the presence of these pathogens. Most patients present with a subacute to indolent course, characterized by progressive, crescendo wound pain, occasionally accompanied by cutaneous draining sinuses. Fever, soft-tissue swelling, and erythema may be absent. Rarely, some may present with acute, fulminant sepsis with high-grade fever, severe pain over the surgical site and soft tissue swelling, erythema and exudates. The infecting organism in this acute form is typically virulent, such as *Staphylococcus aureus*, and it can elicit more systemic inflammatory responses compared to innocuous organisms, for example coagulase-negative staphylococci, *Bacillus* and *Corynebacterium* spp. β-Hemolytic streptococci and aerobic, enteric gram-negative bacilli are also capable of causing mesh-related infections and these pathogens can incite severe inflammatory reactions similar to *Staphylococcus aureus*.

Case presentation 2 (continued)

During the 2 weeks of local surgical site care and intravenous antibiotic therapy, the patient's signs and symptoms of systemic infection resolved. The abdominal surgical site was left open and she was discharged home with intravenous antibiotic and daily surgical site care by a visiting home-care nurse. One month following the hospital discharge, the patient presented with purulent, foul-smelling greenish suppuration from the abdominal wound and the exposed mesh. She is afebrile and hemodynamically stable. The surgical site culture grew Pseudomonas aeruginosa. At this time, you recommend removal of the infected mesh and the surgeon is reluctant to do so.

Based on the results from the combined European and American groups' observations, which included 12 374 cases of hernia repair using mesh, only eight patients developed mesh infection; five of the eight patients required removal of the mesh [49,50]. In a case report series consisting of three patients, the infections were completely eradicated in all the patients after the removal of the infected mesh [50]. Hence, based on these limited observational findings, it appears that patients who experience refractory infections despite repetitive drainage, lavage, and appropriate systemic antibiotic therapy may improve following removal of the prosthetic material. It is improbable that an adequately powered, prospective, randomized trial of conservative therapy versus surgical management for mesh infection will ever take place, given the very low rate of infectious complications and significant risks and morbidity associated with reoperation.

When a patient presents with infection, the decision and the timing of the mesh removal should be tailored to each patient, while considering the benefit and risks associated with repeat surgery in the individual patient. For patients who display evidence of persistent sepsis, while infected with virulent organisms, such as *S. aureus*, and aerobic, enteric gram-negative bacilli, immediate removal of the mesh is likely necessary.

In conclusion, although mesh-related infection is rare, it is a significant complication. The risk of infection can be minimized with strict adherence to aseptic techniques during mesh preparation and implantation, while conforming to current perioperative recommended guidelines for SSI prevention.

Acute diverticulitis

Case presentation 3

A 62-year-old woman with a history of diverticulosis and hypertension presented with a 3-day history of left lower quadrant pain, anorexia, low-grade fever, and chills. There was associated dysuria, urinary urgency, and frequency. On physical examination, blood pressure was 116/62 mmHg; heart rate, 110 beats per minute; temperature 38.2°C. The jugular venous pressure was 2 cm below the sternal angle and the mucous membranes were dry. There were normal bowel sounds, moderate tenderness, and rigidity in the left lower quadrant and suprapubic area. There was no costovertebral angle tenderness.

The white blood cell count was $16.7 \times 10^9/L$; hemoglobin 104 g/L; platelets $407 \times 10^9/L$. Routine biochemical tests and urinalysis were normal. A clinical diagnosis of diverticulitis was made. You admitted the patient for intravenous hydration and for consultation with a general surgeon. You searched the literature to determine optimal evidence-based diagnosis of diverticulitis.

Epidemiology

Acquired colonic diverticular disease is common in industrialized countries, where it is estimated to affect approximately 5–10% of individuals over 45 years of age and nearly 80% of the elderly over 85 [51]. There is a growing evidence that the overall prevalence is increasing and the incidence in patients under 40 years of age is 2–5% [52,53]. The increase in prevalence in younger patients seems to be without regard to a particular socioeconomic or ethnic group [54]. There is a male preponderance for younger patients compared to both sexes being equally affected in the elderly population [4].

Prior to a few decades ago, diverticular disease was exceedingly rare in developing countries and Japan, attributed largely to sufficient dietary fibre consumption [55]. Recent studies indicate its increasing incidence in Africa and Japan with the introduction of westernized diet, which is high in refined carbohydrate and low in fiber [55,56].

Diverticulitis refers to inflammation of diverticulosis and approximately 15–20% of patients with diverticulosis will develop diverticulitis [57]. Up to 20% of patients with diverticulitis are less than 50 years old. There is no clear evidence that younger patients have more severe diverticulitis, as previously thought. There maybe delay in diagnosis due to the atypical age of presentation and subsequent development of complications [54].

Pathogenesis

Colonic diverticulosis occurs due to elevated intraluminal pressure and thinning of the colonic wall [58]. The weakening of the bowel leads to herniation of mucosa and submucosa. Diets high in refined carbohydrate and low in dietary fiber lead to diminished stool bulk, an increase in gastrointestinal transit time and subsequent increase in intraluminal pressure [59]. Diverticulitis ensues when fecal material or undigested food particles lodge in a diverticulum, which can cause obstruction of the diverticulum neck. This results in accumulation of mucus, bacterial overgrowth, and loss of blood supply to the already distended diverticulum. In the majority of cases, the outcome is a microscopic perforation and localized inflammatory process. Hinchey et al. created a useful method to classify inflammatory conditions associated with diverticulitis [60]. Stage I is defined as small, confined pericolonic abscesses, which can lead to larger paracolic abscesses (stage II). Stage III depicts generalized suppurative peritonitis and stage IV is fecal peritonitis. With recurrent episodes of inflammation, fibrosis and stricture of the colonic wall may emerge [61].

Diagnosis of acute diverticulitis

Clinical features

The most common symptom of acute diverticulitis is a gradual onset of constant lower abdominal pain, particularly in the left lower quadrant, as the descending and sigmoid colons are involved in 90% of the cases [62,63]. There may be associated changes in bowel habits, especially in the setting of partial bowel obstruction. Nonspecific symptoms such as anorexia, nausea, and vomiting may accompany abdominal pain. When there is involvement of the bowel segment near the bladder or presence of colovesical fistula then urinary urgency, frequency, or dysuria may occur [61]. No studies were identified which specifically addressed the diagnostic accuracy of the clinical examination for diverticulitis.

Profuse rectal bleeding is unusual in acute diverticulitis but microscopic fecal blood may be present. Often, low-grade fever, mild leukocytosis, and localized lower quadrant abdominal tenderness are found. Presence of peritonitis reflects perforation of peridiverticular abscess or diverticulum. Patients receiving corticosteroids may not reveal evidence of peritonitis despite extensive colonic inflammation or perforation.

Case presentation 3 (continued)

After reviewing the literature with regard to the role of diagnostic imaging studies in the acute setting of suspected diverticulitis, you decide that your patient required a computed tomography (CT). The CT of the abdomen and pelvis with water-soluble contrast reveals pericolic fat inflammation, multiple diverticula, thickening the of the bowel wall. There is also a 3 cm pelvic abscess.

Imaging studies

Since up to 12% of patients with acute diverticulitis may have free intraperitoneal air, it is important to include chest and abdominal radiographs in the initial management of patients presenting with a significant abdominal pain and possible underlying diverticulitis [64].

Helical computed tomography (CT) scans with water-soluble colonic contrast materials have been shown to be very useful in ascertaining the presence of acute diverticulitis, with a positive predictive value of 100% and a negative predictive value of 98% [51,62,63,65]. Owing to the high risk of perforation, colonoscopy and barium enema should be avoided in acute diverticulitis. CT scanning, on the other hand, appears safe and can be performed even in critically ill patients.

The modern multislice CT scans, which provide speed and high-resolution imaging, when performed with rectal, oral (water-soluble), and intravenous contrast have shown to accurately delineate intraperitoneal and colonic diseases [66,67]. Ambrosetti et al. [68] prospectively evaluated 542 consecutive patients presenting with acute left colonic diverticultis with high-resolution CT scans and contrast enema. The authors found the sensitivity of CT to be 98%, compared with contrast enema at 92% ($P < 0.01$), using a reference standard, which included either test being positive, or pathologic evidence of diverticulitis in resected surgical tissue. In addition to superior performance compared to contrast enema (CE) in terms of sensitivity, CT, also correlated with CE, was found to have better capacity to grade the severity of the inflammation with statistically significant differences ($P < 0.02$). This and several studies support the use of CT in evaluating patients with an acute presentation compatible with underlying diverticulitis, who require hospitalization to confirm the diagnosis, to assess the severity of the inflammation and to further direct patient management [63,65,68,69].

Case presentation 3 (continued)

On day 3 of the admission, the patient developed sudden onset of diffuse abdominal pain and vomiting. On examination, she was pale and diaphoretic. There was generalized abdominal guarding and rebound tenderness. A plain film of the abdomen showed increased gas in small and large intestines.

Treatment of acute diverticulitis

Medical management
Approximately 85% of patients with a first attack of acute diverticulitis will respond to conservative management, which consists of intravenous fluid administration, bowel rest, and broad-spectrum antibiotic therapy for 7–10 days [52,71]. No RCTs were identified that have assessed the individual efficacy of these components. Patients with a mild, first episode of acute diverticulitis, who are able to maintain oral hydration, can be treated as outpatients and given oral antibiotics effective against intestinal bacteria, for example ciprofloxacin and metronidazole [51]. Evans [70] analyzed 198 patients admitted with acute sigmoid diverticulitis as confirmed by CT and physical examination. The daily maximum temperature and leukocyte count of the patients with prolonged stays were compared to the patients who were discharged within 4 days. The average maximum temperature and leukocyte count on admission were not statistically different between the two groups. After the first 24 hours of admission, however, there was a statistically significant difference in maximum temperature ($P = 0.004$) between the two groups. The leukocyte count also decreased significantly by hospital day 2 ($P = 0.003$). The author found that the patients with a significant decline in leukocyte count and maximum temperature over the first 48 hours of medical management were predictably discharged early on oral antibiotics. Patients failing to show improvement of leukocytosis and fever at 48 hours required prolonged hospital stays and/or surgery.

The majority of patients admitted to hospital with initial onset of acute diverticulitis will improve within 2–4 days with bowel rest, appropriate intravenous antibiotic, and fluid therapy. The antibiotic therapy should consist of a regimen which reliably targets colonic gram-negative and anaerobic organisms. Several randomized trials demonstrated no statistically significant difference in overall outcomes between various collated antibiotic regimens for intraabdominal infections: ciprofloxacin + metronidazole vs imipenem/cilastatin [71]; piperacillin/tazobactam vs cefotaxime + metronidazole [72]; ertapenem vs ceftriaxone + metronidazole [73]; cefoxitin and gentamacin + clindamycin [74]; piperacillin/tazobactam vs clindamycin + gentamicin [75].

After the resolution of the initial acute attack, patients should be counseled to consume dietary fiber regularly and be advised to undergo colonoscopy to rule out underlying colonic cancer. Approximately 5–15% of the patients treated with medical management will experience recurrent diverticulitis within 2 years [76].

Surgical management
Fifteen percent of patients presenting with acute diverticulitis will require either percutaneous drainage or surgical intervention [71]. Small abscesses (<5 cm in diameter) usually drain spontaneously because of the development of fistulae between colon and the abscess and they generally resolve with antibiotic treatment [77]. Abscesses that are 5–15 cm in diameter can be drained percutaneously under

radiologic guidance. With the administration of appropriate antibiotic therapy and adequate percutaneous drainage, patients in this group frequently improve within 72 hours, as indicated by reduction in pain and normalization of leukocytosis [61,78]. Some of the advantages of percutaneous drainage are rapid control of sepsis, avoidance of general anesthesia for open drainage, and obviating the potential need for a second operation to restore colon contiguity.

Laparotomy is required when abscesses cannot be drained percutaneously due to inaccessibility, mulitiloculation, or lack of clinical response. Resection with primary anastomosis is the operative procedure of choice in such situations, as well as for patients who require definitive surgery even after a successful medical management, unless there are prohibiting factors such as edematous intestinal ends or inadequate bowel preparation [51,61].

The absolute indications for immediate colonic resection are uncontrolled sepsis, visceral perforation, generalized peritonitis, or colonic obstruction [61]. A review of practices and a recent prospective randomized study by Zeitoun et al. [80] determined that primary resection is superior to secondary resection in the treatment of generalized peritonitis related to diverticulitis in terms of immediate mortality and morbidity. In the latter study, 105 patients with sigmoid diverticulitis and generalized peritonitis were randomized to undergo primary or secondary colonic resection. Primary resection resulted in fewer reoperations (2 of 55 vs 9 of 48, $P = 0.02$) and shorter hospital stay (median 15 vs 24 days, $P < 0.05$).

References

1 Perl TM, Cullen JJ, Wenzel RP, et al. Intranasal mupirocin to prevent postoperative *Staphylococcus aureus* infections. N Engl J Med 2002;346 (24):1871–77.

2 Horan T, Culver D, Gaynes R, et al. Nosocomial infections in surgical patients in the United States, January 1986–June 1992. Infect Control Hosp Epidemiol 1993;14:73–80.

3 Ward VP, Charlett A, Fagan J, Crawshaw SC. Enhanced surgical site infection surveillance following caesarean section: experience of a multicentre collaborative post-discharge system. J Hosp Infect. 2008;70(20):166–73.

4 Sands K, Vineyard G, Platt R. Surgical site infections occurring after hospital discharge. J Infect Dis 1996;173:963–70.

5 Reimer K, Gleed C, Nicolle LE. The impact of postdischarge infection on surgical wound infection rates. Infect Control 1987;8:237–40.

6 Burns SJ, Dippe SE. Postoperative wound infections detected during hospitalization and after discharge in a community hospital. Am J Infect Control 1982;10(2):60.

7 Horan TC, Gaynes RP, Martone WJ, et al. CDC definitions of nosocomial surgical site infections, 1992: A modification of CDC definitions of surgical wound infections. Am J Infect Control 1992;20:271–4.

8 Fanning J, Brewer J. Delay of hospital discharge secondary to postoperative fever – is it necessary? J Am Osteopath Assoc 2002;102(12):660–1.

9 Kossoff EH, Vining EP, Pyzik PL, et al. The postoperative course and management of 106 hemidecortications. Pediatr Neurosurg 2002;37(6):298–303.

10 Hager WD. Postoperative infections: prevention and management. In: Rock JA, Thompson JD, eds. TeLinde's Operative Gynecology, 8th ed. Philadelphia: Lippincott-Raven, 1997: pp. 233–43.

11 Dellinger PE. Surgical infections and choice of antibiotics. Townsend: Sabiston Textbook of surgery, 16th ed. Illinois: Saunders Company, 2001: pp. 171–80.

12 Mangram AJ, Horan TC, Pearson ML, et al. Guideline for prevention of surgical site infection, 1999. Centers for Disease Control and Prevention Hospital Infection Control Practices Advisory Committee. Am J Infect Control 1999;27(2):97–132.

13 Jjuuko G, Moodley J. Abdominal wound sepsis associated with gynaecological surgery at King Edward VIII Hospital, Durban. SAJS 2002;40(1):11–14.

14 Jonkers D, Elenbaas T, Terporten P, et al. Prevalence of 90-days postoperative wound infections after cardiac surgery. Eur J Cardiothorac Surg 2003;23:97–102.

15 Bowler PG, Duerden BI, Armstrong DG. Wound microbiology and associated approaches to wound management. Clin Microbiol Rev 2001;14:244–69.

16 Miller MJ, Holmes HT. Specimen collection, transport and storage. In: Murray PR, Baron EJ, Pfaller MA, Tenover FC, Yolken RH, eds. Manual of Clincial Microbiology, 7th ed. Washington, DC. ASM Press, 1999: pp. 33–63.

17 Sayek I. The role of beta-lactam/beta-lactamase inhibitor combinations in surgical infections. Surg Infect (Larchmt) 2001;2 Suppl 1:23–32.

18 Elsakr R, Johnson DA, Younes Z, et al. Antimicrobial treatment of intra-abdominal infections. Dig Dis 1998;16:47–60.

19 Giuliana A, Lewis F Jr, Hadley K, et al. Bacteriology of necrotizing fasciitis. Am J Surg 1977;134:52.

20 Casali RE, Tucker WE, Petrino RA, et al. Postoperative necrotizing fasciitis of the abdominal wall. Am J Surg 1980;140:787.

21 Stamenkovic I, Lew PD. Early recognition of potentially fatal necrotizing fasciitis: Use of frozen-section biopsy. N Engl J Med 1984;310:1689.

22 Tamussino K. Postoperative infection. Clin Obstet Gynecol 2002;45(2):562–73.

23 Stevens DL, Yan S, Bryant AE. J Infect Dis 1993;167(6): 1401–5.

24 Stevens DL, Bryant AE, Hackett SP. Antibiotic effects on bacterial viability, toxin production and host response. Clin Infect Dis 1995;20:S154–7.

25 Stevens DL, Madaras-Kelly KJ, Richards DM. In vitro anti-microbial effects of various combinations of penicillin and clindamycin against four strains of *Streptococcus pyogenes*. Antimicrob Agents Chemother 1998;42:1266–68.

26 Kaul R, McGeer A, Norrby-Teglund A, et al. Intravenous immunoglobulin therapy for streptococcal toxic shock syndrome – A comparative observational study. Clin Infect Dis 1999;28:800–7.

27 Barry W, Hudgins L, Donta ST, et al. Intravenous immunoglobulin therapy for toxic shock syndrome. JAMA 1992;267:3315–16.

28 Lamothe F, D'Amico P, Ghosn P, et al. Clinical usefulness of intravenous human immunoglobulin in invasive group A streptococcal infections: Case report and review. Clin Infect Dis 1995;21:1469–70.

29 Luijendijk RW, Hop WC, van den Tol P, et al. A comparison of suture repair with mesh repair for incisional hernia. N Eng J Med 2000;343(6):392–98.

30 Read RC, Yoder G. Recent trends in the management of incisional herniation. Arch Surg 1989;124:485–8.

31 Manninen MJ, Lavonius M, Perhoniemi VJ. Results of incisional hernia repair: a retrospective study of 172 unselected hernioplasties. Eur J Surg 1991;157:29–31.

32 Birolini C, Utiyama EM, Rodrigues Jr. AJ, Birolini D. Elective colonic operation and prosthetic repair of incisional hernia: does contamination contraindicate abdominal wall prosthesis use? J Am Coll Surg 2000;191:366–72.

33 Anthony T, Bergen PC, Kim LT, et al. Factors affecting recurrence following incisional herniorrhaphy. World J Surg 2000;24:95–101.

34 Kercher KW, Sing RF, Lohr C, Matthews BD, et al. Feature: Successful salvage of infected polytetrafluoroethylene mesh after ventral hernia repair. Ostomy Wound Management. 2002;48(10):40–2,44–5.

35 Bleichrodt RP, Simmermacher RK, van der Lei B, et al. Expanded polytetrafluoroethylene patch versus polypropylene mesh for the repair of contaminated defects of the abdominal wall. Surg Gynecol Obstet 1993;176:18–24.

36 Brown GL, Richardson JD, Malangoni MA, et al. Comparison of prothetic materials for abdominal wall reconstruction in the presence of contamination and infection. Ann Surg 1985;201(6):705–11.

37 McNeeley SG Jr. Hendrix SL, Bennett SM, et al. Synthetic graft placement in the treatment of fascial dehiscence with necrosis and infection. Am J Obstet Gynecol 1998;179:1430–35.

38 Shulman AG, Amid PK, Lichtenstein IL. The safety of mesh repair for primary inguinal hernias: results of 3019 operations from five diverse sources. Am Surg 1992;58:255–7.

39 Berliner SD. Clinical experience with an inlay expanded polytetrafluoroethylene soft tissue patch as an adjunct in inguinal hernia repair. Surg Gynecol Obstet 1993;176:323–6.

40 Gilbert AI, Felton LL. Infection in inguinal hernia repair considering biomaterials and antibiotics. Surg Gynecol Obstet 1993;177:126–30.

41 Thill RH, Hopkins WM. The use of mersilene mesh in adult inguinal and femoral hernia repairs: a comparison with classic techniques. Am Surg 1994;60:553–7.

42 Arnaud JP, Eloy R, Adloff M, et al. Critical evaluation of prosthetic materials in repair of abdominal wall hernias. Am J Surg 1977;133:339–45.

43 Mann DV, Pout J, Havranek E, et al. Late-onset deep prosthetic infection following mesh repair of inguinal hernia. Am J Surg 1998;176:12–14.

44 Stone HH, Fabian TC, Turkleson ML, et al. Management of acute full-thickness losses of abdominal wall. Ann Surg 1981;193:612–18.

45 Boyd WC. Use of marlex mesh in acute loss of the abdominal wall due to infection. Surg Gynecol Obstet 1977;144:251–2.

46 Kaufman Z, Engelberg M, Zager M. Fecal fistula: a late complication of Marlex mesh repair. Dis Colon Rectum 1981;24:543–4.

47 Leber GE, Garb JL, Alexander AI, et al. Long-term complications associated with prosthetic repair of incisional hernias. Arch Surg 1998:133:378–82.

48 Amid PK. Classification of biomaterials and their related complications in abdominal wall hernia surgery. Hernia 1997;1:15–21.

49 Phillips EH, Arregui M, Carroll BJ, et al. Incidence of complications following laparoscopic hernioplasty. Surg Endosc 1995;9(1):16–21.

50 Avtan L, Avci C, Bulut T, Fourtanier G. Mesh infections after laparoscopic inguinal hernia repair. Surg Laparosc Endosc 1997;7(30):192–5.

51 Ferzoco LB, Paptopoulos V, Silen W. Acute diverticulitis. N Engl J Med 1998;338:1521–6.

52 Minardi AJ Jr, Johnson LW, Sehon JK, et al. Diverticulitis in the young patient. Am Surg 2001;67(5):458–61.

53 Acosta JA, Grebenc ML, Doberneck RC, et al. Colonic diverticular disease in patients 40 years old or younger. Am Surg 1992;58:605–7.

54 Konvolinka CW. Acute diverticulitis under age forty. Am J Surg 1994;167:562–5.

55 Madiba TE, Mokoena T. Pattern of diverticular disease among Africans. East Afr Med J 1994;71(10):644–6.

56 Miura S, Kodiara S, Shatari T, et al. Recent trends in diverticulosis of the right colon in Japan: retrospective review in a regional hospital. Dis Colon Rectum 2000;43:1383–9.

57 Stollman NH, Rakin JB. Diverticular disease of the colon. J Clin Gastroenterol 1999;29:241–52.

58 Whiteway J, Morson BC. Pathology of the ageing – diverticular disease. Clin Gastroenterol 1985;14:829–46.

59 Burkitt DP, Walker ARP, Painter NS. Dietary fiber and disease. JAMA 1974;229:1068–74.

60 Hinchey EJ, Schaal PH, Richards GK. Treatment of perforated diverticular disease of the colon. Adv Surg 1978;12:85–109.

61 Boulos PB. Complicated diverticulosis. Best Prac Resear Clin Gastroenterol 2002;16:649–62.

62 Labs JD, Sarr MG, Fishman EK, et al. Complications of acute diverticulits of the colon: improved early diagnosis with computerized tomography. Am J Surg 1988;155:331–6.

63 Rao PM, Rhea JT, Novellin RA, et al. Helical CT with only colonic contrast material for diagnosing diverticulitis: prospective evaluation of 150 patients. Am J Roentgenol 170:1445–9.

64 McKee RF, Deignan RW, Krukowski ZH. Radiological investigation in acute diverticulitis. Br J Surg 1993;80(5):560–6.

65 Neff CC, van Sonnenberg E. CT of diverticulitis: diagnosis and treatment. Radiol Clin North Am 1989;27:743–52.

66 Tsai SC, Chao TH, Lin WY, et al. Abdominal abscesses in patients having surgery: an application of Ga-67 scintigraphic and computed tomographic scanning. Clin Nucl Med 2001;26(9):761–4.

67 Halligan S, Saunders B. Imaging diverticular disease. Best Prac Res Clin Gastroenterol 2002;16(4):595–610.

68 Ambrosetti P, Becker C, Terrier F. Colonic diverticulitis: impact of imaging on surgical management – a prospective study of 542 patients. Eur Radiol 2002;12:1145–9.

69 Buchanan GN, Kenefick NJ, Cohen CR. Diverticulitis. Best Prac Res Clin Gastroenterol 2002 16:4:635–47.

70 Evans J. Does a 48-hour rule predict outcomes in patients with acute sigmoid diverticulitis? J Gastrointest Surg 2008;12(3):577–82.

71 Solokin JS, Reinhart HH, Dellinger EP, et al. Results of a randomized trial comparing sequential intravenous/oral treatment with ciprofloxacin plus metronidazole to imipenem/cilastatin for intra-abdominal infections. The Intra-Abdominal Infection Study Group. Ann Surg 1996;223(3):303–15.

72 Maltezou HC, Nikolaidis P, Lebesii E, et al. Piperacillin/tazobactam versus cefotaxime plus metronidazole for treatment of children with intra-abdominal infections requiring surgery. Eur J Clin Microbiol Infect Dis 2001;20(9):643–6.

73 Yellin AE, Hassett JM, Fernandez A, et al. The 004 intra-abdominal infection study group. Ertapenem monotherapy versus combination therapy with ceftriaxone plus metronidazole for treatment of complicated intra-abdominal infections in adults. Int J Antimicrob Agents 2002;20(3):165–73.

74 Kellum JM, Sugerman HJ, Coppa GF, et al. Randomized, prospective comparison of cefoxitin and gentamicin-clindamycin in the treatment of acute colonic diverticulitis. Clin Ther 1992;14(3):376–84.

75 Shyr YM, Lui WY, Su CH, et al. Piperacillin/tazobactam in comparison with clindamycin plus gentamicin in the treatment of intra-abdominal infections. Zhonghua Yi Xue Za Zhi (Taipei) 1995;56(2):102–8.

76 Ambrosetti P, Robert J, Witzig JA, et al. Acute left colonic diverticulitis: a prospective analysis of 226 consecutive cases. Surgery 1994;115:546–50.

77 Ambrosetti P, Robert J, Witzig JA, et al. Incidence, outcome, and proposed management of isolated diverticulitis. A prospective study of 140 patients. Dis Colon Rectum 1992;35:1072–6.

78 Stabile BE, Paccio E, Van Sonnenberg E, et al. Prospective percutaneous drainage of diverticular abscesses. Am J Surg 1990;159:99–105.

79 Kurkowski ZH, Matheson NA. Emergency surgery for diverticular disease complicated by generalized and faecal peritonitis: a review. Br J Surg 1984;71:921–7.

80 Zeitoun G, Laurent A, Rouffet F, et al. Multicentre randomized clinical trial of primary versus secondary sigmoid resection in generalized peritonitis complicating sigmoid diverticulitis. Br J Surg 2000;87:1366–74.

CHAPTER 17

Infections in the thermally injured patient

Edward E. Tredget, Robert Rennie, Robert E. Burrell & Sarvesh Logsetty

Case presentation

A 37-year-old male pipe fitter was tightening pipes in a petrochemical refining facility when a pipe burst, spewing him with a hot water/liquid ethylene glycol solvent mixture over 40% of his total body surface area (TBSA) including his upper extremities, chest, abdomen, and back. On the burns unit, routine admission wound, nose, rectum, and throat cultures were performed. He was resuscitated with fluids and nutritional support was provided by enteral feeding commenced at 24 hours post burn according to a routine protocol. His wounds were treated with topical silver sulfadiazine cream and his dressing was changed daily in a Hubbard tank hydrotherapy facility. After 5 days in hospital he underwent debridement and split-thickness skin grafting to his upper extremities; 3 days later he became acutely confused, tachypneic, hypotensive (80/60mmHg), and oliguric. The patient was treated empirically with piperacillin 4g intravenously every 8 hours and gentamicin 350mg daily. His blood cultures grew *Pseudomonas aeruginosa* in both vials and methicillin-susceptible *Staphylococcus aureus* and *Enterococcus faecium* in one of two vials. The antibiotics were switched to amikacin 1g daily, ceftazidime 2g every 8 hours, and vancomycin 1g every 12 hours. He required massive fluid resuscitation with crystalloids, fresh frozen plasma, and albumin totaling 35 liters over 30 hours as well as intravenous vasopressors, initially dopamine and dobutamine, but ultimately noradrenalin before he was stabilized and his urine output recovered.

Evidence-Based Infectious Diseases, 2nd edition. Edited by Mark Loeb, Fiona Smaill and Marek Smieja. © 2009 Wiley-Blackwell Publishing, ISBN: 978-1-4051-7026-0

Serious infections remain a common complication in thermally injured patients, contributing substantially to burn morbidity and mortality. Despite advancements in medical and surgical care of burns patients, no significant improvement in mortality has been documented over a 25-year period in one major institution caring for burns patients once bacteremic with *Pseudomonas aeruginosa* [1]. Much of the evidence guiding management of infections in thermally injured patients is based on case series where bacteriologic results have been reported. Therefore a review of the bacteriology of burns is essential to understanding the evidence base for current practice.

Bacteriology of burns patients

The types of bacteria that colonize and infect burns patients, as well as their susceptibilities to antimicrobials, is highly variable between burns units. It is influenced by both the topical antimicrobial and wound care policies of the burns center as well as the approach to usage of systemic antibiotics. In India, Revathi et al. reviewed their experience with 600 infections in burns patients [2] and, similar to many burns centers, found that the most frequent and severe infections were caused by *Pseudomonas* spp followed by *Staphylococcus aureus* and then by other gram-negative organisms including *Klebsiella* spp., *Acinetobacter* spp., *Escherichia coli*, *Enterococcus faecalis*, and *Proteus* sp. In a survey of 176 burn care centers in North America, *P. aeruginosa* was considered the most serious cause of life-threatening infections in thermally injured patients [3]. Similarly, in a 25-year review of *Pseudomonas* bacteremia in burns patients by McManus et al., an overall burn mortality of 77% with *P. aeruginosa* bacteremia was documented, 28% above predicted rates [1].

A comparison of two 10-year periods of gram-negative isolates in pediatric burns patients demonstrated that, in the 1990s, *P. aeruginosa* accounted for 35% of the gram-negative organisms from all sites of infections, as compared with 34% in the 1980s. Most recently, however, *Acinetobacter* spp. have replaced *Klebsiella* spp. as the second most common gram-negative bacteria causing infections in children with burns [4]. Similarly, in an overview of wound isolates in burns centers in the United Kingdom, an increasing prevalence of *Acinetobacter* spp. has been described [5]. It is important to note that *Aeromonas* sp. is an uncommon, but rapidly aggressive gram-negative burn wound pathogen that can lead to early burn wound sepsis (within the first burn week) commonly after patients have been exposed to lake or slough water post injury [6].

In a large case series of established infections in the US army burns center, Pruitt et al. reported that 25% of infections were due to pneumonia, 22% to urinary tract, 26% to primary blood stream infections, and 5% to invasion of the burn wound [7]. Of the 57 documented cases of invasive wound infection that occurred in burns patients treated during the 1986–95 period, there were 26 cases of secondary bacteremia due to *P. aeruginosa*. In this major academic American military burns center where early burn wound excision, avoidance of immersion hydrotherapy, dependence on quantitative and histologic evidence for burn wound infection, and topical sulfamyalon are routine practices, a high rate of yeast and fungal infections occurred in burns of 50% or more of the total body surface area. Most of these fungal infections were in massive burn injuries and were due to *Candida* spp., which on average, colonized the burn wound on post-burn day 30, infected the urinary tract on day 48, and other sites at day 41 [7]. Filamentous fungi such as *Aspergillus* spp. and *Fusarium* spp. have also been reported to cause invasive infection [8]. Predisposition of burns patients to fungal infections has been identified when strong dependence on topical mafenide acetate solutions is used to control gram-negative bacteria in the burn wound [9].

Diagnosis

Clinical presentation

Approximately 400 000 cases of sepsis occur in the US each year with 30–45% mortality [10]. The clinical spectrum of burns patients resembles that of other septic patients [11]. Fever and inflammation following a burn injury is a very common response to localized microbial invasion to the burn wound. However, when the size of the burn increases beyond 15–20% of the total body surface area, release of cytokines and eicosanoid mediators leads to a systemic inflammatory response syndrome (SIRS), in the presence or the absence of a definable bacteriologic infection [11]. With progressive bacterial or fungal colonization of the burn wound, sepsis progressing to multiple organ dysfunction syndrome (MODS) and septic shock may occur. There are, to date, no clinical features that have been found distinguishing a burns patient with SIRS from a septic burns patient without hypotension. A thorough physical examination and septic work-up (blood, wound, and urine cultures; chest radiograph, and urinalysis) is necessary for the initial investigation of the burns patient with symptoms and signs of infection [12].

Evaluation of infected thermally injured patients is a challenge for clinicians. The clinical presentation of infection can range from an acute (such as the patient presented) to a chronic onset. This may range from low-grade cellulitis or minor skin graft infection to fulminant septic shock and widespread infection of skin graft donor site wounds and complete non-take of split-thickness skin grafts in the postoperative period [7]. Classically, bacterial colonization of the burn wound and eschar leads to progressive increases in the numbers of bacteria and penetration of the eschar from superficial to deep into the eschar before invasion into healthy uninjured tissue leads to bacteremia and sepsis [7]. Altered mental status, tachypnea, paralytic ileus, hyper- or hypothermia ($>38.5°C$ or $<36.5°C$), hypotension and oliguria, associated with leukocytosis $>15.0 \times 10^3$ cells/mm^3 or leukopenia $<3.5 \times 10^3$ cells/mm^3, thrombocytopenia $<50 000$ platelets/mm^3, hyperglycemia, and unexplained acidosis are cardinal signs of burn wound sepsis [7]. Local evidence of invasive wound infection includes black or brown patches of wound discoloration, rapid eschar separation, conversion of partial thickness wounds to full thickness injuries, spreading peri-wound erythema, punctate hemorrhagic, subeschar lesions, and, with *P. aeruginosa*, violaceous or black lesions in unburned tissue termed "ecthyma gangrenosum" [13].

Microbiology cultures

Commonly, wound infection is diagnosed clinically and wound swabs of potentially contaminated tissues are obtained. Surface wound cultures are considered only partially representative of the bacterial flora contained within the wound [14]. For this reason, burn wound biopsies have been employed by many burn care centers to allow quantitation of the numbers of bacteria present within the wound where $>10^5$ organisms/g of wet tissue is considered evidence of wound infection, which will prevent successful wound closure surgically [14]. Recently, Steer et al. used parallel cultures from 141 samples in 74 burns patients to demonstrate that recovery of the same set of species of bacteria from a burn wound biopsy versus a surface swab was 54%, and the predictive value of the counts obtained by one method to predict the counts obtained by the other was poor, owing, in part, to wide variation in bacterial densities from simultaneous cultures taken from the same burn wound [14]. Further, in burns $>15\%$ TBSA, quantitative bacteriology by burn wound biopsy or surface swab did not aid in the prediction of sepsis or graft loss [14]. By definition, burn wound invasion leading to bacteremia is a histologic diagnosis where microscopic evidence of invasion of nonburned tissue with bacteria occurs, a finding which McManus found was present in only 36% of biopsies with positive cultures ($>10^5$ organisms/g) [15]. Unfortunately, burn wound biopsies are expensive, invasive because a section of unburned tissue needs to be included with the biopsy, and associated with considerable variability between adjacent sites of the burn wound [16]. These facts together with more aggressive wound debridement, newer topical antimicrobials, and improved nutritional support and intensive care have limited the use of burn wound biopsy in many burns centers [17].

Laboratory diagnosis of infection in the burns patient also includes blood cultures, urine and respiratory cultures, depending on clinical clues such as sepsis, pyuria, and evidence of pulmonary infiltrates.

To date, there is little evidence to support the routine use of blood culture testing in burns patients. Keen et al. in a small retrospective analysis of 47 burns patients found that positive blood cultures were more common in patients who were in shock, had larger burn wounds, were receiving more antibiotics, and who had indwelling catheters [18]. Reduced frequency of blood cultures was not associated with increased length of stay, ventilator days, or mortality [18]. The small size of this study, however, probably precludes the ability to detect differences. Henke et al. conducted a retrospective analysis of 1040 routine blood cultures in 121 surgical patients (including 31 burns patients) [19]: 48 positive blood cultures led to a change in management or therapy in 19 (40%). Of interest is the fact that the mortality rate was highest in burns patients who had positive blood cultures (39%) as compared with those with negative blood cultures (7%) [19].

It is routine practice for many burns units to perform cultures of the burn wounds, throat, nose, and rectum upon admission to identify any unusual or high-risk pathogens. However, there are no data to support this practice. Although many burns centers perform routine weekly cultures on patients with open wounds, there is little evidence to support routine wound cultures and the practice is expensive and timeconsuming [20]. In addition, considerable data suggest that surface swabs of burns and other wounds are often not representative of the major bacteria present in the wound [14–19] and therefore quantitative burn wound biopsy and histology, with their inherent limitations as discussed earlier, is employed in many but not all burns centers.

Prevention of infection

Topical antimicrobials

The burn eschar is a relatively avascular mass of necrotic material in which therapeutic levels of systemically administered antibiotics are difficult to achieve [21]. Topically applied antimicrobials provide high concentrations of drug at the wound surface acting as a barrier to infection and penetrate the eschar to varying extents, significantly delaying the onset of invasive infection [22]. Much of the evidence on the use of topical antimicrobials in thermally injured patients is based on small clinical trials that used bacteriologic primary outcomes or bacteriologic considerations alone. Choice of topical agents often also depends on ease of use and other treatment modalities being offered to burns patients.

Silve sulfadiazine

Silver sulfadiazine is synthesized from silver nitrate and sodium sulfadiazine and is easily applied to burn wounds and does not stain the environment. Although this used to be a common prophylactic topical agent in burns patients, its white, water-soluble cream base interacts with the wound to produce a yellow mucopurulent exudate that needs to be washed off the wound before reapplication every 12 hours as recommended by the supplier [23]. Clinical experience suggests that silver sulfadiazine reduces wound bacterial density and delays colonization with gram-negative organisms but that treatment failures occur frequently in large burns >50% TBSA [24]. Because this agent is of limited spectrum in the large burn and requires hydrotherapy, which is an established risk factor for nosocomial infections, its usefulness in established *Pseudomonas* infections appears to be low, and its use combined with hydrotherapy predisposes major burns patients to early *Pseudomonas* colonization of the burn wound. Systemic absorption and multi-organ toxicity of silver is high in major burns, often unrecognized, and severe in patients with compromised renal function, the kidney being the principal route of excretion of absorbed silver [25].

Silver nitrate

Historically, **silver nitrate** was the first topical agent employed to delay burn eschar colonization based on its effectiveness against most strains of *Pseudomonas* and *Staphylococcus*. New topical agents were then developed to improve on the limitations of silver nitrate, including limited penetration of the burn eschar and environmental staining [26]. However, there has been a resurgence in the use of silver nitrate based on the recognition that, as a solution, it avoids the mucopurulent exudate common with cream-based topicals, and therefore does not require hydrotherapy. In addition, with the use of new skin and dermal substitutes, topical therapy without hydrotherapy is imperative and effective. Finally, eliminating the use of hydrotherapy not only reduces the risk of nosocomial infection (as discussed below) [27], it reduces the frequency of dressing change to once per day, significantly decreasing the dressing-related pain and cold stress endured by patients during hydrotherapy sessions, and also substantially lowers the overall cost of care of both the topical agents required but primarily of the staffing required for twice daily wound care and hydrotherapy sessions [3,27].

Mafenide acetate

Mafenide acetate is a topical burns agent with activity primarily against gram-negative organisms including *Pseudomonas* [24], where its efficacy has been established in vivo based on the Walker burns model in rats, where both topical 5% mafenide acetate solution and 10% cream significantly reduced *Pseudomonas* colonization to <10% organisms/g over 48 hours in standardized full-thickness burns [28]. Using ^{14}C-labeled mafenide acetate, Harrison demonstrated rapid penetration of this topical antimicrobial through burned skin [29]. It has minimal antifungal activity and limited activity against *Staphylococcus aureus*, particularly methicillin-resistant strains. It is formulated as an 11.1% cream or more recently as a 5% solution [28]. Mafenide is a potent carbonic anhydrase inhibitor; hyperchloremic metabolic acidosis limits its application to <20% TBSA; otherwise, severe hyperventilation can develop as respiratory compensation for the metabolic acidosis. For established *Pseudomonas* infections, mafenide acetate solutions can be combined with nystatin for improved antifungal activity and effectiveness in serious infections; it is often alternated every 12 hours with 0·5% AgNO$_3$ or other topical agents [30].

Acticoat

Acticoat is a new topical agent that is a novel nanocrystalline silver complex that has been widely tested and effective in vitro against a broad range of gram-negative and gram-positive organisms including multiply resistant strains [31–33], and it possesses strong antifungal properties [30]. It releases silver in aqueous solutions and therefore must be moistened with sterile water for activity, but thereafter can be left in place for up to 72 hours; it also does not normally require hydrotherapy for wound cleansing before reapplication [17]. In vivo studies have been completed on the antimicrobial barrier properties of the Acticoat dressing [34] as well as on the healing rates of skin graft donor sites [35] and contaminated full-thickness burn wounds [36]. One small randomized controlled trial in patients with major burns suggests that Acticoat treatment may be associated with lower rates of burn wound sepsis and fewer secondary bacteremias [27]. Using a matched pairs design of patients with symmetric wounds, one wound in each of 15 pairs was randomized to receive Acticoat, the other standard therapy (0.5% silver nitrate solution). Five cases of burn wound sepsis based on quantitative wound biopsy cultures ($>10^5$ organisms per gram of tissue), associated with one secondary bacteremia were noted in the Acticoat group compared with 16 positive wound biopsies and five secondary bacteremias with silver nitrate standard therapy. Other small uncontrolled clinical trials have been supportive of its use in burn wounds [37,38].

Other topical agents

Other topical agents for wound care include nitrofurazone, chlorhexidine, providone-iodine, nystatin, cerium nitrate, and combinations of agents, but are of limited proven efficacy and safety in *Pseudomonas* infections as yet [24]. Similarly, infusion of antibiotics under the burn eschar, termed "subeschar lysis," has been performed but has not yet been tested in randomized controlled trials [39].

Surgery

Prompt surgical excision of the burn wound and timely closure have significantly reduced the occurrence of invasive burn wound infection and its related mortality; however, as wound closure is delayed in patients with massive burns, the potential of invasive wound infection remains [40]. Two randomized controlled trials have reported no survival advantage with early total excision as compared with conservative treatment commencing at the day 10–14 post burn [41,42]. However, Tompkins et al. reviewed mortality in adult burns patients from Massachusetts General Hospital during a period prior to early excision and after prompt eschar excision and immediate wound closure. Using logistic regression of 1103 patients over a 10-year period encompassing both surgical approaches, the data showed a reduction in mortality from 24% to 7% ($P < 0.001$) associated with a significant reduction in length of stay in hospital from 32 to 22 days [42]. Staged surgical wound closure beginning within 10 days of injury and continuing at 7-day intervals remains the most common surgical approach to the burn wound at present [41]. The supporting evidence for this approach is limited to observational studies. In one study, this approach was associated with a 6-fold reduction in mortality in patients with burns >50% TBSA, with delayed surgical excision commencing after 7–10 days post injury

[43]. In a single-center retrospective analysis of 3561 burns patients over a 14-year period, Munster et al. reported significant reductions in mortality, length of stay, and cost of care with more aggressive staged surgical excision of the burn wound in the later 7-year period compared with the early era [41]. However, comparison with historical cohorts is a substantial limitation of the study [1]. Large, adequately powered randomized controlled trials are needed to establish optimal timing of surgery. In patients who already have established *Pseudomonas* infection including ecthyma gangrenosum, surgical debridement of infected tissues and temporary wound closure with allograft skin or autograft once the patient has stabilized is considered crucial to survival [13,44,45].

Empiric antibiotic treatment

Unstable septic patients often require empiric therapy usually guided by initial cultures taken on admission. Initial antibiotic therapy is based on these swabs and tailored once further cultures and susceptibilities become available. Leibovici et al. surveyed 296 episodes of gram-negative bacteremia in 286 patients aged 13–99 years and found that thermal trauma, hospital acquisition of the infection, antibiotic treatment before the bacteremic episode, and endotracheal intubation were variables that independently predicted subsequent isolation of a multiresistant strain [46]. In a second group of 144 episodes of gram-negative bacteremia, the predictive index derived from these variables for optimizing empiric treatment maintained good discriminative power and improved empiric antibiotic treatment in 24% of patients [46].

Pseudomonal sepsis is a significant cause of burn-associated mortality and morbidity requiring systemic antimicrobial therapy. McManus found that 10% of all burns patients developed pseudomonal bacteremia [1]. Unfortunately, with the development of multidrug-resistant *Pseudomonas*, the choice of antibiotics for empiric therapy becomes more difficult.

Case presentation (continued)

Septic work-up cultures in the unstable burns patient were positive for *P. aeruginosa*, which was quantified

Continued

Case presentation (continued)

in burn wound biopsies $>10^8$ organisms per gram of tissue, and skin graft donor sites from multiple regions of the body including his chest, back, both lower extremities, face, and scalp, as well as his blood cultures. The organism was resistant to gentamicin, tobramycin, carboxy- and ureidopenicillins. The patient's topical antimicrobial therapy for all infected wounds was switched to mafenide acetate twice daily. Once hemodynamically stable, the patient underwent a series of seven surgical debridements under general anesthetic for infected burn wounds and donor sites, but also for other infected wounds, which were not in the original burn areas but were hematogenously disseminated wounds in the scalp and other areas in which *Pseudomonas* was recovered on culture of the debrided tissue. Early surgical procedures were directed at debridement of *Pseudomonas*-infected tissues and avoidance of creation of any new skin graft donor wounds until reduction of bacterial load had been achieved, evidenced by adherence of fresh allograft skin to the debrided wounds. Despite secondary urine and wound infection with *Candida albicans*, the patient recovered after 77 days of intensive care in the burns unit. He spent 2 months in a rehabilitation hospital before being able to return home; he recommenced his work approximately 1 year after his original injury.

Infection control

Pseudomonas aeruginosa is the most important cause of nosocomial infection in the burns patient. However, only 6–8% of burns patients have rectal colonization [27]. Nosocomial acquisition of *P. aeruginosa* and other gram-negative bacteria arises from contaminated water and aqueous solutions used in Hubbard tanks, ventilators, nebulizers, intravenous solutions, and hemodialysis systems [47]. During wound care, hand-to-hand transmission is considered to be the major preventable mode of transmission.

Both the experimental and observational evidence to support infection control interventions in burns units are extremely limited. Strict handwashing is considered the cornerstone in preventing transmission of antibiotic-resistant organisms. Ongoing surveillance of infections in the burns unit is important to defect new resistant organisms so that infection control precautions can be quickly instituted [48].

Isolation and performing admission swabs for culture of new patients can potentially identify new pathogens, especially those from patients who have received care in another institution [49]. However, there are no comparative studies at present that have validated this. Strict barrier precautions are used in many burns units. On entry into the burns patient's room, all personnel and visitors are required to wear a disposable gown and mask and to wash their hands [50]. For all direct contact with patients sterile gloves are worn. Hands are washed with an antibacterial soap or alcohol-based hand disinfectants, and all protective garments are changed after each patient encounter. Individualized rooms and beds are cleansed and walls washed with a quaternary ammonium disinfectant between patient admissions. Again, however, comparative evidence for various levels of barrier precautions in burns units and terminal cleaning are lacking.

Improperly designed sinks that have short trap drains and deficient splash guards in themselves can be a source of hand and subsequently wound contamination [51,52]. This is very difficult to detect and establish as a mechanism of transmission of nosocomial infection but has been reported [53–55] and corrected by redesign and implementation of appropriate facilities for safe handwashing. Each individual piece of equipment is soaked with full strength (12%) sodium hypochlorite solution if positive surveillance cultures are obtained [1].

Selective decontamination of the gastrointestinal flora of the burns patient has been tried without success to reduce burn wound infection by either direct contact or by bacterial translocation of organisms from the gut [56]. Small numbers of burns patients treated with selective gut decontamination compared with historical controls found lower but not significantly reduced rates of wound colonization and respiratory infection, but a subsequent prospective randomized double-blind study of 23 pediatric burns patients demonstrated comparable rates of colonization and infection as compared with the blinded placebo controls [57].

The role of hydrotherapy in burn wound management

There are no randomized controlled trials that have compared hydrotherapy to no hydrotherapy for burn wound management and its use appears to have developed from a practical desire to wash burn wounds and the need to remove topical antimicrobial creams prior to reapplication of fresh agents. However, observational data of harm related to this therapy exists. Following an outbreak of *P. aeruginosa* linked to hydrotherapy in one burns unit, the incidence of *P. aeruginosa* infections in equal periods of time before and after discontinuation of hydrotherapy was compared [27]. Demographic data showed no difference in burn size, age of patient, duration of hospitalization, or sample size. However, a significant reduction in overall mortality (14 vs 6, $P < 0.05$), septic mortality (8 vs 1, $P < 0.05$), and *Pseudomonas*-associated septic deaths (6 vs 0, $P < 0.05$) was found in the non-hydrotherapy group. There was a significant reduction in the nosocomially acquired organisms (29 vs 18, $P < 0.05$), and in the number of aminoglycoside-resistant strains of *Pseudomonas* sp. (20 vs 4, $P < 0.05$) in the non-hydrotherapy group. Avoidance of hydrotherapy was also associated with a delay in appearance of *Pseudomonas* sp. in the burn wound (10.1 vs 16.5 days) and a delay in the onset of aminoglycoside resistance (10.3 vs 19.5 days), such that the appearance of an aminoglycoside-resistant organism in the burns patient was delayed approximately 16 days longer in the nonhydrotherapy group (20.4 vs 36.0 days) [27]. During the post-hydrotherapy period, an elimination of *Pseudomonas* sp. infection from traditionally clean wounds of the skin graft donor site was achieved (5 or 2.3% vs 0, $P < 0.05$). During the period prior to and after discontinuing hydrotherapy, the cost of care for patients in this burns unit was also analyzed where, from 1987 to 1991, silver sulfadiazine cream and hydrotherapy was routine before hydrotherapy was discontinued and topical 0.5% silver nitrate solution was substituted [58]. By using mathematical modeling to control for the number of burns patients and severity of injury during each period, substantial reduction in overall costs were predicted and savings in excess of the predicted were actually achieved. The majority of reduction in cost of care was not in the expense of the topical antimicrobials employed for wound care (Can$29 623 vs Can$10 145 per month), but in the reduced labor/nursing costs ($112 046 vs $91 256 per month) associated with elimination of hydrotherapy and once daily dressings within the patient's isolation room. An important limitation of this study, however, is the use of an historical cohort for comparison.

Similarly, many burns centers are experiencing an increase in *Acinetobacter* infections that are nosocomial in origin. Wisplinghoff et al. demonstrated that, in 367 patients hospitalized with severe burn injury where *Acinetobacter baumannii* was endemic (attack rate of 7.9%), 29 patients developed bloodstream infections [59]. When compared with 58 noninfected matched controls, the mortality rates were 31% and 14% respectively, and two deaths were directly attributable to *Acinetobacter* infections. Pulsed-field gel electrophoresis demonstrated three common strains, which were multidrug resistant. Multivariate analysis showed that bloodstream infection was independently associated with the severity of burn injury, prior nosocomial colonization at a distant site, and the use of hydrotherapy, again emphasizing the importance of effective infection control in other types of gram-negative infections. In summary, there are no trials that establish the efficacy or benefit of hydrotherapy for burn wounds. However, the substantial risk of cross-contamination of multidrug-resistant bacteria owing to hydrotherapy is well documented. This has led many burns centers to avoid using immersion hydrotherapy [4].

Prognosis

Based on retrospective, multifactorial logistic regression and probit analysis of 1705 burns patients, the mortality and morbidity of burns patients is related to the age of the patient, the total area of the burn wound (TBSA), and the presence or absence of concomitant inhalation injury [43], which resemble the findings of other burns centers [60]. Measures of the severity of injury after burns injury such as burn surface areas are often only broad, insensitive predictors of outcome. This is because of the failure to recognize the importance of inhalation injury and the depth of burn as a reflection of the volume or magnitude of necrotic tissue [61]. For example, superficial sun burns over 90% of the TBSA without inhalation injury can be considered in the same category of severity as full-thickness flame burns after a house fire, where the same TBSA is recorded but the patient also sustained a significant inhalation injury. Despite these limitations, predictive equations derived from one burns center would suggest that the illustrated index case would have a 75% probability of survival, where the total burn surface area, age of the patient, and presence or absence of inhalation injury are independent variables [43].

Inhalation injury and or adult respiratory distress syndrome (ARDS) and sepsis, ranging from SIRS to frank septic shock, are the major causes of mortality in burns patients [62]. Surveys from burns centers identify gram-positive organisms including MRSA as the most frequent cause of burn wound and skin graft infection [63]. However, the evidence suggests that gram-negative bacteria including *K. pneumoniae*, *E. coli*, and *Acinetobacter* spp. as well as *P. aeruginosa* are the major causes of mortality in burns centers. McManus et al. reported that 10% of all burns patients develop *Pseudomonas* bacteremia, carrying a mortality rate of 80% [1,64]. The risk of *Pseudomonas* infection increases substantially in burns >30% of the TBSA.

Emerging data for major burns involving more than 30–35% of the TBSA suggests that they do not necessarily all become infected with *P. aeruginosa* [65]. However, *Pseudomonas* morbidity and mortality may be reduced by measures taken to avoid nosocomial infection or to delay the onset of infection as long as possible [27]. One study of burns patients, using historical controls, suggested that the delay in the onset of resistant infections led to a 9-day or more infection-free period, enough time for surgical procedures to remove potentially infected burns tissue and close wounds with skin grafts [27]. McManus et al. reported similar findings after moving into a new burns center and avoiding transmission of an endemic strain of *Pseudomonas* in the old center by cohort nursing and avoidance of moving patients from the old burns center into the new center [64].

Avoidance of nosocomial *Pseudomonas* infections is most important for patients with larger or deeper wounds, or in those who are older, have inhalation or other risk factors that put them at high risk of death from burn injury [1]. Recently, a review of mortality in burns >50% TBSA demonstrated a 6-fold lower risk of death when a setting with better control of nosocomial infection [51] was compared with historic controls in the same setting at a time when nosocomial infections were more common, and shared practices, facilities, or equipment for wound care (such as hydrotherapy) occurred. Recent improvements in outcomes may be due to additional factors such as earlier surgical care, newer skin substitutes, or better intensive care. However, reports exist where these factors did not significantly improve outcomes over a similar time period [60]. To date, a number of other reports of nosocomial *Pseudomonas* outbreaks in other burns centers have emerged resembling that described herein, where mortality was very high in the infected patients [47,66–69].

In burns centers that use silver nitrate as a topical agent for the burn wounds, thus avoiding hydrotherapy and maintaining high levels of reverse isolation in laminar flow units, the cross-contamination rate with multidrug-resistant organisms is extremely low, 3.2 cases per 1000 patient-days [70]. Other centers where similar isolation is not possible have demonstrated that 74% of burns patients wounds become colonized with *P. aeruginosa*, >95% of which are resistant to multiple antibiotics including gentamicin, when only 4.75% of patients are contaminated at the time of admission [71]. Such dramatic differences in infection rates between burns centers illustrate the broad range of treatment approaches practiced and the difficulty and deficiency of clinical trials addressing isolation procedures and antimicrobial therapy in burns centers.

New preventive strategies: vaccines

The serious nature of infections caused by *P. aeruginosa* has led to concerted efforts by many investigators to develop candidate vaccines for prevention of *Pseudomonas* infections in the burned patient and in persons with cystic fibrosis. Lipolysaccharide (LPS) vaccines conjugated to carriers have been produced. While they showed good immunogenicity in human trials, toxicity from the lipid A portion of the LPS has prevented their use [72,73]. Whilst there have been some studies with flagellar vaccines, their efficacy in humans has not been clearly identified [74,75]. Recently, outer membrane proteins (OMPs) have also been used as targets for *P. aeruginosa* vaccines. In human volunteers, recombinant OMPs expressed in *E. coli* showed good immunogenicity [76,77]. In one recent study in burns patients, a composite OMP vaccine showed promise in reduction of sepsis caused by *P. aeruginosa* [78]. Peptide vaccines are also being investigated. They have been derived from OMPs [79,80] or are being produced synthetically as consensus sequences from pilin proteins [81,82]. These compounds may be conjugated to other proteins (e.g., tetanus toxoid) as haptens, to improve their immunogenicity. These consensus sequence peptides are strongly immunogenic in animal models, and are now undergoing phase I human clinical trials. It is still unknown if any of these candidate vaccine molecules will come into routine clinical use. It has been observed that the immune response following thermal injury may not be optimal [83] and therefore immunogenicity of these vaccines in animals or in healthy persons may not translate into efficacy in the burned patient.

Acknowledgments

The authors acknowledge the research support of the Alberta Heritage Foundation for Medical Research and the Canadian Institute for Health Research, as well as the Firefighters' Burn Trust Fund of the University of Alberta Hospital.

References

1 McManus AT, Mason AD, Jr., McManus WF, Pruitt BA, Jr. Twenty-five year review of *Pseudomonas aeruginosa* bacteremia in a burn center. Eur J Clin Microbiol 1985;4:219–23.

2 Revathi G, Puri J, Jain BK. Bacteriology of burns. Burns 1998;24:347–9.

3 Shankowsky HA, Callioux LS, Tredget EE. North American survey of hydrotherapy in modern burn care. J Burn Care Rehabil 1994;15:143–6.

4 Heggers JP, McCauley R, Herndon DN. Antimicrobial Therapy in Burns patients. Surg Rounds 1992:613–17.

5 Frame JD, Kangesu L, Malik WM. Changing flora in burn and trauma units: experience in the United Kingdom. J Burn Care Rehabil 1992;13:281–6.

6 Barillo DJ, McManus AT, Cioffi WG, et al. Aeromonas bacteremia in burns patients. Burns 1996;22:48–52.

7 Pruitt BA, Jr., McManus AT, Kim SH, Goodwin CW. Burn wound infections: current status. World J Surg 1998;22:135–45.

8 Pruitt BA, Jr. Phycomycotic infections. In: Alexaner JW, ed. Problems in General Surgery. Philadelphia: Lippincott, 1984.

9 Kucan JO, Smoot EC. Five percent mafenide acetate solution in the treatment of thermal injuries. J Burn Care Rehabil 1993;14:158–63.

10 Wendt C, Messer SA, Hollis RJ, et al. Molecular epidemiology of gram-negative bacteremia. Clin Infect Dis 1999;28:605–10.

11 Definitions for sepsis and organ failure and guidelines for the use of innovative therapies in sepsis. In: American College of Chest Physicians/Society of Critical Care Medicine Consensus Conference; 1992: Critical Care Medicine, 1992.

12 Vindenes HA, Ulvestad E, Bjerknes R. Concentrations of cytokines in plasma of patients with large burns: their relation to time after injury, burn size, inflammatory variables, infection, and outcome. Eur J Surg 1998;164:647–56.

13 Bisno AL. Cutaneous infections: microbiologic and epidemiologic considerations. Am J Med 1984;76:172–9.

14 Steer JA, Papini RP, Wilson AP, McGrouther DA, Parkhouse N. Quantitative microbiology in the management of burns patients. I. Correlation between quantitative and qualitative burn wound biopsy culture and surface alginate swab culture. Burns 1996;22:173–6.

15 McManus AT, Kim SH, McManus WF, Mason AD, Jr., Pruitt BA, Jr. Comparison of quantitative microbiology and histopathology in divided burn-wound biopsy specimens. Arch Surg 1987;122:74–6.

16 Williams HB, Breidenbach WC, Callaghan WB, Richards GK, Prentis JJ. Are burn wound biopsies obsolete? A comparative study of bacterial quantitation in burns patients using the absorbent disc and biopsy techniques. Ann Plast Surg 1984;13:388–95.

17 Tredget EE, Shankowsky HA, Groeneveld A, Burrell R. A matched-pair, randomized study evaluating the efficacy and safety of Acticoat silver-coated dressing for the treatment of burn wounds. J Burn Care Rehabil 1998;19:531–7.

18 Keen A, Knoblock L, Edelman L, Saffle J. Effective limitation of blood culture use in the burn unit. J Burn Care Rehabil 2002;23:183–9.

19 Henke PK, Polk HC, Jr. Efficacy of blood cultures in the critically ill surgical patient. Surgery 1996;120:752–9.

20 Miller PL, Matthey FC. A cost-benefit analysis of initial burn cultures in the management of acute burns. J Burn Care Rehabil 2000;21:300–3.

21 Nagesha CN, Shenoy KJ, Chandrashekar MR. Study of burn sepsis with special reference to *Pseudomonas aeruginosa*. J Indian Med Assoc 1996;94:230–3.

22 Moncrief JA, Lindberg RB, Switzer WE, Pruitt BA, Jr. The use of a topical sulfonamide in the control of burn wound sepsis. J Trauma 1966;6:407–19.

23 George N, Faoagali J, Muller M. Silvazine (silver sulfadiazine and chlorhexidine) activity against 200 clinical isolates. Burns 1997;23:493–5.

24 Monafo WW, West MA. Current treatment recommendations for topical burn therapy. Drugs 1990;40:364–73.

25 Sano S, Fujimori R, Takashima M, Itokawa Y. Absorption, excretion and tissue distribution of silver sulphadiazine. Burns Incl Therm Inj 1982;8:278–85.

26 Klasen HJ. A historical review of the use of silver in the treatment of burns. II. Renewed interest for silver. Burns 2000;26:131–8.

27 Tredget EE, Shankowsky HA, Joffe AM, et al. Epidemiology of infections with *Pseudomonas aeruginosa* in burns patients: the role of hydrotherapy. Clin Infect Dis 1992;15:941–9.

28 Murphy RC, Kucan JO, Robson MC, Heggers JP. The effect of 5% mafenide acetate solution on bacterial control in infected rat burns. J Trauma 1983;23:878–81.

29 Harrison HN, Blackmore WP, Bales HW, Reeder W. The absorption of C 14-labeled Sulfamylon acetate through burned skin. I. Experimental methods and initial observations. J Trauma 1972;12:986–93.

30 Wright JB, Lam K, Hansen D, Burrell RE. Efficacy of topical silver against fungal burn wound pathogens. Am J Infect Control 1999;27:344–50.

31 Yin HQ, Langford R, Burrell RE. Comparative evaluation of the antimicrobial activity of ACTICOAT antimicrobial barrier dressing. J Burn Care Rehabil 1999;20:195–200.

32 Wright DG, Hansen DL, Burrell R. The comparative efficacy of two antimicrobial barrier dressings: In vitro examination of two controlled release of silver dressing. Wounds 1998;10:179–88.

33 Wright JB, Lam K, Burrell RE. Wound management in an era of increasing bacterial antibiotic resistance: a role for topical silver treatment. Am J Infect Control 1998;26:572–7.

34 Burrell RE, Heggers JP, Davis GJ, Wright JB. Effect of silver coated dressings on animal survival in a rodent burn sepsis model. Wounds 1999;11(4):64–71.

35 Olson ME, Wright JB, Lam K, Burrell RE. Healing of porcine donor sites covered with silver-coated dressings. Eur J Surg 2000;166:486–9.

36 Wright JB, Lam K, Buret AG, Olson ME, Burrell RE. Early healing events in a porcine model of contamined wounds: effects of nanocrystalline silver on matrix metalloproteinases, cell apoptosis and healing. Wound Repair Regen 2002;10:141–51.

37 Voigt DW, Paul CN. The use of Acticoat silver impregnated telfa dressing in a regional burn and wound care center: The clinician's view. Wounds 2001;13:5–12.

38 Kirsner RS, Orsted H, Wright JB. Matrix metalloproteinases in normal and impaired wound healing: A potential role for nanocrystalline silver. Wounds 2001;13:5–12.

39 Baxter CR, Curreri PW, Marvin JA. The control of burn wound sepsis by the use of quantitative bacteriologic studies and subeschar clysis with antibiotics. Surg Clin North Am 1973;53:1509–18.

40 Herndon DN, Spies M. Modern burn care. Semin Pediatr Surg 2001;10:28–31.

41 Munster AM, Smith-Meek M, Sharkey P. The effect of early surgical intervention on mortality and cost-effectiveness in burn care, 1978–91. Burns 1994;20:61–4.

42 Tompkins RG, Burke JF, Schoenfeld DA, et al. Prompt eschar excision: a treatment system contributing to reduced burn mortality. A statistical evaluation of burn care at the Massachusetts General Hospital (1974–1984). Ann Surg 1986;204:272–81.

43 Tredget EE, Shankowsky HA, Taerum TV, Moysa GL, Alton JD. The role of inhalation injury in burn trauma. A Canadian experience. Ann Surg 1990;212:720–7.

44 Ng W, Tan CL, Yeow V, Yeo M, Teo SH. Ecthyma gangrenosum in a patient with hypogammaglobulinemia. J Infect 1998;36:331–5.

45 Eldridge JP, Baldridge ED, MacMillan BG. Ecthyma gangrenosum in a burned child. Burns Incl Therm Inj 1986;12:578–85.

46 Leibovici L, Konisberger H, Pitlik SD, Samra Z, Drucker M. Predictive index for optimizing empiric treatment of gram-negative bacteremia. J Infect Dis 1991;163:193–6.

47 Kolmos HJ, Thuesen B, Nielsen SV et al. Outbreak of infection in a burns unit due to Pseudomonas aeruginosa originating from contaminated tubing used for irrigation of patients. J Hosp Infect 1993;24:11–21.

48 Roberts SA, Findlay R, Lang SD. Investigation of an outbreak of multi-drug resistant Acinetobacter baumannii in an intensive care burns unit. J Hosp Infect 2001;48:228–32.

49 Cook N. Methicillin-resistant Staphylococcus aureus versus the burns patient. Burns 1998;24:91–8.

50 Marvin J. Burn care protocols-infection control in burn unit. Review of infection control procedure at Jackson Memorial Hospital Burn Center, From Harborview Hospital, Seattle. J Burn Care Rehabil 1987;8:71.

51 Tredget EE, Anzarut A, Shankowsky H, Logsetty S. Outcome and quality of life of massive burn injury: The impact of modern burn care. In: American Burn Association Annual Meeting; 2002; Chicago, Illinois; 2002.

52 Berrouane YF, McNutt LA, Buschelman BJ, et al. Outbreak of severe Pseudomonas aeruginosa infections caused by a contaminated drain in a whirlpool bathtub. Clin Infect Dis 2000;31:1331–7.

53 Doring G, Ulrich M, Muller W, et al. Generation of Pseudomonas aeruginosa aerosols during handwashing from contaminated sink drains, transmission to hands of hospital personnel, and its prevention by use of a new heating device. Zentralbl Hyg Umweltmed 1991;191:494–505.

54 Doring G, Jansen S, Noll H et al. Distribution and transmission of Pseudomonas aeruginosa and Burkholderia cepacia in a hospital ward. Pediatr Pulmonol 1996;21:90–100.

55 Doring G, Horz M, Ortelt J, Grupp H, Wolz C. Molecular epidemiology of Pseudomonas aeruginosa in an intensive care unit. Epidemiol Infect 1993;110:427–36.

56 Manson WL, Westerveld AW, Klasen HJ, Sauer EW. Selective intestinal decontamination of the digestive tract for infection prophylaxis in severely burned patients. Scand J Plast Reconstr Surg Hand Surg 1987;21:269–72.

57 Barret JP, Jeschke MG, Herndon DN. Selective decontamination of the digestive tract in severely burned pediatric patients. Burns 2001;27:439–45.

58 Inkson TI, Shankowsky HA, Brown K, et al. Cost comparison of silver sulfadiazine and silver nitrate for burn wound care. In: American Burn Association meeting, Chicago, Illinois, 1993.

59 Wisplinghoff H, Perbix W, Seifert H. Risk factors for nosocomial bloodstream infections due to Acinetobacter baumannii: a case-control study of adult burns patients. Clin Infect Dis 1999;28:59–66.

60 Ryan CM, Schoenfeld DA, Thorpe WP, et al. Objective estimates of the probability of death from burn injuries. N Engl J Med 1998;338:362–6.

61 O'Keefe GE, Hunt JL, Purdue GF. An evaluation of risk factors for mortality after burn trauma and the identification of gender-dependent differences in outcomes. J Am Coll Surg 2001;192:153–60.

62 Gullo A. Sepsis and organ dysfunction/failure. An overview. Minerva Anesthesiol 1999;65:529–40.

63 Taylor GD, Kibsey P, Kirkland T, Burroughs E, Tredget E. Predominance of staphylococcal organisms in infections occurring in a burns intensive care unit. Burns 1992;18:332–5.

64 McManus AT, McManus WF, Mason AD, Jr., Aitcheson AR, Pruitt BA, Jr. Microbial colonization in a new intensive care burn unit. A prospective cohort study. Arch Surg 1985; 120:217–23.

65 Tredget E, Shankowsky H, Lee J, Swanson T. The impact of nosocomial resistant pseudomonas infections in a burn unit. In: American Burn Association Annual Meeting, Miami, Florida, 2003.

66 Perinpanayagam RM, Grundy HC. Outbreak of gentamicin-resistant *Pseudomonas aeruginosa* infection in a burns unit. J Hosp Infect 1983;4:71–3.

67 Douglas MW, Mulholland K, Denyer V, Gottlieb T. Multi-drug resistant *Pseudomonas aeruginosa* outbreak in a burns unit – an infection control study. Burns 2001;27:131–5.

68 Hsueh PR, Teng LJ, Yang PC, et al. Persistence of a multidrug-resistant *Pseudomonas aeruginosa* clone in an intensive care burn unit. J Clin Microbiol 1998;36:1347–51.

69 Fujita K, Lilly HA, Ayliffe GA. Spread of resistant gram-negative bacilli in a burns unit. J Hosp Infect 1982;3:29–37.

70 Weber JM, Sheridan RL, Schulz JT, Tompkins RG, Ryan CM. Effectiveness of bacteria-controlled nursing units in preventing cross-colonization with resistant bacteria in severely burned children. Infect Control Hosp Epidemiol 2002;23:549–51.

71 Rastegar Lari A, Bahrami Honar H, Alaghehbandan R. *Pseudomonas* infections in Tohid Burn Center, Iran. Burns 1998;24:637–41.

72 Cryz SJ, Jr., Sadoff JC, Cross AS, Furer E. Safety and immunogenicity of a polyvalent *Pseudomonas aeruginosa* O-polysaccharide-toxin A vaccine in humans. Antibiot Chemother 1989;42:177–83.

73 Jones RJ, Roe EA, Gupta JL. Controlled trials of a polyvalent *Pseudomonas* vaccine in burns. Lancet 1979;2:977–82.

74 Doring G, Dorner F. A multicenter vaccine trial using the *Pseudomonas aeruginosa* flagella vaccine IMMUNO in patients with cystic fibrosis. Behring Inst Mitt, 1997.

75 Holder IA, Wheeler R, Montie TC. Flagellar preparations from *Pseudomonas aeruginosa*: animal protection studies. Infect Immun 1982;35:276–80.

76 von Specht BU, Lucking HC, Blum B, et al. Safety and immunogenicity of a *Pseudomonas aeruginosa* outer membrane protein I vaccine in human volunteers. Vaccine 1996;14:1111–17.

77 Mansouri E, Gabelsberger J, Knapp B, et al. Safety and immunogenicity of a *Pseudomonas aeruginosa* hybrid outer membrane protein F-I vaccine in human volunteers. Infect Immun 1999;67:1461–70.

78 Kim DK, Kim JJ, Kim JH, et al. Comparison of two immunization schedules for a *Pseudomonas aeruginosa* outer membrane proteins vaccine in burns patients. Vaccine 2000;19:1274–83.

79 Hughes EE, Gilleland LB, Gilleland HE, Jr. Synthetic peptides representing epitopes of outer membrane protein F of *Pseudomonas aeruginosa* that elicit antibodies reactive with whole cells of heterologous immunotype strains of *P. aeruginosa*. Infect Immun 1992;60:3497–503.

80 Hughes EE, Gilleland HE, Jr. Ability of synthetic peptides representing epitopes of outer membrane protein F of *Pseudomonas aeruginosa* to afford protection against *P. aeruginosa infection* in a murine acute pneumonia model. Vaccine 1995;13:1750–3.

81 Sheth HB, Glasier LM, Ellert NW, et al. Development of an anti-adhesive vaccine for *Pseudomonas aeruginosa* targeting the C-terminal region of the pilin structural protein. Biomed Pept Proteins Nucleic Acids 1995;1:141–8.

82 Cachia PJ, Glasier LM, Hodgins RR, et al. The use of synthetic peptides in the design of a consensus sequence vaccine for *Pseudomonas aeruginosa*. J Pept Res 1998;52:289–99.

83 Lawrence MH, de Riesthal HF, Calvano SE. Changes in memory and naive CD4+ lymphocytes in lymph nodes and spleen after thermal injury. J Burn Care Rehabil 1996;17:1–6.

CHAPTER 18

Infections in healthcare workers

Gregory Rose & Virginia R. Roth

Case presentation 1

A phlebotomist presents to you with a needlestick injury from a patient known to have advanced HIV and hepatitis C infections. She used the needle to draw blood and injected a small amount of blood into her finger accidentally while re-sheathing the needle before disposal. She is fully vaccinated against hepatitis B and had her antibody levels checked within the last 6 months. You counsel her about the risk of transmission of HIV and hepatitis C.

Occupational bloodborne pathogen exposures

It is estimated that American healthcare workers (HCWs) suffer between 300 000 and 460 000 needlesticks and other sharps injuries every year [1]. The American Hospital Association estimates that one case of infection by a bloodborne pathogen can incur expenditures of $1 million or more for clinical care and lost productivity. The cost of follow-up for a high-risk bloodborne pathogen exposure is almost $3000, even when no infection occurs [2]. The World Health Organization estimates that bloodborne pathogen exposures among HCWs are responsible for 66 000 cases of hepatitis B, 16 000 cases of hepatitis C, and 200–5000 cases of human immunodeficiency virus (HIV) annually, as well as a smaller number of other infections such as tuberculosis or malaria [3].

Evidence-Based Infectious Diseases, 2nd edition. Edited by Mark Loeb, Fiona Smaill and Marek Smieja. © 2009 Wiley-Blackwell Publishing, ISBN: 978-1-4051-7026-0

HIV: infection and risk assessment

A summary of 25 case–control studies (22 seroconversions in 6955 exposed people) found that the risk of HIV transmission after percutaneous exposure was 0.32% (95% confidence interval [CI] 0.18–0.45%) and the risk after mucocutaneous exposure was 0.03% (95% CI 0.006–0.19%) [4]. However, the risk of transmission is higher following certain percutaneous exposures [5] (Table 18.1).

A recent Cochrane review [6] identified no randomized controlled trials on the effect of postexposure prophylaxis (PEP) on HIV transmission following occupational exposure. The only case–control study that was included in this review compared HCWs who acquired HIV infection after percutaneous exposure with HCWs who remained HIV-seronegative at least 6 months following occupational exposure [5]. After controlling for risk factors for seroconversion (Table 18.1), HIV infection was 81% less likely in HCWs who received postexposure zidovudine compared with those who did not (95% CI 43–94%). Efficacy of PEP following occupational exposures is

Table 18.1 Risk factors for HIV seroconversion after percutaneous exposure to a known HIV-infected source

	Adjusted odds ratio	95% CI
Deep injury	15	6.0–41
Visible blood on device	6.2	2.2–21
Procedure involving a needle placed in source patient's blood vessel	4.3	1.7–12
Source patient with terminal AIDS	5.6	2.0–16

Source: reference [5].

also extrapolated from the effect of antiretrovirals on perinatal transmission. A retrospective cohort study of 939 infants demonstrated that postnatal zidovudine prophylaxis within 48 hours of birth reduces the incidence of HIV transmission from 26.6% to 9.3%, even in the absence of maternal therapy [7]. The importance of the timing of PEP is supported by primate studies showing that PEP confers no benefit if initiated more than 24 hours postexposure [8,9].

The Cochrane review identified no studies that evaluated the effect of combination antiretroviral therapy for PEP following occupational exposure [6]. Reasons for considering combination therapy in this setting include enhanced treatment effectiveness for HIV-infected patients, enhanced effectiveness in preventing perinatal transmission, reduced risk of emergence of resistant strains, and potential exposure to zidovudine-resistant strains. Adverse effects are reported in over 70% of HCWs started on PEP [10,11]. The Cochrane review found that adverse events were significantly higher with the use of multi-drug regimens, but that discontinuation rates were not significantly different [6]. The Centers for Disease Control and Prevention (CDC) guidelines recommend a basic 4-week regimen of two drugs for most HIV exposures, and an expanded regimen that includes a third drug (usually a protease inhibitor) for HIV exposures that pose an increased risk for transmission (Table 18.1) [12,13].

Rapid HIV testing of the source following occupational exposure can significantly reduce the unnecessary use of PEP, the cost of managing HCWs receiving PEP and its associated side effects, and psychological stress [14,15]. When the source is unknown or cannot be tested, HCWs should be counseled to exercise sexual abstinence or use condoms [16], and not to donate blood, semen, or organs for the first 6–12 weeks following exposure.

Hepatitis B virus infection

Healthcare workers are at risk of occupational exposure to hepatitis B virus (HBV). Unvaccinated HCWs exposed to a source patient that is hepatitis B surface antigen (HBsAg)-positive and HBeAg-positive have a 22–31% risk of developing clinical hepatitis and a 37–62% risk of seroconversion. Unvaccinated healthcare workers exposed to a source patient that is HBsAg-positive, HBeAg-negative have a 1–6% of

developing clinical hepatitis and a 23–37% risk of seroconversion [17].

Effective vaccines are now available to prevent occupational acquisition of HBV, and evidence from a Cochrane review supports occupational health guidelines that all HCWs should be offered HBV vaccination [18]. Since the availability of vaccines, the proportion of acute HBV cases in the United States related to occupational exposure has dropped from 4.5% to 0.5% [19].

Studies reported in the early 1980s showed an overall benefit of plasma-derived HBV vaccine for preventing HBV infection in HCWs (RR 0.51, 95% CI 0.35–0.73), although the differences were not significant for the low-risk HCWs (RR 0.20, 95% CI 0.02–1.70). Recombinant DNA HBV vaccines have been shown to be as safe and immunogenic as the original plasma-derived vaccine [18,20]. Attempts at administering reduced doses of vaccine intradermally have been unsuccessful. Six trials comparing full-dose intramuscular administration of plasma-derived or recombinant DNA HBV vaccine to low-dose intradermal administration have all demonstrated reduced incidence of protective immunity from intradermal administration [18].

There is no evidence that booster doses are necessary to maintain seropositive HBsAb titers [21]. Although not prospectively evaluated, most guidelines recommend serologic testing for hepatitis antibody after a primary immunization course has been completed. Approximately 10% of HCWs may fail to respond to HBV immunization (nonresponders). In one HCW study, factors associated with failure to develop protective levels of HBV antibodies included increasing age, obesity, smoking, and male gender [20]. Persons who do not respond to an initial three-dose vaccine series have a 30–50% chance of responding to a second three-dose series [12,22].

Postexposure vaccination of susceptible HCWs has been shown to be protective against the development of clinical hepatitis [23]. Hepatitis B immune globulin (HBIG) is also effective in preventing clinical infection postexposure [24]; however, HCWs who received HBIG were as likely as those who received immune serum globulin to develop subclinical infection [25]. The effectiveness of combined vaccination and HBIG following exposure has not been evaluated in the occupational setting; however, increased efficacy of this combination compared with HBIG alone in preventing perinatal transmission provides indirect support of this practice [26]. Thus, unvaccinated (or incompletely vaccinated) HCWs should receive a single HBIG dose plus HBV vaccine following a significant exposure [12,27]. For HCWs who remain nonresponders after the second three-dose vaccination series, two doses of HBIG are recommended following a significant exposure [12].

Hepatitis C virus infection

Hepatitis C virus (HCV) is not efficiently transmitted by occupational exposure. The average transmission rate to more than 11 000 exposed HCWs from six countries was 0.5% (95% CI 0.39–0.65) [28]. Transmission occurred through percutaneous or mucosal exposure; no occupational transmission has been documented from intact or nonintact skin exposures [12].

There is no evidence of benefit of postexposure immunoglobulin prophylaxis for HCV and its use is not recommended [12,27]. Similarly, there have been no clinical trials evaluating the efficacy of antiviral agents (e.g., interferon or ribavirin) to prevent HCV infection following occupational exposure, and antivirals are not FDA-approved for this indication [12].

Early therapy of acute HCV has been studied, but heterogeneity of definitions of acute HCV disease and in the antiviral regimens used has made it difficult to interpret the results of these studies. In an open-label study which included 14 HCWs a 24-week course of interferon-α-2b prevented chronic HCV infection in 98% of patients and treatment was well tolerated [29].

A series of related intervention studies by Kamal and colleagues demonstrated no difference between peginterferon-α-2a compared to peginterferon-α-2b, a nonsignificant advantage to the addition of ribavirin, advantage to a longer (i.e., 24-week) course of therapy for genotype 1 virus (whereas 8-week or 12-week regimens sufficed for other genotypes), and an advantage to earlier initiation of therapy (i.e., 8 or 12 weeks after first evidence of biochemical hepatitis with positive HCV viremia demonstrated by PCR) [30–32]. Although uncertainty remains around the optimal antiviral regimen and duration of therapy, these studies demonstrate the importance of early diagnosis and treatment in the prevention of chronic HCV infection.

Current CDC guidelines recommend measuring HCV antibody at 4–6 months to detect infection [12], while European guidelines recommend testing for HCV antibody at baseline, 6 months, and 12 months, as well as alanine aminotransferase monthly for the first 4 months, with HCV PCR performed upon detection of abnormal results [27]. Current guidelines do not establish an optimal approach for treating HCWs occupationally infected with HCV, but it seems reasonable to undertake surveillance for biochemical hepatitis and seroconversion, confirm this with quantitative HCV PCR and genotyping, and then observe 8 to 12 weeks for spontaneous viral clearance before offering therapy for acute HCV with pegylated interferon, with or without ribavirin [33].

Prevention

Risk factors for bloodborne pathogen exposure include less-experienced or less-educated HCWs, HCWs in higher-workload centers, HCW fatigue, and extended duration of workshifts [34–36]. There have been few randomized trials evaluating the effectiveness of interventions to reduce exposures among HCWs. In one systematic review that included 11 randomized trials mostly focusing on surgical procedures, a reduction in sharps injuries and glove perforations was associated with double gloving, use of specialized needles for wound closure, use of safety-engineered devices, and use of a "no-touch" technique during wound closure [37].

A systematic review of 17 intervention studies of needleless or safety-engineered sharps systems demonstrated reduced incidence of percutaneous injury by 22–100% compared to pre-intervention, although involvement of HCWs in the selection and implementation of safety systems was important in the success of harm reduction strategies [38]. Several of these studies also demonstrated cost savings with implementation of safety-engineered devices.

Summary

Harm prevention strategies should incorporate education about safer work practices, particularly for more inexperienced healthcare workers, and incorporate "no-touch" surgical closure techniques and safety-engineered devices. Should a bloodborne pathogen exposure occur, HCW require prompt evaluation and management. For high-risk exposures, combination antiretroviral therapy should be initiated promptly and rapid testing performed on the source patient. There is good evidence to support universal HBV vaccination of HCWs, but weak evidence for postexposure use of HBIG. Occupational exposures to HCV should be managed by surveillance for, and early treatment of, acute disease.

Case presentation 2

At the end of his 24-hour on-call shift, a resident asks his attending staff to look at his rash. It is obviously chickenpox. Infection Control and Occupational Health Services are promptly called for advice regarding management of the resident and his contacts. The resident believed he had chickenpox as a child, but had not been tested further. As a result of exposure to this resident, 15 healthcare workers spent 14 days of paid leave off work and 8 exposed patients were kept in respiratory isolation during the period they were potentially infectious. A recommendation is made for a thorough review of the screening protocols for healthcare workers and policies for vaccine-preventable infections.

Varicella zoster virus infections

Varicella zoster virus (VZV) causes chickenpox or varicella zoster. Although chickenpox is usually self-limited in children, it is generally more severe in adults and immunocompromised persons, with higher rates of pneumonia, encephalitis, and death reported [39]. Individuals at higher risk of complications include pregnant women, premature infants born to varicella susceptible mothers, infants born at less than 28 weeks gestation or weighing ≤1000 g (regardless of maternal immune status) and immunocompromised individuals [40]. The risk of congenital varicella syndrome following maternal infection during the first trimester of pregnancy has been estimated to be 2.2% (95% CI 0–4.6%) [41]. Following primary chickenpox infection, the virus remains dormant in sensory nerve ganglia and may reactivate, resulting in varicella zoster or shingles.

Nosocomial transmission of VZV is well recognized [39,42], and prevention and control measures are costly [43,44]. Thus, control measures in healthcare facilities are strongly recommended [42,45,46]. VZV is transmitted from person to person via direct contact with infected lesions, or airborne spread from either the lesions or respiratory tract secretions [39]. It is generally accepted that patients with localized zoster are less contagious than those with primary chickenpox or disseminated zoster; however, patients with localized zoster have been shown to be the source for extensive environmental contamination and aerosolization [47–49].

Although there have been no controlled clinical trials of the effectiveness of VZV vaccine in HCWs, a long-term prospective follow-up study of vaccinated HCWs showed that the attack rate following household and hospital exposure was reduced from an estimated 90% to 18% and 8% respectively, that all illness was mild to moderate (mean 40 vesicles), and that 96% of HCWs developed antibodies to varicella [50]. Based on these data, current guidelines recommend that all susceptible HCWs be immunized with two doses of standard-dose live attenuated VZV vaccine [39,42,46].

Most adults are immune to VZV because of infection during childhood. The sensitivity of a history of chickenpox for predicting serologic immunity in HCWs ranges from 79% to 100% [51–55], with a high positive predictive value (98–100%) but a negative predictive value of less than 10%. Thus, HCWs who give a history of chickenpox as a child may be considered to be immune [56]. However, those with an uncertain or negative history of chickenpox should have a serologic test to determine susceptibility [39,42,46]. Overall, less than 5% of HCWs in the western world lack serologic immunity to VZV [52–54]; however, HCWs from Africa, the Middle East, and East Asia may be at higher risk (12–19% lack seroprotection) [57]. Serologic testing of all staff with a negative or uncertain history of VZV, and vaccinating those who are seronegative, was found to be a cost-effective strategy by both modeling and clinical studies [58–60]. Post-vaccination serologic testing is not recommended, as 94–99% of adults will develop immunity [61,62].

It is recommended that susceptible HCWs (i.e., seronegative HCWs who have not been vaccinated) be excluded from work from days 8 to 21 following a significant exposure [39,40,42,45,46]. However, there is variation between current guidelines as to what constitutes a significant varicella exposure [39,46,63]. Proposed postexposure strategies for managing these susceptible HCWs have included vaccination, varicella-zoster immune globulin (VZIG), and antivirals. Controlled studies of postexposure prophylaxis using VZV vaccine in HCWs have not been carried out. A review of current evidence suggests that postexposure vaccination of children within 3 days of rash onset of the index case appears to be an effective preventive measure [63]. For the small proportion of contacts that develop infectious VZV despite vaccination, the clinical illness is mild. These data have been extrapolated to support recommendations for postexposure vaccination in healthcare settings, however, pre-employment testing and vaccination remains the preferred approach [39,42,46].

There is no evidence to support the routine use of VZIG in healthy HCWs exposed to chickenpox. VZIG administered within 96 hours after exposure has been shown in observational studies to prevent or modify clinical illness in nonimmune, immunocompromised persons who are exposed to varicella [64–66]. An observational study in neonates found that VZIG reduced the incidence of varicella disease if the mother had chickenpox during the last week of pregnancy [67]. Based on these observational studies, VZIG is recommended postexposure for immunocompromised or pregnant HCWs who are susceptible [39,46]; however, there is no evidence from controlled trials to support this approach. It should be noted that VZIG may extend the incubation period of the virus from 10–21 days to ≥28 days, and this should be taken into account when excluding susceptible, exposed HCWs from work.

There are few studies evaluating the use of acyclovir as postexposure prophylaxis. In one report two varicella-susceptible resident physicians were deliberately exposed to an infected child and then given a 7-day course of acyclovir beginning 9 to 11 days postexposure. Both residents developed limited disease (less than 48 hours' duration, fewer than five lesions) and developed protective immunity by the fourth week postexposure [68]. In two small household studies, 7.4% and 16% of contacts given acyclovir developed disease compared with 77% and 100% of contacts who were not given acyclovir [69,70]; however, acyclovir use was associated with a decreased

rate of seroconversion and approximately half of the contacts remained susceptible to VZV [45]. VZV infection following prophylactic acyclovir use has been reported [71]. Based on current evidence, the prophylactic use of acyclovir is not recommended; postexposure vaccination remains the approach of choice for otherwise healthy susceptible individuals and VZIG is recommended for immunocompromised individuals [39,46].

Summary

Nosocomial transmission of varicella to susceptible HCWs is a risk both to the health of the worker as well as their patients. The key prevention strategy is pre-employment screening of HCWs, and providing vaccination to those susceptible. Postexposure vaccination of susceptible HCWs within 3 days of exposure is a secondary prevention measure. The indications for prophylactic VZIG are very limited, and prophylactic acyclovir is not recommended.

Case presentation 3

You are approached by an emergency department nurse concerned about a patient she treated during her last shift. The patient is an elderly woman who presented with fever, cough, and shortness of breath. The nurse tended to this patient in an open stretcher bay for some time prior to the initial physician assessment, and afterwards was dismayed to learn that the patient had presumed influenza. The nurse, like many of her colleagues, declined influenza vaccine this year citing concern regarding possible adverse reactions, and is now worried about becoming ill. She wants to know what steps can be taken to ameliorate her risk now, and for future exposures.

Influenza-like illness

Influenza

Influenza epidemics and pandemics have had a remarkable societal impact throughout history. One review of the socioeconomic burden of influenza suggests that the indirect costs associated with annual influenza epidemics (including work absenteeism and loss of productivity) are up to 10-fold higher than the direct costs of medical care [72]. Nosocomial influenza is one of the most common pathogens resulting in closure of clinical units, generating additional healthcare costs and impacting patient care [73]. Elderly or chronically ill adults are at increased risk for pneumonia, hospitalization, and death related to influenza; however, healthy HCWs become part of the chain of transmission of influenza during outbreaks, particularly in nosocomial transmission [74].

A Cochrane review assessing the effectiveness of the influenza vaccine demonstrated a 62% reduction in laboratory-confirmed cases of influenza in healthy adults (95% CI 45–73%) for the live aerosol vaccine and an 80% reduction (95% CI 56–91%) for the inactivated parenteral vaccine, but only a modest effect on non-laboratory-confirmed disease ("influenza-like illness", ILI) of 10% and 30% respectively [75]. Vaccination was also associated with a significant reduction in work absenteeism. A recent review of three randomized controlled trials of HCW influenza vaccination revealed conflicting results [76], with one study showing a significant reduction in serologically confirmed influenza of 88% (95% CI 47–97%) but no significant reduction in work absenteeism [77], one study showing no difference in ILI but a significant reduction in work absenteeism due to ILI [78], and the third study showing no significant difference in rates of ILI or work absenteeism [79]. The lack of effect in the third study was explained by a poor match between the vaccine strains and the circulating strains. Vaccination was safe and well-tolerated in all three studies [76].

Another recent Cochrane review found that HCW vaccination significantly reduces ILI in patients (but only when patients are vaccinated too), death from pneumonia, and death from all causes [80]. There was no effect on confirmed influenza cases or lower respiratory tract infection; however, systematic laboratory testing of patients to confirm an influenza diagnosis was not done. An economic evaluation using UK data suggests that HCW vaccination saves approximately £12 in healthcare costs per vaccine administered based on reduced work absenteeism [76]. Thus, several national guidelines strongly recommend annual influenza vaccine for patients and HCWs as a means of preventing transmission in healthcare facilities [42,46].

The uptake of influenza vaccine amongst HCWs varies widely between studies, from as low as 2% [76] to as high as 82% [81]. Two recent reviews found that the major barriers to vaccination were: (1) HCWs' misperception of the need for vaccination; (2) lack of (or perceived lack of) conveniently available vaccine; (3) misperception of vaccine effectiveness; (4) fear of adverse effects; (5) fear that the vaccine would cause influenza; and (6) fear of injections or needles [76,81]. A review of seven controlled studies evaluating the effect of promotional campaigns on HCW influenza vaccination rates yielded variable results, and found that studies performed to date are limited by bias, confounding, incomplete reporting, and lack of long-term follow-up [76]. These studies reported baseline vaccination rates of 5–17% with increases of 5–45% in response to vaccination campaigns. The best-designed study in this review, a cluster-randomized controlled trial, showed no increase in vaccination uptake by HCWs despite an intensive promotional campaign [82]. Thus, uncertainty remains around whether behavioral interventions can improve HCW influenza vaccination coverage in a sustained manner. As a result, some consideration had been given to making influenza vaccination mandatory [83]. In the meantime, for HCWs concerned about side effects, there is good evidence from a placebo-controlled trial that acetaminophen will significantly reduce symptoms of sore arm and nausea associated with the vaccine [84].

There are no controlled trials assessing the effect of antiviral prophylaxis in HCWs [85]. A Cochrane systematic review showed that neuraminidase inhibitor prophylaxis in adults was not effective in preventing ILI, although it did prevent laboratory-confirmed influenza (dose- and agent-dependent: oseltamivir 150 mg per day most efficacious at 73%) [85]. Another Cochrane review showed that amantadine prevented 25% of cases of ILI (95% CI 13–36%) and 61% of laboratory-confirmed influenza A, but was associated with significant gastrointestinal side effects [86]. Based on these findings, current guidelines recommend antiviral prophylaxis for the management of unimmunized HCWs during a nosocomial outbreak; however, vaccination remains the preferred preventive measure [87].

Institutional measures to control ILI – the SARS experience

The role of HCWs in both nosocomial and community-based transmission of ILI was dramatically highlighted during the 2003 severe acute respiratory syndrome (SARS) outbreak [88–90]. Worldwide,

HCWs composed approximately 5% of all SARS cases; however, in some countries (including Vietnam, Singapore, and Canada) HCWs represented over 40% of all cases [90]. In these countries, several factors were associated with transmission of SARS to and from HCWs, and these factors are likely to apply to transmission of other etiologies of ILI. These include HCWs working while ill ("presenteeism"), inadequate use of personal protective equipment (such as gloves, gowns, masks), poor hand hygiene practices, and most fundamentally, a lack of early recognition of the severity and transmissibility of the illness [88,89,91]. Thus, recent guidelines on respiratory hygiene recommend that appropriate precautions (e.g., masking and/or isolating patients) be initiated for all patients ill with ILI at the initial point of healthcare contact (e.g., upon registration or triage), rather than being delayed until after medical assessment [92].

Prevention of other infections in healthcare workers

General measures

Many issues noted in the transmission of SARS to and from HCWs stem from inappropriate attention to previous infection control/occupational health standards, and likely apply to other occupational exposures as well. For example, a case–control analysis of SARS exposure among HCWs in Singapore demonstrated a protective relationship between post-patient contact handwashing and incidence of SARS (OR 0.07; 95% CI 0.008–0.66) [89].

There is evidence among other populations that hand hygiene is a self-protective measure. A cluster-randomized trial among university students noted that a hand hygiene campaign decreased incidence of ILI 20%, with a 43% reduction in absentee days [93]. Similarly, a cluster-randomized study of a hand hygiene campaign among military personnel noted a 40% reduction in outpatient visits for ILI, a 48% reduction in diarrheal illness, and a 44% reduction in lost training time due to illness [94]. A Cochrane systematic review supports the use of handwashing to reduce diarrheal illness in institutional and community settings [95]. Unfortunately HCW compliance with hand hygiene standards is often suboptimal [96], as is compliance with other infection control/occupational health recommendations such as use of

personal protective equipment [97], and avoidance of "presenteeism" (presenting to work while ill) [98].

Other infections

Nosocomial transmission of measles and rubella is well documented [99]. A number of observational studies have shown that serologic screening of HCWs before immunization is cost-effective for measles [100–102]. A history of disease or vaccination can be unreliable [103]. Immunization of HCWs who do not have evidence of immunity against measles, mumps, and rubella is strongly recommended [42,46], with evidence from case–control and cohort studies supporting a vaccine efficacy of greater than 95% [104–106].

Invasive meningococcal disease is associated with a case fatality rate of up to 10%. There are no controlled trials on the effects of prophylactic antibiotics on the incidence of meningococcal disease nor good evidence to identify which contacts should be treated [107]. Although there are reports of transmission of infection to HCWs, nosocomial transmission is extremely rare. In a retrospective survey from England and Wales the risk of invasive meningococcal disease in HCWs was 0.8 per 100 000 HCWs exposed to meningococcal disease, roughly 25 times that in the general population; however, the authors of the study concluded that the excess risk was small [108]. Nonetheless, based on case reports of meningococcal infection in HCWs with unprotected airway exposure to respiratory droplets from patients with meningococcal infection, occupational health guidelines recommend prophylaxis in these settings [42]. There is evidence from randomized trials, using eradication of *Neisseria meningitidis* as the endpoint, to support the use of rifampin, single-dose ceftriaxone, or single-dose ciprofloxacin for PEP [109–110].

Using retrospective data on cases of laboratory-acquired invasive meningococcal disease, the CDC estimated an increased attack rate of 13 per 100 000 population (95% CI 5–29) and recommended that vaccination be considered for laboratory workers working with isolates of *Neisseria meningitidis* [111]. The vaccine, however, will only protect against meningococcal disease caused by serogroups contained in the vaccine.

Summary

There is good evidence, in many instances from controlled trials, to support current guidelines for the screening and immunization of HCWs against vaccine-preventable infections. Infection control standards should be reinforced among HCWs, and control measures put in place early in the care of potentially infectious patients.

Acknowledgments

The authors acknowledge the work of Drs Fiona Smaill and Brian Angus in the first edition, upon which this revised chapter is based.

References

1 Panlilio AL, Orelien JG, Srivastava PU, et al. Estimate of the annual number of percutaneous injuries among hospital-based healthcare workers in the United States, 1997–1998. Infect Control Hosp Epidemiol 2004;25:556–562.

2 Occupational Safety and Health Administration. Record Summary of the Request for Information on Occupational Exposure to Bloodborne Pathogens Due to Percutaneous Injury. (Washington, D.C.: Occupational Safety and Health Administration, May 1999). http://www.osha-slc.gov/html/ndlreport052099.html

3 Prüss-Üstün A, Rapiti E, Hutin Y. Sharps injuries: Global burden of disease from sharps injuries to health-care workers. WHO Environmental Burden of Disease Series, No 3. World Health Organization, Geneva, Switzerland. 2003.

4 Public Health Laboratory Service. Occupational transmission of HIV. Summary of published reports. PHLS, London, UK 1997.

5 Cardo DM, Culver DH, Ciesielski CA, et al. A case-control study of HIV seroconversion in health care workers after percutaneous exposure. Centers for Disease Control and Prevention Needlestick Surveillance Group. N Engl J Med 1997;337:1485–90.

6 Young TN, Arens FJ, Kennedy GE, Laurie JW, Rutherford G. Antiretroviral post-exposure prophylaxis (PEP) for occupational HIV exposure. Cochrane Database Syst Rev. 2007 (1), CD002835, DOI: 10.1002/14651858.

7 Wade NA, Birkhead GS, Warren BL, et al. Abbreviated regimens of zidovudine prophylaxis and perinatal transmission of the human immunodeficiency virus. N Engl J Med 1998;339:1409–14.

8 Tsai CC, Emau P, Sun JC, et al. Post-exposure chemoprophylaxis (PECP) against SIV infection of macaques as a model for protection from HIV infection. J Med Primatol 2000;29:248–58.

9 Le Grand R, Vaslin B, Larghero J, et al. Post-exposure prophylaxis with highly active antiretroviral therapy could not protect macaques from infection with SIV/HIV chimera. AIDS 2000;14:1864–6.

10 Wang SA, Panlilio AL, Doi PA, White AD, Stek M Jr, Saah A. Experience of healthcare workers taking postexposure prophylaxis after occupational HIV exposures: findings of the HIV Postexposure Prophylaxis Registry. Infect Control Hosp Epidemiol 2000;21(12):780–5.

11 Srivastava P, Cardo DM, Panlilio A, Campbell S. Tolerability of antiretroviral agents used by health-care workers (HCWs) as post-exposure prophylaxis (PEP) for occupational exposures to HIV. Int Conf AIDS, 12:626 (abstract no. 246/33171). 1998.

12 Centers for Disease Control and Prevention. Updated US Public Health Service Guidelines for the management of occupational exposures to HBV, HCV, and HIV and recommendations for postexposure prophylaxis. MMWR 2001;50(RR-11):1–52.

13 Centers for Disease Control and Prevention. Updated US Public Health Service guidelines for the management of occupational exposures to HIV and recommendations for postexposure prophylaxis. MMWR 2005;54(RR-9):1–17.

14 King AM, Osterwalder JJ, Vernazza PL. A randomized prospective study to evaluate a rapid HIV-antibody assay in the management of cases of percutaneous exposure amongst health care workers. Swiss Med Wkly 2001; 12:10–13.

15 Landrum ML, Wilson CH, Perri LP, Hannibal SL, O'Connell RJ. Usefulness of a rapid human immunodeficiency virus-1 antibody test for the management of occupational exposure to blood and body fluid. Infect Control Hosp Epidemiol 2005;26(9):768–74.

16 Weller S, Davis-Beaty K. Condom effectiveness in reducing heterosexual HIV transmission. Cochrane Database Syst Rev 2002 (1), CD003255, DOI: 10.1002/14651858.

17 Werner BG, Grady GF. Accidental hepatitis B surface antigen positive inoculations: use of e antigen to estimate infectivity. Ann Intern Med 1982;97:367–9.

18 Chen W, Gluud C. Vaccines for preventing hepatitis B in health-care workers. Cochrane Database Syst Rev 2005 (4), CD000100, DOI: 10.1002/14651858.

19 Centers for Disease Control and Prevention. Hepatitis Surveillance Report Number 60. Atlanta, GA: US Department of Health and Human Services, Centers for Disease Control and Prevention; 2005.

20 Averhoff F, Mahoney F, Colemen P, et al. Immunogenicity of hepatitis B vaccines. Implications for persons at occupational risk of hepatitis B infection. Am J Prev Med 1998; 15:1–8.

21 European Consensus Group on Hepatitis B Immunity. Are booster immunisations needed for lifelong hepatitis B immunity? Lancet 2000; 355:561–565.

22 Hadler SC, Francis DP, Maynard JE, et al. Long-term immunogenicity and efficacy of hepatitis B vaccine in homosexual men. N Engl J Med 1986;315:209–14.

23 Palmović D, Crnjaković-Palmović J. Prevention of hepatitis B virus (HBV) infection in health-care workers after accidental exposure: a comparison of two prophylactic schedules. Infection 1993;21(1):42–5.

24 Veterans Administration Cooperative Study. Type B hepatitis after NSI exposure: prevention with hepatitis B immune globulin. Final report of the Veterans Administration Cooperative Study. Ann Intern Med 1978;88:285–93.

25 Hoofnagle JH, Seeff LB, Bales ZB, et al. Passive-active immunity from hepatitis B immune globulin. Reanalysis of

a Veteran Administration cooperative study of needle-stick hepatitis. Ann Intern Med 1979;91:813–18.

26 Beasley RP, Hwang L-Y, Steven CE, et al. Efficacy of hepatitis B immune globulin for prevention of perinatal transmission of the hepatitis B virus carrier state: final report of a randomized double-blind, placebo controlled trial. Hepatology 1983;3:135–41.

27 Puro V, De Carli G, Cicalini S et al. European recommendations for the management of healthcare workers occupationally exposed to hepatitis B virus and hepatitis C virus. Euro Surveill 2005;10:260–4.

28 Jagger J, Puro V, De Carli G. Occupational transmission of hepatitis C virus. JAMA 2002;288:1469–70.

29 Jaeckel E, Cornberg M, Wedemeyer H, et al. Treatment of acute hepatitis C infection with interferon alfa-2b. N Engl J Med 2001;345:1452–7.

30 Kamal SM, Ismail A, Graham CS, et al. Pegylated interferon alpha therapy in acute hepatitis C: relation to hepatitis C virus-specific T cell response kinetics. Hepatology 2004;39:1721–31.

31 Kamal SM, Fouly AE, Kamel RR, et al. Peginterferon alfa-2b therapy in acute hepatitis C: impact of onset of therapy on sustained virologic response. Gastroenterology 2006;130:632–8.

32 Kamal SM, Moustafa KN, Chen J, et al. Duration of peginterferon therapy in acute hepatitis C: a randomized trial. Hepatology 2006;43:923–31.

33 Varghese GM, Abraham OC, Mathai D. Post-exposure prophylaxis for blood borne viral infections in healthcare workers. Postgrad Med J 2003;79(932):324–8.

34 Ayas NT, Barger KL, Cade BE, et al. Extended work duration and the risk of self-reported percutaneous injuries in interns. JAMA 2006;296:1055–62.

35 Brasel KJ, Mol C, Kolker A, et al. Needlesticks and surgical residents: who is most at risk? J Surg Educ 2007;64:395–8.

36 Clarke SP. Hospital work environments, nurse characteristics, and sharps injuries. Am J Infect Control 2007;35:302–9.

37 Rogers B, Goodno L. Evaluation of interventions to prevent needlestick injuries in health care occupations. Am J Prev Med 2000;18:90–8.

38 Tuma S, Sepkowitz KA. Efficacy of safety-engineered device implementation in the prevention of percutaneous injuries: a review of published studies. Clin Infect Dis 2006;42:1159–70.

39 Marin M, Güris D, Chaves SS, Schmid S, Seward JF; Advisory Committee on Immunization Practices, Centers for Disease Control and Prevention (CDC). Prevention of varicella: recommendations of the Advisory Committee on Immunization Practices (ACIP). MMWR Recomm Rep 2007;56(RR-4):1–40.

40 Stover BH, Bratcher DF. Varicella-zoster virus: infection, control, and prevention. Am J Infect Control 1998;26(3):369–81.

41 Pastuszak AL, Levy M, Schick B, et al. Outcome after maternal varicella infection in the first 20 weeks of pregnancy. N Engl J Med 1994;330:901–5.

42 Centers for Disease Control and Prevention. Immunization of Health-Care Workers: Recommendations of the Advisory

Practices and the Hospital Infection Control Practices Advisory Committee. MMWR 1997;46 (RR-18):1–43.

43 Wreghitt TG, Whipp J, Redpath C, Hollingworth W. An analysis of infection control of varicella-zoster virus infections in Addenbrooke's Hospital Cambridge over a 5-year period, 1987–92. Epidemiol Infect 1996;117(1):165–71.

44 Tennenberg AM, Brassard JE, Van Lieu J, Drusin LM. Varicella vaccination for healthcare workers at a university hospital: an analysis of costs and benefits. Infect Control Hosp Epidemiol 1997;18(6):405–11.

45 Weber DJ, Rutala WA, Hamilton H. Prevention and control of varicella-zoster infections in healthcare facilities. Infect Control Hosp Epidemiol 1996;17:694–705.

46 Health Canada. Prevention and control of occupational infection in health care. CCDR 2002;28S1:1–264.

47 Yoshikawa T, Ihira M, Suzuki K, Suga S, Tomitaka A, Ueda H, Asano Y. Rapid contamination of the environments with varicella-zoster virus DNA from a patient with herpes zoster. J Med Virol 2001;63(1):64–6.

48 Suzuki K, Yoshikawa T, Tomitaka A, Matsunaga K, Asano Y. Detection of aerosolized varicella-zoster virus DNA in patients with localized herpes zoster. J Infect Dis 2004;189(6):1009–12.

49 Josephson A, Gombert ME. Airborne transmission of nosocomial varicella from localized zoster. J Infect Dis 1988;158(1):238–41.

50 Saiman L, LaRussa P, Steinberg SP, et al. Persistence of immunity to varicella-zoster virus after vaccination of healthcare workers. Infect Control Hosp Epidemiol 2001; 22:279–83.

51 Alter SJ, Hammond JA, McVey CJ, Myers MG. Susceptibility to varicella-zoster virus among adults at high risk for exposure. Infect Control 1986;7(9):448–51.

52 Ferson MJ, Bell SM, Robertson PW. Determination and importance of varicella immune status of nursing staff in a children's hospital. J Hosp Infect 1990;15:347–51.

53 Vandersmissen G, Moens G, Vranckx R, et al. Occupational risk of infection by varicella zoster virus in Belgian healthcare workers: a seroprevalence study. Occup Environ Med 2000;57:621–6.

54 Gallagher J, Quaid B, Cryan B. Susceptibility to varicella zoster virus infection in health care workers. Occup Med (Lond) 1996;46:289–92.

55 McKinney WP, Horowitz MM, Battiola RJ. Susceptibility of hospital-based health care personnel to varicella-zoster virus infections. Am J Infect Control 1989;17(1):26–30.

56 Santos AM, Ono E, Weckx LY, Coutinho AP, de Moraes-Pinto MI. Varicella zoster antibodies in healthcare workers from two neonatal units in São Paulo, Brazil – assessment of a staff varicella policy. J Hosp Infect 2004;56(3):228–31.

57 Almuneef MA, Memish ZA, Balkhy HH, et al. Seroprevalence survey of varicella, measles, rubella, and hepatitis A and B viruses in a multinational healthcare workforce in Saudi Arabia. Infect Control Hosp Epidemiol 2006;27:1178–83.

58 Gray AM, Fenn P, Weinberg J, et al. An economic analysis of varicella vaccination for health care workers. Epidemiol Infect 1997; 119:209–20.

59 Gayman J. A cost-effectiveness model for analysing two varicella vaccination strategies. Am J Health Syst Pharm 1998;15:S4–8.

60 Thiry N, Beutels P, Van Damme P, et al. Economic evaluations of varicella vaccination programmes: a review of the literature. Pharmacoeconomics 2003;21:13–38.

61 Kuter BJ, Ngai A, Patterson CM, et al. Safety, tolerability, and immunogenicity of two regimens of Oka/Merck varicella vaccine (Varivax®) in healthy adolescents and adults. Vaccine 1995;13: 967–72.

62 Gershon AA, Steinberg SP, LaRussa P, et al. NIAID Varicella Vaccine Collaborative Study Group. Immunization of healthy adults with live attenuated varicella vaccine. J Infect Dis 1988;158:132–7.

63 Ferson MJ. Varicella vaccine in post-exposure prophylaxis. Commun Dis Intell 2001;25(1):13–15.

64 Balfour HH Jr, Groth KE, McCullough J, et al. Prevention or modification of varicella using zoster immune plasma. Am J Dis Child 1977;131:693–6.

65 Orenstein WA, Heymann DL, Ellis RJ, et al. Prophylaxis of varicella in high risk children: dose response effect of zoster immune globulin. J Pediatr 1981;98:368–73.

66 Zaia J, Levin MJ, Preblud SK, et al. Evaluation of varicella-zoster immune globulin: protection of immunosuppressed children after household exposure to varicella. J Infect Dis 1983;147:737–43.

67 Miller E, Cradock-Watson JE, Ridehalgh MK. Outcome in newborn babies given anti-varicella-zoster immunoglobulin after perinatal maternal infection with varicella-zoster virus. Lancet 1989;2:371–3.

68 White CB, Hawley WZ, Harford DJ, et al. The pediatric resident susceptible to varicella: providing immunity through postexposure prophylaxis with oral acyclovir. Pediatr Infect Dis J 1994;13:743–4.

69 Asano Y, Yoshikawa T, Suga S, et al. Post-exposure prophylaxis of varicella in family contact by oral acyclovir. Pediatrics 1993; 92:219–22.

70 Lin TY, Huang YC, Ning HC, et al. Oral acyclovir prophylaxis of varicella after intimate contact. Pediatr Infect Dis J 1997;16:1162–5.

71 Maeda A, Hisakawa H, Wakiguchi H, Kurashige T. An immunocompetent child with herpes zoster following post-exposure prophylaxis of varicella by oral acyclovir. Acta Paediatr 1999;88(10):1161–2.

72 Szucs T. The socio-economic burden of influenza. J Antimicrob Chemother 1999;44 Suppl B:11–15.

73 Hansen S, Stamm-Balderjahn S, Zuschneid I, et al. Closure of medical departments during nosocomial outbreaks: data from a systematic analysis of the literature. J Hosp Infect 2007;65(4):348–53.

74 Sartor C, Zandotti C, Romain F, et al. Disruption of services in an internal medicine unit due to a nosocomial influenza outbreak. Infect Control Hosp Epidemiol 2002;23(10):615–19.

75 Jefferson TO, Rivetti D, Di Pietrantonj C, et al. Vaccines for preventing influenza in healthy adults. Cochrane Database Syst Rev 2007 (2), CD001269, DOI: 10.1002/14651858.

76 Burls A, Jordan R, Barton P, Olowokure B, Wake B, Albon E, Hawker J. Vaccinating healthcare workers against influenza to protect the vulnerable – is it a good use of healthcare resources? A systematic review of the evidence and an economic evaluation. Vaccine 2006;24(19):4212–21.

77 Wilde JA, McMillan JA, Serwint J, et al. Effectiveness of influenza vaccine in health care professionals: a randomized trial. JAMA 1999;281:908–13.

78 Saxén H, Virtanen M. Randomized, placebo-controlled double blind study on the efficacy of influenza immunization on absenteeism of health care workers. Pediatr Infect Dis J 1999;18(9):779–83.

79 Weingarten S, Staniloff H, Ault M, Miles P, Bamberger M, Meyer RD. Do hospital employees benefit from the influenza vaccine? A placebo-controlled clinical trial. J Gen Intern Med 1988;3(1):32–7.

80 Thomas RE, Jefferson T, Demicheli V, Rivetti D. Influenza vaccination for healthcare workers who work with the elderly. Cochrane Database Syst Rev 2006 (3), CD005187, DOI: 10.1002/14651858.

81 Hofmann F, Ferracin C, Marsh G, Dumas R. Influenza vaccination of healthcare workers: a literature review of attitudes and beliefs. Infection 2006;34(3):142–7.

82 Dey P, Halder S, Collins S, et al. Promoting uptake of influenza vaccination among health care workers: a randomized controlled trial. J Public Health Med 2001;23:346–8.

83 Steckel CM. Mandatory influenza immunization for health care workers – an ethical discussion. AAOHN J 2007;55(1):34–9.

84 Aoki FY, Yassi A, Cheang M, et al. Effects of acetaminophen on adverse effects of influenza vaccination in health care workers. CMAJ 1993;149:1425–30.

85 Jefferson T, Demisheli V, Di Pietrantonj C, et al. Neuraminidase inhibitors for preventing and treating influenza in healthy adults. Cochrane Database Syst Rev 2006 (3), CD001265, DOI: 10.1002/14651858.

86 Jefferson T, Demicheli V, Di Pietrantonj C, et al. Amantadine and rimantadine for influenza A in adults. Cochrane Database Syst Rev 2006 (2), CD001169, DOI: 10.1002/14651858.

87 Fiore A, Shay DK, Haber P, et al. Prevention and control of Influenza: Recommendations of the Advisory Committee on Immunization Practices (ACIP) 2007. MMWR 2007;56(RR-06):1–54.

88 Svoboda T, Henry B, Shulman L, et al. Public health measures to control the spread of the Severe Acute Respiratory Syndrome during the outbreak in Toronto. N Engl J Med 2004;350:2352–61.

89 Teleman MD, Boudville IC, Heng BH, et al. Factors associated with transmission of severe acute respiratory syndrome among health-care workers in Singapore. Epidemiol Infect 2004;132:797–803.

90 World Health Organization. Summary of probable SARS cases with onset of illness from 1 November 2002 to 31 July 2003. World Health Organization Geneva, Switzerland 2004. Online at http://www.who.int/csr/sars/country/table2004_04_21/en/index.html, accessed March 17, 2008.

91 Varia M, Wilson S, Sarwal S, et al. Investigation of a nosocomial outbreak of severe acute respiratory syndrome (SARS) in Toronto, Canada. CMAJ 2003;169:285–92.

92 Siegel JD, Rhinehart E, Jackson M, et al. 2007 Guideline for Isolation Precautions: Preventing Transmission of Infectious Agents in Healthcare Settings, CDC, Atlanta USA, June 2007, available at http://www.cdc.gov/ncidod/dhqp/pdf/isolation2007.pdf. Accessed March 2008.

93 White C, Kolble R, Carlson R, et al. The effect of hand hygiene on illness rate among students in university residence halls. Am J Infect Control 2003;31(6):364–70.

94 Mott PJ, Sisk BW, Arbogast JW, et al. Alcohol-based instant hand sanitizer use in military settings: a prospective cohort study of Army basic trainees. Mil Med 2007;172:1170–6.

95 Ejemot RI, Ehiri JE, Meremikwu MM, Critchley JA. Handwashing for preventing diarrhoea. Cochrane Database Syst Rev 2008;1:CD004265, DOI: 10.1002/14651858.

96 Haas JP, Larson EL. Measurement of compliance with hand hygiene. J Hosp Infect 2007;66:6–14.

97 Manian FA, Ponzillo JJ. Compliance with routine use of gowns by healthcare workers (HCW) and non-HCW visitors on entry into the rooms of patients under contact precautions. Infect Control Hosp Epidemiol 2007;28:337–40.

98 Aronsson G, Gustafsson K, Dallner M. Sick but yet at work. An empirical study of sickness presenteeism. J Epidemiol Community Health 2000;54(7):502–9.

99 Atkinson WL, Markowitz LE, Adams NC, et al. Transmission of measles in medical settings – United States, 1985089. Am J Med 1991;91:320–4S.

100 Ferson MJ, Roberston PW, Whybin LR. Cost-effectiveness of prevaccination screening of healthcare workers for immunity to measles, rubella and mumps. Med J Aust 1994;18:478–82.

101 Sellick JA Jr, Longbine D, Schideling R, et al. Screening hospital employees for measles immunity is more cost-effective than blind immunization. Ann Intern Med 1992;116:982–4.

102 Stover BH, Adams G, Keubler CA, et al. Measles-mumps-rubella immunization of susceptible hospital employees during a community measles outbreak: cost-effectiveness and protective efficacy. Infect Control Hosp Epidemiol 1994;15:18–21.

103 Ziegler E, Roth C, Wreghitt T. Prevalence of measles susceptibility among health care workers in a UK hospital. Does the UK need to introduce a measles policy for its healthcare workers? Occup Med (Lond) 2003;53:398–402.

104 Hennessey KA, Ion-Nedeleu N, Craciun MD, et al. Measles epidemic in Romania, 1996–1998: assessment of vaccine effectiveness by case-control and cohort studies. Am J Epidemiol 1999;150:1250–7.

105 Rivest P, Bedard L, Arruda H, et al. Risk factors for measles and vaccine efficacy during an epidemic in Montreal. Can J Pub Health 1995;86:86–90.

106 Janaszek W, Gay NJ, Gut W. Measles vaccine efficacy during an epidemic in 1998 in the highly vaccinated population of Poland. Vaccine 2003;21:473–8.

107 Correia J, Hart C. Meningococcal disease. BMJ Clinical Evidence. Search date March 2008. BMJ Publishing.

108 Gilmore A, Stuart J, Andrews N. Risk of secondary meningococcal disease in healthcare workers. Lancet 2000;356:1654–5.

109 Schwartz B, Al-Tobaiqi Al-Ruwais A, et al. Comparative efficacy of ceftriaxone and rifampicin in eradicating pharyngeal carriage of group A *Neisseria meningitidis*. Lancet 1988;1:1239–42.

110 Dwarozack DL, Sanders CC, Horowitz EA, et al. Evaluation of single-dose ciprofloxacin in the eradication of *Neisseria meningitidis* from nasopharyngeal carriers. Antimicrob Agents Chemother 1988;32:1740–1.

111 Centers for Disease Control and Prevention. Laboratory-acquired meningococcal disease – United States, 2000. MMWR 2002;51:141–4.

CHAPTER 19
Infections in long-term care

Lindsay E. Nicolle

Case presentation

The nursing staff at a long-term care facility contact you to assess a resident who the ward staff are concerned is "not well." This woman is 85 years old, and requires permanent institutional care because of progressive Alzheimer disease. She is incontinent of urine, but controlled with a toileting program, and is a "wanderer." There is no history from the patient. The nursing staff say she has not been as active as usual, and has been eating poorly for the past several days. The patient has a past history of complete heart block for which a pacemaker was inserted, and congestive heart failure. Her temperature is 37.9°C, respiratory rate 24, pulse a paced rate of 72, and blood pressure 120/80. The physical examination reveals no abnormalities of the skin, bilateral inspiratory crepitations in both lung fields, a mildly elevated JVP, and bilateral pedal edema. The nursing staff say they obtained a urine specimen as the urine was "foul smelling," and a dipstick is positive for leukocyte esterase. They request you to order antimicrobial therapy for urinary infection.

As you are already at the facility, you are requested to assess a second resident. This is a 92-year-old male with obstruction secondary to prostate hypertrophy managed with a chronic indwelling catheter. He is aphasic and hemiplegic following a stroke. The nursing staff notes that his temperature is 38.2°C, and he is "restless." Physical examination reveals poor inspiration bilaterally but no adventitial signs. There are no skin lesions. The nursing staff have also obtained a urine specimen from his Foley drainage bag and this, too, is leukocyte esterase positive. Again, they request an order for antimicrobial therapy.

Evidence-Based Infectious Diseases, 2nd edition. Edited by Mark Loeb, Fiona Smaill and Marek Smieja. © 2009 Wiley-Blackwell Publishing, ISBN: 978-1-4051-7026-0

Long-term care facilities

Long-term care facilities provide long-term residential care for individuals who are unable to function independently. A variety of different facilities serve diverse patient populations including pediatric and adult, psychiatric, and patients requiring long-term interventions such as chronic respirator therapy or chronic hemodialysis. The majority of long-term care facilities, however, provide permanent residential care for elderly, functionally impaired adults. Information characterizing infections in long-term care facilities is primarily relevant to these facilities and residents, and this is the population addressed in this chapter.

The goals of care for long-term care facilities differ from acute care. The long-term care facility is the permanent residence for most of these individuals. The major goal is to maximize quality of life for residents. This includes maintaining optimal medical status, functional capacity, and social activity while preserving resident comfort and dignity. These facilities also differ fundamentally from the acute care facility in being a low-technology environment. The intensity of care and access to both expertise and technology which characterize the acute care facility are not available nor appropriate for long-term care. Patient management and institutional practices should not be imported from acute to long-term care facilities without evidence of benefit for the long-term care facility resident.

Infections in long-term care facilities

Incidence of infections

Infections are common in residents of long-term care facilities [1]. The most frequent endemic infections are lower respiratory tract infections – primarily

Table 19.1 Reported rates of common endemic infections in long-term care facilities

Location [reference]	Rate per 1000 resident days				
	Multiple studies [1]	Idaho, USA [2]	Germany [3]	Italy [4]	Norway [5]
All infections	2.6–9.5	3.73 (1.45–6.96)*	6.0	11.8	5.2
Respiratory	0.46–4.4	1.75 (0.79–2.85)	2.2	2.5	1.4
Urinary	0.1–2.4	0.57 (0–2.28	1.2	3.2	2.0
Skin/soft tissue	<0.1–2.1	1.19 (0.66–2.67)	1.0	2.7	0.5
Gastroenteritis	0–0.9	0.16 (0–0.64)	1.2	1.2	0.4

Source: references [1–5].
* Mean (range) for multiple facilities.

pneumonia – skin and soft-tissue infections, symptomatic urinary tract infections, and gastrointestinal infections (Table 19.1). The incidence and relative frequency of infections have been consistent in reports from developed countries over several decades [1–5]. Wide variations in endemic infection rates, particularly for urinary tract infection or pneumonia, are reported among some studies [1]. This variability is partially attributable to the different patient populations described. For instance, bacteremia rates are higher in facilities providing care for chronic hemodialysis patients with indwelling vascular lines, and the incidence of pneumonia is higher in facilities caring for residents with chronic tracheostomies. Infection rates are lower in psychiatric facilities which care for younger individuals with few comorbidities. Thus, infection rates must be interpreted within the context of the facility population. The reported variation in infection rates is also partially attributable to the use of different definitions for case ascertainment [6]. This is particularly an issue for urinary tract infection, where symptomatic and asymptomatic infection may be confused. A recent report of infections in Idaho, USA, nursing homes using a standard surveillance strategy for definitions and case-finding together with consistent training of data abstractors reported a narrower range of infection rates among facilities, although some interfacility variation remained [2].

Outbreaks of infections also occur frequently in long-term care facilities. The microbial etiology of these outbreaks is wide, and new organisms are continually being implicated (Table 19.2). Respiratory and gastroenteritis outbreaks are most frequent. Influenza viruses [7] and noroviruses [8] are the most common organisms and have the greatest impact.

Scabies and, occasionally, group A streptococcal infection [9] are less common but may cause problematic outbreaks of skin infections.

Factors promoting infection

Many variables contribute to the high incidence of infection in long-term care facility residents. Normal aging changes in organ systems, including the immune system, may promote infection (Table 19.3). A decline in cell-mediated immunity is a consistent accompaniment of aging and contributes to increased rates of reactivation of latent infections such as tuberculosis [10] and varicella zoster virus [11]. Other aging-associated alterations in the immune system have not been associated with infections in long-term care residents. It is likely changes associated with normal aging in other body systems increase the risk of infection, but the relative importance of these compared with other contributing factors is not known.

The most important factors promoting infection are associated chronic diseases and functional disability. These are also the most frequent causes precipitating the need for institutional care. The more functionally impaired elderly – those who are immobile, incontinent, and unable to provide self-care – are at greatest risk of infection [12]. For instance, aspiration is an important precipitating event for pneumonia, and swallowing impairment following a stroke increases the risk of aspiration. Voiding abnormalities accompanying chronic neurologic diseases lead to both incontinence and an increased likelihood of urinary tract infection. Peripheral vascular disease and leg edema both contribute to leg and foot ulcerations and infection. Previous leg vein stripping for coronary artery bypass surgery is a risk for recurrent erysipelas,

Table 19.2 Organisms identified as causes of outbreaks of infection in long-term care facilities

	Viral	Bacterial	Other
Respiratory outbreaks	Influenza A & B* Respiratory syncytial virus* Human metapneumovirus Parainfluenza Coronavirus Adenovirus Rhinovirus	*Mycobacterium tuberculosis* *Streptococcus pneumoniae* *Chlamydia pneumoniae* *Hemophilus influenzae* *Legionella* spp *Bordatella pertussis*	

Gastrointestinal	Norovirus*
	Astrovirus
	Hepatitis B
	Rotavirus
		Salmonella spp*
		Shigella spp
		E. coli O157:H7
		Clostridium difficile
		Foodborne toxin (*S. aureus,*
		    Bacillus cereus, Clostridium
		    perfringens)
		Campylobacter jejuni
		Aeromonas hydrophilia
			Giardia lamblia
			Entamoeba histolytica

Skin/soft-tissue infection		Group A streptococcus +	Fleas Scabies *Trychophyton* spp.

Resistant bacteria		Methicillin-resistant *S. aureus*
		Vancomycin-resistant
		    enterococcus
		Penicillin-resistant *S. pneumoniae*
		TEM-21 producing *Pseudomonas*
		    aeruginosa	

* Most common organisms causing outbreaks.
+ Also causes respiratory infections.

Table 19.3 Some organ system changes with normal aging which may promote infection

System	Aging change	Impact
Pulmonary	↓ cough reflex ↓ elastic tissue ↓ mucociliary transport ↓ IgA secretion	↓ clearing of secretions
Gastrointestinal	impaired oropharynx neuromuscular coordination altered gut motility ↓ mucosal immunity	↑ dysphagia, choking, aspiration ↑ infection
Genitourinary	↑ prostate size (men) hypoestrogenism (women)	obstruction, turbulent urine flow altered vaginal flora
Skin	epidermal thinning ↓ elasticity, vascularity, thermoregulation, melanocytes, Langerhans cells, subcutaneous tissue	↑ injury potential ↓ wound healing
Immune	↓T-cell function ↓ primary humoral response ↑ autoantibiotic ↑ Th$_2$ inflammatory response	↑reactivation latent infections

and immobility contributes to development of decubitus ulcers which may become infected.

Interventions for medical care also promote infection. Invasive devices are increasingly used for management of chronic illness in long-term care facility residents. Chronic indwelling urethral catheters are used to manage voiding for 3–7% of residents [13], and percutaneous feeding tubes, central vascular lines, and chronic tracheostomies are increasingly used for patient management. All invasive devices promote infections specific to the device – urinary infection with chronic indwelling catheters, ventilator-associated pneumonia for patients with chronic tracheostomies, bacteremia when central vascular lines are present, and insertion site infections when percutaneous feeding tubes are used. In addition, polypharmacy is the norm for residents of long-term care, and some common medications such as proton pump inhibitors are associated with an increased risk of infection [14].

Finally, institutionalization itself increases exposure to infectious agents. Staff members and visitors introduce pathogens into the facility. Transmission of infectious agents among residents is facilitated through repeated close interactions of staff and residents in the long-term care environment. It is not surprising that outbreaks occur in this vulnerable population with repeated exposures to pathogens and facilitated transmission of organisms within a closed environment.

Impact of infections

For the infected resident, the discomfort and activity restriction attending an episode of infection is associated with a decreased quality of life. Residents experience accelerated functional decline during the 6 months subsequent to an infection [12]. Whether this deterioration is attributable to infection or the infection is an association of accelerated decline is not known. Infections may also lead to serious complications, such as pneumonia precipitating a myocardial infarction or foot infection requiring amputation. There are adverse impacts for the institution as well including costs for investigation and treatment of the infected resident, and transfer to acute care facilities for care in some cases. Outbreaks of infection are associated with substantial additional costs for treatment and control. Considerable disruption to usual facility activities accompany outbreaks of infection, and all residents are negatively affected irrespective of whether they are themselves infected.

Despite the high frequency of infection, only pneumonia and influenza contribute substantially to resident mortality. Between 6% and 23% of residents who develop lower respiratory infection will die [15], and case fatality rates in influenza outbreaks, even with effective vaccination programs, range from 5% to 55% [6]. Gastrointestinal outbreaks of salmonella infection [14] or E. coli O157:H7, and skin and respiratory outbreaks of group A streptococcal infection [16], are much less common, but when they occur may also be associated with high case-fatality rates.

Diagnosis

General clinical considerations

Infection in a long-term care facility resident may have a clinical presentation similar to younger populations. However, in many cases the diagnosis is not straightforward. Determining whether or not infection is present, or the specific site when infection is suspected, is frequently problematic [17,18]. Clinical assessment is compromised by limited communication when residents have impaired hearing or vision, or decreased mental capacity. Chronic symptoms accompanying comorbid illnesses, such as cough, dyspnea, or venous insufficiency, compromise the interpretation of acute signs and symptoms of infection. Infection may also present with nonspecific findings such as lethargy, decreased appetite, or increased functional impairment [17,19]. Acute delirium is a common presentation of severe infection in this population. These nonspecific signs and symptoms are, however, also frequently attributable to noninfectious problems such as dehydration, adverse drug effects, drug interactions, fecal impaction, or exacerbation of comorbid illness.

The temperature response in elderly individuals is attenuated relative to younger populations [17]. The maximum temperature achieved with infection is, on average, lower and elderly persons are more likely to experience afebrile infection. A temperature of >37.8°C has been reported to provide optimal sensitivity and specificity for identifying infection in long-term care facility residents [20]. Some elderly residents have a relatively hypothermic baseline temperature, and measured temperatures should be interpreted in the context of the individual's usual baseline. Notwithstanding these caveats, episodes of serious systemic infections will usually be accompanied by a documented fever. For instance, in a large series of bacteremias in nursing home residents, only 10% of episodes were afebrile [21].

Laboratory evaluation and diagnostic imaging

Long-term care facilities have restricted access to diagnostic investigations. Diagnostic facilities are usually offsite and clinical specimens must be transported to the laboratory [17,18,22]. The receipt of test results may be delayed. Mobile chest radiographs provide onsite diagnostic imaging for some facilities, but availability is usually restricted to daytime hours [18]. For other diagnostic imaging investigations, the resident must be transferred to another facility.

The peripheral leukocyte count should be interpreted in the context of patient age and disability. Elderly individuals with infections are less likely to demonstrate peripheral leukocytosis than younger patients [17,23]. Evidence of marrow stress is, however, usually evidenced by a left shift with increased bands on the leukocyte differential. A proportional band count of 15%, or an absolute number of ≥1500 bands/mL, correlates with infection in elderly individuals, even with a normal leukocyte count [23].

A critical interpretation of positive microbiology cultures is also essential. Colonization with potentially pathogenic organisms in the absence of infection is common in the oropharynx [1] and for open skin lesions [24,25], and there is a high prevalence of asymptomatic bacteriuria in urine specimens [26]. Cultures should be obtained only when there is a clear clinical indication, and results interpreted in the context of this high prevalence of colonization.

Blood cultures should be requested for elderly residents where a diagnosis of serious systemic infection is considered [17]. They must be collected before the initiation of antimicrobial therapy. The most common source of bacteremia is urinary infection [1,21], with a chronic indwelling catheter the major risk factor for bacteremia [27]. Infected decubitus ulcers and the respiratory tract are other common sources of bacteremia. Urinary infection and infected decubitus ulcers are the source for 70–80% of bacteremic

episodes [21]. When polycrobial bacteremia is identified, an infected pressure ulcer is the most common origin.

Pneumonia

The most useful clinical indicator when a diagnosis of pneumonia is considered is a respiratory rate over 25 breaths per minute. This level of tachypnea had a sensitivity of 90% and specificity of 95% for pneumonia in one study [28]. Other clinical indicators helpful in diagnosing pneumonia include fever, a change in character or quantity of sputum, and increased cough. Oximetry may be a useful test for the diagnosis and evaluation of respiratory tract infection but is not yet accessible in many facilities and has not been critically evaluated for use in this population [17]. Even when a chest radiograph is obtained, the interpretation is not straightforward. Chronic changes, congestive heart failure, chemical pneumonitis, and other findings may be misattributed to pneumonia. There is low interobserver consistency among radiologists in the identification of pneumonia on chest radiographs from long-term care facility residents [29].

Guidelines of the Infectious Diseases Society of America (IDSA) [17] recommend, when a diagnosis of pneumonia is considered in a long-term care facility resident, a respiratory rate should be obtained. If the respiratory rate is ≥25, then pulse oximetry should be obtained, and if pulse oximetry is less than 90%, a chest radiograph should be requested. The utility of this suggested algorithm, or of individual components, has not yet been rigorously evaluated. Consensus guidelines for initiation of antimicrobial therapy in the long-term care facility recommend antimicrobial therapy should be initiated for presumed pneumonia when either: temperature is greater than 38.9°C and there is one of respiratory rate >25 breaths per minute or a productive cough; or temperature is greater than 37.9°C and there is new or increased cough with at least one of pulse >100 beats per minute, delirium, rigors, or a respiratory rate >25 breaths per minute [18]. One consideration in the differential diagnosis of pneumonia is chemical pneumonitis – a common problem in residents following aspiration of gastric contents. It has been proposed that pneumonitis can be differentiated from pneumonia in residents with a positive chest radiograph on the basis of history of witnessed aspiration and duration of symptoms less than 24 hours [30].

The IDSA guidelines also recommend a sputum specimen for culture should be obtained if a diagnosis of pneumonia is made [17]. However, less than 5% of nursing home residents with suspected pneumonia will have a sputum specimen obtained [22]. This limited use of sputum specimens is partially attributable to difficulty in obtaining specimens from residents who are unable or unwilling to cooperate. Even when sputum specimens are obtained, interpretation of positive cultures is problematic because of contamination by gram-negative organisms colonizing the oropharynx, such as *Klebsiella pneumoniae* [1]. These organisms are isolated from the sputum specimen, but are seldom the etiology of infection. However, isolation of gram-negative organisms from sputum specimens drives broad-spectrum antimicrobial use, likely contributing to increased antimicrobial resistance. Sputum specimens may occasionally, however, be helpful in directing antimicrobial therapy, especially if *Streptococcus pneumoniae* is isolated. The collection of sputum specimens or nasopharyngeal aspirates for viral and bacterial culture is essential when there is a potential or confirmed outbreak of respiratory infection.

Thus, pneumonia is a potential diagnosis in the long-term care resident who is febrile and tachypneic. Alternate diagnoses, including congestive heart failure, infection at another site, pulmonary embolus, and pneumonitis should always be considered. The peripheral leukocyte count and differential, and oximetry if available, may be useful to assess the severity of the initial infection and monitor subsequent response to therapy.

Urinary infection

Symptomatic urinary tract infection is diagnosed in residents without indwelling urethral catheters when there are localizing genitourinary signs and symptoms [18,31,32]. Acute onset of symptoms such as frequency, dysuria, or new or increased incontinence support a diagnosis of urinary tract infection. Renal infection is usually accompanied by costovertebral angle pain or tenderness, although this may be difficult to appreciate in the most functionally impaired resident. Fever without localizing findings is unlikely

to be from a urinary source in residents without an indwelling urethral catheter [32]. For residents with a chronic indwelling urethral catheter, however, the most common presentation of symptomatic urinary infection is fever without localizing findings [18]. Hematuria following catheter trauma and catheter obstruction are also both associated with invasive (i.e., febrile) urinary infection. Cloudy or foul-smelling urine are frequently interpreted as urinary infection in residents with or without chronic catheters. These signs may accompany bacteriuria or dehydration [29] but should not, by themselves, be interpreted as symptomatic infection or an indication for antimicrobial therapy [18,31].

A positive urine culture is useful to confirm the diagnosis of urinary infection and identify the specific infecting organism and susceptibilities. This is essential information to assist with appropriate antimicrobial selection. However, 30–50% of residents in long-term care facilities have positive urine cultures at any time [26]. Thus a positive urine culture in the absence of localizing genitourinary findings has a low positive predictive value for the diagnosis of symptomatic urinary infection [32]. Pyuria is a consistent accompaniment of bacteriuria in this population and is also not an indication for antimicrobial therapy in the absence of localizing symptoms [26]. However, a negative urine culture or the absence of pyuria both have high negative predictive values and are useful tests to exclude urinary tract infection [17].

The urine specimen should always be obtained before antimicrobial therapy is initiated, using a collection method which limits contamination. For men, a clean-catch urine specimen can usually be collected, or a specimen obtained from a freshly applied clean condom catheter and leg bag. For incontinent or uncooperative female residents, when a urine specimen is essential for management, in and out catheterization may be necessary. Residents with chronic indwelling catheters uniformly have positive urine cultures. Chronic indwelling urinary catheters are consistently coated with a bacterial biofilm which incorporates three to five different organisms. When symptomatic urinary infection is a diagnostic consideration, the indwelling urethral catheter should be removed and replaced by a new catheter [33]. The urine specimen for culture should be obtained through the new catheter, as this is a sample of bladder urine rather than organisms in the biofilm. Obviously, catheter replacement and specimen collection should occur before antimicrobials are initiated.

Skin infections

The clinical diagnosis of erysipelas – spreading erythema, swelling, and tenderness with a well-demarcated border, usually affecting the face, arm, or leg – is often straightforward. However, acute erythema of the lower leg may occur with venous insufficiency or edema, and these presentations may be misdiagnosed as skin infection. The presence of a pressure ulcer or leg or foot ulcer is clinically apparent. The diagnosis of infection of a chronic ulcer requires the presence of signs such as induration, tenderness, erythema at the margins, or purulent drainage [18].

For clinical presentations consistent with erysipelas, especially in residents with recurrent episodes at the same site, β-hemolytic streptococci are the presumed pathogens, and a specimen for culture is not normally recommended. If purulent drainage is present, a specimen should be obtained for culture prior to initiating antimicrobial therapy. Organisms isolated from a surface swab of mucosa or open skin lesions, however, should not be interpreted as infection without associated signs and symptoms consistent with infection. A culture from a potentially infected ulcer should be obtained after the ulcer is debrided, so a deep swab sampling the base of the ulcer is obtained [25]. When there is necrosis present both aerobic and anaerobic cultures should be requested. Subcutaneous aspiration from the margin of a decubitus ulcer has been suggested as a means to differentiate infection from colonization, with growth from the aspirate presumed evidence for tissue invasion. However, this approach for specimen collection has not been validated, and noninfected ulcers may also have organisms isolated from aspirates [25].

Other skin infections such as varicella zoster (shingles), herpes virus, intertriginous candidiasis, and tinea are usually diagnosed by characteristic clinical presentations. The diagnosis of scabies is sometimes problematic. Prolonged outbreaks of scabies following delayed diagnosis of initial cases in long-term facility residents are repeatedly reported [34,35]. Scrapings to identify the mite are recommended, but may be negative in cases which are subsequently confirmed.

A high index of suspicion is necessary, with dermatologic consultation and biopsy requested when the diagnosis remains uncertain.

Treatment

Antimicrobial use in long-term care
There is intense antimicrobial use in long-term care facilities. Between 22% and 89% of antimicrobial use has been reported to be inappropriate [18], although inappropriate use is a consistent problem in all healthcare settings [36]. Inappropriate use includes treatment of residents presenting with nonspecific symptoms or positive culture results without signs or symptoms to support a diagnosis of infection, or prescription of an antimicrobial regimen inappropriate for the site of infection or infecting organism. Antimicrobial prescriptions are often initiated at the request of nursing staff, without direct physician evaluation of the patient [17]. The limited access to diagnostic tests and complexity in clinical interpretation contribute to overuse of empiric antimicrobial therapy. Broad-spectrum antimicrobial use is frequently initiated because of uncertainty about the diagnosis or concerns about antimicrobial-resistant organisms.

Non-antimicrobial approaches
Potential noninfectious causes should always be considered when residents present with nonspecific signs and symptoms. These nonspecific clinical alterations are unlikely to be attributable to serious infection in the absence of fever [19]. Deterioration of congestive heart failure may explain cough, dyspnea, and tachypnea, and lethargy may be secondary to medication use. "Foul-smelling urine" will frequently respond to rehydration, while fever may be a sign of fecal impaction. Pneumonia must be differentiated from aspiration pneumonitis, which will resolve without antimicrobial therapy [30]. Thus, thoughtful, critical, clinical evaluation is essential for optimal management.

Episodes of fever in long-term care facility residents will often resolve without antimicrobial therapy [37]. When the diagnosis of infection is not definitive and clinical symptoms are of mild or moderate severity, a reasonable approach is to address potential contributing factors such as dehydration or constipation and monitor the clinical status, rather than initiating empiric antimicrobial therapy [18]. This approach, however, has not yet been evaluated in prospective clinical trials. In addition, physicians or nurse practitioners may not be available to provide continuing clinical reassessment, and this may compromise a "wait and see" approach to management [17].

Initiation of antimicrobial therapy

Even with optimal clinical evaluation and monitoring, the decision to initiate antimicrobial therapy is often not clear-cut. Consensus guidelines proposing minimum criteria for initiation of antimicrobial therapy for presumed infections have been developed to address this uncertainty [18]. These proposed guidelines are based on clinical presentation rather than diagnostic tests, so are relevant to the diagnostic uncertainty which often accompanies long-term care facility residents with potential infection.

The utility of these guidelines for urinary infection have been evaluated from the perspective of limiting antimicrobial treatment of asymptomatic bacteriuria [38]. In a randomized, controlled trial, implementation of a multifaceted approach to antimicrobial treatment of urinary infection, including diagnostic and treatment algorithms, together with an intense educational strategy (small-group interactive sessions for nurses, videotapes, written material, outreach visits, and one-on-one interviews with physicians) was associated with a significant decrease in antimicrobials prescribed for suspected urinary infection when compared to usual care homes. However, total antimicrobial use for all indications did not differ between the intervention and usual care homes. This suggests there was a shift of diagnoses for residents with non-localizing presentations, with justification for empiric antimicrobial use based on diagnoses other than urinary infection. This study highlights the complexity of addressing the issue of optimal antimicrobial use in long-term care facilities.

The consensus guideline recommendations for initiating antimicrobial therapy for treatment of pneumonia and other lower respiratory tract infections have also been evaluated as a component of a clinical pathway in a study which randomized long-term care facility residents with pneumonia to management in the long-term care facility or transfer to an acute care facility. Management in the facility was associated with significantly reduced hospitalizations and healthcare costs, and comparable clinical outcomes [39]. A study comparing aspiration pneumonitis with pneumonia reported that presenting symptoms and signs, laboratory tests, severity of illness, or C-reactive protein levels did not distinguish between pneumonia and pneumonitis [30]. The authors propose an algorithm to differentiate these clinical presentations which includes witnessed aspiration of gastric contents, positive chest radiograph, and symptoms <24 hours from the aspiration event. This algorithm requires further evaluation to determine the utility for identifying pneumonitis and, possibly, limiting unnecessary antimicrobial exposure.

For urinary tract infection, antimicrobial therapy should, if possible, be delayed until culture results are available. If symptoms are questionable or mild this is usually a feasible approach. An antimicrobial specific for the infecting organism and susceptibilities may then be selected. Residents with a long-term indwelling catheter who are diagnosed with symptomatic urinary infection should have the catheter replaced and a urine specimen collected through the new catheter before initiation of antimicrobial therapy [33]. In addition to providing a more reliable urine specimen, catheter replacement significantly decreases the time to defervescence and the frequency of early symptomatic relapse after therapy.

Antimicrobial selection

The specific antimicrobial regimen selected is based on the known or presumed site of infection, infecting organism, patient tolerance, renal and hepatic function, and severity of presentation [36]. These principles are similar to those for noninstitutionalized populations of any age. Whenever possible a specific antimicrobial should be selected targeted at a known pathogen. Widespread empiric antimicrobial use should be avoided as it promotes resistance and may limit subsequent therapeutic choices. A conservative approach to selection of an antimicrobial which limits broad-spectrum antimicrobial use as much as possible is suggested by the Society of Healthcare Epidemiology of America (SHEA) guidelines [36]. When any empiric therapy is initiated, the clinical course and relevant microbiology should be reassessed at 48–72 hours to determine whether the regimen should be continued or modified. By this time any culture results obtained prior to antimicrobial therapy will usually be available and the response to initial management can be assessed.

Most elderly long-term care facility residents with lower respiratory tract infection of mild to moderate severity will be effectively treated in the nursing home with relatively narrow-spectrum antimicrobials, as suggested in the SHEA Long Term Care Committee Guidelines [30]. A strategy of reassessment of pneumonia treatment at 72 hours with expanded coverage at that time if response has been inadequate has been shown to be safe and effective [40]. The IDSA guidelines, however, recommend universal empiric treatment with a fluoroquinolone or amoxicillin-clavulanic acid together with azithromycin or clarithromycin [41]. This initial broad-spectrum coverage is proposed to maximize coverage for all potential pathogens. For the few cases where sputum specimens for culture are obtained, a retreat to more specific therapy may then be possible at 72 hours. These recommendations for uniform broad coverage have not, however, been validated in prospective, randomized clinical trials.

Prevention

Resident interventions

Prevention of infections in long-term care facilities can be considered from both the patient and institutional perspective. General patient measures which are recommended to decrease the risk of infection include maintenance of adequate nutrition and optimal management of comorbid illness. Studies to date, however, report no decrease in the frequency of endemic infections in long-term care facility residents with vitamin or mineral supplements [42,43], although one study reported improved immunologic parameters [44]. These findings suggest nutritional supplements should not be recommended for residents of long-term care facilities in developed countries as a strategy to decrease infections. It is evident that optimal management of comorbid illnesses may prevent some infections. For instance, appropriate management of congestive heart failure to limit pedal edema would decrease the risk for leg infections. Following recommended nursing practices for immobile patients will prevent decubitus ulcers. However, given current standards of practice,

whether intensified medical or nursing care can further decrease infections is not known.

The most important specific intervention to prevent infection is yearly influenza vaccination [7]. In a systematic review of the effectiveness of influenza vaccines in elderly people, based on 29 cohort studies in long-term care facilities, immunization with influenza vaccine was found to be 23% effective (95% CI 6–36%) in reducing influenza-like illness when vaccine the match was good, but was not significantly different from no vaccination when the match was poor or unknown [45]. The efficacy of the vaccines against laboratory-confirmed influenza was not significant but there was a large effect of well-matched vaccines in preventing pneumonia (vaccine effectiveness 46%, 95% CI 30–58%), hospital admission for influenza and pneumonia (45%, 95% CI 16–64%), and all-cause mortality (60%, 95% CI 23–79%). Although these findings are more consistent than those in the elderly in the community, where the vaccine was ineffective against influenza-like illness or confirmed influenza but effective against all-cause mortality, concern has been raised about the role of bias in such results [46].

Studies have also repeatedly reported that increased staff vaccination rates are associated with decreased resident mortality during influenza outbreaks [47,48]. Pneumonococcal vaccination is recommended, although clear benefits for residents of long-term care facilities have not been documented [49]. Other specific interventions may be appropriate for selected patients. For instance, prophylaxis with penicillin G or benzathine penicillin G prevents recurrent episodes of erysipelas for residents who experience frequent recurrences, and isoniazid treatment of latent tuberculosis infection prevents reactivation [10].

Infection control

Infection control programs are required for long-term care facilities [50]. The components of these programs include a designated infection control practitioner to oversee and manage the program, and an oversight committee. Specific infection control functions include surveillance of infections, outbreak control, development of infection prevention policies and procedures, education of patients, staff, and visitors with respect to infection prevention, resident and employee health programs to prevent infection, antibiotic review, and meeting legislated requirements for disease reporting. Local regulations and standards for environmental cleaning, laundry, waste management, and food handling must be met.

Studies have not yet been reported to document the effectiveness of these programs. Specific components have been evaluated in some studies. For instance, handwashing with an alcohol rinse or with soap and water does not influence infection rates [51]. Routine glove use is as effective as contact isolation precautions in limiting transmission of antimicrobial-resistant organisms in long-term care facilities [52]. Evaluation of the effectiveness of infection control programs and individual components of these programs has been identified as a priority for research in long-term care facilities [53].

Even with optimal patient management and facility infection control, outbreaks will occur in long-term care facilities. Ensuring that appropriate policies to respond to outbreaks are established proactively is part of the "emergency preparedness" of any facility. These policies should address general approaches to outbreak management with any infectious agent, as well as specific interventions for common organisms including influenza, other respiratory infections, foodborne outbreaks, norovirus outbreaks, scabies, and group A streptococcus. Effective surveillance and control programs which promptly identify residents who are potentially infectious and support rapid institution of effective control measures early in an outbreak will limit adverse effects for residents, staff, and the facility.

When infection control policies for management of potentially infected residents are developed, recommendations for barrier precautions or isolation to limit transmission must be implemented sparingly. Functionally impaired elderly individuals who have restrictions placed on social or physical activity may experience disorientation and further deterioration in functional status. Thus, restrictions should only be considered when there is clearly a danger to other residents or staff and proposed restrictions are effective in decreasing this risk. The approach may be different from recommendations for acute care facilities. For instance, isolation of elderly nursing home residents with shingles would seldom be indicated. Most facility residents will be seropositive for varicella, and management should be through covering active lesions

and glove use by staff members. Similarly, contact precautions do not limit transmission of antimicrobial-resistant organisms, and routine glove use may be a more humane and practical approach [52].

Antimicrobial-resistant organisms

Some long-term care facilities have a high prevalence of antimicrobial-resistant organisms [1,54,55]. MRSA, VRE, and fluoroquinolone-resistant or ESBL-producing gram-negative organisms are of particular concern. The prevalence of resistant organisms is highly variable among facilities, but even in high-prevalence facilities, morbidity attributable to resistant organisms is limited. MRSA and VRE are usually acquired in acute care facilities and introduced into long-term care facilities when residents are transferred, with relatively limited transmission within the facility itself. The approach to preventing transmission of resistant organisms in long-term care facilities is controversial [56]. In the absence of evidence for excess morbidity and mortality, restrictive interventions cannot be advocated. Appropriate hand hygiene should always be followed by staff and residents. In a nonoutbreak situation, restriction of resident participation in social activities, communal dining, or other interactions would not be appropriate solely on the basis of colonization with a resistant organism.

Case presentation (continued)

For the first patient, you diagnose an exacerbation of pulmonary edema and adjust her diuretic medications. Antimicrobials are not initiated, but nursing staff are requested to reassess the patient at 24 and 48 hours. There are no further temperature elevations. Three days later, the urine culture report returns growing E. coli $>10^5$ cfu/mL. However, the patient has returned to her previous clinical status. You interpret the positive urine culture as asymptomatic bacteriuria, and no antimicrobial therapy is initiated.

For the second patient, a chest radiograph is requested. Antimicrobial therapy is not initiated, but the patient's temperature, respiratory rate, and mental status are monitored twice daily. The chest radiograph is obtained the next day and the report, available 48 hours after your evaluation, shows a possible infiltrate behind the heart on the left side.

Continued

Case presentation (continued)

The patient has continued to experience temperatures peaking at 38°C daily, and the respiratory rate is now 28. The urine culture has returned growing an *E. coli* >10⁸, Enterococcus >10⁸, and *P. mirabilis* >10⁸. Your assessment, given the tachypnea and sustained fever, is that the patient has a lower respiratory tract infection, and oral antimicrobial therapy is initiated. The urine culture results are interpreted as consistent with the polymicrobial bacteriuria anticipated for a resident with a chronic indwelling catheter. Over the next 72 hours the temperature returns to normal, the respiratory rate decreases, and the nursing staff report the patient has returned to his former status.

References

1 Nicolle LE, Strausbaugh LJ, Garibaldi RA. Infections and antibiotic resistance in nursing homes. Clin Micro Reviews 1996;9:1–17.

2 Stevenson KB, Moore J, Colwell H, et al. Standardized infection surveillance in long-term care: interfacility comparisons from a regional cohort of facilities. Infect Control Hosp Epidemiol 2005;26:231–8.

3 Engelhart ST, Hanses-Derendorf L, Exner M, et al. Prospective surveillance for healthcare-associated infections in German nursing home residents. J Hosp Infect 2005;60:46–50.

4 Brusaferro S, Regathin L, Silvestro A, et al. Incidence of hospital-acquired infections in Italian long-term care facilities: a prospective six-month surveillance. J Hosp Infect 2006;63:211–15.

5 Erikson HM, Koch AM, Elstrhim P, et al. Heathcare-associated infection among residents of long-term care facilities: a cohort and nested case-control study. J Hosp Infect 2007;65:334–40.

6 McGeer A, Campbell B, Eckert DG, et al. Definition for surveillance of infections in residents of long-term care facilities. Amer J Infect Control 1991;19:1–7.

7 Bradley SF, the Long Term Care Committee of the Society for Healthcare Epidemiology of America. Prevention of influenza in long-term care facilities. Infect Control Hosp Epidemiol 1999;20:629–31.

8 Blanton LH, Adams SM, Beard RS, et al. Molecular and epidemiology trends of caliciviruses associated with outbreaks of acute gastroenteritis in the United States, 2000–2004. J Infect Dis 2006;193:413–21.

9 Jordan HT, Richards CL, Burton DC, et al. Group A streptococcal disease in long-term care facilities: Descriptive epidemiology and potential control measures. Clin Infect Dis 2007;45:742–52.

10 Thrupp L, Bradley S, Smith P, et al. Tuberculosis prevention and control in long-term care facilities for older adults. Infect Control Hosp Epidemiol 2004;25:1097–108.

11 Schmader K. Herpes zoster in the elderly: Issues related to geriatrics. Clin Infect Dis 1999;28:736–9.

12 High KP, Bradley S, Loeb M, et al. A new paradigm for clinical investigation of infectious syndromes in older adults: assessment of functional status as a risk factor and outcome measure. Clin Infect Dis 2005;40:114–22.

13 Nicolle LE. The chronic indwelling catheter and urinary infection in long-term care facility residents. Infect Control Hosp Epidemiol 2001;22:316–21.

14 Bowen A, Newman A, Estivariz C, et al. Role of acid-suppressing medications during a sustained outbreak of *Salmonella enteritidis* infection in a long-term care facility. Infect Control Hosp Epidemiol 2007;28:1202–5.

15 Mylotte JM. Nursing home-associated pneumonia. Clin Geriatr Med 2007;23:553–65.

16 Jordan HT, Richards CL, Burton DC, et al. Group A streptococcal disease in long-term care facilities: Descriptive epidemiology and potential control measures. Clin Infect Dis 2007;45:742–52.

17 Bentley DW, Bradley S, High K, et al. Practice guideline for evaluation of fever and infection in long-term care facilities. Clin Infect Dis 2000;31:640–53.

18 Loeb M, Bentley DW, Bradley S, et al. Development of minimum criteria for the initiation of antibiotics in residents of long-term care facilities: results of a consensus conference. Infect Control Hosp Epidemiol 2001;22:120–4.

19 Berman P, Hogan DB, Fox RA. The atypical presentation of infection in old age. Age Aging 1987;16:201–7.

20 Castle SC, Yeh M, Toledo S, et al. Lowering the temperature criteria improves detection of infections in nursing home residents. Aging Immunol Infect Dis 1993;4:67–76.

21 Mylotte JM, Ammar T, Goodnough S. Epidemiology of bloodstream infection in nursing home residents: Evaluation in a large cohort from multiple homes. Clin Infect Dis 2002;35:1484–90.

22 Mubareka S, Duckworth H, Cheang M, et al. Use of diagnostic tests for lower respiratory infection in long-term care facilities. J Am Geriatr Soc 2007;55:1365–70.

23 Wasserman M, Levinstein M, Keller E, et al. Utility of fever, white blood cells, and differential count in predicting bacterial infections in the elderly. J Am Geriatr Soc 19889;37:537–43.

24 Grahame S, Sim G, Laughren R, et al. Percutaneous feeding tube changes in long term care facility patients. Infect Control Hosp Epidemiol 1996;17:732–6.

25 Nicolle LE, Orr P, Duckworth H, et al. Prospective study of decubitus ulcers in two long term care facilities. Can J Infect Control 1994;9:35–8.

26 Nicolle LE, Bradley S, Colgan R, et al. IDSA guideline for the diagnosis and treatment of asymptomatic bacteriuria in adults. Clin Infect Dis 2005;40:643–54.

27 Muder RR, Brennen C, Wagener MM, et al. Bacteremia in a long-term care facility: a five-year prospective study of 163 consecutive episodes. Clin Infect Dis 1992;14:647–54.

28 McFadden JP, Price RC, Eastwood HD, et al. Raised respiratory rate in dehydrated elderly patients. Clin Endocrinol 1984;20:451–6.

29 Loeb MB, Carusone SBC, Marrie TJ, et al. Interobserver reliability of radiologists' interpretations of mobile chest radiographs for nursing home-acquired pneumonia. J Am Med Dir Assoc 2006;7:416–19.

30 Mylotte JM, Goodnough S, Gould M. Pneumonia versus aspiration pneumonitis in nursing home residents: prospective application of a clinical algorithm. J Am Geriatr Soc 2005;53:755–61.

31 Nicolle LE. Urinary tract infections in the elderly: Symptomatic or asymptomatic? Int J Antimicrob Agents 1999;11:265–8.

32 Orr P, Nicolle LE, Duckworth H, et al. Febrile urinary infection in the institutionalized elderly. Am J Med 1996;100:71–7.

33 Raz R, Schiller D, Nicolle LE. Chronic indwelling catheter replacement prior to antimicrobial therapy for symptomatic urinary infection. J Urol 2000;164:1254–8.

34 de Beer G, Miller MA, Tremblay L, et al. An outbreak of scabies in a long-term care facility: the role of misdiagnosis and the costs associated with control. Infect Control Hosp Epidemiol 2006;27:517–18.

35 Wong SS, Woo PC, Yuen KY. Unusual laboratory findings in a case of Norwegian scabies provided in clue to diagnosis. J Clin Microbiol 2005;43:2542–4.

36 Nicolle LE, Bentley D, Garibaldi R, et al. Antimicrobial use in long-term care facilities. SHEA Long-Term-Care Committee. Infect Control Hosp Epidermiol 2000;21:537–45.

37 Warren JW, Damron D, Tenney JH, Hoopes JM, Deforge B, Muncie HL Jr. Fever, bacteremia, and death as complications of bacteriuria in women with long-term urethral catheters. J Infect Dis 1987;155:1151–8.

38 Loeb M, Brazil K, Lohfeld L, et al. Effect of a multifaceted intervention on number of antimicrobial prescriptions for suspected urinary tract infections in residents of nursing homes: Cluster randomized controlled trial. BMJ 2005;331:669–74.

39 Loeb M, Carusone SC, Goerce R, et al. Effect of a clinical pathway to reduce hospitalizations in nursing home residents with pneumonia: a randomized controlled trial JAMA 2006;295:2503–20.

40 Nicolle LE, Kirshen A, Boustcha E, et al. Treatment of moderate to severe pneumonia in elderly long-term care residents. Infect Dis Clin Pract 1996;5:130–6.

41 Mandell LA, Bartlett JG, Dowell SF, et al. Update of practice guidelines for the management of community-acquired pneumonia in immunocompetent adults. Clin Infect Dis 2003;37:1405–33.

42 Murphy S, West KP Jr, Greenough WB 3rd, Cherot E, Katz J, Clement L. Impact of vitamin A supplementation on the incidence of infection in elderly nursing home residents: a randomized controlled trial. Age Aging 1992;21:435–9.

43 Liu BA, McGeer A, McArthur MA, et al. Effect of multivitamin and mineral supplementation on episodes of infection in nursing home residents: A randomized, placebo controlled study. J Am Geriatr Soc 2007;55:35–42.

44 Langkamp-Henken B, Wood SM, Herlinger-Garcia KA, et al. Nutritional formula improved immune profiles of seniors living in nursing homes. J Am Geriatr Soc 2006;54:1861–70.

45 Jefferson T, Rivetti D, Rivetti A, Rudin M, Di Pietrantonj C, Demicheli V. Efficacy and effectiveness of influenza vaccines in elderly people: a systematic review. Lancet 2005;366:1165–74.

46 Simonsen L, Taylor RJ, Viboud C, Miller MA, Jackson LA. Mortality benefits of influenza vaccination in elderly people: an ongoing controversy. Lancet Infect Dis 2007;7:658–66.

47 Carman WF, Elder AG, Wallace LA, et al. Effects of influenza vaccination of health-care workers on mortality of elderly people in long-term care: a randomized controlled trial. Lancet 2000;355:93–7.

48 Potter J, Stott DJ, Roberts MA, et al. Influenza vaccination of health care workers in long-term care hospitals reduces the mortality of elderly patients. J Infect Dis 1997;175:1–6.

49 Loeb M, Stevenson KB, SHEA Long Term Care Committee. Pneumococcal immunization in older adults. Implications for long-term care facilities. Infect Control Hosp Epidemiol 2004;25:985–94.

50 Smith PW, Rusnak PG. Infection prevention and control in the long-term care facility: SHEA Long-term Care Committee and APIC Guidelines Committee. Infect Control Hosp Epidemiol 1997;18:831–49.

51 Mody L, McNeil SA, Sun R, et al. Introduction of a waterless, alcohol-based hand rub in a long-term care facility. Infect Control Hosp Epidemiol 2003;24:165–71.

52 Trick WE, Weinstein RA, DeMarais PL, et al. Comparison of routine glove use and contact isolation precautions to prevent transmission of multidrug-resistant bacteria in a long-term care facility. J Am Geriatr Soc 2004;52:2003–9.

53 Richards C. Infections in residents of long-term care facilities: An agenda for research. Report of an expert panel. J Am Geriatr Soc 2002;50:570–6.

54 Viray M, Linkin D, Maslow JN, et al. Longitudinal trends in antimicrobial susceptibilities across long-term care facilities: emergence of fluoroquinolone resistance. Infect Control Hosp Epidemiol 2005;26:56–62.

55 Pacio GA, Visintainer P, Maquire G, et al. Natural history of colonization with vancomycin-resistant enterococci, methicillin-resistant Staphylococcus aureus, and resistant gram-negative bacilli among long-term care facility residents. Infect Control Hosp Epidemiol 2003;24:246–50.

56 Richards CL Jr. (2005) Preventing antimicrobial-resistant infections among older adults in long-term care facilities. J Am Med Dir Assoc 2005;6:144–51.

Index

Page number in *italics* represent figures, those in **bold** represent tables.

Acinetobacter spp.
  burn-related infections 280
  ventilator-assisted pneumonia 217
Acinetobacter baumannii 286
ACP Journal Club 2
Aeromonas hydrophilia **304**
Acticoat 283–4
activated protein C 216
active surveillance in MRSA control 242
acyclovir **108**
  genital herpes 153–4
  herpes simplex encephalitis 68
  varicella zoster prophylaxis 295
adenovirus **304**
Aeromonas hydrophilia 12
AIDS dementia complex **197**
albendazole **108**
amantadine 208
amikacin **259**
amoxicillin 151
ampicillin **58**
animal bites 19–21
anthrax 1
antidiarrheals 101–2, 108
antifungals 254–5
antigenic drift 207
antigenic shift 207
antiretroviral therapy 183–7
  adverse reactions 188
  compliance/adherence 185–6
  drug-drug interactions 185
  first-line regimen 183–5
  HAART 178, 183
  side effects 185, 188
  toxicity 186–7
antisecretory agents 102

antivirals 208–9
arboviruses 64, 65
  laboratory tests **67**
Aspergillus spp. 254
astrovirus **304**
asymptomatic bacteriuria 122–3, 309
azithromycin 195
  Chlamydia trachomatis 151
  community-acquired pneumonia 77
  gonorrhoea 150
  syphilis 152

Bacillus spp., mesh-related infections 273
Bacillus cereus **304**
bacitracin 105
BCG vaccination 90–1
blinding 5
bloodborne pathogen exposure 291
  hepatitis B 292–3
  hepatitis C 293
  HIV 291–2, **291**
  prophylaxis 293
bone and joint infections 26–38
  infectious arthritis 26–9
  osteomyelitis in diabetic foot 32–8
  prosthetic joint infection 29–32
Bordetella pertussis **304**
Bradford Hill, Sir Austin 2

Campylobacter spp. 103
Campylobacter jejuni **304**
Candida spp., catheter-related bloodstream
    infections 220
Candida glabrata 222
Candida krusei 222
candidiasis, chronic disseminated 262–3

carbapenem **259**
carboxypenicillin   216
carbuncles   14
CATCH trial   178
catheter-related bloodstream infections
        220–2, *221*
    diagnosis   221–2
    epidemiology   220
    etiology   220
    management   222
    neutropenic patients   261–2
    prevention   220–1
cefazolin   13–14
cefepime   **259**
cefixime   **259**
cefotaxime   57
ceftazidime   **259**
ceftriaxone
    cellulitis   13–14
    community-acquired pneumonia   77
    infective endocarditis   **47**
    meningitis   **57**
    in neutropenic cancer patients   **259**
cellulitis   11–14
cerebrospinal fluid culture in meningitis   58, **59**
cervicitis
    laboratory testing   138–9
    treatment   150–1
    see also sexually transmitted infections
chancroid *see Haemophilus ducreyi*
Charcot foot   18–19
Chlamydia pneumoniae   **304**
Chlamydia trachomatis
    diagnosis   137, **139**, 141
    treatment   150–1
chlorhexidine scrub   235–6
cholera   1
ciprofloxacin
    MRSA control   243
    in neutropenic cancer patients   **259**
    prophylaxis   252
    urinary tract infection   118–19, 127–8
clarithromycin
    diarrhea   **108**
    Mycobacterium avium complex
        prophylaxis   195
clindamycin-primaquine   183
clinical pulmonary infection score   218

Clostridium difficile diarrhea   103–5, 252, **304**
    clinical findings   104
    epidemiology   103–4
    special examinations   104–5
    stool culture   104
    treatment   105
Clostridium perfringens   **304**
cluster randomization   7
co-trimoxazole   182
Cochrane Collaboration   3, 73
colony stimulating factors   255
Colorado tick fever virus   **67**
community-acquired pneumonia   73–9
    admission decision   75
    antimicrobials   77–8
    blood culture   76–7
    burden of illness   73
    chest radiograph   74
    clinical history and physical examination   73–4
    prevention   78–9
    serologies   77
    sputum Gram stain/culture   75–6
    urine legionella antigen   77
    vaccines   78–9
condoms   148
confidence interval   6
confounding factors   5
coronavirus   **304**
corticosteroids
    infectious arthritis   38–9
    meningitis   60–1
    sepsis   216–17
CORTICUS trial   216
Corynebacterium spp., mesh-related infections   273
Coxiella burnetii   45
critical care   213–22
    catheter-related bloodstream infections   220–2
    sepsis   213–17
    ventilator-associated pneumonia   217–19
cryotherapy for genital warts   159
cryptococcal meningitis   192–3
    see also meningitis
Cryptosporidium spp.   **108**
Cyclospora spp.   **108**
cytomegalovirus
    diarrhea   **108**
    encephalitis   66
    laboratory tests   **67**

prophylaxis   196
   stopping   196–7
   treatment   196

Data Base of Abstracts of Reviews of Effects (DARE)   3
debridement   216
decolonization in MRSA control   242–3
diabetes mellitus
   foot infections   18–19
     osteomyelitis   32–8
   glucose control and infection risk   231
diarrhea   98–108
   chronic   106–8
   clinical findings   99, 104, 106
   Clostridium difficile   103–5, 252, **304**
   epidemiology   98–9, 103–4, 106
   HIV-infected patients   **107**
   incidence   **99**
   laboratory findings   99–100
   laboratory tests   106–7
   mortality   103
   nosocomial   103–6
   prognosis   102–3, 108
   special examinations   104–5
   stool culture   100, 104, 106
   traveler's   99
   treatment   100–2, 105, 107–8, **108**
     antidiarrheals   101–2, 108
     antimicrobials   101, 107–8, **108**
     antisecretory agents   102
     fluid management   100–1
diverticulitis, acute   274–7
   clinical features   275
   diagnosis   275–6
   epidemiology   274–5
   imaging studies   275–6
   pathogenesis   275
   treatment   276–7
doxycycline   151

eastern equine encephalitis   64, **64**, **65**
echocardiography in infective endocarditis   43–4
ecthyma gangrenosum   281
efavirenz   184
electroencephalogram in encephalitis   67–8
EMBASE   73
encephalitis   62–9
   causative agents   64

clinical presentation   65–6
   arboviruses   65–6
   enteroviruses   66
   herpes simplex type 1   65
   postinfectious encephalomyelitis   66
   rabies   66
differential diagnosis   63
electroencephalogram   67–8
epidemiology   63, **65**
etiology   63–5
herpes simplex virus   64, **64**, 65
laboratory findings   66–7, **67**
magnetic resonance imaging   67
prevention   68
prognosis   68–9
seasonal virus preference   **64**
treatment   68
Entamoeba spp.   **108**
Entamoeba histolytica   **304**
Enterobacter spp., ventilator-assisted
   pneumonia   217
Enterococcus spp., catheter-related bloodstream
   infections   220
Enterococcus faecalis, burn-related infections   280
enterocolitis, neutropenic   261
enteroviruses   **64**, 66
   laboratory tests   **67**
Epstein-Barr virus
   encephalitis   66
   laboratory tests   **67**
erysipelas   11–14
Escherichia coli   102, **304**
   burn-related infections   280
   in neutropenic cancer patients   258
   surgical site infection   271
   urinary tract infection   118
ethambutol   **108**, 180
evidence-based diagnosis   3–4
evidence-based infectious diseases   1–2
   clinical questions   2–3
evidence-based medicine   1, *2*
evidence-based treatment   4–7
external validity   4

famciclovir
   genital herpes   154
   herpes simplex virus   189
fluconazole   254

fluoroquinolones
    Chlamydia trachomatis   151
    gonorrhoea   150
    prophylaxis   252–4
    urinary tract infection   118–20, 127–8
fosfomycin   118
fungal infection prophylaxis   193–4
furazolidone   **108**
furuncles   14
fusidic acid
    diarrhea   105
    MRSA control   243

ganciclovir   **108**
genital warts
    diagnosis   147–8
    treatment   155, 157–9, **157–8**
gentamicin
    infective endocarditis   **47**
    in neutropenic cancer patients   **259**
Giardia spp.   **108**
Giardia lamblia   **304**
glucose control and infection risk   231
granulocyte-colony stimulating
    factor   37
Guillain-Barré syndrome   66

HAART therapy   178, 183
    drug-drug interactions   185
    side effects   185
    see also antiretroviral therapy
Haemophilus ducreyi
    diagnosis   137, 142–3
    treatment   155, **156**
    ulcer appearance   **138**
Haemophilus influenzae   **304**
    cellulitis   12
    meningitis   57
    prevention   61
    vaccine   56
    see also influenza
hair removal and infection risk   233–4
hand hygiene   210–11, 241–2
healthcare workers, infections in   291–8
    hepatitis B   292–3
    hepatitis C   293
    HIV   291–2, **291**
    influenza-like illness   295–7

occupational bloodborne pathogen
    exposures   291
    prevention   297–8
    varicella zoster   294–5
HEPA filters   251–2
hepatitis B   292–3, **304**
hepatitis C   293
hernia repair, mesh infection   272–4
herpes B virus   **67**
herpes simplex virus
    diagnosis   143–4
    diarrhea   **108**
    encephalitis   64, **64**, 65
    laboratory tests   **67**
    STIs   **138**
    treatment   153–4, 189
    Tzank smear   143
human immunodeficiency virus   177–98
    AIDS dementia complex   197
    antiretroviral therapy   183–7
        adverse reactions   188
        compliance/adherence   185–6
        drug-drug interactions   185
        first-line regimen   183–5
        HAART   178, 183
        side effects   185–8
        toxicity   183–5
    asymptomatic   178
    diagnostic confirmation   177
    diarrhea   **107**
    drug resistance   178
        virus transmission   178–9
    early treatment   177–8
    encephalitis   64, **64**
    exposure risk for healthcare workers   291–2, **291**
    genotypic resistance testing   190
    genotyping   178
    HAART response   178
    and herpes simplex   189
    laboratory tests   **67**
    multiple resistance   191–2
    non-Hodgkin lymphoma   197
    opportunistic infection prophylaxis   187–90,
        192–7, **193**
        cryptococcal meningitis   192–3
        cytomegalovirus infection   196–7
        fungal infections   193–4
        Mycobacterium avium complex   194–5

Pneumocystis jiroveci 182–3
  stopping prophylaxis 189
prognostic features 179
progressive multifocal leukoencephalopathy 197
and STIs *137*
therapeutic drug monitoring 191
and toxoplasmosis 188–90
tuberculosis in 179–82
viral phenotyping 190–1
human metapneumovirus **304**
human papillomavirus 147–8
hydrotherapy 285–6
hyperbaric oxygen 17, 37
hypothermia and infection risk 231–2

imaging studies
  diverticulitis 275–6
  encephalitis 67
  infectious arthritis 27
  meningitis 59–60
  osteomyelitis 35–6
  prosthetic joint infection 30
imipenem **259**
imiquimod **157–8**
impetigo 11
inception cohort 7
infection control 229–43
  in long-term care facilities 310–11
  MRSA 238–43
  surgical site infections 229–38
infectious arthritis 26–9
  antimicrobial therapy 28
  aspiration and lavage 28
  clinical signs and laboratory studies 27
  corticosteroids 28–9
  diagnosis **28**
  imaging 27
  implications for practice 29
  implications for research 29
  microbial culture 27
infective endocarditis 42–50
  antimicrobial therapy 46–7, **47**
  blood culture 43, **45**
  clinical presentation 42–3, **44**
  congestive heart failure 49
  diagnostic criteria 45
  echocardiography 43–4
  embolic events 49

epidemiology 42, *43*
mortality 49–50
prognosis 48–50
surgical intervention 47–8
influenza 206–11, 295–6, **304**
  diagnosis 206–7
  health care workers 296
  laboratory diagnosis 207, **208**
  prevention 209–11, **210**
  prognosis 209
  radiology 207
  symptoms 206–7
  treatment 208–9
  vaccines 209–10, **210**
influenza-like illness 295–7
interferon gamma release assay 86, 91–2
interferon for genital warts **158**
interferon-2b 68
isoniazid 88, 180
Isospora spp. **108**
itraconazole 254

JC polyoma virus **67**

Klebsiella spp., burn-related infections 280
Klebsiella pneumoniae, in neutropenic cancer
  patients 258

La Crosse virus 64, **64**, **65**
Legionella spp. **304**
Legionella pneumophila 77
levels of evidence 4
levofloxacin
  in neutropenic cancer patients 252, **259**
  skin and soft tissue infections 13–14
likelihood ratio 3–4
Listeria monocytogenes, meningitis 57
long-term care facilities, infections in 302–12
  diagnosis 305–6
  factors promoting 303–5, **304**
  impact of 305
  incidence 302–3, **303**
  pneumonia 306–7
  prevention 310–11
    antimicrobial-resistant organisms 311
    infection control 310–11
    resident interventions 310
  skin infections 308

long-term care facilities (*continued*)
  treatment 308–10
    antimicrobials 308
    choice of drug 309–10
    initiation of therapy 309
    non-antimicrobial approaches 308–9
  urinary infection 307–8

mafenide acetate 283
magnetic resonance imaging
  encephalitis 67
  osteomyelitis 35
measles virus encephalitis 64, **64**
MEDLINE 3, 73
men, urinary tract infections in 125–8
meningitis 55–62
  antimicrobials 60
  blood culture 58
  cerebrospinal fluid culture 58, **59**
  clinical presentation 57–8, **58**
  corticosteroids 60–1
  cryptococcal, prophylaxis 193
  differential diagnosis 55–6
  epidemiology 55–7
  etiology 57, **57**
  neuroimaging 59–60
  polymerase chain reaction 59
  preventive therapy 61–2
  prognosis 62
  rapid bacterial antigen testing 58–9
meropenem **259**
mesh-related infections 272–4
methicillin-resistant *S. aureus see* MRSA
metronidazole
  diarrhea 105, **108**
  trichomoniasis 159–60
minocycline
  Chlamydia trachomatis 151
  MRSA control 243
molecular fingerprinting 88
moxifloxacin **259**
MRSA 14–15, 216, 238–43, **304**
  burden of illness 239–40
  clinical presentation 238–9
  community-associated 240–1, **240**
  guidelines 243
  healthcare-associated 240–1
  mortality 239–40

prevention 241–3
  active surveillance 242
  decolonization 242–3
  hand disinfection and contract
    precautions 241–2
  risk factors 241
  soft-tissue infections 14–5
multidrug resistance 7
multiple organ dysfunction syndrome (MODS) 282
mumps virus encephalitis 64, **64**
mupirocin 14
  MRSA control 243
  surgical site infection 235–6
Mycobacterium avium complex 194–5
  drug side effects 195
  prophylaxis 194–5
    stopping 195–6
  treatment 194
Mycobacterium tuberculosis **304**
  in HIV **179–81**
  see also tuberculosis

National Nosocomial Infection Surveillance System
  (NNIS) 57
necrotizing fasciitis 15–18, 271–2
Neisseria gonorrhoeae
  diagnosis **139**, 140, **140**
  treatment 149–50
Neisseria meningitidis 4
  meningitis 57
  prevention 61–2
  vaccine 56
netilmicin
  infective endocarditis **47**
  in neutropenic cancer patients **259**
neuraminidase inhibitors 208, 210
neuroimaging in meningitis 59–60
neutropenia 250–63
  bacterial infections in 258–60
    antibacterial therapy 258–60, **259**
  catheter/line-related infections 261–2
  chronic disseminated candidiasis 262–3
  enterocolitis 261
  febrile 251
    assessment and management 256–8, **257**
    physical examination 256–7, **257**
    risk assessment 257–8
  infection prevention 251–6

adjuvant therapies   255–6
antibacterial agents   252–3
antifungal agents   254–5
protected environments   251–2
nevirapine   184
nitrofurantoin   118
non-Hodgkin lymphoma   197
non-nucleoside reverse transcriptase inhibitors   178, 184
norovirus   **304**
novobiocin in MRSA control   243
nuclear imaging in osteomyelitis   35–6
nucleic acid amplification tests   87
number needed to harm   6
number needed to treat   6

Oscillococcinum   209
oseltamivir   208
osteomyelitis in diabetic foot   32–8
   antimicrobial therapy   36–7
   blood investigations   34
   clinical findings   34
   diagnosis   33–4
   implications for practice   37
   implications for research   37–8
   incidence and prevalence   32
   magnetic resonance imaging   35
   microbiological investigations   34–5, **35**
   nuclear imaging   35–6
   pathology and microbiology   32–3, **33**
   radiography   35
   risk factors for infection/ulceration   33, **34**
   surgical management   36
oxygen therapy and infection risk   232–3

parainfluenza   **304**
Pasteur, Louis   1
pelvic inflammatory disease
   diagnosis   141, **142**
   treatment   151–2
penicillin G
   infective endocarditis   **47**
   syphilis   152–3
pentamidine   182
PICO   2
piperacillin   **259**
Pneumocystis jiroveci   182–3
   diagnosis   182

   prophylaxis   187–8
   stopping prophylaxis   189
   treatment   182–3
      alternative   183
pneumonia
   community-acquired *see* community-acquired pneumonia
   in long-term care facilities   306–7
podophyllotoxin   **157**
polymerase chain reaction   59
posaconazole   254
postinfectious encephalomyelitis   66
   laboratory tests   **67**
Powassan virus   **65**
prognosis
   diarrhea   102–3, 108
   encephalitis   68–9
   evidence-based assessment   7
   infective endocarditis   48–50
   influenza   209
   meningitis   62
   thermal injury-related infections   286–7
   urinary tract infections   120
progressive multifocal leukoencephalopathy   197
prostatitis   126
prosthetic joint infection   29–32
   aspiration of hip   30
   blood investigations   30
   diagnosis   29–30
   histology   30
   imaging   30
   implications for practice   32
   implications for research   32
   microbial culture of specimens   30
   polymerase chain reaction   30
   reference standard   29–30
   sonication of removed prostheses   30
   treatment and outcomes   31
protected environments   251–2
Proteus spp., burn-related infections   280
PROWESS trial   216
Pseudomonas spp., burn-related infections   280
Pseudomonas aeruginosa
   burn-related infections   285
   catheter-related bloodstream infections   220
   cellulitis   12
   in neutropenic cancer patients   258
   ventilator-assisted pneumonia   217

PUBMED   3
pyrazinamide   88, 180

quinacrine   **108**

rabies virus
  encephalitis   64, **64**, 65, 66
  laboratory tests   **67**
radiography
  community-acquired pneumonia   74
  osteomyelitis   35
  tuberculosis   85
randomized controlled trials   1, 4, 5
rapid bacterial antigen testing   58–9
relative risk   6
respiratory syncytial virus   **304**
rhinovirus   **304**
ribavirin   68
rifabutin   88, 194
rifampicin   88, 180
  MRSA control   243
rimantidine   208
rotavirus   **304**

St Louis encephalitis   64, **64**, **65**
Salmonella spp.   **304**
Salmonella enteritidis   103
Salmonella typhimurium   103
sepsis   213–17
  definitions   213
  diagnostic criteria   **214**
  epidemiology   213
  management   213–17
    activated protein C   216
    antimicrobial therapy   215–16
    corticosteroids   216–17
    goal-directed therapy   214–15
    source control   216
  mortality risk   *215*
severe acute respiratory syndrome (SARS)   7, 296–7
sexually transmitted infections   136–63
  chancroid   142–3
  Chlamydia trachomatis   141
  counselling and behavioral interventions   162–3, *163*
  diagnosis   137–8, **137**
  genital warts and human papillomavirus   147–8
  herpes simplex virus   143–4

high-risk populations   162
and HIV infection   *137*
laboratory testing   138–9, **139**
management   149–60
  chancroid   155
  Chlamydia trachomatis   150–1
  genital herpes   153–5, *154*
  genital warts   155–9, **156–8**
  Neisseria gonorrhoeae   149–50
  partners   160
  pelvic inflammatory disease   151–2
  syphilis   152–3
  trichomoniasis   159–60
Neisseria gonorrhoeae   140, **140**
pathogen identification   139–40
pelvic inflammatory disease   141, **142**
population-based screening programs   161–2
prevention   148
syphilis   144–7, **145–6**, *146*, **147**
Trichomonas vaginalis   142
two glass test   139
vaccination   160–1, *161*
Shigella spp.   **304**
Shigella flexneri   103
silver nitrate   283
silver sulfadiazine   282–3
skin/soft tissue infections   11–21
  animal bites   19–21
  cellulitis and erysipelas   11–14
  diabetic foot infections   18–19
  furuncles and carbuncles   14
  impetigo   11
  in long-term care facilities   308
  MRSA   14–15
  necrotizing fasciitis   15–18
  surgery-related *see* surgical site infections
smoking cessation and infection risk   234–5
Snow, John   1
soft-tissue infections, postoperative   270
SPREAD trial   178
sputum Gram stain   75–6
Staphylococcus aureus   **304**
  burn-related infections   280
  catheter-related bloodstream infections   220
  cellulitis   12
  elimination of   235–6
  impetigo   11
  mesh-related infections   273

methicillin-resistant *see* MRSA
  in neutropenic cancer patients 258
  surgical site infections 271
  ventilator-assisted pneumonia 217
Staphylococcus saprophyticus 118
statistical significance 6
Stenotrophomonas maltophilia 217
STIs *see* sexually transmitted infections
streptococcal toxic shock syndrome (STSS) 272
Streptococcus pneumoniae **304**
  meningitis 57
  prevention 61
  vaccine 56
Streptococcus pyogenes
  cellulitis 12
  surgical site infection 271
subeschar lysis 284
surgery-related infections 270–7
  acute diverticulitis 274–7
  mesh infections post-hernia repair 272–4
  necrotizing fasciitis 271–2
  patient evaluation 270–1
  see also surgical site infections
surgical site infections 229–38
  burden of illness 229
  clinical relevance 229
  comprehensive interventions 237–8
  cost 229, **230–1**
  glucose control 231
  hair removal 233–4
  perioperative antimicrobial prophylaxis 236–7, **236**
  perioperative warming 231–2
  risk factors 229, 232
  S. aureus elimination 235–6
  smoking cessation 234–5
  soft tissue 270
  supplemental oxygen 232–3
surgical wound classification **236**
syphilis 144–7, **145–6**, *146*, **147**
  treatment 152–3
  see also Treponema pallidum
systemic inflammatory response syndrome (SIRS) 213, 281

teicoplanin 105
thermal injury-related infections 280–8
  bacteriology of burns patients 280–1
  clinical presentation 281
  diagnosis 281–2
  empiric antibiotic treatment 284–5
  hydrotherapy 285–6
  infection control 285
  microbiology 282
  prevention 282–4
    surgery 284
    topical antimicrobials 282–4
    vaccines 287–8
  prognosis 286–7
ticarcillin **259**
tinidazole **108**
  trichomoniasis 159–60
tobramycin **259**
toxoplasmosis 189–90
  prophylaxis 188–9
Treponema pallidum
  diagnosis 137
  syphilis 144–7, **145–6**, *146*, **147**
  ulcer appearance **138**
trichloroacetic acid 159
Trichomonas vaginalis
  diagnosis 142
  treatment 159–60
trimethoprim-sulfamethoxazole
  MRSA control 243
  urinary tract infection 118, 127–8, 130
Trychophyton spp. **304**
tuberculin skin test 91
tuberculosis 2, 83–92
  BCG vaccination 90–1
  chest radiograph 85
  clinical presentation 85
  directly observed therapy 89
  drug-resistant 90
  epidemiology 83–4
  and HIV 180–1
    diagnosis 180
    prophylaxis 181
    treatment 180–1
  immunologic testing 85–6
  interferon gamma release assays 91–2
  latent, treatment of 92
  microbiologic testing 86
  molecular fingerprinting 88
  mycobacterial culture 87
  nucleic acid amplification tests 87

tuberculosis (*continued*)
  phage-based tests   88
  risk factors   84–5
  serological tests   87–8
  smear examination   86–7
  treatment   88–90
Tzank smear   143

ureidopenicillin   216
urethritis
  laboratory tests   138
  treatment   150–1
  see also sexually transmitted infections
urinary tract infections   115–31
  asymptomatic bacteriuria   122–3
  clinical presentation
    likelihood ratios   **116**
    in men   125
  diagnosis   115–17
    in men   126–7
    severe infections   128–9
  drug resistance   119
  follow-up   121–2
  in long-term care facilities   307–8
  in men   125–8
  pathogenesis   120–1
  prevention   123–5
  prognosis   120
  prostatitis   126
  severe   128–31
    site of care   129
  treatment
    ambulatory patients   118–20
    men   127–8
    response time   131
    severe infections   129–31
urine legionella antigen   77
urine leukocyte esterase   **139**

vaccines
  BCG   90–1

burn-related infections   287–8
community-acquired pneumonia
    78–9
  Haemophilus influenzae   56
  hepatitis B   292–3
  influenza   209–10, **210, 296**
  Neisseria meningitidis   56
  STIs   160–1, *161*
  Streptococcus pneumoniae   56
valacyclovir
  genital herpes   154, *154*
  herpes simplex encephalitis   68
  herpes simplex virus   189
valganciclovir   **108, 196**
vancomycin
  diarrhea   105
  meningitis   **57**
varicella zoster virus
  encephalitis   64, **64**, 66
  in healthcare workers   294–5
  laboratory tests   **67**
ventilator-associated pneumonia
    217–19
  diagnosis   218–19
  epidemiology   217
  management   219
  pathophysiology and microbiology   217
  prevention   217–18
Vibrio cholerae   102
Vibrio vulnificus   12
voriconazole   254

West Nile virus   64, **64, 65**
  laboratory tests   **67**
  western equine encephalitis   64, **64, 65**

Yersinia pseudotuberculosis   103

zanamivir   208–9
zidovudine   178
  side effects   185

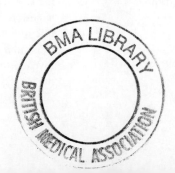
BMA LIBRARY
BRITISH MEDICAL ASSOCIATION